ANNALS OF
THE NEW YORK ACADEMY
OF SCIENCES

Volume 762

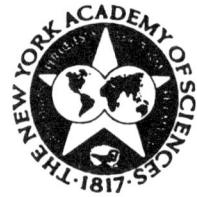

EDITORIAL STAFF

Executive Editor
BILL BOLAND

Managing Editor
JUSTINE CULLINAN

Associate Editor
JOYCE HITCHCOCK

The New York Academy of Sciences
2 East 63rd Street
New York, New York 10021

THE NEW YORK ACADEMY OF SCIENCES
(Founded in 1817)
BOARD OF GOVERNORS, July 1994–September 1995

JOSHUA LEDERBERG, *Chairman of the Board*
HENRY M. GREENBERG, *President*
MARTIN L. LEIBOWITZ, *President-Elect*

Honorary Life Governor
WILLIAM T. GOLDEN

HENRY A. LICHSTEIN, *Treasurer*

Governors-at-Large

ELEANOR BAUM	BARRY R. BLOOM	D. ALLAN BROMLEY
EDWARD COHEN	SUSANNA CUNNINGHAM-RUNDLES	BILL GREEN
SANDRA PANEM	RICHARD A. RIFKIND	DOMINICK SALVATORE
DAVID E. SHAW	WILLIAM C. STEERE, JR.	SHMUEL WINOGRAD

CYRIL M. HARRIS, *Past Chairman*   HELENE L. KAPLAN, *General Counsel* [ex officio]

RODNEY W. NICHOLS, *Chief Executive Officer* [ex officio]

INTERLEUKIN-6-TYPE CYTOKINES

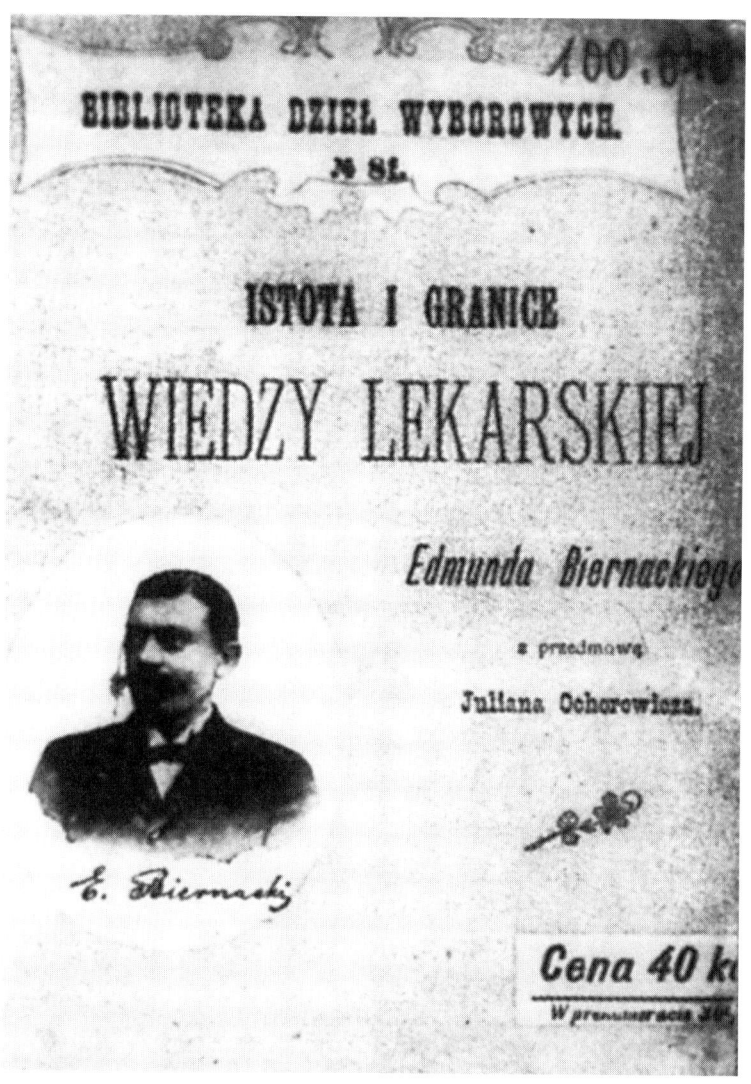

Edmund F. Biernacki (1866–1911), Polish physician and pathologist, head of the Wolski Hospital in Warsaw and, after 1908, professor of the University of Lwow. Dr. Biernacki is best known for his discovery of the incrteased erythrocyte sedimentation rate (ESR) in columns of citrated blood obtained from patients with infectous diseases and rheumatoid arthritis (*Zeitschrift fur Physiologisches Chemie* **19**: 179–224, 1894). In Poland, ESR is known by the acronym OB (objaw Biernackiego = phenomenon of Biernacki).

ANNALS OF THE NEW YORK ACADEMY OF SCIENCES
Volume 762

INTERLEUKIN-6-TYPE CYTOKINES

Edited by Andrzej Mackiewicz, Aleksander Koj, and Pravin B. Sehgal

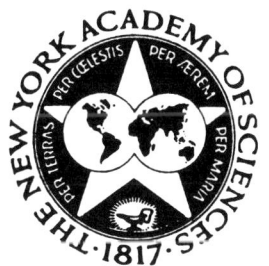

The New York Academy of Sciences
New York, New York
1995

Copyright © 1995 by the New York Academy of Sciences. All rights reserved. Under the provisions of the United States copyright Act of 1976, individual readers of the Annals are permitted to make fair use of the material in them for teaching or research. Permission is granted to quote from the Annals provided that the customary acknowledgment is made of the source. Material in the Annals may be republished only by permission of the Academy. Address inquiries to the Executive Editor at the New York Academy of Sciences.

Copying fees: For each copy of an article made beyond the free copying permitted under Section 107 or 108 of the 1976 Copyright Act, a fee should be paid through the Copyright Clearance Center, 222 Rosewood Drive, Danvers, MA 01923. For articles of more than 3 pages, the copying fee is $1.75.

⊚The paper used in this publication meets the minimum requirements of American National Standard for Information Sciences—Permanence of Paper for Printed Library Materials, ANSI Z39. 48-1984.

COVER: The photograph on the designed cover is of the City Hall of Poznań Poland.
PHOTO CREDIT: Dr. Serguisz Nawrocki.

Library of Congress Cataloging-in-Publication Data

Interleukin-6-type cytokines / edited by Andrezj Mackiewicz, Aleksander Koj, and Pravin B. Sehgal.
    p. cm. — (Annals of the New York Academy of Sciences ; v. 762)
  This volume is the result of a conference held in Poznan, Poland June 19-22, 1994.
  Includes bibliographical references and index.
  ISBN 0-89766-931-2 (alk. paper). — ISBN 0-89766-932-0 (pbk. : alk. paper)
  1. Interleukin-6—Congresses. I. Mackiewicz, Andrzej. II. Koj, A. III. Sehgal, Pravin B. IV. Series.
Q11.N5 vol. 762
[QR185.8.I56]
500 s—dc20
[616.07'9]
                                      95-30188
                                            CIP

MC/PCP
Printed in the United States of America
ISBN 0-89766-931-2 (cloth)
ISBN 0-89766-932-0 (paper)
ISSN 0077-8923

ANNALS OF THE NEW YORK ACADEMY OF SCIENCES

Volume 762
July 21, 1995

INTERLEUKIN-6-TYPE CYTOKINES[a]

Editors and Conference Organizers

ANDRZEJ MACKIEWICZ, ALEKSANDER KOJ, AND PRAVIN B. SEHGAL

CONTENTS

Preface. *By* ANDRZEJ MACKIEWICZ, ALEKSANDER KOJ, AND PRAVIN B. SEHGAL xiii

Welcoming Remarks. *By* J. GADZINOWSKI xv

Part I. The Cytokines

Interleukin-6-Type Cytokines. *By* PRAVIN B. SEHGAL, LING WANG, RAVI RAYANADE, HENG PAN, AND LOLA MARGULIES 1

Transcription Factors NF-IL6 and APRF Involved in gp130-mediated Signaling Pathway. *By* S. AKIRA, Y. NISHIO, T. TANAKA, M. INOUE, T. MATSUSAKA, X.-J. WANG, S. WEI, N. YOSHIDA, AND T. KISHIMOTO 15

LIF and Related Cytokines in the Regulation of Mammalian Development. *By* COLIN L. STEWART AND EMILY CULLINAN 29

Interleukin (IL)-11-mediated Signal Transduction. *By* YU-CHUNG YANG AND TINGGUI YIN 31

In Vivo Properties of Oncostatin M. *By* PHILIP M. WALLACE, JOHN F. MACMASTER, JILL R. RILLEMA, KATHERINE A. ROULEAU, MARCIA B. HANSON, SAMUEL A. BURSTEIN, AND MOHAMMED SHOYAB 42

Signal Transduction through IL-6 Receptor: Involvement of Multiple Protein Kinsases, Stat Factors, and a Novel H7-sensitive Pathway. *By* KOICHI NAKAJIMA, TADASHI MATSUDA, YOSHIO FUJITANI, HIROTADA KOJIMA, YOJIRO YAMANAKA, KAZUTO NAKAE, TAKASHI TAKEDA, AND TOSHIO HIRANO 55

Part II. Expression and Cytokine Networks

Cytokine Networks and Corticosteroid Receptors. *By* A. FALUS, J. BIRÓ, AND É. RÁKÁSZ 71

Regulation of Interleukin-6 Gene Expression by Steroids. *By* ANURADHA RAY, DONG-HONG ZHANG, MARK D. SIEGEL, AND PRABIR RAY 79

Interleukin-11 in Respiratory Inflammation. *By* O. EINARSSON, G. P. GEBA, Z. ZHOU, M. L. LANDRY, R. A. PANETTIERI, JR., D. TRISTRAM, R. WELLIVER, A. METINKO, AND J. A. ELIAS 89

[a] This volume is the result of a conference entitled **Interleukin-6-Type Cytokines** sponsored by the New York Academy of Sciences and the State Committee for Scientific Research, Warsaw, Poland and held in Poznań, Poland June 19–22, 1994.

Do Post-transcriptional Mechanisms Participate in Induction of C-reactive Protein and Serum Amyloid A by IL-6 and IL-1? *By* IRVING KUSHNER, SHUN-LIN JIANG, DONGXIAO ZHANG, GERARD LOZANSKI, AND DAVID SAMOLS 102

Modified Proteins as Possible Signals in the Acute Phase Response. *By* ALEKSANDER KOJ AND AMALIA GUZDEK 108

Part III. Structure-Function Relationships

Interleukin-6 Chaperones in Blood. *By* LESTER T. MAY, MACKEVIN I. NDUBUISI, KIRIT PATEL, AND DORYS GARCIA 120

Development of Human IL-6 Receptor Antagonists. *By* P. J. BRAKENHOFF, FLORIS D. DE HON, AND LUCIEN A. AARDEN 129

The Molecular Design of Human IL-6 Receptor Antagonists. *By* A. LAHM, R. SAVINO, A. L. SALVATI, A. CABIBBO, L. CIAPPONI, A. DEMARTIS, C. TONIATTI, G. PAONESSA, S. ALTAMURA, AND G. CILIBERTO 136

Alanine-scanning Mutagenesis of Human Interleukin-11: Identification of Regions Important for Biological Activity. *By* MARTA CZUPRYN, FRANN BENNETT, JENNIFER DUBE, KATHY GRANT, HUBERT SCOBLE, HEMCHAND SOOKDEO, AND JOHN M. MCCOY 152

Inter-Species Chimeras of Leukemia Inhibitory Factor Define a Human Receptor Binding Site. *By* CATHERINE M. OWCZAREK, MEREDITH J. LAYTON, DONALD METCALF, ROSLYN CLARK, NICHOLAS M. GOUGH, AND NICOS A. NICOLA 165

The Crystal Structure of Murine Leukemia Inhibitory Factor. *By* R. C. ROBINSON, L. M. GREY, D. STAUNTON, D. I. STUART, J. K. HEATH, AND E. Y. JONES 179

Part IV. Receptors and Signal Transducers

Function of Hematopoietin Receptor Subunits in Hepatic Cells and Fibroblasts. *By* CHUN-FAI LAI, KAREN K. MORELLA, YANPING WANG, SATORU KUMAKI, DAVID GEARING, STEVEN F. ZIEGLER, DAVID J. TWEARDY, SUSANA P. CAMPOS, AND HEINZ BAUMANN 189

The Soluble Interleukin-6 Receptor. *By* STEFAN ROSE-JOHN, MARC EHLERS, JOACHIM GRÖTZINGER, AND JÜRGEN MÜLLBERG 207

Membrane-bound and Soluble Interleukin-6 Receptor: Studies on Structure, Regulation of Expression, and Signal Transduction. *By* PETER C. HEINRICH, LUTZ GRAEVE, STEFAN ROSE-JOHN, JENS SCHNEIDER-MERGENER, ELKE DITTRICH, ANDREA ERREN, CLAUDIA GERHARTZ, ULRIKE HEMMANN, CLAUDIA LÜTTICKEN, URSULA WEGENKA, OLIVER WEIERGRÄBER, AND FRIEDEMANN HORN 222

Transcription Factors as Targets of Cytokine Signals. *By* WARREN S.-L. LIAO, SZU-YAO LU, JIANYI HUANG, LI LI, AND ZHANYONG BING . . . 238

Isolation of Two Interleukin-6 Response Element Binding Proteins from Acute Phase Rat Livers. *By* JÜRGEN RIPPERGER, STEFAN FRITZ, KARIN RICHTER, BIRGIT DREIER, KURT SCHNEIDER, KLAUS LÖCHNER, ROLF MARSCHALEK, GERTRUD HOCKE, FRIEDRICH LOTTSPEICH, AND GEORG H. FEY 252

Functional Analysis of IL-6 and IL-6DBP/C/EBPβ by Gene Targeting. *By* ELENA FATTORI, CAROLINA SELLITTO, MANUELA CAPPELLETTI, DOMENICO LAZZARO, DIANA BELLAVIA, ISABELLA SCREPANTI, ALBERTO GULINO, FRANK COSTANTINI, AND VALERIA POLI 262

Part V. *In Vivo* Physiology and Pathology

In Lethally Irradiated Mice Interleukin-12 Protects Bone Marrow but Sensitizes Intestinal Tract to Damage from Ionizing Radiation. *By* R. NETA, S. M. STIEFEL, AND N. ALI 274

Adenovirus Vectors for Cytokine Gene Expression. *By* CARL D. RICHARDS, TODD BRACIAK, ZHOU XING, FRANK GRAHAM, AND JACK GAULDIE .. 282

Interleukin-6-Type Cytokines in Myeloproliferative Disease. *By* ROBERT G. HAWLEY 294

Pleiotropic Defects of IL-6-deficient Mice Including Early Hematopoiesis, T and B Cell Function, and Acute Phase Responses. *By* MANFRED KOPF, ALISTAIR RAMSAY, FRANK BROMBACHER, HEINZ BAUMANN, GIULIA FREER, CHRIS GALANOS, JOSE-CARLOS GUTIERREZ-RAMOS, AND GEORGES KÖHLER 308

Interleukin-6-Type Cytokine-induced Changes in Acute Phase Protein Glycosylation. *By* WILLEM VAN DIJK AND ANDRZEJ MACKIEWICZ 319

Co-ordinate Inhibition of the Production of TNF, IL-1, and IL-6 by Small Molecules. *By* ANTHONY C. ALLISON AND ELSIE M. EUGUI 331

Part VI. Preclinical and Clinical Therapeutics

Interleukin-6: Effects on Tumor Models in Mice and on the Cellular Regulation of Transcription Factor IRF-1. *By* MICHEL REVEL, ANNE KATZ, LEA EISENBACH, MICHAEL FELDMAN, NECHAMA HARAN-GHERA, SHEILA HARROCH, AND JUDITH CHEBATH 342

Clinical Trials with IL-6. *By* JEFFREY S. WEBER 357

Phase IA/IB Evaluation of Mammalian Cell-derived Glycosylated Recombinant Human Interleukin (SIGOSIX) before and after Cytotoxic Chemotherapy. *By* P. S. RITCH, C. KEEVER, J. SCHILLER, S. RIVKIN, P. L. WITT, S. E. GROSSBERG, R. L. TRUITT, H. BURRIS, D. D. VON HOFF, L. VAICKUS, D. DRECHSLER, E. C. BORDEN, A. GALAZKA, J. B. BREITMEYER, AND A. ABDUL-AHAD 359

Interleukin-6-Type Cytokines and Their Receptors for Gene Therapy of Melanoma. *By* ANDRZEJ MACKIEWICZ, MACIEJ WIZNEROWICZ, ELKE ROEB, JERZY NOWAK, TOMASZ PAWLOWSKI, HEINZ BAUMANN, PETER C. HEINRICH, AND STEFAN ROSE-JOHN 361

Interleukin-6-Type Cytokines in Diagnostics and Therapeutics: Roundtable Discussion. *Participants:* AYAD ABDUL-AHAD, HEINZ BAUMANN, JACK A. ELIAS, GEORG FEY, MICHAEL S. GORDON, PETER C. HEINRICH, FRIEDEMANN HORN, ALEKSANDER KOJ, MANFRED KOPF, VALERIA POLI, MICHEL REVEL, PRAVIN B. SEHGAL, PHILIP M. WALLACE, AND JEFFREY S. WEBER 375

Poster Papers

Increase of High Molecular Weight Fibrinogen after Surgery for Renal Cancer. *By* G. ADLER, W. EICHMAN, I. TARGONSKA, AND M. SZCZEPANSKI 388

Interleukin-6 Production in Children with Acute Lymphoblastic Leukemia. *By* A. CHYBICKA, J. BOGUSLAWSKA-JAWORSKA, AND W. JAWORSKI ... 391

Selectin-P (PADGEM, GMP-140)-mediated Adhesion of Human Platelets to Neutrophils *in Vitro* and Immune Complex-induced Peritonitis in Rats is Influenced by Interleukin-8. *By* A. DEMBIŃSKA-KIEĆ, M. BURCHERT, J. DULAK, M. POLUS, M. PAWELEC, A. SIEDLECKI, AND B. A. PESKAR 395

Blood Serum Concentration of C-Reactive Protein and Interleukin-6 in Diagnosis of Neonatal Infection. *By* K. DREWS, J. SZCZAPA, J. ŻAK, R. ANDRZEJEWSKA, L. ŻAK, AND A. MACKIEWICZ 398

Residues 77-95 of the Human Interleukin-6 Protein Are Responsible for Receptor Binding and Residues 41-56 for Signal Transduction. *By* MARC EHLERS, JOACHIM GRÖTZINGER, FLORIS D. DE HON, JÜRGEN MÜLLBERG, JUST P. J. BRAKENHOFF, AXEL WOLLMER, AND STEFAN ROSE-JOHN 400

Interleukin-6 and Interleukin-6 Receptor mRNA Expression in Rat Central Nervous System. *By* R. A. GADIENT AND U. OTTEN 403

ELISA Detection of Circulating Levels of LIF, OSM, and CNTF in Septic Shock. *By* CATHERINE GUILLET, MARYVONNE FOURCIN, SYLVIE CHEVALIER, ANNICK POUPLARD, AND HUGUES GASCAN 407

A Region within the Cytoplasmic Domain of the Interleukin-6 Signal Transducer gp130 Important for Ligand-induced Endocytosis of the IL-6 Receptor. *By* ELKE DITTRICH, CLAUDIA GERHARTZ, STEFAN ROSE-JOHN, JÜRGEN MÜLLBERG, TANJA STOYAN, PETER C. HEINRICH, AND LUTZ GRAEVE 410

Interleukin-6-Type Cytokines Affect Glycosylation of Acute Phase Proteins *in Vitro*. *By* KATARZYNA GRYSKA, ARTUR SLUPIANEK, MARIA LACIAK, HEINZ BAUMANN, AND ANDRZEJ MACKIEWICZ 413

Cytokines and the Activity of Tyrosine Aminotransferase and Superoxide Dismutase in Rat Hepatoma Cells in Culture. *By* AMALIA GUZDEK, KRYSTYNA STALIŃSKA, AND JOANNA BERETA 416

Effects of HGF and RA on the Class 1 and Class 2 Rat Acute Phase Proteins. *By* AMALIA GUZDEK AND ALEKSANDER KOJ 419

Structural and Biological Chracterization of Murine-Human Interleukin-6 Chimeras. *By* A. HAMMACHER, L. D. WARD, J. WEINSTOCK, AND R. J. SIMPSON 422

Renal Mesangial Cells Have the Capacity to Synthesize and React to Leukemia Inhibitory Factor. *By* A. HARTNER, M. GOPPELT-STRÜBE, G. M. HOCKE, G. H. FEY, AND R. B. STERZEL 424

The LIF-Response Element Confers LIF-induced Transcriptional Control in P19 Embryonal Carcinoma Cells. *By* GERTRUD M. HOCKE 426

Pituitary Glycoprotein Hormones and Interleukins Secretion: *In Vitro* and *in Vivo* Human Study. *By* J. KOMOROWSKI, M. PAWLIKOWSKI, AND H. STĘPIEŃ 429

Serum Levels of IL-6 in Mycosis Fungoides, Psoriasis, and Lichen Planus.
By B. TORUNIOWA, D. KRASOWSKA, M. KOZIOT, A. KSIAŻEK, AND
A. PIETRZAK 432

Interleukin-6- and Interleukin-4-related Proteins (C-reactive Protein and
IgE) Are Prognostic Factors of Asbestos-related Cancer. By A. LANGE,
L. KARABON, AND J. TOMECZKO 435

IL-6 Is Present in Sera of Bone Marrow-transplanted Patients in Aplastic
Period, and High Levels of IL-6 During Acute Graft-versus-Host
Disease Are Associated with Severe Gut Symptoms. By L. KARABON,
A. MONIEWSKA, A. LABA, C. SWIDER, AND A. LANGE 439

Plasma Acute Phase Proteins and Metalloproteins in Children with
Neuroblastoma at Diagnosis. By L. LIPIŃSKA, T. IZBICKI, T.
LASKOWSKA-KLITA, AND D. PEREK 443

The Value of Determining the Interleukin-6 Levels in Epithelial Ovarian
Cancer. By J. MARKOWSKA, K. WIKTOROWICZ, Z. SZEWIERSKI, AND
R. MĄDRY 446

Immunohistochemical Localization of Interleukin-6-like Immunoreactivity to
Peripheral Nerve-like Structures in Normal and Inflamed Human Skin.
By K. NORDLIND, C. LIBING, A. A. AHMED, A. LJUNGBERG, AND S.
LIDÉN 450

Kinetics of the Activation of the LIF-Response Factor in M1 Myeloid
Leukemic Cells. By R. P. PIEKORZ, R. BLÄSIUS, G. H. FEY,
AND G. M. HOCKE 452

Interleukin-6 Levels in Sera and Bronchoalveolar Lavages of Patients with
Selected Disorders. By Z. POJDA, J. STRUŻYNA, M. MARUSZYŃSKI, T.
PŁUSA, AND A. JUNG 455

IL-6-Receptor-mediated Growth Inhibition by *All*-trans Retinoic Acid but
not by Interferon-α in Human Myeloma Cells. By KARI PULKKI,
MARKO NEVA, KARI KOSKELA, HANNA OLLIKAINEN, KARI REMES,
AND TARJA-TERTTU PELLINIEMI 457

Purification of the Interleukin-6-inducible Complex II Reveals Two Proteins
Capable of Binding to the IL 6 Response Element. By J. A. RIPPERGER,
S. FRITZ, G. M. HOCKE, AND G. H. FEY 459

TIMP-1 Protein Expression Is Stimulated by IL-1β and IL-2 in Primary Rat
Hepatocytes. By ELKE ROEB, LUTZ GRAEVE, JÜRGEN MÜLLBERG,
SIEGFRIED MATERN, AND STEFAN ROSE-JOHN 462

Changes in IL-6 Receptor Subunit mRNA Expression in Primary Mouse
Hepatocyte Cultures and Murine and Rat Hepatoma Cell Lines. By
HANNA ROKITA, PIOTR PIERZCHALSKI, AND KRYSTYNA STALIŃSKA .. 465

Diurnal Variations of Plasma Interleukin-6 in Man: Methodological
Implications of Continuous Use of Indwelling Cannulae. By WALTHER
SEILER, HILDEGARD MÜLLER, AND CRISTOPH HIEMKE 468

Stoichiometry of the Interleukin-6 High Affinity Receptor Complex. By
L. D. WARD, G. J. HOWLETT, A. HAMMACHER, R. L. MORITZ, AND
R. J. SIMPSON 471

Interleukin-6 Serum Levels in Depressed Patients before and after Treatment
with Fluoxetine. By A. SŁUŻEWSKA, J. K. RYBAKOWSKI, M. LACIAK, A.
MACKIEWICZ, M. SOBIESKA, AND K. WIKTOROWICZ 474

Possible Relationship between Interleukin-6 and Response of
Immunoglobulin E to Surgical Trauma. *By* ANDREW SZCZEKLIK, JACEK
JAWIEŃ, BEDA M. STADLER, JADWIGA RADWAN, WIESŁAWA
PIWOWARSKA, AND ANTONI DZIATKOWIAK 477

Molecular Cloning and Functional Expression of Mouse cDNAs Encoding
the Membrane Receptor and the Soluble Receptor for D-Factor/LIF. *By*
MIKIO TOMIDA 480

Monoclonal Antibodies Define Different Functional Epitopes on gp130
Signal Transducer. *By* SYLVIE CHEVALIER, CLAUDE CLEMENT, OLIVIER
ROBLEDO, BERNARD KLEIN, HUGUES GASCAN, AND JOHN WIJDENES . 482

Functional Reconstitution of IL-6 Signaling in a Myeloid Leukemic Cell
Line. *By* P. WULF, R. P. PIEKORZ, AND G. M. HOCKE 485

Lesion-induced Interleukin-6 mRNA Expression in Rat Sciatic Nerve. *By*
JIAN ZHONG AND ROLF HEUMANN 488

Effect of Interferon-α on Mitotic Index and Corticosterone Secretion in
Early Stage of Adrenal Cortex Regeneration. *By* WOJCIECH
ZIELENIEWSKI 491

Acute Phase Proteins and Interleukin-6 Serum Levels in Patients with
Chronic Arterial Occlusion. *By* WACLAW MAJEWSKI, RYSZARD
STANISZEWSKI, ARTUR SLUPIANEK, ALEKSANDER GORNY, AND
ANDRZEJ MACKIEWICZ 493

Inflammatory Cytokines in Peritoneal Fluid of Women with Endometriosis.
By J. SKRZYPCZAK, P. JEDRZEJCZAK, M. KASPRZAK, E. PUK, AND
M. KURPISZ 496

Increased Resistance of CSF-1-deficient, Macrophage-deficient, TNFα-
deficient, and IL-1α-deficient *op/op* Mice to Endotoxin. *By*
MALGORZATA SZPERL, AFTAB A. ANSARI, ELZBIETA URBANOWSKA,
PRZEMYSLAW SZWECH, PAWEL KALINSKI, AND WIESLAW WIKTOR-
JEDRZEJCZAK 499

Characterization of the IL-6/LIF-Response Factor by Proteolytic Analysis.
By K. SCHNEIDER, J. RIPPERGER, G. H. FEY, AND G. M. HOCKE . . . 502

Acute Phase Response and Interleukin-6 after Operative Laparoscopy and
Microsurgery in Gynecology. *By* KRZYSZTOF DREWS, KRZYSZTOF
SZYMANOWSKI, JANA SKRZPCZAK, PIOTR JĘDRZEJCZAK, AND
TOMASZ ŻAK 505

Acute Phase Proteins in Endometriosis. *By* KRZYSZTOF DREWS, JANA
SKRZYPCZAK, TOMASZ ŻAK, KRZYSZTOF SZYMANOWSKI, AND ANDRZEJ
MACKIEWICZ 508

Subject Index 511

Index of Contributors 519

Financial assistance was received from:

Supporters
- ACADEMY OF MEDICINE, POZNAŃ
- ARES SERONO, SWITZERLAND

- MARIA SKOLDOWSKA-CURIE II FUND
- SYNTEX PHARMACEUTICALS AG, POLAND

Contributors
- ABBOTT LABORATORIES
- ALAB
- AVL DIAGNOSTICA
- BIOMEDICA
- BRISTOL MYERS
- CHEMINST
- CORMAY
- GENZYME CORPORATION-ARCID, POLAND
- GLAXO
- IMMUNEX RESEARCH AND DEVELOPMENT CORPORATION
- JENOPTIC-MERAZET POLSKA
- KEBO-LAB
- MILES INC.
- PFIZER CENTRAL RESEARCH
- POLISH SOCIETY FOR IMMUNOLOGY
- PROSPECTA
- R. W. JOHNSON PHARMACEUTICAL RESEARCH INSTITUTE
- STEFAN BATORY FOUNDATION
- SY-LAB

The New York Academy of Sciences believes it has a responsibility to provide an open forum for discussion of scientific questions. The positions taken by the participants in the reported conferences are their own and not necessarily those of the Academy. The Academy has no intent to influence legislation by providing such forums.

Preface

This meeting may be viewed as the descendant of the conference **Regulation of the Acute Phase and Immune Responses: Interleukin-6** sponsored by The New York Academy of Sciences and the National Foundation for Cancer Research that was held in New York City on December 12–14, 1988 (P.B. Sehgal, G. Greininger, and G. Tosato, Eds., Ann. N.Y. Acad. Sci. **557**: 1–583, 1989). At that meeting the participants agreed that the cytokine previously known under various names—interferon-β_2, B-cell stimulatory factor-2, hybridoma/plastocytoma growth factor, and hepatocyte growth factor—should be referred to as interleukin-6. In the years to follow, interleukin-6 emerged as a principal cytokine controlling the synthesis of acute phase plasma proteins in the liver and the systemic response to inflammation, as well as a contributor to hematopoietic cell proliferation, cell differentiation (B cells), thrombocytopoiesis, and activation of cells of the immune system (T cells and natural killer cells).

In the last few years it has been discovered that other cytokines also possess biological properties very similar to those of interleukin-6. These include leukemia inhibitory factor, interleukin-11, oncostatin M, ciliary neurotrophic factor, and cardiotrophin-1. These cytokines are unrelated to interleukin-6 in primary structure, but all use a common signal-transducing β chain (gp130) in their cell surface receptors. These "interleukin-6-type" cytokines form a group in which the cytokines, although unrelated in the conventional sense, appear to have similar structure and elicit largely similar effects on, for example, the hepatocyte. Several of the interleukin-6-type cytokines are now in early clinical trials in humans. The papers presented at this symposium represent the cutting edge of basic and clinical research in the field of interleukin-6-type cytokines today.

Two additional aspects of this New York Academy of Sciences conference on **Interleukin-6-Type Cytokines** held in Poznań, Poland need to be emphasized.

First, this conference took place in Poland on the hundredth anniversary of the publication of E. Biernacki, a Polish physician, of his discovery of the erythrocyte sedimentation rate and its use as an indicator of acute inflammatory disease (E. Biernacki, *Uber die Beziehung des Plasmas zu den rothen Blutkorperchen und über den Wert verschiedener Methoden der Blutkorperchenvolumbestimmung* Zeitschrift f. physiologische Chemie **19**, 1894). In 1994, we recognize that the production and activity of interleukin-6-type cytokines during inflammation is the basis for the phenomenon reported by Biernacki in 1894.

Second, this is the first New York Academy of Sciences conference to be held in Central or Eastern Europe. We greatly appreciate the efforts of the Conference Director, Mrs. Geraldine Busacco, and of Ms. Sherryl Greenberg (Conference Coordinator), Ms. Lynn Serra, and Ms. Xanthe Ellis of the Conference Department of the New York Academy of Sciences for their superb professionalism in putting together this conference in a place rather remote from New York City.

We also wish to express our gratitude to the cosponsor of this conference, the State Committee for Scientific Research (Warsaw), the Maria Sklodowska-Curie Joint Fund II of the U.S.-Polish Joint Commission, and the local organizers in Poznań, in particular The Academy of Medicine, who worked hard to make this conference a success. Furthermore, we heartily acknowledge the assistance of Dr. Maria Łaciak, without whose help this conference would not have been possible. We also thank Ms. Małgorzata Mackiewicz for transcribing the tapes of all the oral discussion periods. Finally, we express our appreciation of the speakers and other participants who made an especial effort to put forward their best and newest science at this conference.

****

This volume is dedicated to the memory of Dr. Igor Tamm (1922–1995) of The Rockefeller University, a teacher and colleague to several generations of virologists and cell biologists.

ANDRZEJ MACKIEWICZ
ALEKSANDER KOJ
PRAVIN B. SEHGAL

Welcoming Remarks

J. GADZINOWSKI

Rector, University School of Medical Sciences
61-878 Poznań, Poland

On behalf of the authorities of the University School of Medical Sciences I am honored to welcome you. This town, Poznań, is nearly 1000 years old. Our University is a little younger, however, but has strong medical roots. At the moment we have nearly 200 full professors, 1000 academic teachers, and 3500 students in the various faculties: medicine, dentistry, pharmacy, and health sciences. All together, the University contains nearly 10,000 people. So, in the name of this quite big, local community, I am pleased to wish you a very good conference and a very pleasant stay in Poznań.

Interleukin-6-Type Cytokines[a]

PRAVIN B. SEHGAL,[b-f] LING WANG,[b] RAVI RAYANADE,[b]
HENG PAN,[d] AND LOLA MARGULIES[d]

[b]*Department of Cell Biology & Anatomy*
[c]*Department of Medicine*
[d]*Department of Microbiology & Immunology*
New York Medical College
Valhalla, New York 10595

INTRODUCTION

On December 14, 1988 at a New York Academy of Sciences conference held in New York City[1] a consensus emerged among all of the investigators who had independently discovered a fascinating and exciting new cytokine to call this cytokine "interleukin-6" (IL-6). IL-6 participated in the regulation of the acute phase and immune responses.[1] Some of the terms that were subsumed under the name IL-6 were interferon-β_2 (IFN-β_2), 26-kD protein, B-cell stimulatory factor 2 (BSF-2), hybridoma/plasmacytoma growth factor (HPGF/HGF), hepatocyte stimulating factor (HSF), interleukin-HP1 (IL-HP1), monocyte-granulocyte inducer type 2 (MGI-2), and cytotoxic T-cell differentiation factor (CDF).[1] IL-6 continues to be re-discovered by investigators. A recent example is the identification of "human fibroblast-derived growth inhibitor (hFDGI) for early-melanoma cells" as IL-6.[2]

In 1991 IL-6 came of age, and was honored by two conferences organized by Metcalf[3] and by Revel[4] that dealt in considerable detail with this polyfunctional cytokine. Also in 1991 it became clear that IL-6 was only one of several apparently structurally unrelated cytokines that exerted their biological effects via activation of the same signal-transducing β chain in their cell membrane receptor (the gp130). Thus the common targeting of cytokines such as IL-6, leukemia inhibitory factor (LIF) and other cytokines through gp130 was particularly highlighted in October 1991 by Metcalf with the help of the CIBA Foundation.[3] Very rapidly it has become apparent that a group of cytokines that include IL-6, LIF, oncostatin M (OM), interleukin-11 (IL-11), ciliary neurotrophic factor (CNTF), and cardiotrophin-1 (CT-1) use a common β chain, the gp130, as part of their receptor signal-transduction mechanism. The cell surface receptor for each of these cytokines includes distinct α chain components that, as a simple approximation, determine the high-affinity access of the ligand to the signal transducing chain(s). The detailed receptor chemistry for interaction

---

[a] Supported by Research Grant AI-16262 from the National Institutes of Health, Research Grant IM-701 from the American Cancer Society, and a contract from the National Foundation for Cancer Research.

[e] This manuscript is dedicated to Elyse S. Goldweber, Josephine Lauriello, Larry Jainchill, Loy Daniels, Gerald M. LaBush, Suzanne E. Andrews, Kimberly A. Sorrentino, Peter S. Marx, Pramila Warke, Manohar V. N. Shirodkar, and the many friends on my "team" without whom this work would have been impossible.

[f] Address correspondence to: Dr. P. B. Sehgal, Dept. of Cell Biology & Anatomy, Basic Science Building, New York Medical College, Valhalla, NY 10595; Tel: 914-993-4196, FAX: 914-993-4825.

TABLE 1. The Cytokines

Interleukin-6-type cytokines (receptor contains common gp130 β chain)
 Interleukin-6 (IL-6)
 Interleukin-11 (IL-11)
 Leukemia inhibitory factor (LIF)
 Oncostatin M (OM)
 Ciliary neurotrophic factor (CNTF)
 Cardiotrophin-1 (CT-1)
Interleukin-12 (IL-12) (architectural similarity with the binary IL-6/sIL-6R complex)

---

with and activation by each of these cytokines at the cell surface is the subject of intense investigation and is dealt with in a number of chapters in this volume.

We now had a semantic problem. The need for a simple term that would collectively allow one to refer to the group of six cytokines that involve gp130 in their signal transduction was brought into sharp focus as this conference was in its planning stages. Dr. Andrzej Mackiewicz conducted extensive informal polling. As a result of this polling, together with comments from numerous reviewers recruited by the Conference Committee of the New York Academy of Sciences, we have made bold to use the term "IL-6-type cytokines" to collectively refer to these cytokines (TABLE 1). Drs. Heinz Baumann, Carl Richards, and Jack Gauldie have been instrumental in forcing us to think about these cytokines in a collective fashion.[5] The ability of these cytokines to stimulate acute-phase plasma protein synthesis in appropriate hepatoma lines in a qualitatively similar manner is a property ascribable to the fact that their receptors contain the same gp130 signal-transducing chain.

In a way interleukin-12 (IL-12) also needs to be thought of as a relative of the IL-6-type cytokines, in that the two chains of the IL-12 ligand are reminiscent of the binary complex of IL-6 bound to its soluble p80 (IL-6R) component. A consideration of IL-12 and some of its biological effects is presented by Neta[5] in this volume.

INTERLEUKIN-6

Although all of the IL-6 type cytokines can elicit, for example, stimulation of plasma protein synthesis in hepatocyte cultures reminiscent of the acute-phase response, the key question that had to be asked was which is the key cytokine that mediates the acute-phase response *in vivo*? The answer to this question is provided in two chapters in this volume by Kopf *et al.*[7] and Poli *et al.*[8] who investigated the acute-phase response in IL-6 knockout mice. The answer is clear. IL-6 is the key systemic alarm signal. In the homozygous IL-6 knockout mouse, the systemic acute-phase plasma protein response to injury (*e.g.* a sterile turpentine abscess) is blunted.[7]

The working hypothesis for research in this laboratory has had the perspective that rapid and marked induction of IL-6 is crucial to its role as the major systemic alarm signal that alerts the body to the presence of tissue damage or injury of any kind. Almost every noxious stimulus induces IL-6 gene expression in many different cell types. In fact the molecular dissection of the IL-6 promoter reveals it to be responsive to activation by all three signal transduction pathways—protein kinase C, cAMP/ protein kinase A and calcium ionophore (FIG. 1). The multiple response elements MRE-I and MRE-II in the IL-6 promoter represent the common and overlapping DNA targets for a variety of different activation pathways.[9] The efficient induction of the IL-6 promoter depends upon the cooperative interactions of several transcription

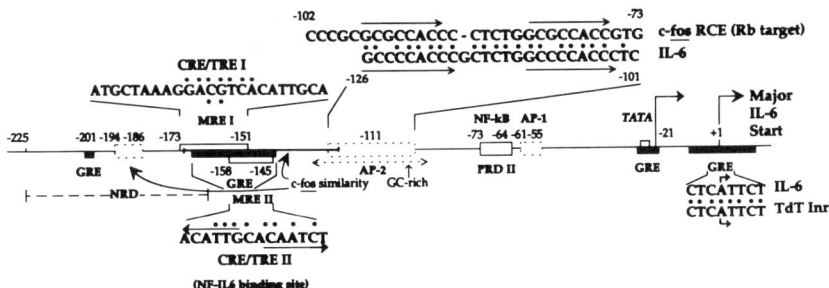

FIGURE 1. Schematic representation of positive and negative transcription regulatory elements in the 5'-flanking region of the human IL-6 gene. Solid lines (either boxes or arrows) indicate DNA regulatory elements that have already been functionally implicated in IL-6 gene expression, while those marked by broken lines or boxes are based on DNA sequence analyses. The inducible transcription start sites were derived by S1 nuclease mapping (ratio of major +1 to minor −21 was 99:1.[1] The presence of a negative regulatory domain (NRD) between −225 and −165 was inferred from 5' deletion results. The typical GACGTCA CRE/TRE motif in MRE I and the nucleotides in the novel CRE/TRE in MRE II which match with nucleotides in the CRE identified in bovine cytochrome $P450_{17\alpha}$ promoter are highlighted by solid circles. The mutation of the CG residues (open circles) to GT reduces the responsiveness of MRE I to TPA and forskolin; similarly point mutations in MRE II reduce inducibility to these agents. PRDII refers to the NF-κB-like domain in the β-interferon promoter. Inr refers to the initiator RNA start site motif as functionally characterized in the terminal deoxynucleotidyltransferase (TdT) gene. RCE is the Rb-repressible DNA target in the c-*fos* promoter. (Adapted from Ray et al., 1990.[9])

factors including C/EBP family members and NF-κB.[10] Ray et al.[11] in this volume discuss the cooperative interactions of transcription factors involved in IL-6 induction and their modulation by glucocorticoids and estrogens.

Consistent with the presence of a strongly inducible promoter, IL-6 is readily found in the peripheral circulation at concentrations that would be sufficient to elicit biological effects (e.g. on hepatocytes). May et al.[12] in this volume discuss the novel finding that IL-6 in the human circulation can occur in a "chaperoned" state as high molecular mass complexes. In this form the associated proteins appear to modulate the systemic availability and function of IL-6.

There has been spectacular progress in the dissection of the IL-6 induced signal-transduction pathways activated through the gp130 β chain of the IL-6 receptor. Several chapters in this volume represent a careful blow-by-blow account of the role of Tyr-kinases and stat protein family members in IL-6 triggered signal transduction. The generality of these signaling events is emphasized by the observations that several of the IL-6 type cytokines as well as other completely unrelated cytokines such as the interferons use the same pathways. [For some of us it is personally interesting that IL-6 research has brought us back to signal-transduction pathways used by the interferons.] The link between IL-6 effects at the cell membrane (Tyr-phosphorylation of gp130 and stat3) and the activation of target promoters such as those of the acute-phase plasma proteins still needs to be demonstrated in a robust manner.

Two areas of IL-6 research that are under investigation in the authors' laboratory are briefly reviewed in the following two sections. The first relates to the discovery that p53 can regulate not only the IL-6 promoter but also the βfibrinogen enhancer, and the second deals with the practical application of IL-6 measurements as a diagnostic and prognostic tool in the hands of the obstetrician.

MODULATION OF HEPATIC IL-6 RESPONSE BY p53

p53 is a cellular transcription regulatory factor.[13–15] Wild-type (wt) p53 can *enhance* transcription from a set of promoters that contain DNA-binding sites for p53, whereas wt p53 can *repress* many promoters that do not contain direct p53-DNA binding sites. Mutations in p53 alter the ability of this molecule to modulate transcription. p53 mediates its effects by interacting with a variety of cellular and viral proteins (TABLE 2). Up to now the biological functions of p53 have been discussed in the context of cell proliferation, apoptosis, and repair of radiation-induced DNA damage.[13–18] Our discovery that p53 physically interacts with the C/EBP family transcription factors (see below) has led us to ask a novel question: can the transcription factor p53 modulate the response of cells to cytokines in a context distinct from considerations of cell proliferation? Can mutations in p53 alter the response of tumor cells to cytokines (or biological response modifiers in general)? Do alterations in p53 affect cytokine-induced gene expression in hepatoma cells? And, very generally, does the transcription factor p53 participate in regulating non-immunological or immunological aspects of the "acute-phase" response of the host to infection and neoplasia? For the first time we are asking questions about the place of p53 as a transcription factor in the "acute" response cascade triggered by cytokines as distinct from the effects of p53 on cell proliferation. What is the role of p53 as a modulator of cytokine synthesis and the differentiated-cell response to cytokines?

We depart from all previous investigations in that we have begun to examine the effect of p53 species on cytokine function in a context different from the control of cell proliferation. Can mutations in p53 alter the cascade of plasma protein gene expression elicited by IL-6 type cytokines in *hepatoma* cells? We propose that the disruptive influence of mutations in p53 on gene expression and cell physiology is amplified by targeted interference with cytokine-elicited signal-transduction pathways that, in turn, regulate expression of numerous other genes.

Studies summarized in this section describe how the work with p53 was initiated in this laboratory several years ago[19] and how it connected with our long-standing interests in IL-6 and C/EBPβ.[20,21] We also briefly summarize new experiments that form the basis for the interference that p53 species may modulate IL-6-responsive plasma protein gene expression in hepatoma cells, and that lay the foundation for the suggestion that p53 species may modulate the function of C/EBPα, β and δ in hepatoma cell lines.

TABLE 2. Proteins that Bind to p53

Adenovirus E1B
Papillomavirus E6
Hepatitis B HBX
Heat shock protein 70 (hsc70)
Murine double minute-2 (MDM-2)
Wilms' tumor-1 (WT-1)
TATA-binding protein (TBP), and thus TFIID
CAAT-binding factor (CBF)
Transcription-coupled DNA repair factor ECCR3
C/EBPα, β, δ (our data)

TABLE 3. IL-6/CAT and Other Reporter Constructs Used

Plasmid	Comment
pIC225	-225 to $+13$ IL-6/CAT
pmRCE-1	pIC225 with CG to GT mutation in MRE-1 at $-161, -162$
pmRCE-2	pIC225 with TG to CA mutation in MRE-2 at $-153, -154$ in C/EBP site
pmNF-κB	pIC225 with GGG to AAT mutation in NF-κB site at $-71, -72, -73$
pInrC	-60 to $+13$ IL-6 TATA and Inr site/CAT
pAR12TKC	IL-6 MRE (-173 to -145) in pTKC$_{-105}$
pTKC$_{-105}$	-105 herpes TK with CAAT box (C/EBP-binding site)/CAT
pTKC$_{-80}$	-80 herpes TK with CAAT box deleted/CAT
p50-2	2×50-bp p53-binding element from MCK/CAT
pCH110	SV40 early enhancer-promoter/βgal (used occasionally)
pRSVβgal	RSV LTR/βgal (used routinely)

From Margulies and Sehgal, 1993.[20]

Studies with p53 and the IL-6 Promoter That Led to the Identification of C/EBPβ as a Target for p53 Modulation

The hypothesis that p53 and Rb might be involved in regulating IL-6 synthesis first arose in the spring of 1990 when we noted the similarity between the c-*fos* Rb-control element (RCE) and the region in the IL-6 promoter DNA from -126 to -101 (FIG. 1). Soon thereafter we found in transient transfection experiments that both wt p53 and wt Rb repressed human IL-6 promoter constructs.[19] However, because the effects of p53 species were particularly marked and consistently reproducible, we have concentrated our current efforts to studying the effects of p53 species on IL-6 biology.

Modulation of the Activity of IL-6 Promoter Constructs by Cotransfection of Expression Vectors for wt or Mutant p53 Species

Although wt p53 (human and murine) strongly repressed the IL-6 promoter in pIC225 (TABLE 3), the mutants SCX3 and c5 (TABLE 4) no longer repressed this promoter, and the mutants Val-135 and Phe-132 consistently enhanced IL-6 promoter activity at both 32.5°C and 37°C (FIG. 2). The IL-6 MRE (-145 to -173) confers cytokine responsiveness on the herpesvirus thymidine kinase promoter (TK$_{-105}$). This construct, pAR12TKC (TABLE 3), was used in assays designed to investigate the effect of p53 species on the isolated IL-6 MRE. Human and murine wt p53 species strongly repressed expression from the reporter construct pAR12TKC, but the mutants SCX3 and c5 did not. However, strong upregulation of pAR12TKC by both p53 Val-135 and Phe-132 was observed at both temperatures.

Effect of p53 Val-135 on Reporter Construct p50-2 (in HeLa and CV1 Cells)

We tested the effect of Val-135 on reporter construct p50-2 in these cells. This reporter construct contains two copies of a 50-bp p53-binding DNA element from within the muscle-specific creatine kinase promoter (MCK).[22] Zambetti *et al.*[23] have shown that p50-2 transfected into rat fibroblasts was upregulated by wt p53 and by

TABLE 4. p53 and Other Expression Vectors Used[a]

Plasmid	Comment
p53-SN3	human p53, wt
p53-SCX3	human p53, transforming mutant (Val143 to Ala)
pCMVNc9	murine p53, wt
pCMVc5	murine p53, transforming mutant (Glu168 to Gly; Met234 to Ile)
p53Val135	murine p53, transforming mutant with "ts" phenotype, Harvey sarcoma virus LTR promoter
p53Phe132	murine p53, transforming mutant, "non-ts" phenotype, Harvey sarcoma virus LTR promoter
pNF-IL6	human NF-IL6 (alias C/EBPβ) in vector pCDM8
pCMV	Vector control derived from p53-SN3 by removal of p53 cDNA insert; used as a control to adjust total transfected DNA amounts
pCDM8	CMV promoter vector with expression cloning site intact
pSVneo	Additional control plasmid used to adjust total transfected DNA amounts in experiments with p53 Val135 or p53 Phe132

From Margulies and Sehgal, 1993.[20]

[a] Driven by cytomegalovirus (CMV) early enhancer/promoter unless otherwise stated.

Val-135 at 32.5° but less so at 39°C. As expected, wt p53 enhanced expression from p50-2 at both 32.5° and 37°C. Strikingly, in HeLa cells, Val-135 resulted in a higher level of activation of p50-2 than did wt p53 at both temperatures. Although Val-135 was not ts in HeLa cells, additional experiments using both the p50-2 and IL-6 reporter constructs verified that p53 Val-135 was clearly "ts" in CV1 cells in our hands. These experiments made it clear that the ts phenotype of p53 Val-135 was cell-type and promoter-dependent (TABLE 5).[21]

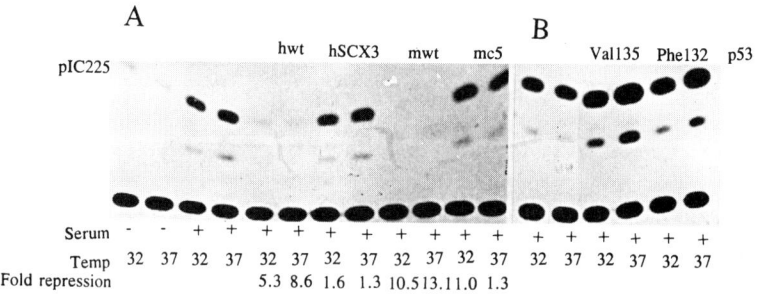

FIGURE 2. Modulation of the IL-6 promoter (−225 to +13) in construct pIC225 in HeLa cells cotransfected by various p53 expression vectors at different temperatures. HeLa cell cultures in 100-mm plastic petri dishes were transfected with pIC225 (10 μg) and pRSVβgal (5 μg) together with each of various p53 expression vectors (5 μg each) or with 5 μg of the pCMV (*panel A*) or pSVneo (*panel B*) control DNA. Cultures were incubated in the absence of serum (−) or the presence of serum (+) at 32.5°C or 37°C. CAT assays were performed by normalizing between groups using βgal activity. Fold-repression and fold-activation were calculated with respect to the serum-treated controls at the corresponding temperature. (From Margulies and Sehgal, 1993.[20])

TABLE 5. Summary: Cell-type and Promoter-dependent Variations in the Effects of p53 Val-135

Reporter Construct	Cell Type	p53 Species		
		wt[a]	Val-135 32.5°C	Val-135 37°C
pMCK	CV1	↑↑↑↑[b]	⇌	⇌
	Hela	↓↓	⇌	↑↑
p50-2	CV1	↑↑↑	↑↑	⇌
	HeLa	↑↑	↑↑	↑↑
pIC225	CV1	↓↓	↑↑	⇌
	HeLa	↓↓	↑	↑

From Sehgal and Margulies, 1993.[21]
[a] Same phenotype at both 32.5 and 37°C.
[b] ↑, activation; ↓, repression; ⇌, minimal effect.

Mechanism of Modulation of the IL-6 Promoter by p53 Species

a) The DNA Target

In preliminary experiments we used the DNA-binding-immunoprecipitation assay employing ^{32}P-labeled segments of IL-6 promoter DNA, extracts from HeLa cells transfected with p53 expression vectors, and various anti-p53 monoclonal antibodies (PAb421, P1801, and PAb420), but were unable to detect specific binding of IL-6 promoter DNA fragments to p53-containing complexes. Therefore, we focused our effort towards a series of functional assays in order to gain insight into the mechanism(s) by which p53 species affect the function of the human IL-6 promoter.

An evaluation of the effects of p53 species on a series of point-mutation constructs engineered within the context of the intact IL-6 promoter in pIC225 (-225 to $+13$) was informative (TABLE 3).[20] Whereas mutations in the NF-kB site (pmNF-kB) and the MRE-1 element (pmRCE-1) reduced overall chloramphenicol acetyltransferase(CAT) signal strength derived from the IL-6 promoter in HeLa cells, they did not affect the ability of the reporter to be modulated by p53 species (repression by wt p53, upregulation by Val-135). In contrast, a point mutation in MRE-2 in the C/EBPβ (alias NF-IL6) binding site (pmRCE-2) blocked modulation by p53. Additionally, the core IL-6 Inr/CAT construct pInrC was neither repressed nor upregulated by p53 species. Taken together, the data pointed to the requirement for an intact C/EBPβ site for modulation by p53 species.

b) Modulation of Transcription Factor C/EBPβ alias NF-IL6 Function by p53 Species

As a direct extension of the DNA target studies, we evaluated the ability of p53 species to affect C/EBPβ function.[20] C/EBPβ upregulated the IL-6 promoter in pIC225. However, wt human p53 but not its mutant SCX3, inhibited C/EBPβ-mediated activation of pIC225 in a dominant manner. Thus, transcription factor C/EBPβ was a functional target for repression by wt p53 in HeLa cells. TABLE 6 shows that C/EBPβ function is further upregulated by Val-135 and Phe-132 provided that the reporter constructs have an intact C/EBP-binding site.[20] TABLE 6, experiment A shows that pIC225, but not the C/EBPβ-site mutant pmRCE-2, was upregulated

TABLE 6. DNA Sequence Requirements for the Effects of Mutant p53 Species and of C/EBPβ on the IL-6 and TK Promoters

Reporter Construct	Fold Increase in CAT Activity[a]				
	C/EBPβ	p53 Phe-132		p53 Val-135	
			+ C/EBPβ		+ C/EBPβ
Experiment A[b]					
pIC225	2.8	1.5	4.4	1.6	9.9
pmRCE-2	0.9	0.9	0.9	1.0	0.9
Experiment B					
pTK$_{-105}$C	13.1	3.8	77.2	3.5	68.9
pTK$_{-80}$C	1.3	1.1	2.0	1.1	1.7

From Margulies and Sehgal, 1993.[20]

[a] Values for % conversion of radiolabeled chloramphenicol to the acetylated forms in control cultures were 1.83, 0.64, 1.0 and 0.55% in cultures transfected with pIC225, pmRCE-2, pTK$_{-105}$C and pTK$_{-80}$C, respectively.

[b] In experiment A, HeLa cells were transfected with pIC225 (10 μg) or the C/EBPβ-binding site mutant pmRCE-2 (2.5 μg). In experiment B, HeLa cells received pTKC$_{-105}$ (2.5 μg) or the C/EBPβ-binding site deletion mutant pTKC$_{-80}$ (2.5 μg). In addition each culture received pRSVβgal (5 μg) together with various p53 expression vectors (5 μg each) and the additional inclusion of the C/EBPβ expression vector pNF-IL6 in the transfection (10 μg). Control DNA plasmids used included pCMV (10 μg) to match the CMV-driven plasmid pNF-IL6 and pSVneo (5 μg) to match the p53 vectors; thus, all the cultures received the same amount of DNA in each transfection.

by C/EBPβ in conjunction with Val-135 and Phe-132. The inability of Val-135 or Phe-132 to affect pmRCE-2 even in the presence of exogenously expressed C/EBPβ, indicates that this transcription factor and its cognate binding site in the IL-6 promoter DNA are part of a major mechanism accounting for upregulation of the IL-6 promoter by p53 Val-135 and Phe-132. This inference was confirmed by the data in TABLE 6, experiment B which demonstrate dramatic transcriptional activation effects of C/EBPβ in association with p53 Val-135 or Phe-132 on the herpesvirus TK promoter provided that the reporter construct included the C/EBP-binding site (pTKC$_{-105}$), but not when this site was deleted (pTKC$_{-80}$).

Although wt p53 repressed the IL-6 promoter, specific tumor-derived mutations in p53 (e.g. Val-135 and Phe-132) upregulated this promoter. The p53 "ts" mutant Val135 upregulated the IL-6 promoter at both 32.5° and 37°C in HeLa cells (TABLE 5).[20,21] This phenotype defines a "gain in function" mutation in p53 because under no experimental conditions did Val-135 or Phe-132 display the repression phenotype that is characteristic of wt p53 with respect to the the human IL-6 promoter in these cells. Modulation of the function of transcription factor C/EBPβ by wt p53 (inhibition) and by Val-135 (enhancement) was identified as a mechanism for the effects of p53 species on IL-6 gene expression. The discovery that p53 species modulate C/EBPβ function, for the first time, raised the possibility that mutations in p53 could also contribute to alterations in the responsiveness of tumor cells to different cytokines in a manner independent of the regulation of cell proliferation. That p53 species functionally modulate the transcription factor C/EBPβ ties p53 into a large body of work that relates to the response of cells to cytokines and to cell differentiation in general. How do wt p53 and its various mutants behave in hepatoma cell lines with respect to plasma protein gene promoters?

Transient Transfection Studies in Hepatoma Cell Lines Showing That p53 Species Modulate IL-6- and C/EBP-responsive Gene Expression

We tested the ability of p53 to affect plasma protein gene expression in Hep3B and HepG2 cells treated with IL-6. The choice of the plasma protein gene promoter rat βfibrinogen (βFibCAT)[24] for our initial experiments was based on the fact that fibrinogen species have been intensively studied for response to cytokines (IL-6, LIF, OM, CNTF, IL-11) and to C/EBPα, β and δ species in hepatoma cell lines, and that the particular βFibCAT construct used ["βFb(2xIL6-RE)CAT"][24] was a "matched" construct with respect to p50-2. Both βFibCAT and p50-2 contain two copies of the respective enhancers upstream of the major late adenovirus type 2 promoter (therefore same TATA box). Do p53 species modulate the IL-6- and C/EBP-activated pathway(s)? The answer is yes.

The βFib/CAT reporter was activated by IL-6 in Hep3B and HepG2 cells. This activation was blocked by human (SN3) and murine (Nc9) wt p53 species. Mutations in p53 either no longer repressed βFib/CAT or enhanced the activity of the reporter construct. The data clearly established the fact that p53 species can modulate the response of liver cells to IL-6. Plasma protein gene expression is a target for p53 species.

Is the function of C/EBP species also affected by p53 species in hepatoma cells? The answer is yes. It has been shown previously that the βFb(2xIL6-RE)CAT reporter,[24] although it contains the CTGGGA Type II IL-6 responsive element, is also responsive to C/EBPα, β and δ. In our hands the βFib/CAT reporter was activated by cotransfection with different C/EBPα, β and δ expression plasmids in HepG2 cells. Wt p53 inhibited βFib/CAT activation by C/EBP species whereas mutations in p53 either had little effect or enhanced expression. As a key control the reporter p50-2 was activated by wt p53 and C/EBP species in the same cells.

Protein-Protein Interactions between Different C/EBP Species and Different p53 Species

The functional experiments suggest the hypothesis that one mechanism by which p53 (wt and its mutants) may modulate transcription is through interaction with the members of the transcription factor C/EBP family. This hypothesis was tested in direct biochemical experiments. We prepared ^{35}S-methionine-labeled C/EBP α, β or δ using a coupled transcription/translation system (T7/SP6 promoters and reticulocyte lysates; the Promega TNT system), and recombinant murine wt p53 in the baculovirus expression system. The reagents were used to demonstrate cross-precipitation of C/EBPα, β or δ species but not a control protein (luciferase) by wt murine p53. In these experiments radio-labeled C/EBP species were incubated with p53 at room-temperature for 30 minutes, the proteins were cross-linked in solution using dithio-bis(succinimidyl propionate)(DSP)(5 mM), blocking of DSP by ethanolamine (0.1 M), and precipitation. The p53 preferentially precipitated the labeled C/EBP species but not the control luciferase protein as detected by reversal of cross-link and SDS-PAGE.

We propose that the transcription factor p53 is involved in modulating the host "acute phase" response to infection and injury. The mechanistic basis for this hypothesis may be the interaction between p53 and C/EBP species. Indeed, several predictions of this hypothesis can be tested for biological relevance in the p53 −/− mouse, and in cell lines derived from such knockout animals. Such studies are in progress. As a further corollary, we propose that mutations in p53 alter the response of tumor cells to IL-6-type cytokines. This corollary hypothesis leads to several predictions that can also be tested by evaluating p53 status in clinical materials and clinical response data in cancer patients administered IL-6-type cytokines (or administered cells expressing receptors for IL-6-type cytokines).

DIAGNOSTIC AND PROGNOSTIC VALUE OF AMNIOTIC FLUID IL-6 MEASUREMENTS

Over the last five years we have investigated IL-6 levels in human body fluids in a variety of clinical situations. These include studies of serum IL-6 levels in patients administered TNF or endotoxin, of serum, cerebrospinal fluid and synovial fluid in patients with systemic bacterial infections or with compartmentalized infections and various arthritides, of serum IL-6 in patients with graft-vs-host disease following bone marrow transplantation, and in patients with psoriasis (reviewed in ref. 25). There is one clinical situation where we have now accumulated compelling data testifying to the diagnostic and prognostic value of IL-6 measurement in a body fluid: in amniotic fluid in premature preterm labor. In several studies[26-30] carried out in collaboration with Drs. Roberto Romero, Anthony C. Allison and their colleagues, we have documented marked elevations of amniotic fluid IL-6 in patients in preterm premature labor (PTL) refractory to tocolysis (a therapeutic regimen designed to inhibit labor contractions that includes administration of ritodrine, a β-adrenergic agent) (FIG. 3).

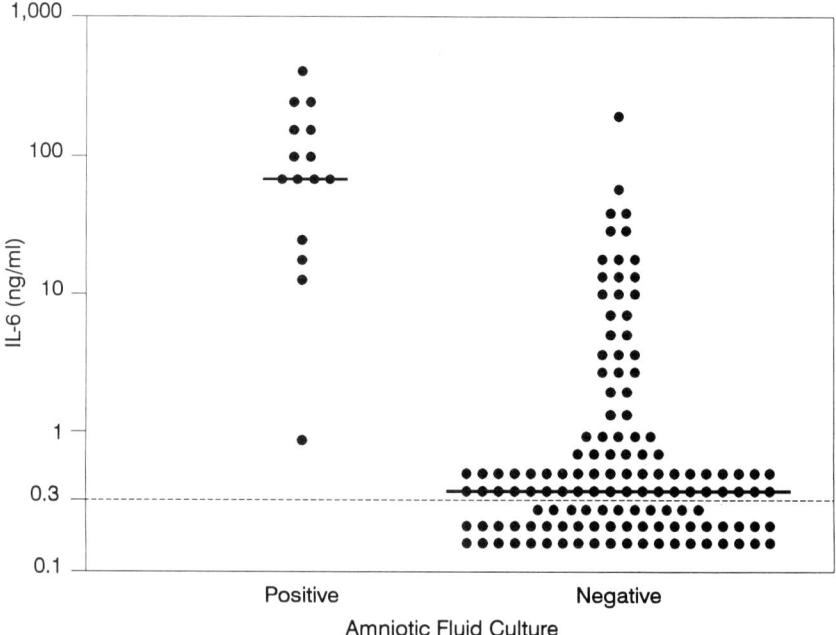

FIGURE 3. Amniotic fluid interleukin-6 concentrations (IL-6, ng/ml) in patients in preterm labor with intact membranes. Patients with a positive amniotic fluid culture had a significantly higher median amniotic fluid IL-6 concentrations than patients with a negative culture (median, 91.2 ng/ml; range, 0.9–437 ng/ml vs. median, 0.4 ng/ml; range, <0.3–195 ng/ml; respectively; $p < 0.0001$, Wilcoxon test for censored data). (From Romero et al., 1993.[28])

TABLE 7. Comparison of Diagnostic Indices of Amniotic Fluid Gram Stain and Interleukin-6 Concentrations in the Diagnosis of Positive Amniotic Fluid Culture

	Gram Stain	Amniotic Fluid IL-6 ($\geq$11.3 ng/ml)	Amniotic Fluid IL-6 and Gram Stain
Sensitivity	73.3% (11/15)	93.3% (14/15)	100% (15/15)
Specificity	100% (131/131)[a]	91.6% (120/131)	91.6% (120/131)
Positive predictive value	100% (11/11)	56.0% (14/25)	57.7% (15/26)
Negative predictive value	97.0% (131/135)	99.1% (120/121)	100% (120/120)

From Romero et al., 1993.[28]
[a] $p < 0.005$

IL-6 elevation was found to have the greatest sensitivity and the Gram stain the greatest specificity in the prediction of a positive amniotic fluid culture (TABLE 7). A combination of amniotic fluid Gram-stain and IL-6 had 100% sensitivity. Amniotic fluid IL-6 levels are the best predictor of outcome in preterm labor.[28–30] In this setting, amniotic fluid IL-6 levels >11 ng/ml were associated with rapid preterm delivery without exception (FIG. 4). In turn, such high levels were related to the presence of intraamniotic infection. If the IL-6 levels were <2 ng/ml there was an 85% chance of salvaging the pregnancy to term using conservative management. Similar conclusions were reached by us in several studies in patients with premature

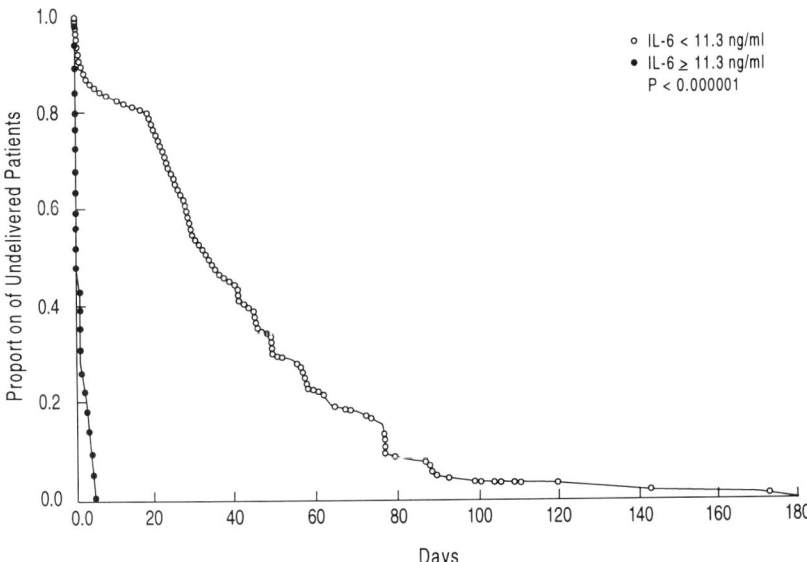

FIGURE 4. Survival analysis of the amniocentesis-to-delivery interval according to amniotic fluid interleukin-6 (IL-6) concentrations with different cut off levels. This panel displays the amniocentesis to delivery interval in patients with an amniotic fluid IL-6 above/equal to or below 11.3 ng/ml (median, 0.5 days; range, 0.1 to 6 days [n = 25] vs. median, 30 days; range, 0.3 to 175 days [n = 121]; $p < 0.000001$). (From Romero et al., 1993.[28])

TABLE 8. Relationship of Various Independent Variables with the Occurrence of Neonatal Morbidity/Mortality Analyzed by Logistic Regression

Independent Variables	Odds Ratio	95% Confidence Limits	p Value
Amniotic fluid interleukin-6 concentration[a]	13.84	2.96–64.66	0.001
Cervical dilatation	1.03	0.65–1.62	NS
Gestational age at admission	0.86	0.72–1.03	NS
Amniotic fluid glucose concentration[a]	0.97	0.19–4.72	NS
Amniotic fluid Gram stain	5.04	0.21–120.90	NS
Amniotic fluid white blood cell count[a]	4.97	0.68–36.30	NS

From Romero et al., 1993.[29]

[a] Variables were dichotomized: amniotic fluid IL-6 (<11.3 ng/ml vs ≥11.3 ng/ml), amniotic fluid white blood cell count (< 50 cells/mm^3 vs ≥50 cells/mm^3, and amniotic fluid glucose (≤14 mg/dl vs >14 mg/dl).

[b] NS = not significant.

rupture of membranes (PROM). Overall, amniotic fluid IL-6 was the best prognostic indicator of outcome—of premature delivery and infection, including neonatal morbidity (TABLE 8).[26–30]

Our very extensive studies of amniotic fluid IL-6 in PTL and PROM patients (n = 500) provide the strongest identification of a clinical situation where rapid IL-6 analysis in a tertiary referral setting can provide information to the obstetrician that is valuable in clinical management.[26–30] We have devised a rapid 60-minute ELISA for IL-6 for these studies. We have confirmed and extended our observations in a collaboration with Dr. Nergesh Tejani in the Department of Obstetrics at the New York Medical College. These studies in a tertiary referral setting have already generated intense interest in the Maternal-Fetal Medicine Community, and the testing of amniotic fluid IL-6 measurements in obstetric practice is now under serious evaluation.

CONCLUSIONS

One hundred years ago Biernacki[31] working here in Poland, in Warsaw, drew attention to the diagnostic value of what we now know to be the erythrocyte sedimentation rate (ESR). An increase in the sedimentation (of erythrocytes) in columns of oxalated blood was a feature of pregnancy, infections and many other illnesses. One hundred years ago, Biernacki had already noted that the increased sedimentation was correlated with an increase in the fibrin concentration. Indeed, through the efforts of Fåhræus,[32] Avery and his school who coined the term "acute phase" response (reviewed in 33), and a large number of investigators (reviewed in refs. 1, 34) we now know the increase in ESR to be the result of alterations in plasma protein composition, which is in turn ascribable to the induction and function of IL-6-type cytokines. It is most fitting that one hundred years after Biernacki, the structure and function of IL-6-type cytokines be discussed here in Poland.

[Note added in proof: The newly characterized cytokine cardiotrophin-1 (CT-1) that causes cardiac myocyte hypertrophy, neuronal cell differentiation, and inhibition of M1 myeloid cell proliferation turns out to belong to the IL-6–type cytokine family and uses gp130 as the signal transducing chain in its cell surface receptor[35,36].]

ACKNOWLEDGMENTS

We thank Mr. Kirit Patel and Mr. Giacomo Vinces for excellent technical help. We also thank Drs. Lester T. May, Frank Landsberger, and Mary Rifkin and the late Dr. Igor Tamm for numerous helpful discussions.

REFERENCES

1. SEHGAL, P. B., G. GRIENINGER & G. TOSATO, Eds. 1989. Regulation of the acute phase and immune responses: Interleukin-6. Ann. N. Y. Acad. Sci. **557:** 1–583.
2. LU, C., M. F. VICKERS & R. S. KERBEL. 1992. Interleukin 6: a fibroblast-derived growth inhibitor of human melanoma cells from early but not advanced stages of tumor progression. Proc. Natl. Acad. Sci. USA **89:** 9215–9219.
3. METCALF, D. 1992. Polyfunctional cytokines: IL-6 and LIF. Ciba Foundation Symposium **167:** 1–279. John Wiley & Sons, Chichester.
4. REVEL, M. 1992. IL-6: Physiopathology and Clinical Potentials. Serono Symposium **88:** 1–296. Raven Press, New York.
5. BAUMANN, H., J. GAULDIE & C. RICHARDS. 1994. The cellular and molecular regulation of the acute inflammatory response. J Cell. Biochem. Supplement **18B:** 309–330.
6. NETA, R., S. M. STIEFEL & N. ALI. 1995. In lethally irradiated mice interleukin-12 protects bone marrow but sensitizes intestinal tract to damage from ionizing radiation. Ann. N. Y. Acad. Sci. **762:** 274–281. This volume.
7. KOPF, M., A. RAMSAY, F. BROMBACHER, H. BAUMANN, G. FREER, C. GALANOS, J.-C. GUTIERREZ-RAMOS & G. KÖHLER. 1995. Pleiotropic defects of IL-6-deficient mice including early hematopoiesis, T and B cell function, and acute phase responses. Ann. N. Y. Acad. Sci. **762:** 308–318.
8. FATTORI, E., C. SELLITTO, M. CAPPELLETTI, D. LAZZARO, D. BELLAVIA, I. SCREPANTI, A. GULINO, F. COSTANTINI & V. POLI. 1995. Functional analysis of IL-6 and IL-6DBP/C/EBPβ by gene targeting. Ann. N. Y. Acad. Sci. **762:** 262–273. This volume.
9. RAY, A., K. S. LAFORGE & P. B. SEHGAL. 1990. On the mechanism for the efficient repression of the interleukin-6 promoter by glucocorticoids: Enhancer, TATA-box and RNA start site (Inr motif) occlusion. Mol. Cell. Biol. **10:** 5736–5746.
10. SEHGAL, P. B. 1992. Regulation of IL-6 gene expression. Res. Immunol. **143:** 724–734.
11. RAY, A., D-H ZHANG, M. D. SIEGEL & P. RAY. 1995. Regulation of Interleukin 6 gene expression by steroids. Ann. N. Y. Acad. Sci. **762:** 79–88. This volume.
12. MAY, L. T., M. I. NDUBUISI, K. PATEL & D. GARCIA. 1995. Interleukin-6 chaperones in blood. Ann. N. Y. Acad. Sci. **762:** 120–128. This volume.
13. VOGELSTEIN, B. & K. W. KINZLER. 1992. p53 function and dysfunction. Cell **70:** 523–526.
14. KOSHLAND, D. E. & E. CULOTTA. 1993. p53 sweeps through cancer research. Science **262:** 1958–1961.
15. OLINER, J. D. 1993. Discerning the function of p53 by examining its molecular interactions. BioEssays **15:** 703–707.
16. LEVINE, A. J., J. MOMAND & C. A. FINLAY. 1991. The p53 tumor supressor gene. Nature **351:** 453–456.
17. HOLLSTEIN, M., D. SIDRANSKY, B. VOGELSTEIN & C. C. HARRIS. 1991. p53 mutations in human cancers. Science **253:** 49–54.
18. MICHALOVITZ, D., O. HALAVEY & M. OREN. 1991. p53 mutations: Gains or losses. J. Cell. Biochem. **45:** 22–29.
19. SANTHANAM, U., A. RAY & P. B. SEHGAL. 1991. Repression of the interleukin-6 promoter by p53 and the retinoblastoma susceptibility gene product Rb. Proc. Natl. Acad. Sci. USA **88:** 7605–7609.
20. MARGULIES, L. & P. B. SEHGAL. 1993. Modulation of the human interleukin-6 (IL-6) promoter and transcription factor C/EBPβ (NF-IL6) activity by p53. J. Biol. Chem. **268:** 15096–15100.

21. SEHGAL, P. B. & L. MARGULIES. 1993. Cell type- and promoter-dependent ts phenotype of p53 Val[135]. Oncogene **8:** 3417–3419.
22. WEINTRAUB, H., S. HAUSCHKA & S. J. TAPSCOTT. 1991. The MCK enhancer contains a p53-responsive element. Proc. Natl. Acad. Sci. USA **88:** 4570–4571.
23. ZAMBETTI, G. P., J. BARGONETTI, K. WALKER, C. PRIVES & A. J. LEVINE. 1992. Wild-type p53 mediates positive regulation of gene expression through a specific DNA sequence element. Genes & Develop. **6:** 1143–1152.
24. BAUMANN, H., S. MARINKOVIC-PAJOVIC, K. A. WON, V. E. JONES, S. P. CAMPOS, G. P. JAHREIS & K. K. MORELLA. 1992. The action of interleukin 6 and leukaemia inhibitory factor on liver cells. CIBA Found. Symp. **167:** 100–114.
25. SEHGAL, P. B. 1990. Interleukin-6 in infection and cancer. Proc. Soc. Exp. Biol. Med. **195:** 183–191.
26. ROMERO, R., C. AVILA, U. SANTHANAM & P. B. SEHGAL. 1990. Amniotic fluid interleukin-6 in preterm labor: Association with infection. J. Clin. Invest. **85:** 1392–1400.
27. SANTHANAM, U., C. AVILA, R. ROMERO, H. VIGUET, N. IDA, S. SAKURAI & P. B. SEHGAL. 1991. Cytokines in normal and abnormal parturition: Elevated amniotic fluid IL-6 levels in women with premature rupture of membranes associated with intrauterine infection. Cytokine **3:** 1–9.
28. ROMERO, R., W. SEPULVEDA, J. S. KENNEY, L. E. ARCHER, A. C. ALLISON & P. B. SEHGAL. 1993. Amniotic fluid interleukin-6 determinations are of both diagnostic and prognostic value in preterm labor. Am. J. Reprod. Immunol. **30:** 167–183.
29. ROMERO, R., B. H. YOON, M. MAZUR, R. GOMEZ, M. P. DIAMOND, J. S. KENNEY, M. RAMIREZ, P. L. FIDEL, Y. SOROKIN, D. COTTON & P. B. SEHGAL. 1993. The diagnostic and prognostic value of amniotic fluid white blood cell count, glucose, interleukin-6, and Gram stain in patients with preterm labor and intact membranes. Am. J. Obstet. Gynecol. **169:** 805–816.
30. ROMERO, R., B. H. YOON, M. MAZUR, R. GOMEZ, M. GONZALEZ, M. P. DIAMOND, P. BAUMANN, H. ARANEDA, J. S. KENNEY, D. B. COTTON & P. B. SEHGAL. 1993. A comparative study of the diagnostic performance of amniotic fluid glucose, white blood cell count, interleukin-6, and Gram stain in the detection of microbial invasion in patients with preterm premature rupture of membranes. Am. J. Obstet. Gynecol. **169:** 839–851.
31. BIERNACKI, E. 1894. Über die Beziehung des Plasmas zu den rothen Blutkorperchen und über den Wert verschiedener Methoden der Blutkorperchenvolumbestimmung. Zeitschrift f. physiologische Chemie **19:**179–224.
32. FÅHRAEUS, R. 1921. The suspension stability of the blood. Acta. Med. Scand. **55:** 1–228.
33. MCCARTY, M. 1982. Historical perspective on C-reactive protein. Ann. N. Y. Acad. Sci. **389:** 1–10.
34. KUSHNER, I., J. E. VOLANAKIS & H. GEWURZ, Eds. 1982. C-reactive protein and the plasma protein response to tissue injury. Ann. N. Y. Acad. Sci. **389:** 1–482.
35. PENNICA, D., K. L. KING, K. J. SHAW, E. LUIS, J. RULLAMAS, S.-M. LUOH, W. C. DARBONNE, D. S. KNUTZON, R. YEN, K. R. CHIEN, J. B. BAKER & W. I. WOOD. 1995. Expression cloning of cardiotrophin 1, a cytokine that induces cardiac myocyte hypertrophy, Proc. Natl. Acad. Sci. USA. In press.
36. PENNICA, D., K. J. SHAW, T. A. SWANSON, M. W. MOORE, D. L. SHELTON, K. A. ZIONCHECK, A. ROSENTHAL, T. TAGA, N. F. PAONI & W. I. WOOD. 1995. Cardiotrophin-1: Biological activities and binding to the leukemia inhibitory factor receptor/gp130 signalling complex. J. Biol. Chem. In press.

Transcription Factors NF-IL6 and APRF Involved in gp130-mediated Signaling Pathway[a]

S. AKIRA,[b] Y. NISHIO,[b] T. TANAKA,[b,c] M. INOUE,[b]
T. MATSUSAKA,[b] X.-J. WANG,[b] S. WEI, N. YOSHIDA,[d] AND
T. KISHIMOTO[c]

[b]*Institute for Molecular and Cellular Biology*
Osaka University
1-3 Yamadaoka
Suita, Osaka 565, Japan

[c]*Department of Medicine III*
Osaka University Medical School
2-2 Yamadaoka
Suita, Osaka 565, Japan

[d]*Research Institute*
Osaka Medical Center for Maternal and Child Health
Izumi, Osaka 590-02, Japan

INTRODUCTION

Growth and differentiation of hematopoietic, lymphopoietic, and neural systems are regulated by various kinds of soluble mediators called cytokines. These molecules exert their biological effects through specific receptors expressed on the cell surfaces. Recently, many cytokines and their receptors have been cloned and characterized. Functional pleiotropy and redundancy, two characteristics of cytokines, may now be explained on the basis of the molecular structure of cytokine receptors.[1] Most cytokine receptors consist of multiple chains, *i.e.*, ligand-binding receptors specific for each cytokine, and signal transducers common to several cytokines. Homo- or heterodimerization of receptor molecules by ligand binding triggers the association and activation of intracellular tyrosine kinases. However, the intracellular mechanisms which link receptor activation to cellular responses are still poorly understood.

One approach to elucidate the molecular basis for receptor-activated transcriptional induction by cytokines is the identification of *cis*-responsive elements within genes and the corresponding transcription factors that respond to cytokine signals. One of the best characterized of these systems is that of the acute phase protein genes. During inflammation there are significant alterations in the serum levels of several plasma proteins, known as acute phase proteins.[2,3] Several cytokines have been found to directly induce acute phase proteins in the liver. These include IL-6, IL-1, TNF, leukemia inhibitory factor (LIF), transforming growth factor β, oncostatin M (OM), ciliary neurotrophic factor (CNTF) and IL-11. Among these cytokines, IL-6 is the most important inducer for the majority of acute phase proteins. The IL-6 receptor

---

[a] This work was supported by grants from the Ministry of Education of Japan and from the Human Frontier Science Program.

TABLE 1. IL-6 Response Elements Identified in Acute Phase Protein Genes

Type 1 Elements		Type 2 Elements	
rat AGP	TTGTGCAAG	rat AGP	CTGGGAA
	TGGCACAAT	human α_1-antitrypsin	CTGGGAT
mouse	TTGCGCAAG	human α_1-antichymotrypsin	CTGGTAA
	TGGCACAAT	rat α-fibrinogen	CTGGAAA
rat angiotensinogen	TTGGGAAAT	β-fibrinogen	CTGGGAA
human CRP	TGGCGCAAA	γ-fibrinogen	CTGGGAA
human C3	TTGAGAAAT	human CRP	TTGGAAA
human hemopexin	TGATGTAAT	human haptoglobin	CTGGAAA
human haptoglobin	TGAAGCAAG	rat T-kininogen	CTGGGTA
	TTACGAAAT	rat α_2-macroglobulin	CTGGGAA
mouse SAA	TTATGCAAG		CTGGAAA
	TGGAGCAAT	mouse SAA	GTGGGAT
Consensus	TTNNGNAAT		CTGGGAA
	(G) (G)		(A)

system consists of a ligand-binding receptor and the signal-transducing molecule gp130. The receptor systems for LIF, OM, CNTF, and IL-11 also utilize gp130 for initiating signal transmission.

Site-directed mutagenesis studies of the promoter regions of hepatic acute phase proteins have revealed the existence of two types of IL-6-response elements (IL-6REs), designated Type 1 and Type 2 IL-6REs (TABLE 1).[4,5] Type 1 IL-6REs, characterized by the consensus sequence T(T/G)NNGNAA(T/G), are present in the promoter regions of the genes for C-reactive protein, haptoglobin, hemopexin, and α_1-acid glycoprotein. This element binds members of the C/EBP family, of which NF-IL6 (also called C/EBPβ, AGP/EBP, LAP, and IL-6DBP) and NF-IL6β (also called C/EBPδ) have been shown to be implicated in the regulation of acute phase protein genes by IL-6.[6-8] NF-IL6 is activated as a consequence of phosphorylation by ras-regulated MAP kinases.[9] The other type of promoter elements, Type 2, consists of the hexanucleotide motif, CTGGGA and is present in the control region of fibrinogen, α_1-acid glycoprotein, T kininogen, α_2-macroglobulin, C-reactive protein and the haptoglobin genes. A nuclear factor, called acute phase response factor (APRF), binds the hexanucleotide.[10] Activation and tyrosine phosphorylation of APRF occurs in the cytoplasm within minutes after stimulation by IL-6, after which this factor is translocated to the nucleus. Recent cloning of cDNA encoding APRF has revealed that APRF is related to IFN-stimulated gene factor 3(ISGF3) families involved in IFN signaling pathway.[11] Success in molecular cloning of transcription factors binding to the IL-6 responsive elements has begun to open the black box of cytokine signaling pathways.

NF-IL6

NF-IL6 Is a Member of C/EBP Family

NF-IL6 was initially identified as a nuclear factor binding to a 14 bp palindromic sequence (ACATTGCACAATCT) within an IL-1–responsive element in the human IL-6 gene.[12] The gene encoding NF-IL6 was cloned from a λgt 11 cDNA expression library of LPS-stimulated human peripheral monocytes by a south-western method.[6] Interestingly, the cloned NF-IL6 contained a region highly homologous to the C-terminal portion of C/EBP, the first nuclear factor proposed to contain a leucine zipper structure.[13] The highly homologous region includes a basic domain and a leucine zipper structure essential for DNA binding and dimerization, respectively. NF-IL6 recognizes the same nucleotide sequences as C/EBP. Both proteins recognize a variety of the divergent nucleotide sequences with different affinity and the consensus sequence is T(T/G)NNGNNAA(T/G). However, expression of these two proteins is quite different. C/EBP is expressed in liver and adipose tissues and is presumed to regulate several hepatocyte- and adipocyte-specific genes. By contrast, NF-IL6 is expressed at an undetectable or a minor level in all normal tissues, but it is drastically induced by stimulation of LPS, IL-1, TNF or IL-6, indicating that NF-IL6 may be involved in acute phase, immune and inflammatory responses.

NF-IL6 Binds to Type 1 IL-6-response Elements in Acute Phase Protein Genes

Two types of IL6 *cis*-acting response elements have been identified in hepatic acute phase protein genes; one (Type 2 IL-6RE) is the hexanucleotide CTGGGA and the other (Type 1 IL-6RE) is a group of the sequences which seem to be dissimilar to each other but recognized by the same set of proteins, including the IL-6–inducible protein (IL-6–dependent DNA-binding protein, IL-6DBP). Type 1 IL-6RE sequences include the recognition sequence of NF-IL6. Actually, recombinant NF-IL6 binds to these IL-6REs. A cDNA coding for IL-6DBP was cloned and it turned out a rat homologue of human NF-IL6.[7] When the NF-IL6 gene was introduced into a hepatoma cell line Hep3B, basal production as well as IL-6–mediated induction of haptoglobin were significantly augmented, suggesting that NF-IL6 works on the endogenous gene for haptoglobin as a positive transcription factor.[14] Expression of NF-IL6 and C/EBP is reciprocally regulated by IL-6 in the liver. NF-IL6 mRNA is rapidly and drastically induced after IL-6 stimulation, preceding the induction of haptoglobin mRNA, whereas constitutively expressed C/EBP mRNA decreases dramatically after IL-6 treatment.[15] A reciprocal expression of NF-IL6 and C/EBP in the presence of IL-6 may explain the induction of the positive acute phase proteins and the decrease of the negative acute phase proteins including albumin as observed in inflammation.

Macrophage-specific Expression of NF-IL6

NF-IL6 is drastically and abundantly induced in all tissues after stimulation with LPS or inflammatory cytokines such as IL-1, TNF, and IL-6. Many cytokines, including IL-1, TNF, IL-6, IL-8 and G-CSF, are released from macrophages by LPS, or inflammatory cytokines. This evidence implies that NF-IL6 may be involved in the genes activated in macrophages. In fact, NF-IL6 binding motifs were identified in the functional regulatory regions of the genes for G-CSF, TNF, IL-1, IL-6, IL-8, lysozyme, and nitric oxide synthase. In several leukemic cell lines capable of differentiating to mature macrophages, NF-IL6 mRNA increased markedly along with macrophage differentiation, although C/EBPmRNA remained constant.[16]

Several lines of recent evidence have demonstrated that C/EBP is an important regulatory factor in adipocyte differentiation. First, C/EBP mRNA increases markedly during differentiation of 3T3-L1 preadipocytes to adipocytes. Premature expression of C/EBP impedes cell proliferation and accentuates differentiation in the presence of adipogenic hormones.[17] Furthermore, C/EBP can *trans*activate the promoters of the adipocyte-specific genes, 422(aP2), SCD1 and GLUT4 (insulin-responsive glucose transporter).[18] It is known that treatment of adipocytes with TNF causes a dramatic morphological dedifferentiation of adipocytes and a decrease in transcription of the adipocyte specific genes. In this case adipocyte-differentiated 3T3-L1 cells exhibit a rapid TNF-induced decrease in C/EBP protein level and a reciprocal increase in NF-IL6, preceding TNF-induced phenotypic de-differentiation of the cells.[19] Taken together, these facts indicate an important role of the acute phase–induced change in the NF-IL6/C/EBP ratio in determining the expression of those genes whose products are positively or negatively regulated in inflammatory and acute phase responses.

Phosphorylation of NF-IL6 by a Ras-dependent MAP Kinase Cascade

NF-IL6 is a phosphoprotein. Phosphoamino acid analysis shows that phosphorylation occurs on the serine and threonine residues. By transient expression of a series of site-directed mutants of NF-IL6 and subsequent phosphopeptide mapping, three phosphorylated residues were identified; Ser-231 and Thr-235, both located within the serine-rich domain (SRD) adjoining bZIP, and Ser-325 located within the leucine zipper (FIG. 1). Closer inspection of NF-IL6 phosphorylation sites revealed the presence of the consensus sequence for MAP kinase in the region immediately surrounding Thr-235 (SSPPGTPSP). In fact, a synthetic peptide containing Thr-235 was phosphorylated *in vitro* by purified MAP kinases. MAP kinases, also known as the extracellular signal-regulated kinases (ERKs), are a family of serine/threonine kinases that are activated very rapidly in response to many extracellular stimuli, including insulin, nerve growth factor, epidermal growth factor, platelet-derived growth factor, IL-2, IL-6, activators of protein kinase C, and antigen stimulation of T cells. Recently it has been demonstrated that MAP kinases are activated through a Ras-Raf-MAPKK (MEK)-MAP kinase cascade.[20]

When vectors expressing NF-IL6 and/or oncogenic p21^{ras} were cotransfected with an IL-6 promoter–luciferase gene reporter construct, simultaneous expression of both NF-IL6 and oncogenic p21^{ras} resulted in a dramatic synergistic stimulation of the reporter gene. Two dimensional phosphopeptide mapping showed that oncogenic p21^{ras} expression dramatically augmented the phosphorylation on Thr-235 of NF-IL6. Furthermore, substitution of Ala for Thr-235 resulted in the loss of ras-dependent activation of NF-IL6. These results demonstrated that ras-dependent activation of NF-IL is mediated through phosphorylation of Thr-235 by MAP kinases.[9]

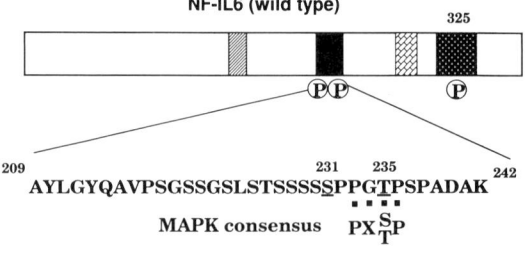
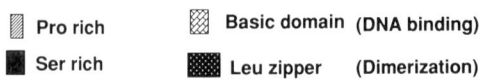

FIGURE 1. Phosphorylation sites of NF-IL6.

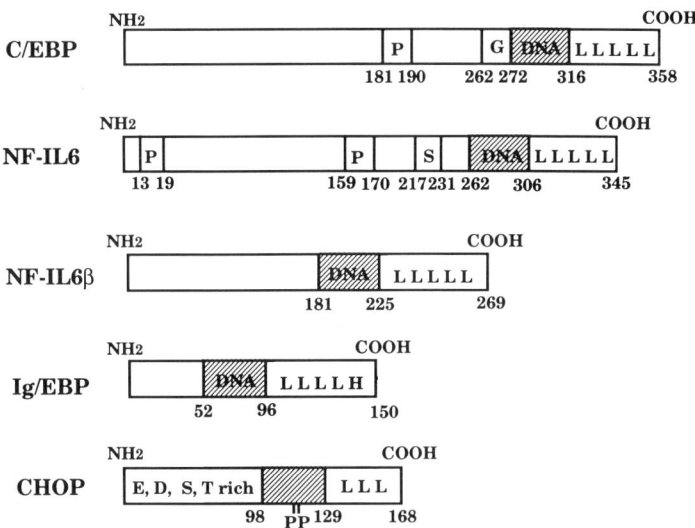

FIGURE 2. C/EBP family members. P: Pro rich, G: Gly rich, S: Ser rich, E: Glu, D: Asp, T: Thr.

It has been also demonstrated that C/EBPβ, the mouse homologue of human NF-IL6, is phosphorylated within the leucine zipper in response to increased intracellular calcium concentrations via the activation of a calcium-calmodulin–dependent kinase.[21] In addition, cAMP-mediated phosphorylation of NF-IL6 was shown to be associated with nuclear translocation and transcriptional activation.[22] Recently, LAP, the rat homologue of NF-IL6, has been shown to be activated through phosphorylation of the N-terminal domain by PKC.[23] Thus, NF-IL6 is found to be activated via several different signaling pathways.

C/EBP Family Members

There are five members of the C/EBP family (FIG. 2). These include C/EBP, NF-IL6 (also known as LAP, IL-6DBP, AGP/EBP), Ig/EBP-1, NF-IL6β(C/EBPδ), and CHOP-10 (also known as gadd153).[6–8,13,24–28] C/EBP is expressed in adipose, liver, and placental tissues, which play a vital role in energy metabolism. The expression of NF-IL6 and NF-IL6β is normally suppressed but drastically and rapidly induced in many tissues by LPS or several inflammatory cytokines including IL-1, TNF and IL-6. Ig/EBP-1 mRNA is ubiquitously expressed and most abundant in the early stage of the B lymphocyte. CHOP-10 is specifically induced under the condition of growth arrest and/or DNA damage. These members of C/EBP family recognize the same nucleotide sequences except for CHOP-10. The formation of heterodimeric complexes between members of the C/EBP family has also been demonstrated. Because CHOP-10 contains several amino acid substitutions in the highly conserved regions present in all bZIP proteins, dimers can be formed between CHOP-10 and other C/EBP family members, but the heterodimers cannot bind to the C/EBP binding consensus.

Cooperative Interaction of NF-IL6 and NF-κB in Gene Expression

It has become increasingly evident that combinatorial effects of transcription factors are very important in gene regulation. Both NF-IL6 binding site and NF-κB binding site are frequently present in the promoter region of the genes involved in inflammatory and immune responses. In the case of the IL-6 gene, studies with the deletion mutants demonstrated that these two sites are essential for the expression of IL-6. Also in the IL-8 gene, the sequence between -94 and -71 bp, composed of two regulatory elements, NF-κB binding site(-80 to -71 bp) and NF-IL6 binding site (-94 to -81 bp), is minimally essential and sufficient to permit the inducibility of the IL-8 gene expression by IL-1, TNF or PMA.[29] The interaction of NF-IL6 and NF-κB binding sites are observed in several other genes such as the serum amyloid A1, serum amyloid A3, complement C3, α_1-acid glycoprotein, angiotensinogen and G-CSF genes. Recently, an interesting result indicating a direct protein-protein interaction between NF-IL6 and NF-κB has been presented.[30] A λgt11 expression library was screened using radiolabeled NF-κB p50 as a probe in order to obtain transcription factors interacting with p50. This screening has led to the isolation of NF-IL6 cDNA clones in addition to several clones of the NF-κB/rel family members. Subsequent studies have provided evidence for functional and physical interaction between NF-IL6 and NF-κB.[31,32] Protein-protein interaction has also been demonstrated between NF-IL6 and glucocorticoid receptor,[33] and between NF-IL6 and p53.[34]

Generation of NF-IL6 $-/-$ Mice by Gene Targeting

To know the specific regulatory role of NF-IL6 *in vivo*, NF-IL6 $-/-$ mice were generated by gene targeting in embryonic stem cells.[42] The NF-IL6 targeting vector was constructed by inserting a neomycine resistance gene into the bZip domain of the NF-IL6 gene (FIG. 3). Two lines of mice carrying the mutation at the NF-IL6 locus have been generated from independently isolated ES cell lines. Homozygous mutant mice were obtained from heterozygous parents below the expected Mendelian ratio, suggesting prenatal mortality, but newborn mice appeared normal, and presented no significant increase in mortality rate under specific pathogen-free (SPF) conditions. However, NF-IL6 $-/-$ mice presented a high susceptibility to *Listeria* infection. When NF-IL6 $-/-$ and control mice were infected intraperitoneally with 5×10^2 colony-forming units (CFU) (50% lethal dose of wild-mice is 1×10^6 CFU) of L. *monocytogenes*, all NF-IL6 $-/-$ mice died within 5 days after challenge with *Listeria*. Histopathological examination showed multiple foci of microabscesses in the liver and spleen of NF-IL6 $-/-$ mice. Electromicroscopic observation revealed escape of a large number of the pathogens from phagosome to cytoplasm in activated macrophages from NF-IL6 $-/-$ mice. These results demonstrate an essential role of NF-IL6 in intracellular killing of *Listeria* by macrophages. Furthermore, it has been demonstrated that G-CSF induction by macrophages and fibroblasts is impaired in NF-IL6 $-/-$ mice.

APRF

Molecular Cloning of APRF

Nuclear extracts were prepared from mouse liver at various time points after IL-6 injection, and analyzed by electrophoretic mobility shift assay (EMSA) using a

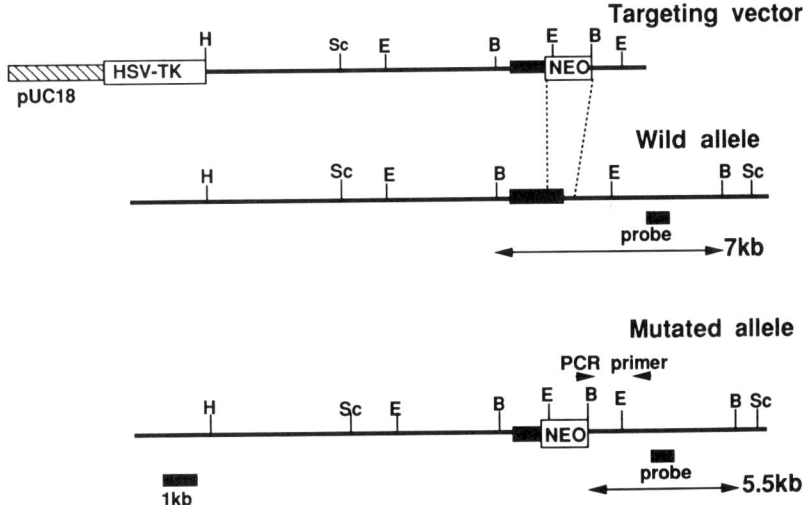

FIGURE 3. NF-IL6 targeting vector. The NF-IL6 targeting vector was constructed by inserting a neomycine resistance gene derived from pMCpoly A into the bZip domain of the NF-IL6 gene with simultaneous deletion of 0.5 kb of DNA containing the leucine zipper domain and 3′ untranslated region, and placing the herpes simplex virus thymidine kinase gene X kb upstream of the NF-IL6 gene for negative selection against nonhomologous integration events. The targeting vector was transfected into ES embryonic stem cells by electroportation, and transfectants were selected with G418.

^{33}P-labeled rat α_2-macroglobulin APRE (acute phase response element [5′-CTTCTGGGAATTCC-3′]) as a probe. APRF binding activity reached a maximum by 5 min after injection of IL-6 and subsequently declined by 1 hour. In addition, binding activity was abolished by addition of anti-phosphotyrosine monoclonal antibodies, indicating that APRF itself was phosphorylated on tyrosine residues. APRF was purified from a pool of mouse liver nuclear extracts using DNA affinity chromatography. The purified material contained a major polypeptide with a molecular weight of 95 kD, which was phosphorylated on tyrosine residues and was not detected in extracts of untreated cells. The 95 kD protein band was excised from the gel and digested with a lysylendopeptidase; several partial amino sequences were obtained. Based on the amino acid sequences, cDNA encoding mouse APRF was cloned. APRF is encoded by a single mRNA of 4.8 kb. APRF transcripts were ubiquitously expressed and further induced with IL-6 stimulation. Mouse APRF encodes an open reading frame encoding 770 amino acids predicting a protein of 88 kD. A GenBank data base search revealed that the cDNA sequence of mouse APRF has a high degree of homology to a human ISGF3 p91/84 (52.5% identity) or p113 (37.5%). Human APRF showed 99% identity with its mouse counterpart (Eight out of 770 amino acids differ between mouse and human APRFs). FIGURE 4 shows the alignment of the amino acid sequences of human APRF with that of p91. p91 and p113 have a heptad-leucine repeat in the N-terminus and a functional SH2 domain in the C-terminus.[35] These structures are completely conserved within APRF. p91 is phosphorylated on Tyr701 after cells are treated with IFN-γ, IFN-α, or EGF. A tyrosine residue flanked by similar amino acid sequences can be found at the corresponding location in APRF.

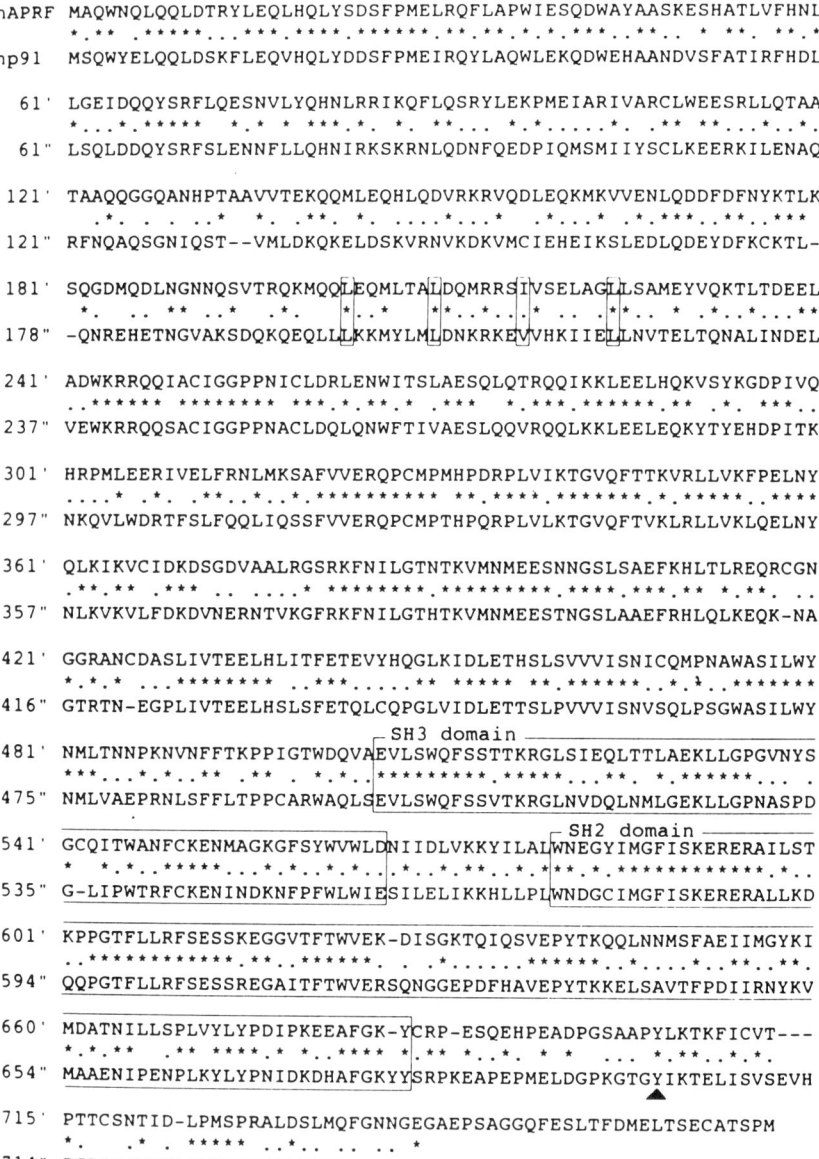

FIGURE 4. Sequence comparison of Human APRF and p91. Asterisks and dots indicate identical and related amino acids, respectively. The heptad-leucine residues in the amino-terminal region are shown in boxes. A closed triangle indicates the phosphorylation site of p91. (Taken from ref. 11.)

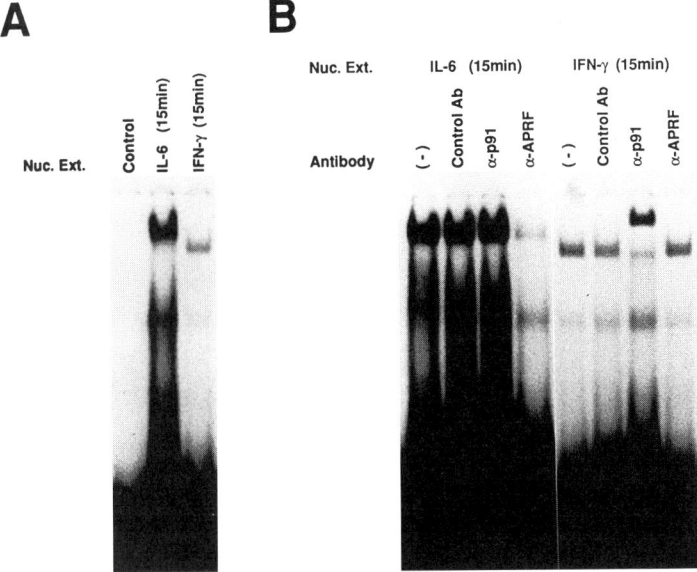

FIGURE 5. Identification of APRF by specific antibodies. Nuclear extracts from control mice or mice treated with either IL-6 or mIFN-γ (15 min after intravenous injection) were preincubated with antibodies indicated, and subjected to EMSA. (Taken from ref. 11.)

Polyclonal antibodies were raised against a synthetic peptide corresponding to the region between amino acids 626–640 in APRF. When added to EMSA reaction, anti-APRF antibody, but not unrelated control antibody, blocked the formation of the complex between IL-6–treated liver nuclear extracts and APRE, confirming that the isolated cDNA represents APRF (FIG. 5). Anti-p91 antibody did not affect the complex. In contrast, the complex activated by treatment with IFN-γ was recognized by anti-p91 antibody but not by anti-APRF antibody. Taken together, these results indicate that APRF is a major component of the complex formed between IL-6–treated liver nuclear extracts and APRE and that p91 is not involved in the formation of this complex. Conversely, APRF is not involved in the formation of the complex between IFN-γ–treated extracts and APRE.

Tyrosine Phosphorylation of APRF in Response to IL-6, LIF, OM, and CNTF, Whose Receptors Share gp130

Nuclear extracts from mouse liver were prepared before and after IL-6 treatment and immunoprecipitated with the anti-APRF–specific antibodies (FIG. 6A). The precipitated proteins were resolved by SDS-PAGE and immunoblotted with specific monoclonal anti-phosphotyrosine antibodies. After treatment of mouse liver with IL-6, tyrosine phosphorylation of the APRF protein was detected in the nucleus within 5 min, persisted for over 30 min, and disappeared by 1 h, similar to the kinetics of APRF-binding activities detected by EMSA. The amount of APRF protein in the nuclear extracts was examined by immunoblotting with anti-APRF antibody. The

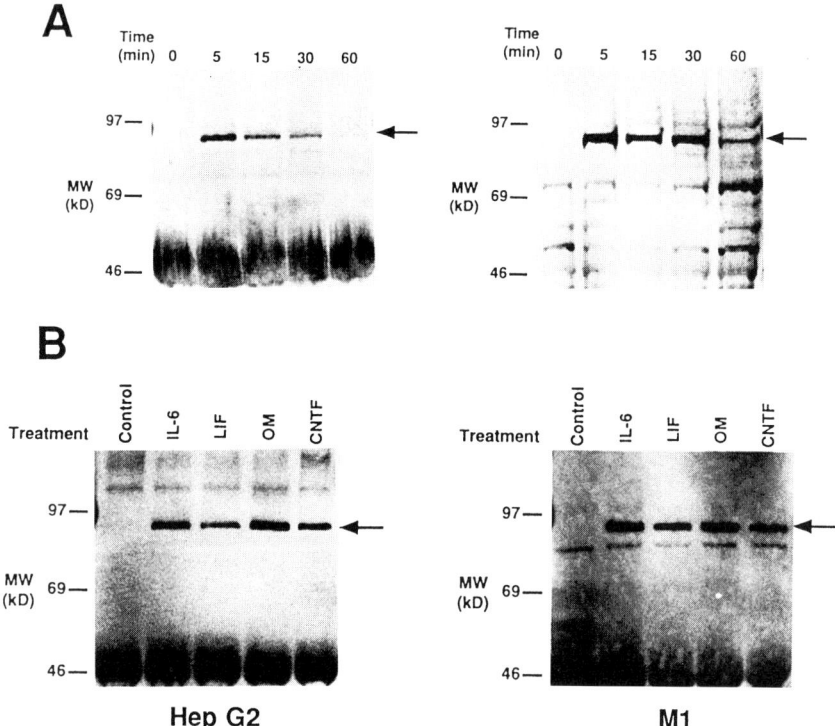

FIGURE 6. Tyrosine phosphorylation of APRF. **A,** *Left panel:* Time course of tyrosine-phosphorylated APRF. Nuclear extracts from the mouse livers were immunoprecipitated with APRF specific antibody, separated by SDS-PAGE, and subjected to immunoblotting with anti-phosphotyrosine monoclonal antibody, 4G10. *Right panel:* Immunoblotting of crude nuclear extracts with APRF specific antibody. APRF is arrowed in both panels. **B,** Whole cell lysates from Hep G2 cells and M1 cells, untreated or treated with IL-6, LIF, OM, or CNTF for 15 min were immunoprecipitated with anti-APRF and immunoblotted with 4G10. (Taken from ref. 11.)

time course of APRF protein phosphorylation corresponded well with that of the amount of APRF protein present in the nuclei. These results indicate that the APRF protein is rapidly tyrosine phosphorylated and translocated into the nucleus in response to IL-6.

IL-6, LIF, CNTF, OM, IL-11 make up a family of cytokines whose receptors share the IL-6 signal-transducing protein gp130. APRF was also tyrosine phosphorylated in response to LIF, OM, and CNTF in HepG2 cells as well as in M1 cells, a mouse myeloid precursor cell line that undergoes growth arrest and terminal differentiation to macrophages in response to IL-6 or LIF (FIG. 6B). These findings indicate that APRF is phosphorylated and activated in response to gp130-mediated signals in various cell types.

Cytokines Activate Different ISGF3 Family Members

Following IFN-α treatment, three subunits (p113, p91, and p84) of an IFN-α induced transcription factor, ISGF3, become phosphorylated on tyrosine, migrate into the nucleus, and assemble into a complex together with p48, a DNA-binding protein that specifically binds to the ISRE (interferon-stimulated response element).[36–38] In contrast, IFN-γ stimulates tyrosine phosphorylation of cytoplasmic p91 but not of p113 or p84, and phosphorylated p91 binds directly to the GAS element.[39] IL-6 type cytokines induce tyrosine phosphorylation of APRF (also known as Stat3).[11,40] A number of other cytokines including IL-3, IL-4, IL-5, and GM-CSF have been shown to induce activation of ISGF-like transcription factors.[41] However, the complexes activated by these cytokines do not seem to contain either the p91 or p113 components of ISGF3 or APRF, suggesting the existence of other members of the ISGF3 family. Although a variety of cytokine receptors do not have intrinsic kinase activities, several experiments have demonstrated the involvement of non-receptor protein tyrosine kinases of the Jak family including Tyk2, Jak1, and Jak2.[41] Although the exact mechanism which results in the activation of ISGF3 family members in cytokine signal pathways is still unclear, it is most plausible that the observed diversity in cellular responses to different cytokines can be mediated by the selective activation of different ISGF3 family members.

CONCLUSIONS

Cloning of two transcription factors binding to the IL-6 response elements in the acute phase protein genes has disclosed the existence of ras-dependent and ras-independent pathways in IL-6 signaling (FIG. 7). NF-IL6 is phosphorylated and activated via a Ras-MAP kinase cascade, whereas APRF is directly phosphorylated

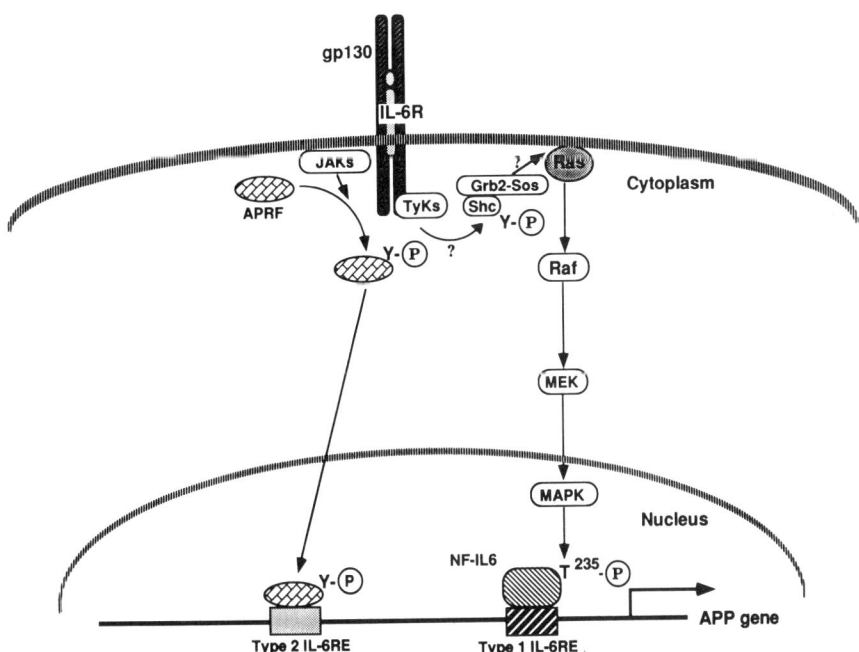

FIGURE 7. Signal transduction through gp130.

by tyrosine protein kinases (Jaks) in the cytoplasm, followed by translocation of this factor to the nucleus. However, many important questions still remain to be answered. The molecules connecting gp130 to Ras have been not identified. Direct activation of APRF by Jaks has not been demonstrated. Besides acute phase protein induction in hepatocytes, IL-6 has both growth-stimulatory and -inhibitory effects depending on the cell type. It is not known whether each or both of these two pathways is actually involved in these functions.

NF-IL6 knock out mice have been generated. Targeting of the NF-IL6 gene demonstrates an essential role of NF-IL6 in intracellular bactericidal activities by macrophages. Future identification of the genes regulated by NF-IL6 will uncover the microbicidal mechanisms by which macrophages control the proliferation of intracellular pathogens.

ACKNOWLEDGMENT

We thank Ms. K. Kubota for her excellent secretarial assistance.

REFERENCES

1. KISHIMOTO, T., T. TAGA & S. AKIRA 1994. Cell **76**: 253–262.
2. KUSHNER, I. 1982. Ann. N.Y. Acad. Sci. **389**: 39–48.
3. KOJ, A. 1985. The Acute-Phase Response to Injury and Infection. A. H. Gordon and A. Koj, Eds. Vol. 10:139–144. Amsterdam/New York: Elsevier.
4. BAUMANN, H., K. R. PROWSE, S. MARINKOVIC, K. A. WON & G. P. JAHREIS. 1989. Ann. N.Y. Acad. Sci. **557**: 280–295.
5. AKIRA, S. & T. KISHIMOTO. 1992. Immunol. Rev. **127**: 25–50.
6. AKIRA, S., H. ISSHIKI, T. SUGITA, O. TANABE, S. KINOSHITA, Y. NISHIO, T. NAKAJIMA, T. HIRANO & T. KISHIMOTO. 1990. EMBO. J. **9**: 1897–1906.
7. POLI, V., F. P. MANCINI & R. CORTESE. 1990. Cell **63**: 643–653.
8. KINOSHITA, S., S. AKIRA & T. KISHIMOTO. 1992. Proc. Natl. Acad. Sci. USA **87**: 1473–1476.
9. NAKAJIMA T., S. KINOSHITA, T. SASAGAWA, K. SASAKI, M. NARUTO, T. KISHIMOTO & S. AKIRA. 1993. Proc. Natl. Acad. Sci. USA **90**: 2207–2211.
10. WEGENKA, U. M., J. BUSHMANN, C. LÜTTICKEN, P. C. HEINRICH & F. HORN. 1993. Mol. Cell. Biol. **13**: 276–288.
11. AKIRA, S., Y. NISHIO, M. INOUE, X.-J. WANG, S. WEI, T. MATSUSAKA, K. YOSHIDA, T. SUDO, M. NARUTO & T. KISHIMOTO. 1994. Cell **77**: 63–71.
12. ISSHIKI, H., S. AKIRA, O. TANABE, T. NAKAJIMA, T. SHIMAMOTO, T. HIRANO & T. KISHIMOTO. 1990. Mol. Cell. Biol. **10**: 2757–2764.
13. LANDSCHULZ, W. H., P. F. JOHNSON, E. Y. ADASHI, B. J. GRAVES & S. L. MCKNIGHT. 1988. Genes Dev. **2**: 786–800.
14. NATSUKA, S., H. ISSHIKI, S. AKIRA & T. KISHIMOTO. 1991. FEBS Lett. **291**: 58–62.
15. ISSHIKI, H., S. AKIRA, T. SUGITA, Y. NISHIO, S. HASHIMOTO, T. PAWLOWSKI, S. SUEMATSU & T. KISHIMOTO. 1991. New Biol. **3**: 63–70.
16. NATSUKA, S., S. AKIRA, Y. NISHIO, S. HASHIMOTO, T. SUGITA, H. ISSHIKI & T. KISHIMOTO. 1992. Blood **79**: 460–466.
17. UMEK, R. M., A. D. FRIEDMAN & S. L. MCKNIGHT. 1991. Science **251**: 288–291.
18. CHRISTY, R. J., V. W. YANG, J. M. NTAMBI, D. E. GEIMAN, W. H. LANDSCHULZ, A. D. FRIEDMAN, Y. NAKABEPPU, T. J. KELLY & M. D. LANE. 1989. Genes Dev. **3**: 1323–1335.
19. RON, D., A. R. BRASIER, R. E. MCGEHEE & J. F. HABENE. 1992. J. Clin. Invest. **89**: 223–233.
20. PELECH, S. L. & J. S. SANGHERA. 1992. Science **257**: 1355–1356.

21. WEGNER, M., Z. CAO & M. G. ROSENFELD. 1992. Science **256:** 370–373.
22. METZ, R. & E. ZIFF. 1991. Genes Dev. **5:** 1754–1766.
23. TRAUTWEIN, C., C. CAELLES, P. VAN DER GEER, T. HUNTER, M. KARIN & M. CHOJKIER. 1993. Nature **364:** 544–547.
24. DESCOMBES, P., M. CHOJKIER, S. LICHTSTEINER, E. FALVEY & U. SCHIBLER. 1990. Genes Dev. **4:** 1541–1551.
25. CHANG, C. J., T. T. CHEN, H. Y. LEI, D. S. CHEN & S. C. LEE. 1990. Mol. Cell. Biol. **10:** 6642–6653.
26. ROMAN, C., J. S. PLATERO, J. SHUMAN & K. CALAME. 1990. Genes Dev. **4:** 1404–1415.
27. CAO, Z., R. M. UMEK & S. L. MCKNIGHT. 1991. Genes Dev. **5:** 1538–1552.
28. RON, D. & J. F. HABENER. 1992. Genes Dev. **6:** 439–453.
29. MUKAIDA, N., Y. MAHE & K. MATSUSHIMA. 1990. J. Biol. Chem. **265:** 21128–21133.
30. LECLAIR, K.-P., M.-A. BLANAR & P.-A. SHARP. 1992. Proc. Natl. Acad. Sci. USA **89:** 8145–8149.
31. STEIN, B., P. C. COGSWELL & A. S. BALDWIN, JR. 1993. Mol. Cell. Biol. **13:** 3964–3974.
32. MATSUSAKA, T., K. FUJIKAWA, Y. NISHIO, N. MURAKIDA, K. MATSUSHIMA, T. KISHIMOTO, S. AKIRA. 1993. Proc. Natl. Acad. Sci. USA **90:** 10193–10197.
33. NISHIO, Y., H. ISSHIKI, T. KISHIMOTO & S. AKIRA. 1993. Mol. Cell. Biol. **13:** 1854–1862.
34. MARGULIES, L. & P. B. SEHGAL. 1993. J. Biol. Chem. **268:** 15096–15100.
35. FU, X.-Y. 1992. Cell **70:** 323–335.
36. FU, X.-Y., D. S. KESSLER, S. A. VEALS, D. E. LEVY, J. E. DARNELL, JR. 1990. Proc. Natl. Acad. Sci. USA **87:** 8555–8559.
37. KESSLER, D. S., S. A. VEALS, X.-Y. FU & D. E. LEVY. 1990. Genes Dev. **4:** 1753–1765.
38. SCHINDLER, C., X.-Y. FU, T. IMPROTA, R. AEBERSOLD & J. E. DARNELL, JR. 1992. Proc. Natl. Acad. Sci. USA **89:** 7836–7839.
39. SCHINDLER, C., K. SHUAI, V. R. PREZIOSO & J. E. DARNELL, JR. 1992. Science **257:** 809–813.
40. ZHONG, Z., Z. WEN & J. E. DARNELL, JR. 1994. Science **264:** 95–98.
41. IHLE, J. N., B. A. WITTHUHN, F. W. QUELLE, K. YAMAMOTO, W. E. THIERFELDER, B. KREIDER & O. SILVENNOINEN. 1994. Trends Biochem. Sci. **19:** 222–227.
42. TANAKA, T., S. AKIRA, K. YOSHIDA, M. UMEMOTO, Y. YONEDA, N. SHIRAFUJI, H. FUJIWARA, S. SUEMATSU, N. YOSHIDA & T. KISHIMOTO. 1995. Cell **80:** 353–361.

DISCUSSION OF THE PAPER

P. B. SEHGAL (*New York Medical College, Valhalla*): In the listeria model have you looked at the appearance of cytokines in the NF-IL6 knock-out mice challenged with listeria?

S. AKIRA: Yes, all the cytokines are induced normally.

SEHGAL: Are they in the circulation?

AKIRA: We examined the serum level for TNF and INF-γ—both were induced normally. Other cytokines we measured only by quantitative RT-PCR.

SEHGAL: I have another more general question, which probably has a slightly historic flavor. If IL-6 and interferons activate similar signal transduction molecules, how come IL-6 has no anti-viral activity?

AKIRA: I think that a specific Stat family member is differentially activated between IL-6 and interferons. Stat3 is activated by IL-6 but not IFN-γ whereas Stat1 is activated by IFN-γ but not IL-6.

SEHGAL: Yes. Would Dr. Revel like to comment on that?

M. REVEL (*Weizmann Institute, Rehovot, Israel*): I would like to make a comment and ask a question of Dr. Akira. The comment is the following: we also thought that IL-6 will activate Stat91 in the other cells, in epithelial cells and also in B-9 hybridoma cells. The fact is that in HepG2 cells you do not see it; we also actually see it less in these cells. The other fact is that interferons can also activate the APRF complex. So, the specificity that you are describing may not be as strong as you want to describe. The question I would like to ask you is: what do you believe to be the function of the leucine zipper in the Stat proteins?

AKIRA: We have no data about it, but the Darnell group thinks that this is used for heterodimer or homodimer formation. We are now performing extensive mutagenesis studies of APRF. They will answer this question.

A. RAY (*Yale University School of Medicine, New Haven, CT*): Are Stat-91 and APRF phosphorylated by different Jak-kinases? I mean, is it very specific at a still higher level? It is extremely specific in terms of, on the one hand, IFN-γ and EGF signaling, and, on the other hand cytokine signaling, and is this specificity conferred by Jak-kinases?

AKIRA: The specificity may not be conferred by Jak-kinases. In our cotransfection assays either Jak1 or Jak2 can phosphorylate APRF.

RAY: Does EGF treatment of cells phosphorylate APRF?

AKIRA: Yes, EGF phosphorylates APRF, but other cytokines such as IL-2, -3, -4, -5, -7, do not. APRF is phosphorylated by IL-6-type cytokines and G-CSF.

H. BAUMANN (*Roswell Park Cancer Institute, Buffalo, NY*): You propose that the activation of the MAP kinases by any agent will activate your NF-IL6 or C/EBPβ. That in turn will activate the haptoglobin gene. Will activation of MAP kinase by another hormone like PDGF or EGF or insulin activate haptoglobin?

AKIRA: I do not think so.

BAUMANN: But your model shows a prominent role for MAP kinase and the control of acute phase plasma proteins. A MAP kinase, of course, is a target for many hormones. Will that be used, or is it a specific MAP kinase pathway you propose?

AKIRA: I do not know.

BAUMANN: You do not know. My other question is: the APRE you use, is that the target for C/EBPβ or NF-IL6?

AKIRA: No, it is different.

BAUMANN: So, would that sequence inserted into a reporter gene be activated by IL-6 treatment? Is it functional as a regulatory element or is it only serving as a binding site?

AKIRA: I do not understand the question.

BAUMANN: The APRE or SIE sequence you use as a target for APRF, does it serve as a regulatory element responsive to IL-6?

AKIRA: Yes, of course, APRE is responsive to IL-6.

BAUMANN: My last question. You use HepG2 cells to demonstrate the activation of APRF, but not p91. However, treatment of HepG2 cells will activate both Stat1 and -3 in the hands of the Darnell group. You did not see any activation of Stat1 or equivalent?

AKIRA: No, in our system we do not detect this.

BAUMANN: So, there are different HepG2 cells.

AKIRA: In the gel-shift assay we detect only the slowly migrating band. We do not detect the fast band, which corresponds to the complex formed by Stat1.

BAUMANN: So, you do not see p91 activation in HepG2 cells.

AKIRA: Certainly. We do not see that in our system. Perhaps stimulation with too large amounts of IL-6 induced two bands in HepG2 cells in other systems.

R. NETA (*Armed Forces Radiobiology Research Institute, Bethesda, MD*): What effect does that have on neutrophils in mice lacking G-CSF?

AKIRA: They are not decreased. Impairment of G-CSF induction is observed only in macrophages and fibroblasts but not in other cell types from NF-IL6 knockout mice.

LIF and Related Cytokines in the Regulation of Mammalian Development

COLIN L. STEWART AND EMILY CULLINAN

Roche Institute of Molecular Biology
Roche Research Center
340 Kingsland Street
Nutley, New Jersey 07110

Leukemia Inhibitory Factor (LIF) is a member of the group of cytokines, that include interleukin-6, oncostatin M (OSM) and Ciliary Neurotrophic Factor (CNTF). Among LIF's many functions, a principal one is in regulating the development of the early mammalian embryo. This it does by regulating implantation of the embryo by controlling receptivity of the uterus and cell proliferation in the embryo. We analyzed LIF expression in human tissues and we find a similar pattern of expression to that seen in the mouse. A detailed analyzis revealed LIF to be highly expressed in the endometrial glands during the secretory or post-ovulatory phase of the menstrual cycle implying that LIF has a similar function in regulating implantation in the human as in the mouse. We have also analyzed the patterns of CNTF and OSM expression in humans and we find their expression occurs in tissues in which LIF expression is absent, suggesting they may be substituting for LIF in tissues in which it is not produced.

DISCUSSION OF THE PAPER

P. B. SEHGAL (*New York Medical College, Valhalla*): The expression of LIF in endometrial epithelial cells is very reminiscent of staining for IL-6. Do you know whether the LIF is actually secreted in a vectorial fashion in the apical or the basal side?

C. L. STEWART: I am sorry, I would love to answer this question. I was asked a similar question at a meeting 2 years ago. Unfortunately, we do not yet know the answer; we would like to have an effective RIA or ELISA assay so that we could at least look at uterine secretions of either the mouse or the human. We have not been able to do that yet.

SEHGAL: In the case of IL-6, Dan Carson and Andy Jakobs in Houston have figured out that for polarized uterine epithelium most of the IL-6 is secreted in the apical side with a little on the basal side. Another thing that I find curious in their experiments is that the addition of IL-6 inhibits blastocyst attachment and outgrowth. I wonder whether any similar experiments have been done with other IL-6-type cytokines.

STEWART: These sorts of experiments are perhaps more appropriate in the human. The problem with doing these sorts of experiments in the rodent is that often when you start explanting tissues from the *in vivo* environment to the *in vitro* environment deregulation of cytokine expression occurs, resulting in the cells expressing cytokines that they don't usually express *in vivo*. One thing that comes up very rapidly following explantation of any tissue is in fact LIF. So, whether this would also occur in the appropriate organ culture conditions, I do not yet know.

M. REVEL (*Weizmann Institute, Rehovot, Israel*): A couple of years ago, we published that IL-6 is produced in the trophoblast, and then there was some work using anti-IL-6Ab showing that it inhibits production of HCG by the trophoblast. Can you relate this observation to your finding in the double knock-outs?

STEWART: We have been working in the mouse. No one has found or yet identified a murine equivalent of HCG. It might be something like a prolactin molecule; this is not entirely clear.

C. RICHARDS (*McMaster University, Hamilton, Ont., Canada*): I am interested in the mechanism by which LIF may impact the implantation. There has been a study showing that at least *in vitro* LIF will induce expression of tissue inhibitor of metalloproteinases, TIMP. I am just wondering if you have actually looked at TIMP expression in the system.

STEWART: Not yet. We would like to analyze LIF-deficient blastocysts to determine whether they express TIMP; however, G. Schulz at the University of Calgary has in fact been looking at UPA plasminogen-activator expression and some other proteolytic enzymes in blastocysts in culture. And he has some evidence that in fact LIF can upregulate these proteolytic enzymes, which would be consistent with the invasive nature of the trophoblast.

M. KOPF (*Max-Planck-Institut für Immunobiologie, Freiburg, Germany*): Have you looked at bone development in these LIF-deficient mice?

STEWART: Not yet.

KOPF: To find out why they are smaller?

STEWART: We do not have any clear idea why they are smaller, but we have two current theories. One is that the circulatory or the capillary network around the pituitaries has some unusual features. A few years ago investigators from Genentech published a paper (Ferrara *et al.*, 1992. Proc. Natl. Acad. Sci. **89**: 698.) indicating that there are some critical factors that seem to be involved in how these capillaries grow around the pituitary. They showed that the factor was in fact LIF. Now whether in fact that implies that the capillary network around the pituitary is somehow abnormal and that that could affect growth hormone secretion or other growth hormones, I do not yet know. Another possibility, which we are also looking into at the moment, is that LIF is known to inhibit apoptosis. In certain neuronal cell cultures, M. Nobel has made that suggestion that perhaps, given the widespread expression of LIF, apoptosis will be at very low levels in many tissues. Maybe what is happening is that the increased level of apoptosis is caused by the absence of LIF, which I find very provocative.

KOPF: You have gotten the IL-6-deficient mice from Dr. Valeria Poli. You may have noticed that these are also smaller. We have not bred them as far as you have. I wonder whether there are even more pronounced dwarfs.

STEWART: The double knock-outs are so difficult to derive in reasonable numbers that we have not done any growth studies yet.

KOPF: It is interesting that the IL-6-deficient mice are smaller later in age though not at an early age. Only later.

Interleukin (IL)-11–mediated Signal Transduction[a]

YU-CHUNG YANG[b-d] AND TINGGUI YIN[b,d]

[b]Department of Medicine (Hematology/Oncology)
[c]Department of Biochemistry/Molecular Biology
[d]Walther Oncology Center
Indiana University School of Medicine
975 W. Walnut Street, IB540
Indianapolis, Indiana 46202

INTRODUCTION

Interleukin (IL)-11 is a bone marrow fibroblast–derived cytokine[1] with a variety of *in vitro* biological activities within the hematopoietic, lymphopoietic, hepatic, adipose, bone, and neuronal systems.[2] *In vivo* administration of IL-11 in animals[3,4] and humans[5] has demonstrated the thrombopoietic effect of this cytokine. The expression of the human IL-11 gene, which is localized at 19q13.3–13.4,[6] can be controlled at both transcriptional[7] and posttranscriptional[8] levels in various IL-11-expressing cell lines. Transcriptional control of IL-11 gene expression is mainly regulated through JUN/AP-1 interactions.[7] Posttranscriptional control is regulated by elements other than AUUUA motifs present in the 3′-noncoding region of the IL-11 mRNAs.[8] A possible role of tyrosine kinases in the stabilization of the IL-11 mRNAs following IL-1 stimulation has been proposed.[8]

Biochemical crosslinking studies have identified a 151 kD protein as the potential candidate for the IL-11 ligand-binding subunit.[9] Because of the overlapping biological activities of IL-11 and cytokines such as IL-6, LIF, OSM, and CNTF, it was not surprising to find that these cytokines share a common signal transducer, gp130.[10–13] In order to understand the mechanisms contributing to the common and unique biological activities of these growth factors, we set out to investigate the role of various signaling molecules, including different kinases (Jak family kinases, MAP kinases, pp90[rsk], H7-sensitive kinases, and src-family kinases), second messengers (diacylglycerol, arachidonic acid, and phosphatidic acid), transcriptional factors (mainly Stat family transcriptional factors) and primary response gene expression in IL-11–mediated signal transduction. FIGURE 1 depicts the proposed order of various molecules involved in the signaling pathways mediated by gp130 family cytokines in mouse preadipocytes.

PROTEIN KINASES INVOLVED IN IL-11 SIGNALING

It has been shown that activation of protein tyrosine phosphorylation and primary response gene expression plays an important role in growth factor–mediated signal

---

[a] This work is supported by U.S. Public Health Service Grants RO1HL48819 and RO1DK43105 (to Y-C.Y.) and a Fellowship from American Heart Association, Indiana Affiliated Inc. (to T.Y.). Y.-C.Y. is a Scholar of the Leukemia Society of America.

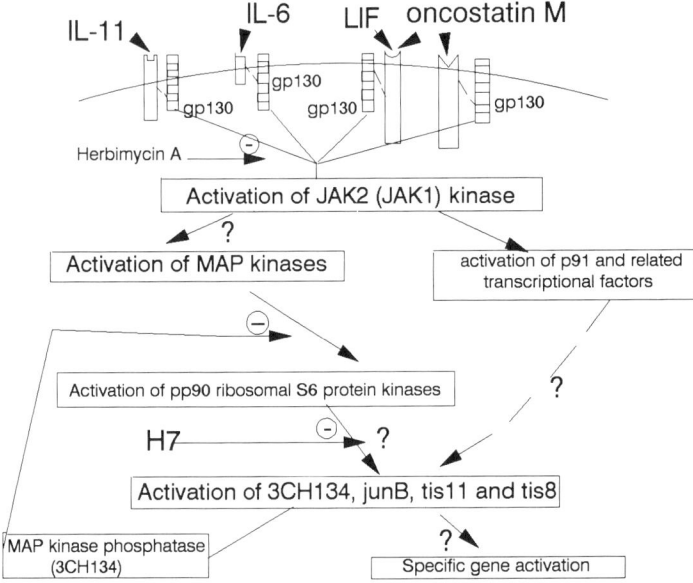

FIGURE 1. Possible signal transduction pathways mediated by IL-11, IL-6, LIF and oncostatin M in 3T3-L1 preadipocytes.

transduction.[14,15] We have examined protein tyrosine phosphorylation and primary response gene expression in several IL-11 responsive cell lines including 3T3-L1 (a mouse preadipocyte cell line), T10 (an IL-6- or IL-11-dependent mouse plasmacytoma cell line), B9-TY1 (an IL-6 or IL-11-dependent mouse hybridoma cell line), H-35 (a rat hepatoma cell line) and TF-1 (a human factor–dependent erythroleukemic cell line). Since IL-11 has many biological activities in common with IL-6, LIF, and OSM, we also compared tyrosine phosphorylation and primary response gene expression mediated by these cytokines in mouse preadipocyte cell line, 3T3-L1. Using different kinase inhibitors, we have shown that tyrosine kinases and H7-sensitive kinases are involved in the signal transduction pathways mediated by these cytokines.[16,17] Consistent with studies in IL-6 and LIF systems,[18,19] H7-sensitive kinases are involved in the more downstream steps than tyrosine kinases along the signaling pathways.

Participation of Jak Family Tyrosine Kinases

Jak family tyrosine kinases have been shown to be involved in the signal transduction mediated by erythropoietin,[20] IL-3,[21] growth hormone,[22] and interferons.[23,24] Since the molecular weight of one of the tyrosine-phosphorylated proteins induced by IL-11, IL-6, LIF and OSM is 130 kD, which is close to the molecular weight of Jak family kinases, we examined the identity of the 130 kD protein with Jak family kinases. Combined immunoblotting with antiphosphotyrosine and anti-Jak2 confirmed that Jak2 is tyrosine phosphorylated following stimulation with gp130 family cytokines.[25] It was also found that tyrosine kinase Jak2 physically associates with gp130 and the *in vitro* kinase activity of Jak2 is greatly enhanced following stimulation with IL-11.[25] Similar observations have been reported for the other members of gp130 family cytokines.[26–28]

Activation of Mitogen-activated Protein Kinases (MAPKs) and Ribosomal S6 Protein Kinases

MAPKs and ribosomal S6 protein kinases have been shown to be activated by a variety of growth factors and mitogens.[29] We have demonstrated that IL-11, IL-6, LIF, and OSM can trigger the activation of MAPKs and the 85–92 kDa ribosomal S6 protein kinases (pp90^{rsk}). We also showed that preincubation of cells with a tyrosine kinase inhibitor, herbimycin A, but not with a serine/threonine kinase inhibitor, H7, blocks activation of MAPKs and pp90^{rsk}. Interestingly, H7, but not herbimycin A, inhibits pp90^{rsk} activity in the *in vitro* kinase assays. These results suggest that pp90^{rsk} is one of the potential candidates for the H7-sensitive protein kinase(s), which is critical for the activation of primary response genes induced by these cytokines (ref. 30; also see below).

Involvement of H7-sensitive Kinases

To dissect the sequential steps involved in IL-11 signaling, we have examined the effects of various inhibitors and activators of different kinases on protein tyrosine phosphorylation and primary response gene expression mediated by IL-11 and related cytokines. Consistent with the previous observations in the IL-6 and LIF systems,[18,19] tyrosine kinases and unidentified H7-sensitive kinases are crucial in IL-11-mediated signal transduction. Our *in vitro* kinase assay results obtained in the presence of H7 indicated that H7 may act on downstream signaling pathways of pp90^{rsk} by inhibiting the pp90^{rsk} activity and suggest that pp90^{rsk} be one of the H7-sensitive protein kinases involved in the expression of primary response genes induced by gp130 family cytokines. In addition to pp90^{rsk}, nuclear run-on studies performed in the presence of H7 have suggested that various H7-sensitive kinases may control the expression of primary response genes at either the transcriptional or posttranscriptional level (TABLE 1). The identification of these H7-sensitive kinases will be essential in the understanding of crosstalks between nuclear and cytoplasmic signaling molecules.

Activation of src-Family Protein Tyrosine Kinases

Src-family tyrosine kinases have been shown to be important for cytokine-mediated signal transduction.[31] 3T3-L1 cells express constitutive level of fyn, src, and yes, and

TABLE 1. Effects of H7 on IL-11-induced Expression of tis8, tis11 and junB in Mouse 3T3-L1 Cells

	Steady-state mRNA Level			Nuclear Run-on Assay		
	Control	IL-11	IL-11+H7	Control	IL-11	IL-11+H7
tis8	−[a]	++	−	−	++	−
tis11	−	+++	−	−	+++	+
junB	−	++++	−	−	++	++

[a] −: no signal; +: expression signal.

each of these kinases can be activated by IL-11 to various extents.[32] Yes and src are activated within the first 10 seconds and 30 seconds, respectively. IL-11–stimulated cells also revealed increased phosphatidylinositol 3-kinase (PI3K) activity. Increased activity of PI3K was seen from antiphosphotyrosine and anti-p62^{yes} immunoprecipitations but not from anti-p60^{src} immunoprecipitations. Immunoprecipitation studies with anti-PI3K revealed that the amount of p60^{src} associated with PI3K does not change significantly with the activation of p60^{src} or PI3K by IL-11. However, the level of p62^{yes} associated with PI3K increased with the activation of p62^{yes} or PI3K. The role of src-family kinases of gp130 family cytokines have been reported previously in other cell types.[33,34]

SECOND MESSENGER(S) INVOLVED IN IL-11 SIGNALING

We have investigated the role of lipid second messengers in IL-11–mediated signal transduction. It was found that IL-11 can increase phosphatidic acid formation through the activation of phospholipase D.[35] In addition, endogenously raised or exogenously added PA can enhance tyrosine phosphorylation of two proteins of 44 kD (p44) and 47 kD (p47), whereas tyrosine phosphorylation of other proteins was not affected in IL-11–treated mouse 3T3-L1 cells. PA stimulation of tyrosine phosphorylation of p44 and p47 was not observed with other phospholipid-derived second messengers including DAG, arachidonic acid, and lysophosphatidic acid. Among various PA species, dipalmitoyl PA was found to be effective for enhancing tyrosine phosphorylation of p44. Furthermore, stimulation of a synthetic substrate for MAP kinase by IL-11- or PA-induced cell lysate and immunoreactivity of p44 and p47 with anti-MAP kinase monoclonal antibodies identified these proteins as members of MAP kinase family. These studies suggest that one of the cellular signaling mechanisms of IL-11 involves the activation of phospholipase D to produce the second messenger PA. The increased level of PA enhances tyrosine phosphorylation of p44 and p47, which belong to the members of MAP kinase family, and thus transduces some of the mitogenic signals of IL-11 in 3T3-L1 cells. The involvement of second messengers for other members of gp130 family cytokines and their relationships to other signaling molecules will require further investigation.

TRANSCRIPTIONAL FACTOR(S) INVOLVED IN IL-11 SIGNALING

Stat91 and related proteins are cytoplasmic proteins which were originally identified as interferon activated transcriptional factors.[36] In untreated cells, Stat91 and related proteins are present in cytoplasm and are in inactive forms. Upon stimulation with interferons, Stat91 and related proteins are tyrosine phosphorylated and translocated to the nucleus and function as transcriptional factors to activate a set of genes. Recent studies have shown that Stat91 and related proteins can also be activated by other growth factors such as EGF.[37] Interestingly, tyrosine phosphorylation and activation of Stat91 and related proteins have been linked to Jak family tyrosine kinases.[36] Since IL-11, IL-6, LIF and OSM significantly activated Jak family tyrosine kinases,[23–26] we examined whether IL-11 can induce tyrosine phosphorylation of Stat91 and related proteins. Using antibodies against Stat91, we were able to show that Stat91 is tyrosine phosphorylated and translocated to nucleus following IL-11

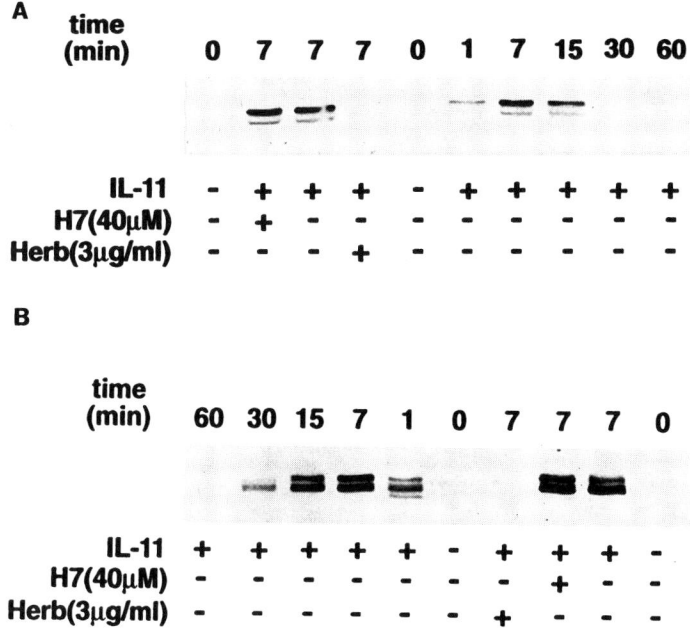

FIGURE 2. Tyrosine phosphorylation of Stat91 and related 89 kilodalton proteins induced by IL-11 in 3T3-L1 cells. The confluent 3T3L1 cells were preincubated without or with 3 μg/ml of herbimycin A for overnight or with H7 (40 μM) for 30 minutes. Cells were then stimulated with 500 ng/ml of IL-11 for indicated periods of time. Cytoplasmic (**A**) and nuclear (**B**) extracts were incubated with anti-Stat91 antibodies for 2 hours on ice. Protein A-Agarose beads were then added and samples were rotated for 1 hour at 4°C. The immunoprecipitates were separated by 7.5% SDS-PAGE and transferred onto PVDF membranes. The membranes were immunoblotted with anti-phosphotyrosine antibodies.

treatment in 3T3-L1 mouse preadipocytes (FIG. 2). The events which IL-11 stimulates tyrosine phosphorylation and nuclear translocation of Stat91 occurred within 1 minute, peaked by 7 minutes and disappeared after 30 minutes. We have observed that IL-11 induces tyrosine phosphorylation of 89 kD proteins which can be immunoprecipitated by anti-Stat 91 antibodies. The kinetics of tyrosine phosphorylation and nuclear translocation of 89 kD proteins is similar to that of Stat91. Interestingly, immunoblotting with anti-Stat91 failed to detect 89 kD proteins, suggesting that 89 kD proteins are antigenically different from Stat91 but may form a stable complex with Stat91. The significance of tyrosine phosphorylation and nuclear translocation of Stat91 and 89 kD proteins induced by IL-11 requires further investigation.

As shown in FIGURE 2, H7 treatment of 3T3-L1 had no effect on tyrosine phosphorylation and the compartmentation of Stat91, suggesting that the activation of primary response genes requires transcriptional factors other than Stat91. Analysis of *cis*- and *trans*-elements required for the primary response gene expression and the participation of H7-sensitive kinases and Stat91 in transcriptional activation will be essential in the understanding of nuclear signaling events mediated by these cytokines.

ACTIVATION OF PRIMARY RESPONSE GENES BY IL-11

We have examined the expression of primary response genes in different IL-11 responsive cell lines stimulated by IL-11. In H35 and 3T3-L1 cells, tis8, tis11 and junB were activated; in B9TY-1 and T10 cells, tis11, tis21 and junB were activated and in TF-1 cells, only junB was activated following stimulation. Nuclear run-on results have demonstrated that transcriptional activation is the major mechanism for the increased steady-state mRNA levels of these primary response genes. The expression of these genes, however, can be affected by H7 at either the transcriptional or posttranscriptional level (TABLE 1).

Recent studies have shown that 3CH134, an immediate early gene, encodes a protein with phosphatase activity.[36] It has been demonstrated that the gene product of 3CH134 is a phosphatase with dual specificity that can specifically dephosphorylate and inactivates MAP kinases both *in vitro* and *in vivo*.[36,37] Based on our observation that MAP kinases are involved in the signaling pathways mediated by IL-11, IL-6, LIF, and OSM in mouse 3T3-L1 cells, we tested whether 3CH134 can be activated by IL-11 stimulation. Our results indicated that IL-11 significantly induces expression of 3CH134 gene by Northern blot analysis (FIG. 3). The time course studies showed that induction of 3CH134 occurred within 5 minutes, peaked by 10–15 minutes and significantly declined by 30 minutes following stimulation. Depletion of protein kinases C by pretreatment of cells with TPA for 40 hours did not significantly reduce

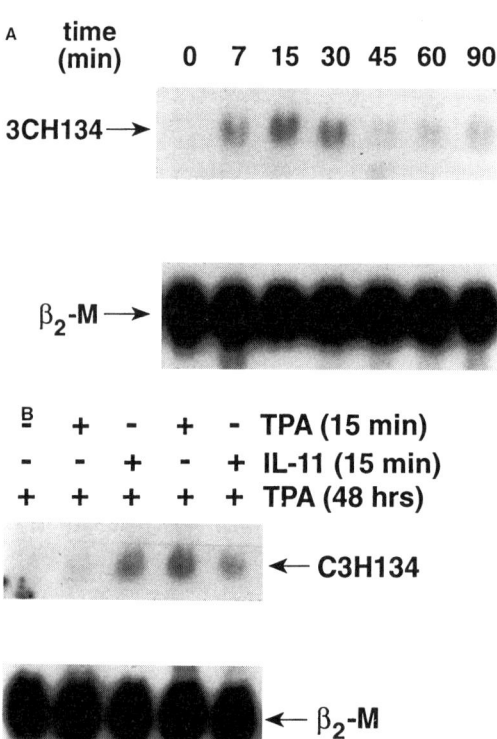

FIGURE 3. Analysis of 3CH134 gene expression induced by IL-11. (A) Kinetic studies of 3CH134 gene expression. Confluent 3T3-L1 cells were stimulated with 500 ng/ml of IL-11 for indicated periods of time. Total RNA was isolated and separated with formaldehyde-agarose gel. RNA was transferred to nitrocellulose membranes and hybridized with 3CH134 cDNA or beta2-microglobulin cDNA as an internal control. (B) 3T3-L1 cells were pretreated without or with 300 ng/ml of TPA for 48 hours. Cells were then stimulated with 500 ng/ml of IL-11 or 300 ng/ml of TPA for 15 minutes as indicated. Total RNA was isolated and analyzed as described in A.

the expression of 3CD134, suggesting that PKC may not be involved in the induced expression of 3CH134 by IL-11. However, expression of 3CH134 triggered by IL-11 can be inhibited by pretreatment of cells with a tyrosine kinase inhibitor herybimycin A or serine/threonine kinase inhibitor H7. These results strongly indicated that tyrosine kinases and H7-sensitive kinases are essential for 3CH134 expression induced by IL-11. Induction of 3CH134 expression stimulated by IL-11 suggested that MAP kinase phosphatase may be actively involved in the signaling pathways mediated by IL-11.

CONCLUSIONS

It has become clear from recent development in the cytokine field that the sharing of receptor complexes may explain some of the biological redundancy of different cytokines.[40] In the analysis of signaling pathways mediated by gp130 family cytokines including IL-11, IL-6, LIF, and OSM, we indeed have found similarities in signaling steps mediated by these cytokines. It is clear that there are crosstalks and selections among different signaling pathways to result in specific gene expression in different cell types. Although the Jak/Stat pathway is involved in the signaling of gp130 family cytokines, the identification and characterization of H7-sensitive kinases will further our understanding on the connection of cytoplasmic and nuclear signaling events.

It has been suggested that the differences in biological activities of cytokines with common receptor components may be in part due to the absence of ligand binding subunits present on particular cell types.[40] In our analysis of signal transduction pathways mediated by gp130 family cytokines, we have observed qualitative and quantitative differences in the activation of certain signaling pathways. For example, we have found differences in tyrosine phosphorylation mediated by IL-11, IL-6, LIF and OSM within the same cell type.[16,30] Similar observations have been reported in other cell systems.[41] The identification of signaling pathways unique to each of the cytokines will be crucial to explain differences in biological functions of cytokines on different cell types.

SUMMARY

IL-11 is a multifunctional cytokine biologically related to IL-6, leukemia inhibitory factor (LIF), oncostatin M (OSM) and ciliary neurotrophic factor (CNTF). It has been shown that these cytokines can utilize common signal transducer, gp130. We have demonstrated that Jak tyrosine kinases, MAP kinases and $pp90^{rsk}$ are highly activated by IL-11 and related cytokines. In addition, we have identified $pp90^{rsk}$ as one of the H7 sensitive protein kinases critical for primary response gene expression induced by IL-11. Furthermore, activation of 3CH134 (a MAP kinase phosphatase) gene by IL-11 suggested that a MAP kinase phosphatase may be involved in IL-11-mediated signal transduction. Our data also suggested that tyrosine phosphorylation of Stat91 and related transcriptional factors is involved in IL-11 signaling but is not sufficient for the activation of primary response genes such as JunB, tis11, tis8 and MAP kinase phosphatase in mouse preadipocytes. The understanding of signal transduction pathways mediated by IL-11 and related cytokines may help to define the common and unique biological properties of these growth factors.

ACKNOWLEDGMENTS

The authors would like to thank Drs. Douglas Fuhrer, Rafat Siddiqui, and Liu Yang for contributing their unpublished results; Drs. Andrew Larner and Xin-Yuan Fu for anti-p91 and Dr. Lester Lau for 3CH134 cDNA.

REFERENCES

1. PAUL, S. R., F. BENNET, J. A. CALVETTI, K. KELLEHER, C. R. WOOD, R. M. O'HARA, JR., A. C. LEARY, B. SIBLEY, S. C. CLARK, D. A. WILLIAMS & Y.-C. YANG. 1990. Molecular cloning of a cDNA encoding interleukin 11, a stromal cell-derived lymphopoietic and hematopoietic cytokine. Proc. Natl. Acad. Sci. USA **87:** 7512–7516.
2. YANG, Y-C. 1993. Interleukin-11: An overview. Stem cells, **11:** 474–486.
3. NEBEN, T. Y., J. LOEBELENZ, L. HAYES, K. MCCARTHY, J. STOUDIMIRE, R. SCHAUB & S. J. GOLDMAN. 1993. Recombinant human interleukin-11 stimulates megakaryocytopoiesis and increases peripheral platelets in normal and splenectomized mice. Blood **81:** 901–908.
4. DU, X. X., T. NEBEN, S. GOLDMAN & D. A. WILLIAMS. 1993. Effects of recombinant human interleukin-11 on hematopoietic reconstitution in transplant mice: Acceleration of recovery of peripheral blood neutrophils and platelets. Blood **81:** 27–34.
5. GORDON, M. S., L. BATTIATO, R. HOFFMAN, E. BREEDEN, W. J. MCCASKILL-STEVENS, B. KUCA, J. KAYE & G. W. SLEDGE, JR. 1993. Subcutaneously (SC) administered recombinant human interleukin-11 (Neumega rhIL-11 growth factor; rhIL-11) prevents thrombocytopenia following chemotherapy (CT) with cyclophosphamide (C) and doxorubicin (A) in women with breast cancer (BC). Blood **89:** 318a.
6. MCKINLEY, D., Q. WU, T. YANG-FENG & Y.-C. YANG. 1992. Genomic sequence and chromosomal location of human interleukin (IL)-11 gene. Genomics **13:** 814–819.
7. YANG, L. & Y.-C. YANG. 1994. Regulation of interleukin (IL)-11 gene expression in IL-1 induced primate bone marrow stromal cells. J. Biol. Chem. **269:** 32732–32739.
8. YANG, L. & Y.-C. YANG. 1994. Posttranscriptional regulation of interleukin (IL)-11 gene expression in IL-1α induced primate bone marrow stromal cells.
9. YIN, T., K. MIYAZAWA & Y.-C. YANG. 1992. Characterization of interleukin-11 receptor and protein tyrosine phosphorylation induced by interleukin-11 in mouse 3T3-L1 cells. J. Biol. Chem. **267:** 8347–8351.
10. GEARING, D. P., M. R. COMEAU, D. J. FRIEND, S. D. GIMPEL, C. J. THUT, J. MCGOURTY, K. K. BRASHER, J. A. KING, S. GILLIS, B. MOSLEY, S. F. ZIEGLER & D. COSMAN. 1992. The IL-6 signal transducer, gp130: An oncostatin M receptor and affinity converter for the LIF receptor. Science **255:** 1434–1437.
11. IP, N. Y., S. H. NYE, T. G. BOULTON, S. DAVIS, T. TAGA, Y. LI, S. J. BIRREN, K. YASUKAWA, T. KISHIMOTO, D. J. ANDERSON, N. STAHL & G. D. YANCOPOULOS. 1992. Cell **69:** 1121–1132.
12. LIU, J., A. MODRELL, A. ARUFFO, J. S. MARKEN, T. TAGA, M. MURAKAMI, K. YASUKAWA, T. KISHIMOTO & M. SHOYAB. 1992. J. Biol. Chem. **267:** 16763–16766.
13. YIN, T., T. TAGA, M. L.-S. TSANG, K. YASUKAWA, T. KISHIMOTO & Y-C. YANG. 1993. Involvement of interleukin-6 signal transducer gp130 in IL-11 mediated signal transduction. J. Immunol. **151:** 2555–2561.
14. L. C. CANTELY, K. R. AUGER, C. CARPENTER, B. DUCKWORTH, A. GRAZIANI, R. KAPELLER & S. SOLTOFF. 1991. Oncogenes and signal transduction. Cell **64:** 281–302.
15. HERSCHMAN, H. R. 1991. Primary response genes induced by growth factors and tumor promoters. Annu. Rev. Biochem. **60:** 281–319.
16. YIN, T. & Y.-C. YANG. 1993. Interleukin-11 mediated signal transduction pathways: comparison with those of IL-6. *In* Growth Factors, Peptides and Receptors. T. W. Moody, Ed. New York: Plenum Press. :323–33.
17. YIN, T. & Y-C. YANG. 1993. Protein tyrosine phosphorylation and activation of primary response genes by interleukin-11 in B9-TY1 cells. Cell Growth Differentiation **4:** 603–608.

18. NAKAJIMA, K. & R. WALL. 1991. Interleukin-6 signals activating junB and tis11 gene transcription in a B cell hybridoma. Mol. Cell. Biol. **11:** 1409–1418.
19. LORD, K. A., A. ABDOLLAHI, S. M. THOMAS, M. DEMARCO, J. S. BRUGGE, B. HOFFMAN-LIEBERMANN & D. A. LIEBERMANN. 1991. Leukemia inhibitory factor and interleukin-6 triggers the same immediate early response including tyrosine phosphorylation, upon induction of myeloid leukemia differentiation. Mol. Cell. Biol. **11:** 4371–4379.
20. WITTHUHN, B. A., F. W. QUELLE, O. SILVENNOINEN, T. YI, B. TANG, O. MIURA & J. N. IHLE. 1993. JAK2 associates with the erythropoietin receptor and is tyrosine phosphorylated and activated following stimulation with erythropoietin. Cell **74:** 227–236.
21. SILVENNOINEN, O., B. A. WITTHUHN, F. W. QUELLE, J. L. CLEVELAND, T. YI & J. N. IHLE. 1993. Structure of the JAK2 protein tyrosine kinase and its role in IL-3 signal transduction. Proc. Natl. Acad. Sci. USA **90:** 8429–8433.
22. ARGETSINGER, L. S., G. S. CAMPBELL, X. YANG, B. A. WITTHUHN, O. SILVENNOINEN, J. N. IHLE & C. CARTER-SU. 1993. Identification of JAK2 as a growth hormone receptor-associated tyrosine kinase. Cell **74:** 237–244.
23. MULLER, M., J. BRISCOE, C. LAXTON, D. GUSCHIN, A. ZIEMIECKI, O. SILVENNOINEN, A. G. HARPUR, G. BARBIERI, B. A. WITTHUHN, C. SCHINDLER, S. PELLEGRINI, A. F. WILKS, J. N. IHLE, G. R. STARK & I. M. KERR. 1993. The protein tyrosine kinase JAK1 complements defects in interferon-alpha/beta and gamma signal transduction. Nature **366:** 129–135.
24. WATLING, D., D. GUSCHIN, M. MULLER, O. SILVENNOINEN, B. A. WITTHUHN, F. W. QUELLE, N. C. ROGERS, C. SCHINDLER, G. R. STARK, J. N. IHLE & I. M. KERR. 1993. Complementation by the protein tyrosine kinase JAK2 of a mutant cell line defective in the interferon-gamma signal transduction pathway. Nature **336:** 166–170.
25. YIN, T., K. YASUKAWA, T. TAGA, T. KISHIMOTO & Y-C. YANG. 1994. Identification of a 130 kilodalton tyrosine phosphorylated protein induced by interleukin-11, interleukin-6, leukemia inhibitory factor and oncostatin M as JAK2 kinase, which associates with gp130 signal transducer. Exp. Hematol. **22:** 467–472.
26. LUTTICKEN, C., U. M. WEGENKA, J. YUAN, J. K. BUSCHMANN, T. TAGA, T. KISHIMOTO, G. BARIERI, S. PELLEGRINI, M. SENDTNER, P. C. HEINRICH & F. HORN. 1994. Association of transcription factor APRF and protein kinase JaK 1 with IL-6 signal transducer gp130. Science **263:** 89–92.
27. STAHL, N., T. G. BAULTON, T. FARRUGGELLA, N. Y. IP, S. DAVIS, B. A. WILTHUHN, F. W. QUELLE, O. SILVENNOINEN, G. BARIERI, S. PELLEGRINI, J. N. IHLE & G. D. YANCOPOULOS. 1994. Association and activation of JAK-Tyk kinases by CNTF-LIF-OSM-IL-6 β Receptor Components. Science **263:** 92–95.
28. NARAZAKI, M., B. A. WITTHUHN, K. YOSHIDA, O. SILVENNOINEN, K. YASUKAWA, J. N. IHLE, T. KISHIMOTO & T. TAGA. 1994. Activation of JAK2 kinase mediated by the interleukin 6 signal transducer gp130. Proc. Natl. Acad. Sci. USA. **91:** 2285–2289.
29. BLENIS, J. 1993. Signal transduction via the MAP kinases: proceed at your own RSK. Proc. Natl. Acad. Sci. USA **90:** 5889–5892.
30. YIN, T. G. & Y-C. YANG. 1994. Involvement of MAP kinase and pp90^{rsk} activation in signaling pathways shared by interleukin-11, interleukin-6 leukemia inhibitory factor and oncostatin M in mouse 3T3-L1 cells. J. Biol. Chem. **269:** 3731–3738.
31. BOLEN, J., P. THOMPSON, E. EISMAN & I. HORAK. 1991. Expression and interactions of the src-family of tyrosine protein kinases in T lymphocytes. Adv. Cancer Res. **57:** 103–149.
32. FUHRER, D. K. & Y-C. YANG. 1994. Activation of src-family protein tyrosine kinases and phosphatidylinositol-3 kinase in 3T3-L1 mouse preadipocytes by interleukin-11. Submitted.
33. BOULTON, T., M. STAHL & G. D. YANCOPOULOS. 1994. Ciliary neurotrophic factor/leukemia inhibitory factor/interleukin-6/oncostatin M family of cytokines induces tyrosine phosphorylation of a common set of proteins overlapping those induced by other cytokines and growth factors. J. Biol. Chem. **269:** 11648–11655.
34. ERNST, M., D. GEARING & A. DUNN. 1994. Functional and biochemical association of hck with the LIF/IL-6 receptor signal transducing subunit gp130 in embryonic stem cells. EMBO J. **13:** 1574–1584.

35. SIDDIQUI, R. A. & Y-C. YANG. 1994. Interleukin-11 induces phosphatidic acid formation and activates MAP kinase in mouse 3T3-L1 cells. Cell. Signal. In press.
36. DARNELL, JR., J. E., I. M. KERR & G. R. STARK. 1994. Jak-Stat pathways and transcriptional activation in response to IFNs and other extracellular signalling proteins. Science **264:** 1415–1421.
37. FU, X. Y. & J. J ZHANG. 1993. Transcriptional factor p91 interacts. With the epidermal growth factor receptor and mediates activating of the c-fos gene promoter. Cell **74:** 1135–1145.
38. CHARLES, C. H., H. SUN, L. F. LOU & N. K. TONKS. 1993. The growth factor inducible immediate-early gene 3CH134 encodes a protein-tyrosine phosphatase. Proc. Natl. Acad. Sci. USA **90:** 5292–5296.
39. SUN, H., C. H. CHARLES, L. F. LOU & N. K. TONKS. 1993. MKP-1 (3CH134), an immediate early gene product, is a dual specificity phosphatase that dephosphorylates MAP kinase *in vivo.* Cell **75:** 487–493.
40. KISHIMOTO, T., T. TAGA & S. ARIKA. 1994. Cytokine signal transduction. Cell **76:** 253–262.
41. TANIGAWA, T., N. ELWOOD, D. METCALF, D. CARY, E. DELUCA, N. A. NICOLA & C. G. BEGLEY. 1993. The SCL gene product is regulated by and differentially regulates cytokine responses during myeloid leukemic cell differentiation. Proc. Natl. Acad. Sci. USA **90:** 7864–7868.

DISCUSSION OF THE PAPER

M. REVEL (*Weizmann Institute, Rehovot, Israel*): Thank you Dr. Yang, and also for clearing up that Stat proteins cannot be involved in the activation of the early genes. Those are proteins which are involved in the effect of interferons, which depress the jun and early genes, so it is important that you clarified that this goes with another mechanism and does not involve Stat91 and the proteins of the same family.

H. BAUMANN (*Roswell Park Cancer Institute, Buffalo, NY*): Your cross-linking with the receptor, does that allow you to tell whether or not you have gp130 recruited, or is it only one gp130 plus the receptor which binds to IL-11?

Y-C. YANG: What I can say is that in the IL-6 system, when Dr. Kishimoto's group did the cross-linking experiment one can see only the gp80, the ligand-binding subunit, but not the gp130. I should say that it is very difficult to answer your question at this point.

BAUMANN: It is only because there was an update in terms of Kishimoto's analysis, and I think that Professor Heinrich has done that too. He found binding of two gp130 and even the higher complexes, which will verify the complexity. And the other question is: in your herbimycin treatment how long before you have challenged these cells with IL-11? Was it several hours or just a few minutes?

YANG: Herbimycin treatment was overnight.

BAUMANN: It is an important issue about what it has to do with Dr. Akira's Stat. You mentioned that IL-11 treatment will lead to the activation of p91, which we equate to Stat91. Did you see the same activation of p91 when you treat cells with IL-6?

YANG: Yes. But we are dealing with two different things here. We mainly study adipocytes, which is the cell type difference between my study and Dr. Akira's. And for those of you who are interested in anti-p91, when we first tried anti-p91 we obtained it from Dr. X-Y. Fu's laboratory and also a commercial antibody from Signal Transduction; with these we did not see tyrosine phosphorylation of p91. It was only when we used Dr. Andrew Larner's that we could detect p91 phosphorylation. So I think that there might be differences in what we are seeing.

BAUMANN: But one has to realize that the IL-6 receptor on adipocyte is structurally identical to the one on liver cell or HepG2 cell. They are not different receptors. So the recruitment of Jak2 as well as Jak1 and probably Tyk-2 will be the same.

REVEL: I do not think that anybody doubts that IL-6 can activate p91.

In Vivo Properties of Oncostatin M

PHILIP M. WALLACE,[a,c] JOHN F. MACMASTER,
JILL R. RILLEMA, KATHERINE A. ROULEAU,
MARCIA B. HANSON, SAMUEL A. BURSTEIN,[b] AND
MOHAMMED SHOYAB[d]

[a]*Bristol-Myers Squibb*
Pharmaceutical Research Institute
3005 First Avenue
Seattle, Washington 98121

[b]*W.K. Warren Medical Research Institute*
Department of Medicine
University of Oklahoma Health Sciences Center
Oklahoma City, Oklahoma 73190

Oncostatin M (OM) is a 28 kD glycoprotein originally purified from the conditioned media of phorbol 12-myristate 13-acetate–treated U937 cells, based on its ability to inhibit the human melanoma cell line, A375.[1] OM is structurally and functionally related to the family of hematopoietic and neurotrophic cytokines whose members include leukemia inhibitory factor (LIF), interleukin-6 (IL-6), interleukin-11 (IL-11), ciliary neurotrophic factor (CNTF), and cardiotrophin.[2–5] OM shares properties with all members of this family of proteins, but is most closely related structurally and functionally to LIF.[2,6] The genes encoding these two molecules exist within 20 kb of each other on human chromosome 22,[7–10] leading to the suggestion that these molecules are the result of a gene duplication.[9] IL-6 and IL-11 seem to be more closely related functionally to each other than OM, with more actions described within the lymphoid system.[2,11,12] CNTF is a more distant relative with a limited receptor distribution[13–15] and a smaller spectrum of activities.[16]

The cellular receptors for these factors also form a family of related proteins that share structural similarities.[3] These multi-component complexes each contain the IL-6 signal transduction subunit (gp130).[17–23] OM binds at least two distinct receptor complexes.[24,25] OM and LIF compete for binding to the high-affinity LIF receptor,[24] composed of the low-affinity LIF receptor and gp130.[26] Although this receptor is shared by the two cytokines, OM binds with a reduced affinity compared to LIF.[24,26] A second OM-specific receptor complex exists[24,25,27,28] which binds OM with both high- and low-affinity interactions.[25,27] OM binds directly to gp130 with low affinity, and therefore gp130 appears to be the low affinity OM receptor found on some cells.[23,29,30] High-affinity binding most likely results from the association of gp130 with a high-affinity–converting subunit, as has been described for LIF.[29] A putative affinity converting subunit that combines with gp130 to produce high affinity OM binding has recently been described in a preliminary form.[31] Though gp130 is necessary it is apparently not sufficient for functional OM receptors.[23,26]

---

[c] Author to whom correspondence should be addressed: Tel: (206) 727-3735; Fax: (206) 727-3603.
[d] *Present address:* Department of Pathobiology, F-167 Health Science Building, SC-38, University of Washington, Seattle, WA 98195.

The overlapping properties of the IL-6–like cytokines presumably arise from the presence of gp130 in each of their receptors.[32,33] However, there are unique properties and signal transduction pathways which are engaged when these receptors bind their ligands.[6,25] *In vitro*, OM acts on a wide variety of cells and elicits a multitude of biological responses including: growth modulation,[34-38] leukemia cell differentiation,[28] LDL receptor up regulation,[39] stimulation of plasminogen activator,[40,41] induction of hematopoietic factors,[42,43] induction of acute phase proteins,[44,45] inhibition of embryonic stem cell differentiation,[46] and induction of tissue-inhibitor of metalloproteinases-1.[47,48] Of these properties, many are shared with the other related cytokines, though others as yet have only been ascribed to OM.[39,42,43]

To further understand the role of OM in normal and pathological states and to identify potential clinical utilities, we undertook studies evaluating the *in vivo* properties of OM.

RESULTS AND DISCUSSION

Blood Clearance and Tissue Distribution of OM

As a prelude to studying the *in vivo* properties of OM, we investigated the toxicity and pharmacokinetics of the molecule. Recombinant human OM expressed by Chinese hamster ovary cells was used in all the studies described below.[49] OM was administered either intravenously (i.v.) or intraperitoneally (i.p.) at 1.3 mg/kg/day (~30 μg/day) on each of 5 successive days with weight loss (~10%) as the only overt sign of toxicity. In other studies OM has been administered at 30 μg/day either i.p., i.v., or subcutaneously (s.c) for 15 days to normal and myelosuppressed mice without lethality and with only minimal weight loss. Nude mice bearing tumors secreting OM showed a rapid erythema localized at the tumor site which then spread to all the parts of the animals and persisted until the animals died from cachexia. The histological examination of the organs of these animals showed few abnormalities; however, the spleen exhibited extramedullary hematopoiesis with increased numbers of megakaryocytes compared to normal animals. The erythema could be reproduced by implantation of slow-release pumps secreting OM. At the dose tested (10 μg/day for 7 days) the lesion was localized within 1 cm of the pumps and was rapidly reversible upon removal of the OM. Histologically the skin from the area of erythema showed no significant inflammatory infiltrate.

Clearance studies with i.v. injection of recombinant human OM in mice showed a $t_{1/2} \alpha$ = 4 minutes. This was followed by a second clearance phase occurring over the next 1–4 hours with a $t_{1/2} \beta$ = 45 minutes (FIG. 1). OM was rapidly accumulated by the liver and kidney with 50%/g and 55%/g of the protein found in these organs at 10 minutes (FIG. 2A). This corresponds to 19% of the total injected material in the kidney and 60% in the liver. At one hour <3%/g of the radioactivity remained in the liver, implying that the OM is metabolized (FIG. 2B). Although the blood at one hour contained a significant amount of radioactivity, analysis by gel electrophoresis and trichloroacetic acid precipitation showed this to be low molecular weight material (<5kD). Furthermore, serum samples contained no biologically active OM (data not shown). Mammalian OM contains carbohydrates recognized by the lectin concanavalin A and thus would be expected to be recognized by liver carbohydrate receptors. However, the rapid clearance cannot be blocked by saturating carbohydrate clearance pathways suggesting other clearance mechanisms. The liver uptake is more likely mediated via OM binding receptors known to be present on liver cells.[50,51]

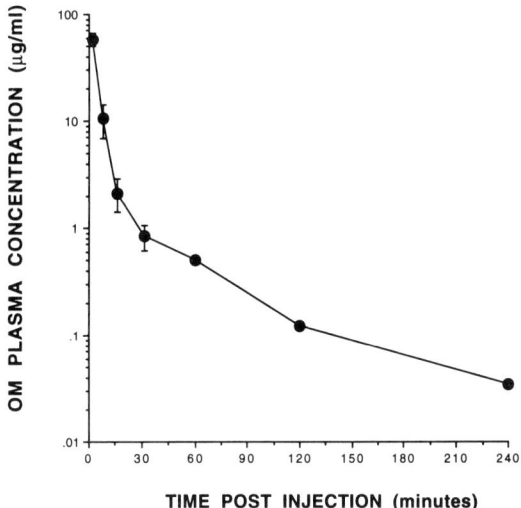

FIGURE 1. Blood clearance of Oncostatin M. Human recombinant Oncostatin M (100 µg) was injected i.v. via the tail vein into C3H/HeJ mice (3 mice/time point). Mice were bled from the retro-orbital sinus and plasma samples collected at the time points indicated. Plasma concentrations of OM were determined by comparison to a standard curve using an OM-specific ELISA. Control studies showed no interference in measurement occurred in the presence of plasma. Shown are the plasma concentrations of OM ± standard deviation (SD).

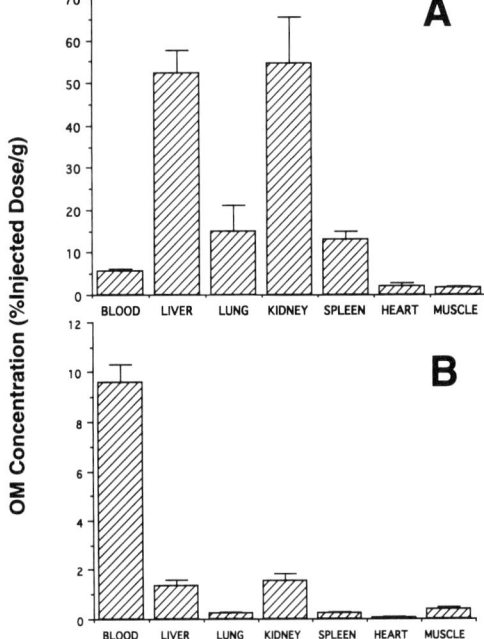

FIGURE 2. Tissue distribution of Oncostatin M. Groups of four Balb/c mice were injected intravenously with ^{125}I-OM. The radiolabeled OM retained biological activity as assessed by a radioreceptor assay. At 10 minutes (**A**) and 1 hour (**B**) post injection mice were bled, sacrificed and tissues excised. Radioactivity in the organs was measured using a gamma counter. The % injected dose/g ± SD is shown.

These clearance characteristics are very similar to the results obtained for IL-6,[52] LIF,[53] and CNTF.[54]

Thrombopoietic Activity of OM

Daily injection of OM for 7 days over a large dose range results in an increase in the circulating levels of platelets in mice (TABLE 1).[55] The hematopoietic effects were seemingly limited to the megakaryocyte lineages as no significant changes occurred in red blood cell (RBC) or white blood cell (WBC) levels. However, changes in plasma volumes accompanying the onset of an acute phase response may have masked any increases in the absolute number of circulating cells.

In vitro studies were performed to further understand the mechanism of the change in platelet levels following OM treatment. Murine bone marrow cells were treated with OM, IL-6, and WEHI conditioned media (CM, a source of murine IL-3) alone, or in combinations. Cells were plated in semi-solid media, cultured, and megakaryocytic colonies enumerated 4–5 days later. Although OM was found not to have any intrinsic colony-forming activity, OM increased the enumerable megakaryocyte colonies in combination with the WEHI CM. This activity was similar to that found with IL-6. A combination of IL-6 or OM was neither additive nor synergistic (FIG. 3).[55]

The interpretation of experiments with human OM in the mouse is complicated because neither a murine OM molecule nor a murine OM-specific receptor have yet been described in the literature. Therefore the thrombopoietic properties of OM were investigated in non-human primates. Treatment of rhesus monkeys with OM showed

TABLE 1. Comparison of the Effects of OM and IL-6 on Circulating Blood Cell Levels in Normal Mice

		Days Post Initiation of Treatment			
	Treatment	0	7	15	21
Platelets	OM 30 μg/day	1032	1585	1351	1275
($\times 10^3$ μl^{-1})	OM 3 μg/day	1061	1370	1328	1350
	OM 1 μg/day	1053	1304	1308	1261
	IL-6 30 μg/day	1160	1357	1146	1222
	IL-6 3 μg/day	1181	1365	1157	1190
	Control	1033	1117	1188	1183
WBC	OM 30 μg/day	8.8	7.9	7.5	7.1
($\times 10^3$ μl^{-1})	OM 3 μg/day	8.1	6.7	8.4	7.4
	OM 1 μg/day	7.4	6.9	8.2	8.8
	IL-6 30 μg/day	8.6	7.0	8.2	8.4
	IL-6 3 μg/day	7.4	7.7	7.4	7.0
	Control	8.5	7.5	8.1	8.4
RBC	OM 30 μg/day	8.6	8.8	9.0	9.0
($\times 10^6$ μl^{-1})	OM 3 μg/day	8.9	7.9	9.4	8.9
	OM 1 μg/day	8.6	8.2	9.4	9.1
	IL-6 30 μg/day	9.4	9.2	9.0	9.5
	IL-6 3 μg/day	9.5	8.8	8.6	9.0
	Control	8.8	8.1	8.5	8.7

Mice (five animals per treatment group) were injected intravenously with PBS/BSA containing recombinant human OM or recombinant human IL-6 daily for seven days. Control mice received diluent alone. Blood was collected via the orbital sinus and complete blood counts were determined using the Serono-Baker Series 9000 hematology analyzer.

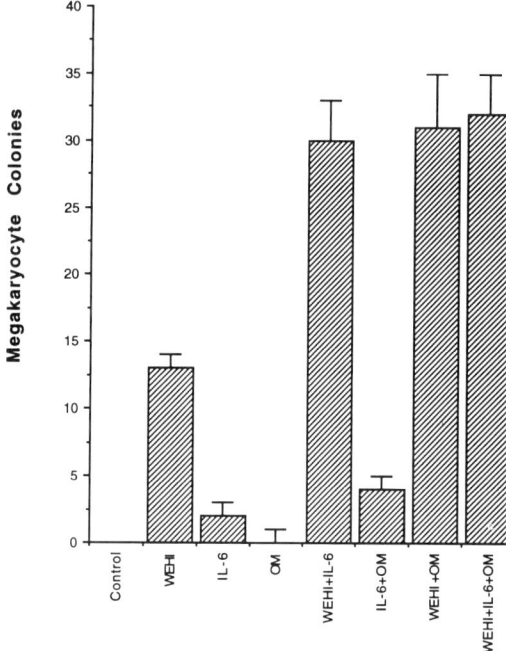

FIGURE 3. Effect of OM on the growth of megakaryocyte colonies. Marrow cells were enriched for progenitors on 1.077 g/cm^3 Ficoll gradient, followed by a 2-h plastic adherence. Megakaryocytic colony-forming cells (CFU-MK) were assayed by culturing the enriched marrow cells (2×10^4 cells/ml) in IMDM rendered semi-solid with 0.9% methylcellulose. Cultures were supplemented with 15% horse serum, 1×10^{-5}M β-mercaptoethanol, and combinations of 10% WEHI-3 conditioned medium (a source of murine IL-3), IL-6 (100 ng/ml) and OM (100 ng/ml). Megakaryocyte colonies ($\geq$3 cells/colony) were enumerated following 5–6 days incubation at 37°C in a 95% air–5% CO_2 tissue culture incubator.[74]

a dose-dependent increase in circulating platelet levels and no significant changes in RBCs or WBCs (TABLE 2). This is in contrast to large animal, and clinical, studies with IL-6 or IL-11, in which similar changes in platelet levels are accompanied by anemia.[56–60]

TABLE 2. Effects of OM on Circulating Blood Cells of Normal Non-Human Primates

Treatment		Days Post Initiation of Treatment			
		0	8	15	24
OM 30 μg/kg bid	WBC ($\times 10^{-3}$ μL)	4.7	5.4	7.7	7.7
	RBC ($\times 10^{-6}$ μL)	5.0	4.7	4.6	5.1
	PLT ($\times 10^{-3}$ μL)	458	780	853	325
OM 90 μg/kg bid	WBC ($\times 10^{-3}$ μL)	9.2	2.8	7.8	5.2
	RBC ($\times 10^{-6}$ μL)	3.9	4.6	4.6	4.7
	PLT ($\times 10^{-3}$ μL)	244	809	893	242
Control	WBC ($\times 10^{-3}$ μL)	10.5	4.2	8.0	7.5
	RBC ($\times 10^{-6}$ μL)	5.5	4.9	4.5	4.4
	PLT ($\times 10^{-3}$ μL)	345	445	326	298

Rhesus monkeys (*Macaca mulata*) were injected with OM in PBS containing 1% autologous serum at the indicated dose or diluent alone for the controls. Animals were treated on days 1–3 and 5–7. Blood samples were collected by bleeding via the femoral artery. Complete blood counts were determined with a Serono-Baker Series 9000 hematology analyzer using human discriminators.

Palliation of Radiation and Drug-induced Thrombocytopenia by OM

The effects of OM on thrombopoiesis are not limited to normal animals. OM can accelerate the platelet recovery of animals rendered thrombocytopenic by either radiation or cytotoxic insult. Following exposure to either 250 or 500 cGy of gamma irradiation mice suffer from thrombocytopenia. Treatment of animals with OM at the 250 cGy dose reduces the nadir of thrombocytopenia and accelerates the recovery to normal platelet levels. At the higher irradiation dose, OM also is capable of ameliorating the duration of the resultant thrombocytopenia. At 500 cGy untreated mice also suffer from anemia; however OM prevents this anemia (data not shown). OM also alleviated the reduction in circulating platelet levels caused by treatment with a single injection at the maximum tolerated dose (MTD) of the anti-cancer agent mitomycin C. Both the nadir and the duration of the ensuing thrombocytopenia was reduced in the OM-treated animals (TABLE 3). Similar results on platelet levels were found when the mitomycin C was administered in a multiple dose regimen at the MTD on days 1, 5 and 9 of 2 mg/kg/day.

Induction of Acute Phase Proteins by OM

OM injection also causes an increase in circulating levels of the acute phase reactants haptoglobin (data not shown) and serum amyloid A (SAA) (FIG. 4). In an inflamma-

TABLE 3. Palliation of Thrombocytopenia by OM

Treatment	Days to Normal Platelet Counts	Days to Nadir	Nadir Platelet Level ($\times 10^{-3}$ μl)	Days Platelets Below 50%
250 RADS[a]	27	12	325	8
250 RADS[a] + OM[b]	17	12	557	2
500 RADS[a]	27	12	223	12
500 RADS[a] + OM[b]	17	8	203	8
MMC[c] 6 mg/kg	26	12	304	13
MMC[c] 6 mg/kg + OM[d]	19	9	496	4
MMC 2 mg/kg q4d × 3	34	16	227	16
MMC 2 mg/kg q4d × 3 + OM[e]	28	16	360	7

Female C3H/HeJ mice (8–10 weeks old) obtained from The Jackson Laboratory (Bar Harbor, ME) were rendered thrombocytopenic with either gamma irradiation or mitomycin C (MMC) injection. Mice were injected i.v. with 100 μl of OM in PBS/BSA or PBS/BSA. Animals were bled via the retro-orbital sinus and complete blood counts, including platelet counts, were obtained using a Serono-Baker 9000 automated cell counter.

[a] Groups of 5 animals were irradiated from a ^{137}Cs source (J. S. Shepherd & Associates, San Fernando, CA) at a rate of 259 cGy/minute.

[b] Animals were treated daily with OM at a dose of 15 μg/day for 15 days starting 1 day post irradiation.

[c] MMC was injected i.v. in saline. A maximum tolerated dose of MMC for normal mice was used.

[d] Mice were injected i.v. with OM (7.5 μg) twice daily for 3 days then rested for one day, followed by two further similar courses of OM.

[e] Mice were injected s.c. with OM (7.5 μg) twice daily on days 1–15. A maximum tolerated dose of MMC for normal mice was used.

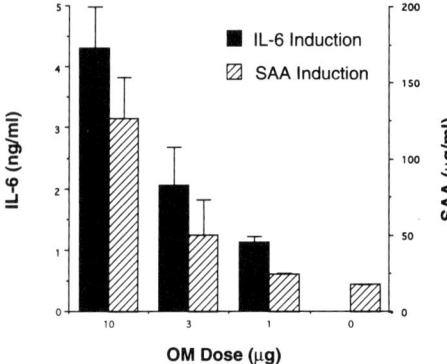

FIGURE 4. Induction of IL-6 and serum amyloid A (SAA) by OM. Mice (3/group) were injected intravenously with OM in PBS/BSA at the indicated dose or with PBS/BSA only. Mice were then bled and plasma samples collected at either 1 hour for the IL-6 or 6 hours for the SAA studies. Plasma concentration of IL-6 and SAA were determined by ELISA (BioSource International, Camarillo, CA) and compared to standard curves. Shown are the plasma concentrations ± SD.

tory response, the acute phase reactants are an early consequence of tissue damage. Secretion of OM by macrophages is consistent with a role for OM in normal inflammatory responses, as tissue macrophages and blood monocytes are thought to initiate the production of acute phase reactants.[61] However, it is clear that many positive and negative regulators of the acute phase response exist, including the other IL-6–like cytokines IL-6, IL-11, LIF and CNTF.[61] Effects of OM on acute phase reactants have also been observed in both dogs and primates, as evidenced by increases in fibrinogen levels (dogs and primates) and SAA (primates) (P. Wallace, unpublished observations).

Induction of IL-6 by OM

Although OM can exert direct effects on both megakaryocytopoiesis and the regulation of acute phase proteins, a second mechanism of augmentation may occur indirectly, via IL-6. OM injection into endotoxin-resistant C3H/HeJ mice results in a dose-dependent induction of IL-6 (FIG. 4). IL-6 is rapidly induced and reaches peak levels at ~75 minutes post-injection. This induction may be mediated via the shared OM/LIF receptor as these findings can be reproduced by recombinant murine and human LIF, injected into this same strain of mice (J. MacMaster, manuscript in preparation). IL-6 induction in response to OM was indistinguishable in splenectomized and normal animals. This is in contrast to LPS treatment in which the predominant organ for the production of IL-6 is the spleen. Northern blot analysis of the organs of mice treated with OM demonstrated that IL-6 messenger RNA was rapidly induced in both the kidney and lung (J. R. Rillema, unpublished results). IL-6 has been shown *in vitro* and *in vivo* to be capable of both inducing acute phase proteins, and altering thrombopoiesis.[56,62,63] Thus, IL-6 induction may play a role in the changes that occur in the levels of platelets and acute phase proteins following OM treatment. However, IL-6 induction is unlikely to be the sole mediator of the thrombopoietic effects of OM. *In vitro* studies of OM in semi-solid media indicate direct effects of OM on megakaryocyte colonies. Furthermore, a maximal effective dose of IL-6 in mice resulted in a significantly smaller increase in circulating platelet number than is seen with OM (TABLE 1). Also, *in vitro,* acute phase proteins can be induced by OM.[44,45] The interactions between OM and IL-6 are further complicated by the finding that OM acts as an IL-6 antagonist.[30] The contributions of IL-6 to the changes observed *in vivo* should be clarified by studies of the effects of OM on IL-6–deficient mice.[64]

CONCLUSIONS

These results shed some light on the therapeutic potential and normal physiological functions of OM. The restorative effects of OM on the hematopoietic insults following radiation or cytotoxic drug treatment suggest the use of this protein in the treatment of thrombocytopenia associated with cancer therapy. The beneficial effects of OM in the treatment of malignancies may not be limited to hematopoietic effects since OM is capable of inhibiting tumor growth directly in a variety of cell lines derived from solid tumors of human origin.[35] Furthermore, *in vitro* studies have found that OM up regulates TIMP-1, an inhibitor of cancer cell metastasis.[65] These other properties of OM, in addition to effects on thrombopoiesis, suggest a role for OM in the management of malignant disease. As each of the members of the IL-6 type family of cytokines exert overlapping sets of properties, the clinical indications of each also overlap. Therefore, the most appropriate use of these molecules in a clinical setting may be determined by the associated toxicities and side-effects.

The role of OM in normal development and homeostasis and its contribution to pathologies is unclear. The actions of OM suggest an involvement in limiting the tissue damage of an inflammatory response, regulating tissue repair, and coordinating the return to homeostasis. Thus, OM can be classified as an anti-inflammatory cytokine. The expression of OM by macrophages[50] and activated T-cells[66] supports the notion that OM would be present at sites of inflammation. The induction of TIMP-1, plasminogen activator, and acute phase reactants and the inhibition of pro-inflammatory cytokines would be expected to result in a process of tissue remodeling and the return toward normality. The effects of OM on thrombopoiesis and erythropoiesis would also seem consistent with responses to injury. Elucidation of the physiological role of OM in normal hematopoiesis is complicated by the extensive array of other proteins that are able to regulate the growth and maturation of megakaryocytes and the production of platelets.[67] This will most easily be addressed by genetically engineering mice incapable of producing OM.

Many of the properties of OM are shared with IL-6, LIF and IL-11. This raises the question of the necessity for each of these molecules as independent products of evolutionary development. Subtle differences in their properties and/or different patterns of tissue expression may provide each with a highly specialized function. Alternatively, these molecules may work in concert with sequential expression of the proteins allowing a smooth transition in some functions whilst maintaining other functions constant. A final possibility is that within the family of proteins there is redundancy in each of the biological activities possessed. This seems unlikely as mice with the genes for IL-6, LIF or CNTF rendered nonfunctional have abnormalities not compensated for by the other family members.[68–70]

Ectopic expression of OM would be expected to result in concordant adventitious expression of a variety of inflammatory mediators for example, acute phase reactants and IL-6. Overexpression of acute phase reactants and IL-6 have been implicated in a variety of disease accompanying chronic inflammation.[11,71] Also, OM has been found to be a growth factor for AIDS-related Kaposi's sarcoma cells *in vitro*.[34,36] Thus OM may also play a role in the pathogenesis of such diseases. Furthermore, genes resident on chromosome 22 are associated with several diseases.[7,72] Such abnormalities may be due to alteration in the OM gene, as has been found for the adjacent LIF gene and meningioma.[73] Therefore antagonists of OM may also have therapeutic potential. Thus, further studies of OM should result in the development of new medicines.

ACKNOWLEDGMENTS

We wish to extend our thanks to Ana Wieman for typing the manuscript, to Greg Bruce and Chris Clegg for their comments on the manuscript, and especially to the conference organizers for their efforts in arranging an excellent scientific meeting.

REFERENCES

1. ZARLING, J. M., M. SHOYAB, H. MARQUARDT, M. B. HANSON, M. N. LIOUBIN & G. J. TODARO. 1986. Oncostatin M: A growth regulator produced by differentiated histiocytic lymphoma cells. Proc. Natl. Acad. Sci. USA **83:** 9739–9743.
2. ROSE, T. M. & A. G. BRUCE. 1991. Oncostatin M is a member of a cytokine family that includes leukemia-inhibitory factor, granulocyte colony-stimulating factor, and interleukin 6. Proc. Natl. Acad. Sci. USA **88:** 8641–8645.
3. BAZAN, J. F. 1990. Structural design and molecular evolution of a cytokine receptor superfamily. Proc. Natl. Acad. Sci. USA **87:** 6934–6938.
4. PENNICA, D., K. L. KING, K. R. CHIEN, J. B. BAKER & W. I. WOOD. 1994. Cardiotrophin-1, a novel cytokine that induces cardiac myocyte hypertrophy. Cytokine **6:** 577 (Abstract).
5. BROWN, M.S. & J. L. GOLDSTEIN. 1986. A receptor-mediated pathway for cholesterol homeostasis. Science **232:** 34–47.
6. PIQUET-PELLORCE, C., L. GREY, A. MEREAU & J. K. HEATH. 1994. Are LIF and related cytokines functionally equivalent. Exp. Cell Res. **213:** 340–347.
7. GIOVANNINI, M., L. SELLERI, G. G. HERMANSON & G. A. EVANS. 1993. Localization of the human oncostatin M gene (OSM) to chromosome 22q12, distal to the Ewing's sarcoma breakpoint. Cytogenet. Cell Genet. **62:** 32–34.
8. GIOVANNINI, M., M. DJABALI, D. MCELLIGOTT, L. SELLERI & G. A. EVANS. 1993. Tandem linkage of genes coding for leukemia inhibitory factor (LIF) and oncostatin M (OSM) on human chromosome 22. Cytogenet. Cell Genet. **64:** 240–244.
9. ROSE, T. M., M. J. LAGROU, I. FRANSSON, B. WERELIUS, O. DELATTRE, G. THOMAS, P. J. DE JOHN, G. J. TODARO & J. P. DUMANKSI. 1993. The genes for oncostatin M (OSM) and leukemia inhibitory factor (LIF) are tightly linked on human chromosome 22. Genomics **17:** 136–140.
10. JEFFERY, E., V. PRICE & D. P. GEARING. 1993. Close proximity of the genes for leukemia inhibitory factor and oncostatin M. Cytokine **5:** 107–111.
11. HIRANO, T., S. AKIRA, T. TAGA & T. KISHIMOTO. 1990. Biological and clinical aspects of interleukin 6. Immunol. Today **11:** 443–449.
12. YIN, T., P. SCHENDEL & Y.-C. YANG. 1992. Enhancement of in vitro and in vivo antigen-specific antibody responses by interleukin 11. J. Exp. Med. **175:** 211–216.
13. TAGA, T. & T. KISHIMOTO. 1992. Cytokine receptors and signal transduction. FASEB J. **6:** 3387–3396.
14. BAZAN, F. J. 1991. Neuropoietic cytokines in the hematopoietic fold. Neuron **7:** 197–208.
15. IP, N. Y., J. MCCLAIN, N. X. BARREZUETA, T. H. ALDRICH, L. PAN, Y. LI, S. J. WIEGAND, B. FRIEDMAN, S. DAVIS & G. D. YANCOPOULOS. 1993. The alpha component of the CNTF receptor is required for signaling and defines potential CNTF targets in the adult and during development. Neuron **10:** 89–102.
16. STOCKLI, K. A., LOTTSPEICH, M. SENDTNER, P. MASIAKOWSKI, P. CARROLL, R. GOTZ, D. LINDHOLM & H. THOENEN. 1989. Molecular cloning, expression and regional distribution of rat ciliary neurotrophic factor. Nature **342:** 920–923.
17. IP, N. Y., S. H. NYE, T. G. BOULTON, S. DAVIS, T. TAGA, Y. LI, S. J. BIRREN, K. YASUKAWA, T. KISHIMOTO, D. J. ANDERSON, N. STAHL & G. D. YANCOPOULOS. 1992. CNTF and LIF act on neuronal cells via shared signaling pathways that involve the IL-6 signal transducing receptor component gp130. Cell **69:** 1121–1132.
18. GEARING, D. P., S. F. ZIEGLER, M. R. COMEAU, D. FRIEND, B. THOMA, D. COSMAN, L. PARK & B. MOSLEY. 1994. Proliferative responses and binding properties of hematopoi-

etic cells transfected with low-affinity receptors for leukemia inhibitory factor, oncostatin M, and ciliary neurotrophic factor. Proc. Natl. Acad. Sci. USA **91:** 1119–1123.
19. LIU, J., B. MODRELL, A. ARUFFO, J. S. MARKEN, T. TAGA, K. YASUKAWA, M. MURAKAMI, T. KISHIMOTO & M. SHOYAB. 1992. Interleukin-6 signal transducer gp130 mediates oncostatin M signaling. J. Biol. Chem. **267:** 16763–16766.
20. TAGA, T., M. NARAZAKI, K. YASUKAWA, T. SAITO, D. MIKI, M. HAMAGUCHI, S. DAVIS, M. SHOYAB, G. D. YANCOPOULOS & T. KISHIMOTO. 1992. Functional inhibition of hematopoietic and neurotrophic cytokines by blocking the interleukin 6 signal transducer gp130. Proc. Natl. Acad. Sci. USA **89:** 10998–11001.
21. HIRANO, T., T. MATSUDA & K. NAKAJIMA. 1994. Signal transduction through gp130 that is shared among the receptors for the interleukin 6 related cytokine subfamily. Stem Cells **12:** 262–277.
22. NISHIMOTO, N., A. OGATA, Y. SHIMA, Y. TANI, Y. OGAWA, M. NAKAGAWA, H. SUGIYAMA, K. YOSHIZAKI & T. KISHIMOTO. 1994. Oncostatin M, leukemia inhibitory factor, interleukin 6 induce the proliferation of human cells via the common signal transducer, GP130. J. Exp. Med. **179:** 1343–1347.
23. LIU, J., B. MODRELL, A. ARUFFO, S. SCHARNOWSKE & M. SHOYAB. 1994. Interactions between Oncostatin M and the IL-6 signal transducer, gp130. Cytokine **6:** 272–278.
24. GEARING, D. P. & A. G. BRUCE. 1992. Oncostatin M binds the high-affinity leukemia inhibitory factor receptor. New Biol. **4:** 61–65.
25. THOMA, B., T. A. BIRD, D. J. FRIEND, P. GEARING & S. K. DOWER. 1994. Oncostatin M and leukemia inhibitory factor trigger overlapping and different signal through partially shared receptor complexes. J. Biol. Chem. **269:** 6215–6222.
26. BAUMANN, H., S. F. ZIEGLER, B. MOSLEY, K. K. MORELLA, S. PAJOVIC & D. P. GEARING. 1993. Reconstitution of the response to leukemia inhibitory factor, oncostatin M, and ciliary neurotrophic factor in hepatoma cells. J. Biol. Chem. **268:** 8414–8417.
27. LINSLEY, P. S., M. B. HANSON, D. HORN, N. MALIK, J. C. KALLESTAD, V. OCHS, J. M. ZARLING & M. SHOYAB. 1989. Identification and characterization of cellular receptors for the growth regulator, oncostatin M. J. Biol. Chem. **264:** 4282–4289.
28. BRUCE, A. G., I. H. HOGGATT & T. M. ROSE. 1992. Oncostatin M is a differentiation factor for myeloid leukemia cells. J. Immunol. **149:** 1271–1275.
29. GEARING, D. P., M. R. COMEAU, D. J. FRIEND, S. D. GIMPEL, C. J. THUT, J. MCGOURTY, K. K. BRASHER, J. A. KING, S. GILLIS, B. MOSLEY, S. F. ZIEGLER & D. COSMAN. 1992. The IL-6 signal transducer, gp130: An oncostatin M receptor and affinity converter for the LIF receptor. Science **255:** 1434–1437.
30. SPORENO, E., G. PAONESSA, A. L. SALVATI, R. GRAZIANI, P. DELMASTRO, G. CILIBERTO & C. TONIATTI. 1994. Oncostatin M binds directly to gp130 and behaves as interleukin-6 antagonist on a cell line expressing gp130 but lacking functional oncostatin M receptors. J. Biol. Chem. **269:** 10991–10995.
31. MOSLEY, B., C. DELMUS, D. FRIEND, B. THOMA & D. COSMAN. 1994. The oncostatin-M specific receptor: Cloning of a novel subunit related to the LIF receptor. Cytokine **6:** 554 (Abstract).
32. YIN, T. & Y.-C. YANG. 1994. Mitogen-activated protein kinases and ribosomal S6 protein kinases are involved in signaling pathways shared by interleukin-11, interleukin-6, leukemia inhibitory factor, and oncostatin M in mouse 3T3-L1 cells. J. Biol. Chem. **269:** 3731–3738.
33. ZHANG, X. G., J-J. GU, Z-Y. LU, K. YASUKAWA, G. D. YANCOPOULOS, K. TURNER, M. SHOYAB, T. TAGA, T. KISHIMOTO, R. BATAILLE & B. KLEIN. 1994. Ciliary neurotropic factor, interleukin 11, leukemia inhibitory factor, and oncostatin M are growth factors for human myeloma cell lines using the IL-6 signal transducer GP 130. J. Exp. Med. **177:** 1337–1342.
34. NAIR, B. F. C., A. L. DEVICO, S. NAKAMURA, T. D. COPELAND, Y. CHEN, A. PATEL, T. O'NEIL, S. OROSZLAN, R. C. GALLO & M. G. SARNGADHARAN. 1992. Identification of a major growth factor for AIDS-Kaposi's sarcoma cells as oncostatin M. Science **255:** 1430–1432.
35. HORN, D., W. C. FITZPATRICK, P. T. GOMPPER, V. OCHS, M. BOLTON-HANSEN, J. ZARLING, N. MALIK, G. J. TODARO & P. S. LINSLEY. 1990. Regulation of cell growth by recombinant oncostatin M. Growth Factors **2:** 157–165.

36. MILES, S. A., O. MARTINEZ-MAZA, A. REZAI, L. MAGPANTAY, T. KISHIMOTO, S. NAKAMURA, S. F. RADKA & P. S. LINSLEY. 1992. Oncostatin M as a potent mitogen for AIDS-Kaposi's sarcoma-derived cells. Science **255:** 1432–1434.
37. BARTON, B. E., J. V. JACKSON, F. LEE & J. WAGNER. 1994. Oncostatin M stimulates proliferation in B9 hybridoma cells: Potential role of oncostatin M in plasmacytoma development. Cytokine **6:** 147–153.
38. GROVE, R. I., C. EBERHARDT, S. ABID, C. MAZZUCCO, J. LIU, P. KIENER, G. TODARO & M. SHOYAB. 1993. Oncostatin M is a mitogen for rabbit vascular smooth muscle cells. Proc. Natl. Acad. Sci. USA **90:** 823–827.
39. GROVE, R. I., C. E. MAZZUCCO, S. F. RADKA, M. SHOYAB & P. A. KIENER. 1991. Oncostatin M up-regulates low density lipoprotein receptors in HepG2 Cells by a novel mechanism. J. Biol. Chem. **27:** 18194–18199.
40. BROWN, T. J., J. M. ROWE, M. SHOYAB & P. GLADSTONE. 1990. Oncostatin M: A novel regulator of endothelial cell properties. *In* Molecular Biology of Cardiovascular System. UCLA Symposium on Molecular and Cellular Biology (new series). R. R. Schneider, Ed. 195–206. New York: Wiley-Liss.
41. HAMILTON, J. A., T. LEIZER, D. S. PICCOLI, K. M. ROYSTON, D. M. BUTLER & M. CROATTO. 1991. Oncostatin M stimulates urokinase-type plasminogen activator activity in human synovial fibroblasts. Biochem. Biophys. Res. Commun. **180:** 652–659.
42. BROWN, T. J., J. LIU, C. BRASHEM-STEIN & M. SHOYAB. 1993. Regulation of granulocyte colony-stimulating factor and granulocyte-macrophage colony-stimulating factor expression by Oncostatin M. Blood **82:** 33–37.
43. BROWN, T. J., J. M. ROWE, J. LIU & M. SHOYAB. 1991. Regulation of IL-6 expression by oncostatin M. J. Immunol. **147:** 2175–2180.
44. RICHARDS, C. D., T. J. BROWN, M. SHOYAB, H. BAUMANN & J. GAULDIE. 1992. Recombinant oncostatin M stimulates the production of acute phase proteins in HepG2 cells and rat primary hepatocytes in vitro. J. Immunol. **148:** 1731–1736.
45. RICHARDS, C. D. & M. SHOYAB. 1993. The role of Oncostatin M in the acute phase response. *In* Acute Phase Proteins: Molecular Biology, Biochemistry and Clinical Applications. A. Mackiewicz, I. Kushner & H. Baumann, Eds. :321–327. CRC Press, Inc.
46. ROSE, T. M., D. M. WELFORD, N. L. GUNDERSON & A. G. BRUCE. 1994. Oncostatin M (OSM) inhibits the differentiation of pluripotent embryonic cells in vitro. Cytokine **6:** 48–54.
47. RICHARDS, C. D., M. SHOYAB, T. J. BROWN & J. GAULDIE. 1993. Selective regulation of metalloproteinase inhibitor (TIMP-1) by oncostatin M in fibroblasts in culture. J. Immunol. **150:** 5596–5603.
48. RICHARDS, C. D. & A. AGRO. 1994. Interaction between oncostatin M, interleukin 1 and prostaglandin E2 in induction of IL-6 expression in human fibroblasts. Cytokine **6:** 40–47.
49. MALIK, N., D. GRAVES, M. SHOYAB & A. F. PURCHIO. 1992. Amplification and expression of heterologous oncostatin M in Chinese hamster ovary cells. DNA Cell Biol. **11:** 453–459.
50. GROVE, R. I., C. MAZZUCCO, N. ALLEGRETTO, P. A. KIENER, G. SPITALNY, S. F. RADKA, M. SHOYAB, M. ANTONACCIO & G. A. WARR. 1991. Macrophage-derived factors increase low density lipoprotein uptake and receptor number in cultured human liver cells. J. Lipid Res. **32:** 1889–1897.
51. HILTON, D. J., N. A. NICOLA & D. METCALF. 1991. Distribution and comparison of receptors for leukemia inhibitory factor on murine hemopoietic and hepatic cells. J. Cell. Physiol. **146:** 207–215.
52. CASTELL, J. V., T. GEIGER, V. GROSS, T. ANDUS, E. WALTER, T. HIRANO, T. KISHIMOTO & P. C. HEINRICH. 1988. Plasma clearance, organ distribution and target cells of interleukin-6/hepatocyte-stimulating factor in the rat. Eur. J. Biochem. **177:** 357–361.
53. HILTON, D. J., N. A. NICOLA, P. M. WARING & D. METCALF. 1991. Clearance and fate of leukemia-inhibitory factor (LIF) after injection into mice. J. Cell. Physiol. **148:** 430–439.
54. DITTRICH, F., H. THOENEN & M. SENDTNER. 1994. Ciliary neurotrophic factor: Pharmacokinetics and acute-phase response in rat. Ann. Neurol. **35:** 151–163.

55. WALLACE, P. M., J. F. MACMASTER, J. R. RILLEMA, S. A. BURSTEIN & M. SHOYAB. 1994. Thrombocytopoietic properties of Oncostatin M. In press.
56. BURSTEIN, S. A., T. DOWNS, P. FRIESE, S. LYNAM, S. ANDERSON, J. HENTHORN, R. B. EPSTEIN & K. SAVAGE. 1992. Thrombocytopoiesis in normal and sublethally irradiated dogs: Response to human interleukin-6. Blood **80:** 420–428.
57. SELIG, C., L. KREJA, H. MULLER, E. SEIFRIED & W. NOTHDURFT. 1994. Hematologic effects of recombinant human interleukin-6 in dogs exposed to a total-body radiation dose of 2.4 Gy. Exp. Hematol. **22:** 551–558.
58. WEBER, J., H. GUNN, J. YANG, D. PARKINSON, S. TOPALIAN, D. SCHWARTZENTRUBER, S. ETTINGHAUSEN, D. LEVITT & S. A. ROSENBERG. 1994. A phase I trial of intravenous interleukin-6 in patients with advanced cancer. J. Immunother. **15:** 292–302.
59. GORDON, M. S., L. BATTIATO, R. HOFFMAN, E. BREEDEN, W. J. MCCASKILL-STEVENS, B. KUCA, J. KAYE & G. W. SLEDGE, JR. 1993. Subcutaneously (SC) administered recombinant human interleukin-11 (Neumega™ rhIL-11 growth factor; rhIL-11) prevents thrombocytopenia following chemotherapy (CT) with cyclophosphamide (C) and doxorubicin (A) in women with breast cancer (BC). Blood **82:** 1255 (Abstract).
60. GORDON, M. S., G. W. SLEDGE JR., L. BATTIATO, E. BREEDEN, R. COOPER, W. J. MCCASKILL-STEVENS, B. KUCA, J. KAYE & R. HOFFMAN. 1993. The in vivo effects of subcutaneously (SC) administered recombinant human interleukin-11 (Neumega™ rhIL-11 growth factor; rhIL-11) in women with breast cancer (BC). Blood **82:** 1977 (Abstract).
61. BAUMANN, H. & J. GAULDIE. 1994. The acute phase response. Immunol. Today **15:** 74–80.
62. HEINRICH, P. C., J. V. CASTELL & T. ANDUS. 1990. Interleukin-6 and the acute phase protein. Biochem. J. **265:** 621–636.
63. GEIGER, T., T. ANDUS, J. KLAPPROTH, T. HIRANO, T. KISHIMOTO & P. C. HEINRICH. 1988. Induction of rat acute-phase proteins by interleukin 6 *in vivo*. Eur. J. Immunol. **18:** 717–721.
64. KOPF, M., H. BAUMANN, G. FREER, M. FREUDENBERG, M. LAMERS, T. KISHIMOTO, R. ZINKERNAGEL, H. BLUETHMANN & G. KOHLER. 1994. Impaired immune and acute-phase responses in interleukin-6-deficient mice. Nature **368:** 339–342.
65. ALVAREZ, O. A., D. F. CARMICHAEL & Y. A. DECLERCK. 1990. Inhibition of collagenolytic activity and metastasis of tumor cells by a recombinant human tissue inhibitor of metalloproteinases. J. Natl. Cancer Inst. **82:** 589–595.
66. BROWN, T. J., M. N. LIOUBIN & H. MARQUARDT. 1987. Purification and characterization of cytostatic lymphokines produced by activated human T lymphokines. J. Immunol. **139:** 2977–2983.
67. GORDON, M. S. & R. HOFFMAN. 1992. Growth factors affecting human thrombocytopoiesis: Potential agents for treatment of thrombocytopenia. Blood **80:** 302–307.
68. ESCARY, J. L., J. PERREAU, D. DUMENIL, S. EZINE & P. BRULET. 1993. Leukaemia inhibitory factor is necessary for maintenance of haematopoietic stem cells and thymocyte stimulation. Nature **363:** 361–364.
69. STEWART, C. L., P. KASPAR, L. J. BRUNET, H. BHATT, I. GADI, F. KONTGEN & S. J. ABBONDANZO. 1992. Blastocyst implantation depends on maternal expression of leukaemia inhibitory factor. Nature **359:** 76–79.
70. MASU, Y., E. WOLF, B. HOTLMANN, M. SENDTNER, G. BREM & H. THOENEN. 1993. Distruption of the CNTF gene results in motor neuron degeneration. Nature **365:** 27–32.
71. STEEL, D. M. & A. S. WHITEHEAD. 1994. The major acute phase reactants: C-reactive protein, serum amyloid P component and serum amyloid A protein. Immunol. Today **15:** 81–88.
72. RUTTLEDGE, M. H., Y. G. XIE, F. Y. HAN, M. PEYRARD, V. P. COLLINS, M. NORDENSKJOLD & J. P. DUMANSKI. 1994. Deletions on chromosome 22 in sporadic meningioma. Genes Chromosom. Cancer **10:** 122–130.
73. PERGOLIZZI, R. G. & E. H. ERSTER. 1994. Analysis of chromosome-22 loci in meningioma—Alterations in the leukemia inhibitory factor (LIF) locus. Mol. Chem. Neuropathol. **21:** 189–217.

74. ISHIBASHI, T., H. KIMURA, T. UCHIDA, S. KARIYONES, P. FRIESE & S. A. BURSTEIN. 1989. Human interleukin 6 is a direct promoter of maturation of megakaryocytes in vitro. Proc. Natl. Acad. Sci. USA **86:** 5953–5957.

DISCUSSION OF THE PAPER

C. RICHARDS (*McMaster University, Hamilton, Ont., Canada*): Is there a specific oncoM receptor in the mouse as well as human cells?

P. WALLACE: To my knowledge, there is no characterized receptor. There are a couple of biological activities that have not been reproduced to my knowledge by LIF, which would imply that there is something specific.

A. KOJ (*Jagiellonian University, Krakow, Poland*): You have mentioned that oncostatin inhibits cholesterol synthesis. Do you have any clue how it works? How this effect is exerted?

WALLACE: I certainly know that the pathway is somewhat unusual. OM stimulation of LDL uptake and increased receptor expression occurs in a cholesterol-independent manner. Some of the details of the signal transduction pathway have been described, but not in as much detail as for other effects.

M. REVEL (*Weizmann Institute, Rehovot, Israel*): The effect on the red blood cells is very impressive, and in relation to IL-6 when you can see the depression of red blood cells, but in that case it has been shown that there is a reticulosis. So there is an increase in formation of new red blood cells with IL-6. Have you studied the reticulosis after OM treatment?

WALLACE: Yes. If you look histologically you clearly see this effect on erythroid lineages. We have not characterized it in the sense of the type of red blood cells looking for early progenitors. We have done histology, and you can see the erythroid lineages are affected. I should point out that even though there is no net effect on red blood cells there is a significant increase in plasma volume related to the induction of acute-phase response, and that if the level still remains normal, one would infer that there is an increase in red blood cells.

Signal Transduction through IL-6 Receptor: Involvement of Multiple Protein Kinases, Stat Factors, and a Novel H7-sensitive Pathway[a]

KOICHI NAKAJIMA, TADASHI MATSUDA, YOSHIO FUJITANI,
HIROTADA KOJIMA, YOJIRO YAMANAKA, KAZUTO NAKAE,
TAKASHI TAKEDA, AND TOSHIO HIRANO[b]

Division of Molecular Oncology
Biomedical Research Center
Osaka University Medical School
2-2 Yamadaoka
Suita, Osaka, 565, Japan

INTRODUCTION

IL-6 is a cytokine regulating the immune response, hematopoiesis and inflammation. IL-6 exhibits its multiple effects in a variety of cells[1-4] through the IL-6 receptor (IL-6R). IL-6R consists of an IL-6 specific receptor subunit (IL-6Rα)[5] and a signal-transducer gp130 (β-chain).[6] Both of them belong to the cytokine receptor superfamily[7] and the latter is shared by the receptor systems for ciliary neurotrophic factor (CNTF), leukemia inhibitory factor (LIF), oncostatin M (OSM) and IL-11 as a signal-transducing receptor subunit.[8-11] Although the cytoplasmic region of neither IL-6Rα nor gp130 has an intrinsic tyrosine kinase domain, IL-6 induces activation of tyrosine kinase(s) and tyrosine phosphorylation of various cellular proteins including gp130 itself.[11-16]

We identified an IL-6 response element in the *junB* gene promoter and showed that the element, termed JRE-IL6, contains at least two DNA motifs, an Ets binding site (JEBS) and a CRE-like site both of which are required for IL-6–induced expression of the *junB* gene.[17] We further demonstrated that the IL-6 signal transduction pathway to the JRE-IL6 is a Ras-independent one involving a novel H7-sensitive pathway distinct from ones using protein kinase C, cyclic AMP dependent kinase or Ca^{2+}/calmodulin-dependent kinases.[17] The IL-6 signal transduction pathway is similar to those activated by interferon (IFN) in that IFN activates a variety of IFN inducible genes through directly phosphorylating the tyrosine residues of the signal transducer and activator of transcription (Stat) family proteins including Stat2 (p113), Stat1α (p91) and Stat2β (p84) without using second messengers or Ras-mediated

---

[a] This work was supported in part by Grants-in-Aid for Scientific Research from the Ministry of Education Science and Culture in Japan, grants from the Ministry of Welfare and Health in Japan, Senri Life Science Foundation, the Yamanouchi Foundation for Research on Metabolic Disorders, Osaka Foundation for Promotion of Clinical Immunology and the Ryoichi Naito Foundation for Medical Research.

[b] Address correspondence to Dr. Toshio Hirano; 2-2 Yamadaoka, Tel: 81-6-879-3880; Fax 81-6-879-3889.

pathways.[18–20] Much evidence showed that this type of pathway involves a family of protein tyrosine kinase(s), Jak1, Jak2 and Tyk2[21–24] and is activated by cytokines and growth factors in addition to IFNs, such as IL-3, growth hormone, erythropoietin, IL-6, CNTF, and EGF.[24–29] The activated Stat factors translocate to the nucleus, form complexes and bind to the sequence of IFN-stimulated response element (ISRE), IFN-γ–activated site (GAS) or related sites, depending on which factors are activated.[18,20] Indeed another IL-6 response elements (RE), called type II IL-6 RE or acute phase RE (APRE) present in the IL-6-inducible gene promoters such as $α_2$ macroglobulin, haptoglobin, β-fibrinogen and $α_1$-acidglycoprotein,[30–33] bear DNA-sequence similarity with those of high affinity site of SIE (c-*sis* inducible element) of c-*fos*[34–36] and GASs of Ly6E[37] or FcγR,[38] to which Stat1α and Stat1-related proteins can bind. Very recently it was shown that phosphorylated APRE binding factor (APRF) was antigenically and functionally related to Stat1.[39] Furthermore, APRE binding proteins, APRFs, were recently characterized and purified to homogeneity from IL-6-stimulated rat liver,[40] or from mouse liver, and its cDNA was cloned.[41] The cloned APRF cDNA revealed that one of APRFs was identical with Stat3, which was independently cloned by Zhong *et al.*[42]

Here we describe that the common IL-6 signaling pathway activates the two IL-6 REs, JRE-IL6 and type II IL-6 RE (APRE), through the multiple IL-6–inducible Stat3 and Stat3-related proteins. We suggested that an H7-sensitive pathway, presumably a serine/threonine kinase, is required for the Stat-related proteins to be transcriptionally active. Furthermore, in addition to the IL-6–induced activation of Jak1 and Jak2 tyrosine kinases that were constitutively associated with gp130, we showed that gp130-stimulation activated a novel 72 kD Stat-associated tyrosine kinase (p72^{sak}). The results showed that the IL-6–induced signal transduction pathway includes the activation of multiple tyrosine kinases, Stat factors and a novel H7-sensitive pathway.

RAS-INDEPENDENT SIGNALING PATHWAY LEADING TO THE ACTIVATION OF AN IMMEDIATE EARLY GENE, *junB* THROUGH gp130: INVOLVEMENT OF A NOVEL H7-SENSITIVE PATHWAY

The induction of the *junB* gene by IL-6 was observed in a wide range of cells, including a murine hybridoma cell line, human myeloma cell lines, a murine hematopoietic cell line and hepatoma cell lines and myeloleukemic cell lines.[13,43] We showed that the IL-6 responsive element of the *junB* gene (JRE-IL6) contains a putative ETS binding site (JEBS) and a CRE-like site and both sites were required for IL-6–induced activation of the JRE-IL6 (FIG. 1).[17] Both IL-6 and forskolin (FK), activator for PKA activated the JRE-IL6, although neither TPA nor Ca ionophore A23187 did. The IL-6–induced activation of JRE-IL6 was inhibited by H7 but not W7. H7 sensitive pathway does not include PKC, because TPA did not activate the JRE-IL6 and the depletion of PKC activity had no effect on the IL-6-induced activation of the JRE-IL6. In contrast to the IL-6 signal that required both the JEBS and the CRE-like site as target sites, FK required only the CRE-like site for its action. Furthermore, the expression of a dominant negative CREB severely impaired FK-induced JRE-IL6 activation, but had no effect on IL-6–induced activation of the JRE-IL6, indicating that IL-6 signal is distinct from PKA signal. None of the exogenous expression of activated Ha-Ras, activated c-Raf-1 or NF-IL6 (C/EBPβ/IL-6DBP/LAP) had significant effects on the JRE-IL6, nor altered the IL-6 signals activating the JRE-IL6. Furthermore, expression of the dominant-negative form of Raf-1 did not inhibit the IL-6–induced activation of the JRE-IL6. On the basis of these results, we con-

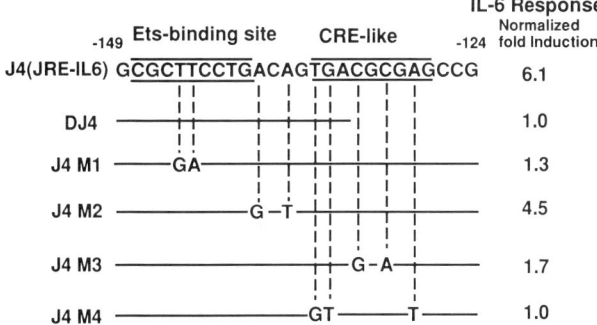

FIGURE 1. The IL-6 responsive element of the *junB* gene (JRE-IL6) consists of an Ets binding site (JEBS) and a CRE-like site. (The data were taken from Nakajima et al.[17])

cluded that IL-6–induced signal transduction pathway activating the JRE-IL6 is a novel H7-sensitive pathway distinct from those utilizing PKC, PKA, Ca^{2+}/CM-dependent kinases, Ras, c-Raf, or NF-IL6.[17]

JEBS-BINDING FACTORS DISTINCT FROM Ets-FAMILY PROTEINS MAY BE MEDIATOR(S) OF IL-6 SIGNAL TRANSDUCTION

Although we showed that JEBS in the *junB* gene promoter perfectly matched with a consensus binding site for Ets1/2 and there is a constitutive factor(s) weakly binding

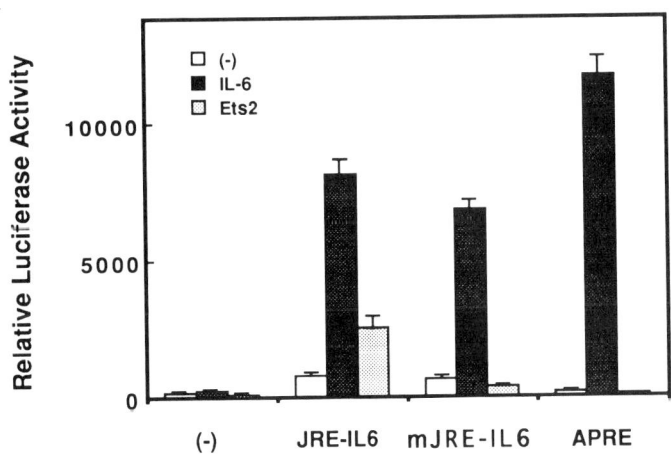

FIGURE 2. Involvement of factors other than the Ets family proteins in the IL-6 signal transduction pathways. Luciferase reporter plasmids containing the minimal *junB* promoter driven by either three repeats of JRE-IL6, three repeats of mutated JRE-IL6(mJRE-IL6), or four repeats of type II IL-6 RE(APRE) and pEFLacZ were transfected into HepG2 cells. Cells were stimulated with 100 ng/ml IL-6 for 5 h.

to the JEBS in the HepG2 nuclear extracts,[17] it is not known whether an Ets family protein is really a mediator of IL-6 signals to the IL-6 response element. To determine the role of the JEBS and to get further insight into the nature of the JEBS binding protein(s) involved in the IL-6 signals, we first compared the responsiveness to IL-6 and to exogenously expressed Ets2 of the wild type and those of the mutant JRE-IL6 having a disrupted core motif of JEBS (from GGAA to GTAA). In agreement with the crucial role of the GGA motif for the binding of Ets family proteins, exogenous Ets2 activated JRE-IL6–driven reporter gene expression but not the expression of the reporter gene driven by the mutated JRE-IL6. However, the responsiveness of the mutated JRE-IL6 to IL-6 was comparable to that of the wild type JRE-IL6 (FIG. 2). IL-6 but not Ets2 efficiently activated another IL-6 response element (type II IL-6 RE also called APRE) containing a GGAA motif, found in the promoters of some acute phase reactant genes (FIG. 2). The results suggest that an unidentified factor(s) with different specificity other than those of the Ets family proteins may be a mediator(s) of IL-6 signals to the two IL-6 response elements.

IL-6–INDUCED DNA BINDING FACTORS INCLUDE STAT FAMILY PROTEINS(S) THAT RECOGNIZE BOTH JRE-IL6 AND APRE OF α_2 MACROGLOBULIN

To identify the JEBS-binding factor(s), we did electromobility shift assay (EMSA) using a synthetic oligonucleotide containing only a JEBS and IL-6–stimulated HepG2 nuclear extracts. We also tested the oligonucleotides containing an APRE of rat α_2 macroglobulin.[31] IL-6 stimulation of HepG2 resulted in the rapid appearance of DNA binding factors which bound to both JEBS and APRE with similar mobility.[44] Moreover these IL-6–inducible DNA binding proteins for both sites appeared within minutes both in the cytoplasm and in the nucleus. Although these two IL-6 response elements have only minimal similarity outside the GGAA region, the results of kinetic pattern and cellular localization suggested that the same or very similar proteins might act on the both sites. These binding sites, in particular APRE of α_2 macroglobulin, are similar to the binding sites for transcription factor Stat1 or other related proteins, including GAS of Ly6E,[37] and high affinity site c-*fos* SIE.[35] As shown in FIGURE 3A, the IFNα/β-induced DNA binding proteins indeed bound to the α_2 macroglobulin APRE with mobilities similar to those of IL-6–inducible proteins (indicated as A and B). The IFN-γ–induced factor (IFN-γ–activated factor, GAF), containing Stat1α, made a complex with this site (indicated as B and shown in FIG. 3C). The binding specificity of IL-6–induced JEBS and APRE binding proteins were tested in EMSAs using excess amount of unlabeled competitor oligonucleotides containing either human α_2 macroglobulin APRE, rat α_2 macroglobulin APRE, JEBS, mutated JEBS(JEBSM), Ly6E GAS, or GBP GAS. Only results of EMSA using ^{32}P-labeled APRE oligonucleotides as probes were shown in FIGURE 3B, because essentially the same results were obtained with labeled JEBS oligonucleotides being used as probes. All of the tested sites except for mutated JEBS and GBP GAS competed for binding of IL-6 RE binding complexes with different efficiencies (FIG. 3B). APRE from human α_2 macroglobulin had the highest affinity, while Ly6E GAS and JEBS had lower affinity for the IL-6–inducible complexes. It is noted that GBP GAS site has very low affinity for the IL-6 RE binding proteins, suggesting that this site has different binding specificity in spite of being a binding site for Stat1. Thus these IL-6–induced IL-6 RE binding proteins appear to have similar but slightly different binding specificity to those of Stat1-related proteins activated by multiple cytokines.[45]

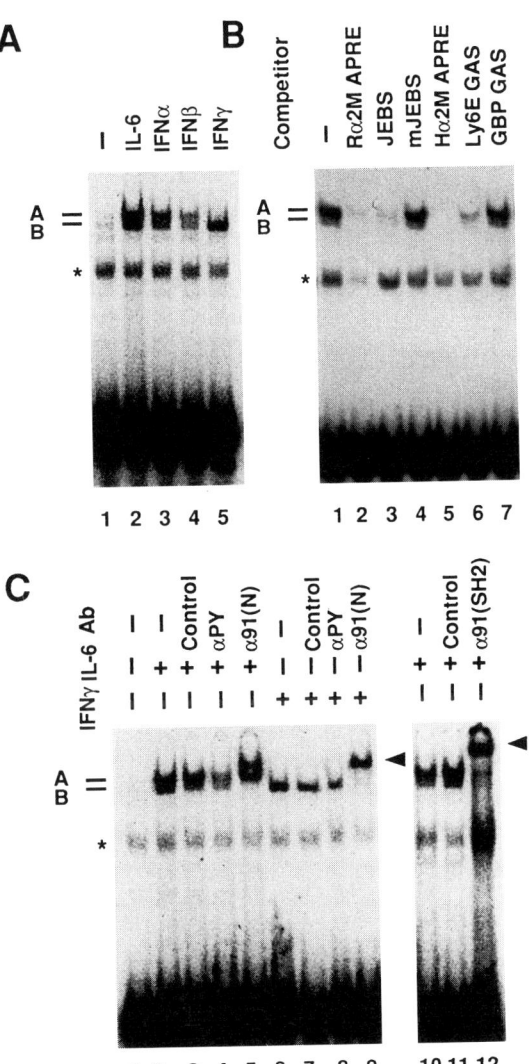

FIGURE 3. IL-6 binding complexes may contain Stat1 and related proteins. **A:** Nuclear extracts from HepG2 cells treated with either 100 ng/ml IL-6, 1000 μ/ml IFN-α, 1000 μ/ml IFN-β, or 100 ng/ml IFN-γ for 15 min were used in an EMSA with the rat α_2 macroglobulin IL-6 RE(APRE) oligonucleotide. Specific complexes are indicated as A and B. A non-specific complex is indicated by an asterisk. **B:** The indicated oligonucleotides corresponding to IL-6 REs (rat α_2 macroglobulin APRE, JEBS, and human α_2 macroglobulin APRE), GAS sequences (Ly6E and GBP) and mutated JEBS (mJEBS, CAGGAAG to CAGGCCG) were added in a 50-fold molar excess. **C:** IL-6 RE binding proteins were characterized by using mAb to phosphotyrosine (lanes 4 and 8, 4G10 mAb), anti-p91(N) mAb (lanes 5 and 9), rabbit anti-p91(SH2) (lane 12). An mAb with irrelevant specificity (lane 3 and 7) or preimmune sera (lane 11) was used as control. (The data of FIG. 3b were taken from Fujitani et al.[44])

To test whether JEBS and APE binding complexes contain Stat1-related proteins, we used two different anti-p91 Ab in EMSAs. Polyclonal anti-p91 Ab against an SH2 domain of stat1α [anti-p91(SH2)(46)] recognized and supershifted the JEBS binding complex(es) (data not shown) and both A and B of APRE-binding complexes (FIG. 3C lane 12), whereas anti-p91 mAb against a N-terminal region of stat91 [anti-p91(N)] recognized and supershifted only complex B of APRE-binding complexes and IFN-γ–activated complex (FIG. 3C lanes 5 and 9). These results imply that JEBS binding protein(s) and APRE binding complexes are very similar or the same and these IL-6–inducible DNA binding complexes contain Stat1-related proteins.

MOLECULAR CLONING OF A cDNA ENCODING A NEW STAT FAMILY PROTEIN, STAT3/APRF, FROM IL-6 RESPONSIVE CELL LINE

Next, we took two approaches to identify in the IL-6 RE binding proteins. First we tried to purify DNA binding proteins using DNA-affinity columns containing concatamerized APRE oligonucleotides. The second was a direct cloning of a cDNA clone encoding a new member of the Stat family protein using the PCR method. For the second approach, we made a partial cDNA library with the RT-PCR method using polyA+ RNA from HepG2 cells and a pair of degenerative primers covering the two conserved stretches of aminoacids between stat1α and stat2. After excluding clones encoding a part of stat1α or stat2 from cDNA clones using other primer sets specific to either stat1α or stat2, we found a clone encoding a part of new stat family protein. We screened a human placenta cDNA library with thus obtained partial cDNA, and obtained a clone containing a 2.2 kb cDNA insert. The clone showed sequence similarities with Stat1α throughout the entire region of the coding sequences. We also found that the clone had a missing portion of about 250 aminoacids at the N-terminus when compared with Stat1α. To test whether the clone really encodes one of the IL-6–inducible Stat family proteins, we raised a rabbit antiserum against a peptide (CIDKDSG DVAALRGS) corresponding to a central region of the human Stat clone. The antiserum reacted with 92 kD tyrosine phosphorylated protein in IL-6–stimulated HepG2 cells and with multiple proteins with a molecular weight range of 85 to 92 kD in IL-6-stimulated rat liver nuclear extracts. The major one was 89 kD molecule.[44] During performing these experiments, we learned that the cDNA clone was identical with Stat3/APRF.[41,42] Therefore, the results with the use of the antiserum, that is, anti-Stat3/APRF, suggested that multiple Stat3-related proteins were tyrosine-phosphorylated in response to IL-6. This notion was further verified by using purified APRE binding proteins as reported in the following section.

PURIFIED APRFs REACTIVE WITH ANTI-STAT3 CAN BIND TO THE JEBS OF JRE-IL-6

To characterize and attempt to identify the molecules assembling the IL-6–induced DNA binding protein complexes, we proceeded to purify the DNA binding proteins. For this purpose, we used rat liver nuclear extracts stimulated with IL-6 by injecting human rIL-6 intraperitoneally. At first we performed anion exchange chromatography using Q Sepharose. The active fractions were pooled, precipitated with 53% ammonium sulfate, and subjected to gel filtration chromatography using Superdex200. As shown in FIGURE 4, A and B, the fractions corresponding to molecular weights of around 200 kD had the highest DNA-binding activity with the same mobility as those of crude nuclear extracts. Considering that Stat1 and its family proteins are around or less than 100 kD in size, the DNA binding complexes seemed to be composed of multiple molecules.

The IL-6–induced DNA binding proteins were purified directly from crude nuclear extracts through three rounds of DNA affinity chromatography using Sepharose 4B-oligonucleotides containing human α_2 macroglobulin APRE. Oligonucleotides containing mutated APRE were also used to remove non-specifically bound proteins and proteins bound to the flanking regions of the APRE. As shown in FIGURE 5,

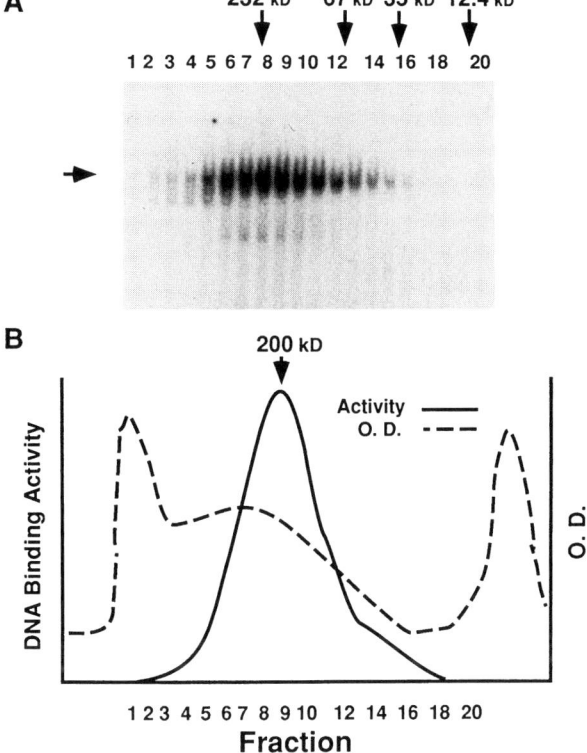

FIGURE 4. Gel filtration chromatography of IL-6 RE binding proteins. Active fractions from anion exchange chromatography column (Q Sepharose, Pharmacia) were precipitated with 53% ammoniumsulphate and applied to a Superdex 200 column. Result of an EMSA is shown in **A**. DNA binding activities were measured by densitometry analysis and the data are plotted with O.D. profile in **B**.

purified IL-6 RE-binding proteins were composed of multiple proteins with sizes 94, 91, 89, and 85. These proteins (indicated by arrows in lane 1, FIG. 5), were phosphorylated on tyrosine residues in agreement with the role of tyrosine phosphorylation in activation of these factors. Among them, 89 kD proteins were most abundant. Both anti-p91(N) mAb and anti-p91(SH2)Ab easily recognized 94 and 91 kD proteins. Since the molecular weight of IFN-γ–activated Stat1α was 94 kD in our hand and anti-Stat3 antiserum reacted with the major 89 kD molecule and minor 91 and 85 kD but not 94 kD molecules, suggesting that the 89 kD molecule is rat Stat3. To further confirm this, we determined partial amino acid sequence of three fragments which were obtained by digesting the purified 89 kD protein with lysylendopeptidase. We totally determined 28 amino acid residues, all of which were identical with those of mouse APRE/Stat3,[41] showing that purified 89 kD protein is rat Stat3. We further showed that purified Stat3 can bind to the JEBS of JRE-IL-6.[44]

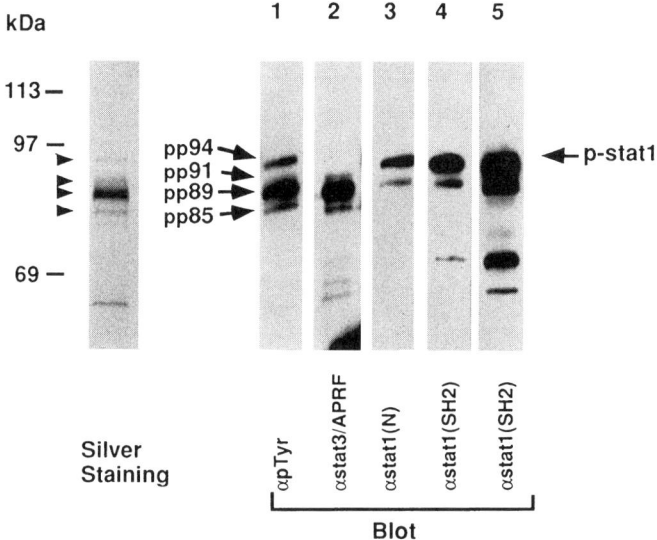

FIGURE 5. Purification of IL-6 RE binding proteins by DNA affinity chromatography. Purified IL-6-induced IL-6 RE binding-proteins were separated by SDS-PAGE and analyzed by silver staining and blotting with various antibodies. Antibodies used are as follows; anti-phosphotyrosine mAb (lane 1), anti-stat3 (lane 2), anti-p91 (N) (lane 3) and rabbit anti-p91(SH2) (lanes 4 and 5). (The data were taken from Fujitani et al.[44])

TYROSINE PHOSPHORYLATION OF STAT3-RELATED PROTEINS ARE ESSENTIAL FOR THE PROTEINS TO MAKE COMPLEXES WITH IL-6 RE

Tyrosine phosphorylation has been shown to be critical for the Stat family proteins to assemble complexes and bind to the corresponding sites.[18–20] We tested whether the IL-6–inducible DNA binding proteins really require tyrosine phosphorylation to make DNA-protein complexes by using anti-phosphotyrosine antibody and tyrosine phosphatase. Anti-phosphotyrosine monoclonal antibody reduced the DNA-protein complexes of A and B (FIG. 3c, lane 4). As shown in FIGURE 6, treatment of crude nuclear extracts from IL-6-stimulated HepG2 cells with tyrosine phosphatase abolished the DNA binding activities of the two complexes (lane 5), while tyrosine phosphatase inhibitor, sodium orthovanadate, prevented the effect of tyrosine phosphatase treatment (lane 4). These results suggest the crucial role of tyrosine phosphorylation in the assembly of DNA protein complexes and are consistent with these proteins being stat family proteins.

COMMON IL-6 SIGNALS ACTIVATING THE TWO IL-6 REs INVOLVE AN UNIDENTIFIED H7-SENSITIVE PATHWAY DISTINCT FROM RAS-, RAF-MEDIATED PATHWAYS

In the previous work,[17] we showed that the IL-6 signal transduction pathway leading to the activation of the JRE-IL6 does not use the RAS- or Raf-mediated

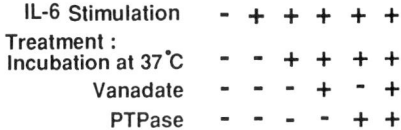

FIGURE 6. Tyrosine phosphorylation is crucial for the assembly of IL-6-induced DNA-binding complexes. Nuclear extracts treated with tyrosine phosphatase (lanes 5 and 6) from yersinia enterocolica in the absence (lane 5) or presence of 1 mM vanadate (lane 6) were used.

pathways but use an H7-sensitive pathway(s) distinct from protein kinase C or cyclic AMP-dependent kinase. We have investigated whether the same pathway is working on the APRE by using a variety of expression vectors, including activated Ras, activated Raf-1, and dominant negative form of Raf-1, and various activators such as TPA and Forskolin, as we did previously.[17] We did not see any difference in the characteristics of signals activating the both IL-6 REs (data not shown).

In agreement with the crucial role of tyrosine phosphorylation in the activation of Stat1-related proteins by IL-6, staurosporine, known as a potent inhibitor for both tyrosine kinases and serine/threonine kinases, efficiently inhibited the IL-6-induced transcriptional activation of both the JRE-IL6-driven and APRE-driven reporter genes (FIG. 7A). Moreover serine/threonine kinase inhibitor H7 with a broad specificity[47] inhibited the IL-6-induced activation of the two IL-6 RE-driven promoters (FIG. 7B). H9,[48] a derivative of H7 had similar inhibitory effect, though higher concentrations were needed than with H7 (FIG. 7B). The inhibitory effect of H7 or H9 was specific and seemed to take place at the transcriptional level, because neither inhibitor at doses used in this study, even when used for longer periods up to 12h, changed the basal activity of the *junB* promoter. To get insight into the mechanisms of inhibitions, we did EMSAs using HepG2 nuclear extracts stimulated with IL-6 in the presence of inhibitors. As shown in FIGURE 7C, staurosporine inhibited the IL-6-induced DNA binding activities by 50% at 100 nM or by around 85% at 500 nM (FIG. 7C, lanes 3 and 4), while H7 even at 100 μM did not inhibit the activities (FIG. 7C lane 5). Neither H7 nor H9 at 100 μM inhibited the IL-6-induced tyrosine phosphorylation of cellular proteins in agreement with no inhibitory effect of H7 on the IL-6-induced DNA binding proteins. Therefore these results suggested that H7

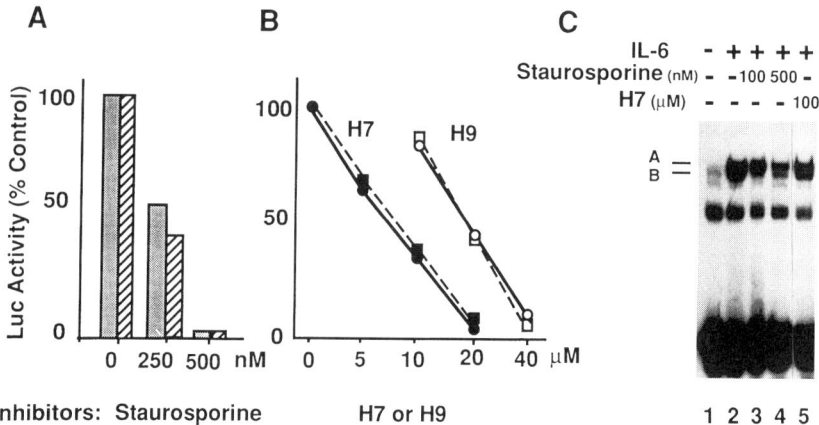

FIGURE 7. The effect of protein kinase inhibitors, staurosporine, H7, or H9 on IL-6–induced transcription and on IL-6–induced DNA binding activity. A and B: HepG2 cells were transfected with the minimal *junB* promoter-luciferase reporter gene construct containing either JRE-IL6 or type II IL-6 RE(α_2 macroglobulin APRE) and pEFLacZ, cultured for 40 h, and treated with staurosporine, H7 or H9 at the indicated concentration. After 15 min, the transfected HepG2 cells were stimulated with 100 ng/ml IL-6 for 5 h, and luciferase and β-galactosidase activities were measured. C: Nuclear extracts from HepG2 pretreated with staurosporine or H7 at indicated concentrations for 15 min and stimulated with IL-6 for 15 min were assayed for IL-6 RE DNA binding activity in an EMSA.

and H9 inhibited the IL-6–induced transcriptional activation of the reporter genes without affecting the IL-6 induction of the DNA binding proteins.

INVOLVEMENT OF MULTIPLE TYROSINE KINASES IN IL-6 RECEPTOR–MEDIATED SIGNALS

Recent studies have shown that IL-6 activates Jak kinase that may be constitutively associated with gp130 in hepatocytes and COS cells transfected with the expression vectors encoding gp130 and Jak kinase.[28,39] We asked the question whether IL-6 signals induce tyrosine phosphorylation of Jak1 and Jak2 tyrosine kinases in a variety of cell lines. As shown in FIGURE 8, IL-6 signals induced tyrosine phosphorylation of Jak1 in a myeloma cell line, U266, while Jak2 in HepG2, a murine hybridoma cell line, MH60 and a murine myeloleukemic cell line, Y6. On the other hand, the stimulation of gp130 with IL-6 plus soluble IL-6Rα in the transfectant of pro-B cell line, BAF-B03 which expresses murine gp130 (BAFm130) resulted in the tyrosine-phosphorylation of both Jak1 and Jak2 (FIG. 8) as previously reported.[15] The results showed that the species of Jak kinase activated by IL-6 was different among various cells. This may be one of the mechanisms by which IL-6 exerts a variety of activities in various kind of cells, although how IL-6 activates different Jak family kinases through the same receptor remains to be elucidated. Next, we examined the direct interaction between gp130 and Jak kinases. After lysis of BAFm130 cells in a mild detergent, the immunoprecipitate with anti-murine gp130 monoclonal antibody, HMβ1, was found to contain both Jak1 and Jak2 proteins (FIG. 9), indicating that

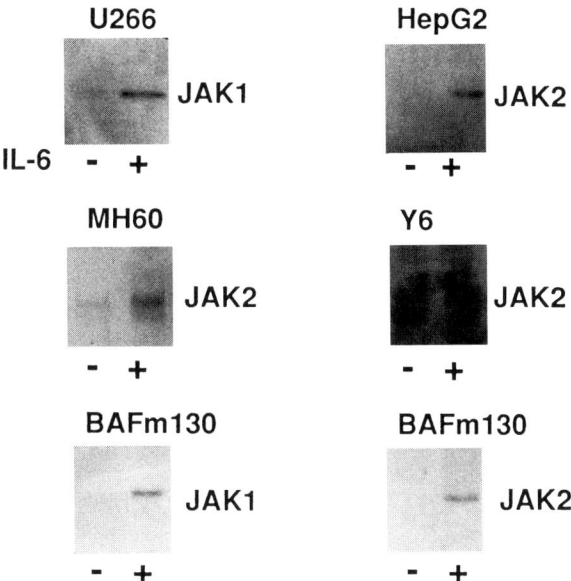

FIGURE 8. IL-6-induced tyrosine-phosphorylation of Jak1 and Jak2 in a variety of cell lines.

Jak kinase is associated with gp130.[15] Furthermore, the association of Jak protein with gp130 was observed even in non-stimulated BAFm130 cells, showing that Jak kinase is constitutively associated with gp130. This was in agreement with the previous report by Lütticken et al.[39] who showed the constitutive association of Jak and gp130 in hepatocytes or that reported by Stahl et al.[28] in COS cells.

To further delineate necessary molecules for the activation of Stat proteins, we investigated the molecules that associate with Stat proteins. We found that the immu-

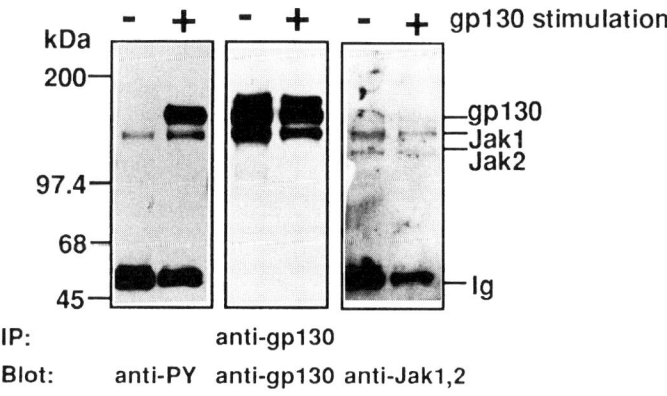

FIGURE 9. Constitutive association of Jak1 and Jak2 with gp130.

noprecipitate with anti-Stat antiserum of the cell lysates obtained from BAFm130 cells stimulated with IL-6 and soluble IL-6Rα included tyrosine-phosphorylated molecules with molecular weights of 150, 90 and 72 kD.[16] The results showed that the stimulation with IL-6 and soluble IL-6Rα induced tyrosine phosphorylation of Stat family proteins, Stat-associated 150 and 72 kD molecules. Furthermore, we showed that *in vitro* kinase activity in the fraction corresponding to the molecular weight of 72 kD was augmented by the stimulation with IL-6 and soluble IL-6Rα and completely inhibited by staurosporine but not H7. Phospho amino acid analysis of the phosphorylated 72 kD molecule revealed that a tyrosine residue was mainly phosphorylated. All results suggested that the 72 kD molecule is a protein tyrosine kinase that associates with Stat proteins and is able to be activated by gp130 stimulation.[16] We termed the 72 kD molecule Stat-associated 72 kD tyrosine kinase (p72^{sak}) and showed that p72^{sak} is distinct from Btk, Tec or Syk. Since IL-6 together with soluble IL-6Rα generates signalings through gp130 in BAFm130 cells and gp130 is shared among the receptors for the IL-6-related cytokine subfamily, such as leukemia inhibitory factor, oncostatin M, IL-11 and ciliary neurotrophic factor,[11] p72^{sak} is probably involved in the signal transduction pathway for these IL-6-related cytokines. Much evidence has shown that Jak family tyrosine kinase is essential for the activation of Stat family proteins in IFN-mediated signal transduction. Jak tyrosine kinase may directly activate Stat proteins,[49,50] although this possibility still remains to be examine. p72^{sak} may directly activate Stat proteins or modulate the function of Stat proteins activated by Jak tyrosine kinase. Alternatively, p72^{sak} may activate other signal transduction molecules distinct from Stat proteins. In this case, Stat proteins act as a signal transducing transcriptional factor on the one hand and as an adaptor protein like Grb2 and Shc on the other hand. In any case, our results provide the new aspect for the delineation of the Stat-mediated signal transduction pathway through cytokine receptors.

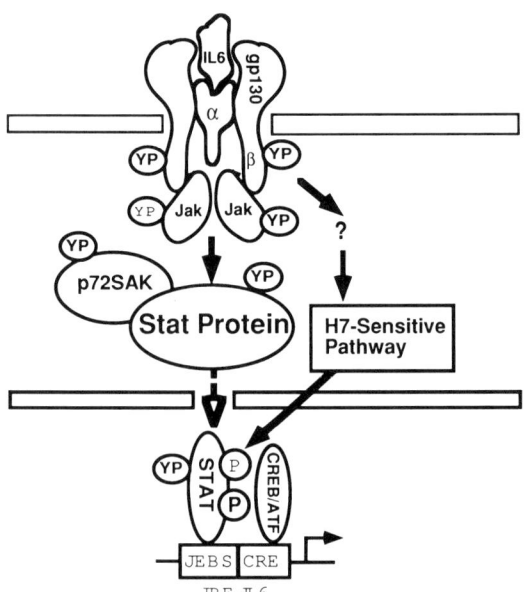

FIGURE 10. Involvement of multiple tyrosine kinases and H7-sensitive pathway in Stat-mediated signal transduction through IL-6 receptor.

CONCLUSION

We showed that i) IL-6 rapidly induced DNA binding activities acting on the two IL-6 REs, JRE-IL6 and Type II IL-6 RE (APRE), ii) IL-6 induced DNA binding proteins contained multiple tyrosine-phosphorylated proteins with major molecules of 89 kD that were considered to be Stat3 or Stat3-related molecules, iii) the common Ras-independent IL-6 signals activate the transcriptional activity of the both IL-6 REs through activating stat family proteins. Moreover we showed that PTK activity was crucial for inducing the assembly of DNA-protein complexes, while another H7 and H9-sensitive process is required for the Stat family proteins bound to the DNA to be transcriptionally active, and iv) Jak1, Jak2 and Sak (p72^{sak}) tyrosine kinases were activated by IL-6 stimulation and both Jak1 and Jak2 are constitutively associated with gp130. The schematic model of IL-6 receptor-mediated signal transduction pathway is illustrated in FIG. 10.

ACKNOWLEDGMENTS

We thank Drs. T. Sudo and M. Naruto for their kind help for the determination of the partial amino acid sequences. We thank Dr. X.-Y. Fu and J. N. Ihle for their generous gifts of rabbit anti-p91(SH2) and anti-Jak sera, respectively. We thank Ms. R. Masuda and M. Tsuda for their excellent secretarial assistance.

REFERENCES

1. SEHGAL, P. B., G. GRIENGER & G. TOSATO, Eds. 1989. Regulation of the acute phase and immune responses: Interleukin-6. Ann. N.Y. Acad. Sci. **557**: 1.
2. VAN SNICK, J. 1990. Interleukin-6: An overview. Annu. Rev. Immunol. **8**: 253.
3. HIRANO, T. 1992. The biology of interleukin-6. Chem. Immunol. **51**: 53.
4. HIRANO, T. & T. KISHIMOTO, Eds. 1992. Molecular biology and immunology of interleukin-6. Res. Immunol. **143**: 723.
5. YAMASAKI, K., T. TAGA, Y. HIRATA, H. YAWATA, Y. KAWANISHI, B. SEED, T. TANIGUCHI, T. HIRANO & T. KISHIMOTO. 1988. Cloning and expression of the human interleukin-6 (BSF-2/IFNβ2) receptor. Science **241**: 825.
6. HIBI, M., M. MURAKAMI, M. SAITO, T. HIRANO, T. TAGA & T. KISHIMOTO. 1990. Molecular cloning and Expression of an IL-6 signal transducer, gp130. Cell **63**: 1149.
7. BAZAN, J. F. 1989. A novel family of growth factor receptors: A common binding domain in the growth hormone, prolactin, erythropoietin and IL-6 receptors, and the p75 IL-2 receptor b-chain. Biochem. Biophys. Commun. **164**: 788.
8. IP, N. Y., S. H. NYE, T. G. BOULTON, S. DAVIS, T. TAGA, Y. LI, S. J. BIRREN, K. YASUKAWA, T. KISHIMOTO, D. J. ANDERSON, N. STAHL & G. D. YANCOPOULOS. 1992. CNTF and LIF act on neuronal cells via shared signaling pathways that involve the IL-6 signal transducing receptor component gp130. Cell **69**: 1121.
9. GEARING, D. P., M. R. COMEAU, D. J. FRIEND, S. D. GIMPEL, C. J. THUT, J. MCGOURTY, K. K. BRASHER, J. A. KING, S. GILLIS, B. MOSLEY, S. F. ZIEGLER & D. COSMAN. 1992. The IL-6 signal transducer, gp130: An oncostatin M receptor and affinity converter for the LIF receptor. Science **255**: 1434.
10. YIN, T., TAGA, M. L.-S. TSANG, K. YASUKAWA, T. KISHIMOTO & Y.-C. YANG. 1993. Involvement of IL-6 signal transducer gp130 in IL-11-mediated signal transduction. J. Immunol. **151**: 2555.
11. HIRANO, T., T. MATSUDA & K. NAKAJIMA. 1994. Signal transduction through gp130 that is shared among the receptors for the interleukin 6 related cytokine subfamily. Stem Cells. **12**: 262.

12. MURAKAMI, M., M. HIBI, N. NAKAGAWA, T. NAKAGAWA, K. YASUKAWA, K. YAMANISHI, T. TAGA & T. KISHIMOTO. 1993. IL-6-induced homodimerization of gp130 and associated activation of a tyrosine kinase. Science **260:** 1808.
13. NAKAJIMA, K. & R. WALL. 1991. Interleukin-6 signals activating *junB* and TIS11 gene transcription in a B-cell hybridoma. Mol. Cell. Biol. **11:** 1409.
14. MURAKAMI, M., M. NARAZAKI, M. HIBI, H. YAWATA, K. YASUKAWA, M. HAMAGUCHI, T. TAGA & T. KISHIMOTO. 1991. Critical cytoplasmic region of the Interleukin 6 signal transducer gp130 is conserved in the cytokine receptor family. Proc. Natl. Acad. Sci. USA **88:** 11349.
15. MATSUDA, T., Y. YAMANAKA & T. HIRANO. 1994. Interleukin-6-induced tyrosine phosphorylation of multiple proteins in murine hematopoietic lineage cells. Biochem. Biophys. Res. Commun. **200:** 821.
16. MATSUDA, T. & T. HIRANO. 1994. Association of p72 tyrosine kinase with stat factors and its activation by interleukin-3, interleukin-6, and granulocyte colony-stimulating factor. Blood **83:** 3457.
17. NAKAJIMA, K., T. KUSAFUKA, T. TAKEDA, Y. FUJITANI, K. NAKAE & T. HIRANO. 1993. Identification of a novel interleukin-6 response element containing an Ets-binding site and a CRE-like site in the *junB* promoter. Mol. Cell. Biol. **13:** 3027.
18. SCHINDLER, C., K. SHUAI, V. R. PREZIOSO & J. E. DARNELL JR. 1992. Interferon-dependent tyrosine phosphorylation of a latent cytoplasmic transcription factor. Science **257:** 809.
19. FU, X.-Y. 1992. A transcription factor with SH2 and SH3 domains is directly activated by an interferon a-induced cytoplasmic protein tyrosine kinase(s). Cell **70:** 323.
20. SHUAI, K., C. SCHINDLER, V. R. PREZIOSO & J. E. DARNELL, JR. 1992. Activation of transcription by IFN-g: tyrosine phosphorylation of a 91-kD DNA binding protein. Science **258:** 1808.
21. WILKS, A. F., A. G. HARPUR, R. R. KURBAN, S. J. RALPH, G. ZURCHER & A. ZIEMIECKI. 1991. Two novel protein-tyrosine kinases, each with a second phosphotransferase-related catalytic domain, define a new class of protein kinase. Mol. Cell. Biol. **11:** 2057.
22. HARPUR, A. G., A.-C. ANDRES, A. ZIEMIECKI, R. R. ASTON & A. F. WILKS. 1992. JAK2, a third member of the JAK family of protein kinases. Oncogene **7:** 1347.
23. FIRMBACH-KRAFT, I., M. BYERS, T. SHOWS, R. DALLA-FAVERA & J. J. KROLEWSKI. 1990. Tyk2, prototype of a novel class of non-receptor tyrosine kinase genes. Oncogene **5:** 1329.
24. SILVENNOINEN, O., B. A. WITTHUHN, F. W. QUELLE, J. L. CLEVELAND, T. YI & J. N. IHLE. 1993. Structure of the murine Jak2 protein-tyrosine kinase and its role in interleukin 3 signal trasnduction. Proc. Natl. Acad. Sci. USA **90:** 8429.
25. VELAZQUEZ, L., M. FELLOWS, G. R. STARK & S. PELLEGRINI. 1992. A protein tyrosine kinase in the interferon a/b signalling pathway. Cell **70:** 313.
26. ARGETSINGER, L. S., G. S. CAMPBELL, X. YANG, B. A. WITTHUHN, O. SILVENNOINEN, J. N. IHLE & C. CARTER-SU. 1993. Identification of Jak2 as a growth hormone receptor-associated tyrosine kinase. Cell **74:** 237.
27. WITHUHN, B. A., F. W. QUELLE, O. SILVENNOINEN, T. YI, B. TANG, O. MIURA & J. N. IHLE. 1993. JAK2 associates with the erythropoietin receptor and is tyrosine phosphorylated and activated following stimulation with erythropoietin. Cell **74:** 227.
28. STAHL, N., T. G. BOULTON, T. FARRUGGELLA, N. Y. IP, S. D. BRUCE, A. WITTHUHN, F. W. QUELLE, O. SILVENNOINEN, G. BARBIERI, S. PELLEGRINI, J. N. IHLE & G. D. YANCOPOULOS. 1994. Association and activation of Jak/Tyk kinases by CNTF/LIF/OSM/IL6 b-receptor components. Science **263:** 92.
29. SHUAI, K., A. ZIEMIECKI, A. F. WILKS, A. G. HARPUR, H. B. SADOWSKI, M. Z. GILMAN & J. E. DARNELL, JR. 1993. Polypeptide signaling to the nucleus through tyrosine phosphorylation of Jak and stat proteins. Nature **366:** 580.
30. HATTORI, M., L. J. ABRAHAM, W. NORTHEMANN & G. H. FEY. 1990. Acute-phase reaction induces a specific complex between hepatic nuclear proteins and the interleukin 6 response element of the rat a2-macroglobulin gene. Proc. Natl. Acad. Sci. USA **87:** 2364.
31. WEGENKA, U. M., J. BUSCHMANN, C. LUTTICKEN, P. HEINRICH & F. HORN. 1993. Acute-phase response factor, a nuclear factor binding to acute-phase response elements, is rapidly activated by interleukin-6 at the posttranslational level. Mol. Cell. Biol. **13:** 276.

32. DALMON, J., M. LAURENT & G. COURTOIS. 1993. The human b fibrinogen promoter contains a hepatocyte nuclear factor 1-dependent interleukin-6 responsive element. Mol. Cell. Biol. **13:** 1183.
33. WON, K.-A. & H. BAUMANN. 1990. The cytokine response element of the rat a1-acid glycoprotein gene is a complex of several interacting regulatory sequences. Mol. Cell. Biol. **10:** 3965.
34. HAYS, T. E., A. M. KITCHEN & B. H. COCHRAN. 1987. Inducible binding of a factor to the c-*fos* regulatory region. Proc. Natl. Acad. Sci. USA **84:** 1272.
35. WAGNER, B. J., T. E. HAYES, C. J. HOBAN & B. H. COCHRAN. 1990. The SIF binding element confers sis/PDGF inducibility onto the c-fos promoter. EMBO J. **9:** 4477.
36. SADOWSKI, H. & M. Z. GILMAN. 1993. Cell-free activation of a DNA-binding protein by epidermal growth factor. Nature **363:** 79.
37. KHAN, K. D., K. SHUAI, G. LINDWALL, S. MAHER, J. E. DARNELL, JR. & L. M. BOTHWELL. 1993. Induction of the Ly-6A/E gene by interferon a/b and g requires a DNA element to which a tyrosine-phosphorylated 91-kD protein binds. Proc. Natl. Acad. Sci. USA **90:** 6806.
38. PEARSE, R. N., R. FEINMAN, K. SHUAI, J. E. DARNELL, JR. & J. V. RAVETCH. 1933. Interferon g-induced transcription of the high-affinity Fc receptor for IgG requires assembly of a complex that includes the 91-kD subunit of transcription factor ISGF3. Proc. Natl. Acad. Sci. USA **90:** 4314.
39. LUTTICKEN, C., U. M. WEGENKA, J. YUAN, J. BUSCHMANN, C. SCHINDLER, A. ZIEMIECKI, A. G. HARPUR, A. F. WILKS, K. YASUKAWA, T. TAGA, T. KISHIMOTO, G. BARBIERI, S. PELLEGRINI, M. SENDTNER, P. C. HEINRICH & F. HORN. 1994. Association of transcription factor APRF and protein kinase Jak1 with the interleukin-6 signal transducer gp130. Science **263:** 89.
40. WEGENKA, U. M., C. LÜTTICKEN, J. BUSCHMANN, J. YUAN, F. LOTTSPEICH, W. MULLER-ESTERL, C. SCHINDLER, E. ROEB, P. C. HEINRICH & F. HORN. 1994. The interleukin-6-activated acute-phase response factor is antigenically and functionally related to members of the signal transducer and activator of transcription (STAT) family. Mol. Cell. Biol. **14:** 3186.
41. AKIRA, S., Y. NISHIO, M. INOUE, X-J. WANG, S. WEI, T. MATSUSAKA, K. YOSHIDA, T. SUDO, M. NARUTO & T. KISHIMOTO. 1994. Molecular cloning of APRF, a novel IFN-stimulated gene factor 3 p91-related transcription factor involved in the gp130-mediated signaling pathway. Cell **77:** 63.
42. ZHONG, Z., Z. WEN & J. E. DARNELL, JR. 1994. Stat3: A STAT family member activated by tyrosine phosphorylation in response to epidermal growth factor and interleukin-6. Science **264:** 95.
43. ORITANI, K., T. KAISHO, K. NAKAJIMA & T. HIRANO. 1992. Retinoic acid inhibits interleukin 6-induced macrophage differentiation and apoptosis in a murine hematopoietic cell line, Y6. Blood **80:** 2298.
44. FUJITANI, Y., K. NAJAJIMA, H. KOJIMA, K. NAKAE, T. TAKEDA & T. HIRANO. 1994. Transcriptional activation of the IL-6 response element in the JunB promoter is mediated by multiple stat family proteins. Biochem. Biophys. Res. Commun. **202:** 1181.
45. LARNER, A. C., M. DAVID, G. M. FELDMAN, K. IGARASHI, R. H. HACKETT, D. S. A. WEBB, S. M. SWEITZER, E. F. PETRICOIN III & D. S. FINBLOOM. 1993. Tyrosine phosphorylation of DNA binding proteins by multiple cytokines. Science **261:** 1730.
46. FU, X.-Y. & J.-J. ZHANG. 1993. Transcription factor p91 interacts with the epidermal growth factor receptor and mediates activation of the c-*fos* gene promoter. Cell **74:** 1135.
47. HIDAKA, H., M. INAGAKI, S. KAWAMOTO & Y. SASAKI. 1984. Isoquinoline sulfonate, novel and potent inhibitors of cyclic nucleotide dependent protein kinase and protein kinase C. Biochemistry **23:** 5036.
48. INAGAKI, M., M. WATANABE & H. HIDAKA. 1985. N-(2-aminoethyl)-5-isoquinolinesulfonamide, a newly synthesized protein kinase inhibitor, functions as a ligand in affinity chromatography. J. Biol. Chem. **260:** 2922.
49. SHUAI, K., G. R. STARK, I. M. KERR & J. E. DARNELL, JR. 1993. A single phosphotyrosine residue of stat91 required for gene activation by interferon-g. Science **261:** 1744.

50. SILVENNOINEN, O., J. N. IHLE, J. SCHLESSINGER & D. E. LEVY. 1993. Interferon-induced nuclear signalling by Jak protein tyrosine kinases. Nature **366:** 583.

DISCUSSION OF THE PAPER

M. REVEL (*Weizmann Institute, Rehovot, Israel*): How do you explain that APRF is able to bind to the GRE of the junB? Looking at the sequences, one does not find the GAS consensus, which is the target for the Stat protein binding including APRF. So, how can you explain that you get such a strong purification?

T. HIRANO: The JEBS does not contain a typical GAS consensus sequence but the sequence of the JEBS and that of rat α_2-macroglobulin APRF binding site are very similar. We purified the binding protein utilizing the α_2-macroglobulin APRE and showed that purified protein specifically bound to the JEBS.

H. BAUMANN (*Roswell Park Cancer Institute, Buffalo, NY*): Dr. Hirano, you mentioned the 5' region for junB as a regulatory site. Did you test the reported 3' region in conjunction or separately?

HIRANO: We did not examine the 3' region.

BAUMANN: This is the one which has been published, I think in MCB, regarding the serum element, which is after the polyadenylation site. The next question is: you have so many phosphorylation sites. Tyrosine phosphorylations which occur at multiple sites on the receptor. So, I am surprised that one has not already identified known SH-2 or SH-3 domain containing protein or src-kinases, which obviously must somehow interact too. Do you have some idea which of the known src-related kinases do actually interact with gp130?

HIRANO: I have no data showing that gp130 can bind src-family. At the moment, we have some preliminary data showing that several nonreceptor type tyrosine kinases other than Jak and src-family are activated by gp130-stimulation.

G. FEY (*University of Erlangen-Nürnberg, Erlangen, Germany*): I would like to come back to the tissue specificity of your p72 new src-kinase. You said that you find it in a pro-B cell line but not in hepatoma cells. Do you also see it in early T-cell progenitor cells?

HIRANO: It is an interesting question. We would like to answer the question when we will make an antibody against p72sak.

FEY: Well, I guess that settles my second question. I was wondering what happens to it in early fetal liver cells that are hematopoietic cells; but I think that unless you have that antibody you would not be able to answer this question.

Cytokine Networks and Corticosteroid Receptors

A. FALUS,[a] J. BIRÓ, AND É. RÁKÁSZ

Department of Biology
Semmelweis Medical University
1445 Budapest, Hungary

The reciprocal interaction between the interleukin-6 (IL-6) and functionally related other inflammatory cytokines as well as the hypothalamo-pituitary-adrenal axis represents a separate facet of complex web of regulatory neuroendocrino-immunological interactions. The activation of the hypothalamo-pituitary-adrenal axis results in increased production of glucocorticoids with anti-inflammatory activity. Glucocorticosteroids are among the most effective drugs used in the therapy of the inflammatory (*e.g.*, rheumatic diseases).[1] The mechanisms by which they accomplish their antiinflammatory effects involve numerous pathways, including that of the modulation of the influence of the inflammatory cytokines IL-1β, IL-6 and TNF-α.

Glucocorticosteroids decrease the level of these cytokines in the peripheral blood via transcriptional and posttranscriptional routes,[2] and prolong their impact on the target cells through the elevation of the expression of their receptors.[3]

These steroids like the other members of the steroid hormone family exert their effects mainly through specific receptors.[4] The receptors are localized in the cytoplasm, anchored to microtubules by two heat shock proteins in the inactive state.[5] After ligand binding the activated receptors dimerize, translocate into nucleus, and act as transcription factors.[6] At high concentrations, glucocorticosteroids downregulate the expression of their own receptor, attenuating hormone responsiveness in this way.[7]

IL-1β, IL-6 and TNF-α regulate glucocorticoid production at different stages, as well. Although data are still controversial, IL-1β and IL-6 seem to elevate serum adrenocorticotropic hormone (ACTH) level indirectly through the stimulation of the corticotropin-releasing hormone (CRH)-secreting neurons in the hypothalamus and directly as intrapituitary-releasing factors.[8] Data concerning the central site of action of the TNF-α are conflicting, showing positive and negative, or no effect at all on ACTH secretion by anterior pituitary cells *in vitro*.[9-11]

However, so far no information is available on whether these cytokines exert any direct effect on the level of glucocorticosteroid binding (or the glucocorticosteroid receptor) of the target cells.

Our present data provide evidence that IL-1β, IL-6 and TNF-α elevate the glucocorticosteroid binding in human monocytic, lymphoid, and hepatoma-derived tumor cell lines U937, CESS and HEPG-2. Scatchard analysis suggests that while the number of glucocorticoid receptors increases, the affinity of the binding decreases. Presently, we have no idea on the level the cytokine action, but mRNA studies seem to exclude that pretranslational effects are involved.

---

[a] Address correspondence to András Falus, Ph.D., D.Sc. at 1445 Budapest P.O. Box 370

MATERIALS AND METHODS

Cell Culture Medium

Cell culture medium consisted of RPMI-1640, 10% fetal calf serum, 2 mM glutamine, 2 g/l $NaHCO_3$, 5000 U/l penicillin G sodium, 5 mg/l streptomycin sulfate and 12.5 µg/l amphotericin B. All of the reagents were obtained from Gibco (Paisley, Renfrewshire, U.K.)

Cell Lines

CESS, an IgG-secreting, EB-virus-positive cell line, U937, a promonocytic-histiocytic cell line in the monoblastic stadium, and HepG2, a hepatoma-derived cell line were used as the objects of these experiments. A total of $4-5 \times 10^6$ cells were incubated in the presence of varying concentrations of human recombinant IL-1β, IL-6 and/or TNF-α (Sigma Chemical Co. St Louis, MO) for 24 hours at 37°C, 5% CO_2.

Assay of Steroid Binding

Glucocorticosteroid binding was determined by the method of "whole cell uptake".[12] Cells were washed 3 times with SSC (0.15 M NaCl, 0.015 M Na-citrate pH 7.4) at 0°C, then duplicate samples of $1.5-2 \times 10^6$ cells were incubated in medium RPMI-1640 in the presence of 7.2×10^{-8} M (1,2,4,(n)-3H]triamcinolone acetonide (Amersham, Buckinghamshire, U.K.), without (for determination of total binding) or with (for determination of unspecific binding) a 500-fold molar excess of unlabeled triamcinolone acetonide (Sigma Chemical Co., St. Louis, MO) at 37°C for 40 minutes. Incubation was performed with vigorous shaking. Then, the excess of the triamcinolone acetonide was removed by washing 3 times with SSC at 0°C. Washed cells were solubilized in toluene-based scintillation cocktail containing 30% Triton X-100. Specific binding was calculated as the difference between total and unspecific binding. The counts were normalized to 1000 cells, and the results were expressed as percentage of the value of the untreated cells. In Scatchard analysis at least 5 points were tested and the data were evaluated by a special Scatchard program by computer.

mRNA Studies

Northern blot analysis was performed using total cellular RNA applying guanidine thiocyanate lysates from U937 cells. For hybridization P32-labeled BamH1-EcoRI inserts from a cDNA (PSTC GR 3-795) clone has been used (kindly provided by Dr. S. Rusconi).

Statistical Analysis

Values shown are means and standard error of the means. Students t-test was used in calculating p values.

RESULTS

The Basal Level of Glucocorticosteroid Binding

Comparing the basal level of the glucocorticosteroid binding (GCSB) of the cell lines we found the highest GCSB in HepG2—$6.13 \pm 2.34 \times 10^{-14}$ Mol GCSB/10^6 cells. The same values in CESS and U937 were $1.68 \pm 0.41 \times 10^{-14}$ and $1.4 \pm 0.57 \times 10^{-14}$ GCSB Mol/10^6, respectively. Considering that one receptor binds only one molecule glucocorticosteroid, these data mean $66\,700 \pm 25500$, $18\,500 \pm 6450$ and $15\,500 \pm 6300$ glucocorticosteroid receptors/cell, respectively.

For comparison normal human leukocytes contain approximately 2–8000 glucocorticosteroid binding sites showing great individual variance.[17] Steroid binding assays were performed in these experiments only at a single concentration of labeled triamcinolone, so we are allowed to make comparisons only between relative values.[14]

Effect of the Three Cytokines on the Glucocorticosteroid Binding

In U937 (FIG. 1.), CESS (FIG. 2.) and HepG2 (FIG. 3.) IL-1β, IL-6 and TNF-α elevated glucocorticosteroid biding in a dose-dependent manner at a concentration range 5–100 U/ml. The extent of the change showed a definite variance in the different cell lines, but the tendency of the effects was the same in each. Furthermore, we observed the most profound effect after the IL-6 and TNF-α treatment in the hepatoma cell line, with about 2.8-fold rise by IL-6 and 2-fold increase by TNF-α (FIG. 3.).

The results of the Scatchard analysis of the effect of TNF-α and IL-6 on the glucocorticosteroid receptors of U937 cells are demonstrated in TABLE 1. These data

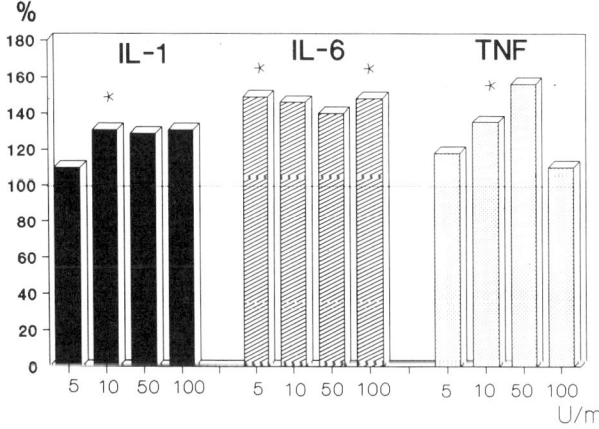

FIGURE 1. Effect of cytokines on GCSB sites of U937 monocytoid cell line. Effect of IL-1β, Il-6 and TNF-α on glucocorticosteroid binding in U937 cell line. The cells were incubated in the presence of different concentrations of the cytokines for 24 hours. The data presented are means of six separate experiments. For the sake of clarity SEM values are not shown (all are under 8%). * = $p < 0.05$ (Student t-test)

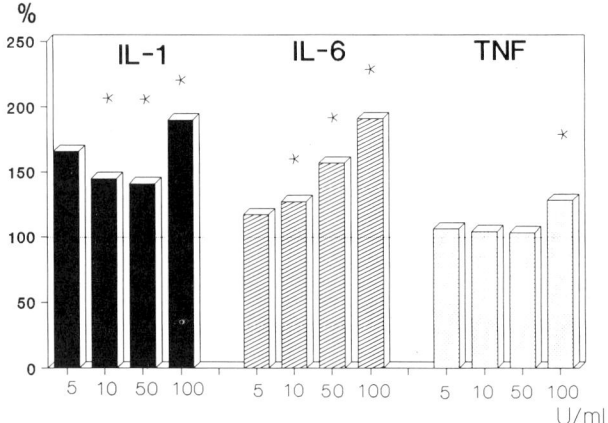

FIGURE 2. Effect of cytokines on GCSB sites of CESS β-lymphoma cell line. Same as FIGURE 1, with CESS cells (four separate experiments) * = $p < 0.05$ (Student t-test)

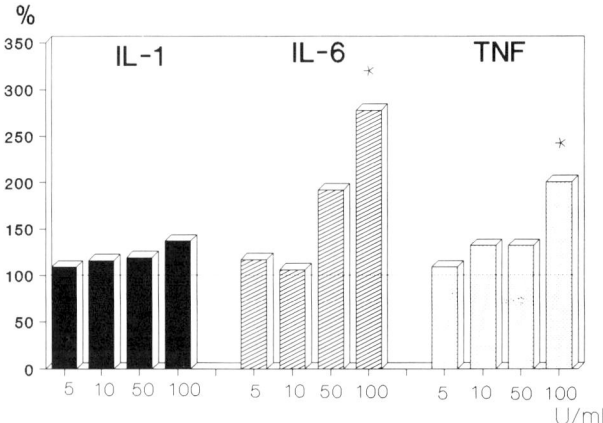

FIGURE 3. Effect of cytokines on GCSB sites of HepG2 hepatoma cell line. Same as FIGURE 1, with HepG2 cells (three separate experiments). * = $p < 0.05$ (Student t-test)

TABLE 1. The Effect of 100 U/ml IL-6 or TNF-α on Glucocorticosteroid Binding by U937 Cells

	Binding Sites/Cell (thousands)	Kd (nmol)
Control (n = 4)	15.3 ± 7.1	3.2 ± 0.9
100 U/ml IL-6 (n = 3)	30.95 ± 11.2	8.84 ± 1.3
100 U/ml TNF-α (n = 3)	49.5 ± 19.4	9.39 ± 1.5

suggest an approximately 2- or 3.3 times more binding sites after IL-6 or TNF-α treatments, respectively. However, there is a parallel drop of affinity in both cases.

Northern blot analysis of glucocorticoid receptor expression showed no detectable change in the mRNA level of U937 cell after 24 hour incubation with either 100 U/ml IL-6 or 100 U/ml TNF-α (results not shown).

DISCUSSION

Although numerous studies have been focused on the effects exerted by glucocorticoids and on the glucocorticoid receptor and its gene itself, examinations of the regulation of the expression of glucocorticosteroid receptor gene are rather sparse. The inhibition of glucocorticosteroid receptor expression by glucocorticosteroids at pharmacological concentrations is well known.[11] There are data showing that cAMP and prostaglandin E2 upregulate glucocorticosteroid receptor expression,[15] but additional factor exhibiting any direct effect on glucocorticosteroid receptor expression remained to be explored.

The cytokines IL-1β, IL-6 and TNF-α released during systemic and local inflammation in elevated amount enhance glucocorticosteroid production via elevation of CRH and/or ACTH level.[13] The glucocorticosteroids reduce IL-1β, IL-6 and TNF-α level sharply in the peripheral blood inhibiting the inflammatory overshoot by this way.[3,5] Moreover, glucocorticosteroids augment the effects of these cytokines as permissive factors by elevating the expression of IL-1β, IL-6 and TNF-α receptors on the target cells.[6,7] The results of a previous study in our laboratory[16] and this study complete the knowledge of the regulation loop by showing that IL-1β, IL-6 and TNF-α in certain circumstances may elevate sensitivity toward glucocorticosteroids by increasing the glucocorticoid binding and in case of IL-1β, translocation of the activated receptors in the cells investigated.

Present data are the first to demonstrate that these cytokines increase glucocorticosteroid binding. We used interleukins in concentration range 5–100 U/ml since the level of IL-1β, IL-6 and TNF-α in inflamed synovium is close to these values. These data are based on experiments accomplished by ELISA and bioactivity assays as well.[17,18]

In those pathological cases and peculiar compartments where the level of one of the three cytokines is predominant and local imbalances in the ratios of the cytokines might occur (*e.g.*, IL-6 in most arthritis), the stimulatory effect exerted by this cytokine on glucocorticosteroid binding may be dominant.[17]

We have no evidence yet to ascertain the mechanisms by which IL-1β, IL-6, and TNF-α accomplish their effect on glucocorticosteroid binding. Data available in the literature show that IL-1β reduces binding of the TNF-α, possibly through decreasing the expression of the TNF-α receptor(s).[19] Consequently, any possible antagonisms observed between these cytokines exerted on glucocorticosteroid binding and glucocorticosteroid receptor level might be due to the modulation of the receptor expression of each other.

Since the nuclear factor NF-kB is involved in molecular pathways used by IL-1β, IL-6, and TNF-α alike, the role of this transactivation factor in the upregulation of glucocorticosteroid receptor gene cannot be excluded either.[20]

At present we do not have any real, acceptable explanation for the simultaneous rise in the number and drop in the affinity of glucocorticosteroid receptors after the cytokine action. Moreover, the lack of the change in the level of glucocorticosteroid receptor transcripts suggest that conformation or subunit assembly, rather than the actual number of *de novo* synthesized glucocorticosteroid receptor is elevated. The decrease of the affinity values raises further questions on the biological significance of this phenomenon.

Further molecular studies will hopefully elucidate the exact mechanism of cytokine regulation on the glucocorticosteroid receptor expression of cells with different inflammatory lesions.

SUMMARY

The role of the inflammatory cytokines on glucocorticosteroid binding (GCSB) and glucocorticosteroid receptor (GR) level was studied. We incubated a B cell line —CESS—, a promonocytic cell line —U937— and a hepatoma cell line —HepG2— in the presence of varying concentrations of IL-1β, IL-6 and TNF-α for 24 hours. Glucocorticosteroid binding was determined by the method of "whole cell uptake," and characterized by Scatchard analysis. A considerable increase in the glucocorticosteroid binding was induced by all the three cytokines. Northern analysis of the glucocorticoid receptor expression demonstrates that the action of the cytokines is likely not pretranslational.

Present data suggest that local imbalance in the ratio of these three cytokines in different pathological cases might influence the glucocorticosteroid sensitivity of the lymphocytes, monocytes and hepatocytes as target cells.

REFERENCES

1. WEISS, M. M. 1991. Corticosteroids in rheumatoid arthritis. EULAR Bull. **1:** 8–15.
2. BOUMPAS, D. T., J. PALIOGIANNI, E. D. ANASTASSION & J. E. BALOW. 1991. Glucocorticosteroid action on the immune system: molecular and cellular aspects. Clin. Exp. Rheum. **9:** 413–423.
3. SNYERS, I., L. DE WIT & J. CONTENT. 1990. Glucocorticoid up-regulation of high affinity interleukin 6 receptors on human epithelial cells. Proc. Natl. Acad. Sci. USA **87:** 2838–2842.
4. GEHRING, U. 1986. Genetics of glucocorticoid receptors. Mol. Cell. Endocrinol. **48:** 89–96.
5. AKNER, G., K. G. SUNDQVIST, M. DENIS, A. C. WIKSTRÖM & J. A. GUSTAFSSON. 1990. Immunocytochemical localization of glucocorticoid receptor in human gingival fibroblasts and evidence for a colocalization of glucocorticoid receptor with cytoplasmic microtubules. Eur. J. Cell Biol. **53:** 390–401.
6. MULLER, M. & R. RENKAWITZ. 1991. The glucocorticoid receptor. Biochim. Biophys. Acta **1088:** 171–182.
7. BURNSTEIN, K. L. & D. L. BELLINGHAM, C. M. JEWELL, F. E. POWELL-OLIVER & J. A. CIDLOWSKY. 1991. Autoregulation of glucocorticoid receptor gene expression. Steroids **56:** 52–58.
8. HERMUS, A. R. M. M. & C. G. J. SWEEP. 1990. Cytokines and the hypothalamic-pituitary-adrenal axis. J. Steroid Biochem. Mol. Biol. **337:** 867–871.
9. MILENKOVIC, L., V. RETTORI, G. SNYDER, B. BEUTLER & S. MCCANN. 1989. Cachectin alters anterior pituitary hormone release by a direct action in vitro. Proc. Natl. Acad. Sci. USA **86:** 2418–2422.
10. SHARP, B., S. MATTA, P. PETERSON, R. NEWTON, C. CHAO & K. MCALLEN. 1989. Tumor necrosis factor is a potent ACTH secretagogue: Comparison to interleukin-1. Endocrinology **124:** 3131–3133.
11. KEHRER, P., D. TURNILL, J.-M. DAYER, A. MULLER & R. GAILLARD. 1988. Human recombinant IL-1 beta and alpha, but not recombinant tumor necrosis factor alpha

stimulate ACTH release from rat anterior pituitary cells in vitro in a prostaglandin E2 and cAMP independent manner. Neuroendocrinology, **48:** 160–166.
12. JUNKER, K. 1983. Glucocorticoid receptors of human mononuclear leukocytes in vitro. J. Clin. Endocrinol. Metab. **57:** 506–512.
13. CIDLOWSKI, J. A., D. L. BELLINGHAM, F. E. POWELL-OLIVER, D. B. LUBAHN & M. SAR. 1990. Novel antipeptide antibodies to the human glucocorticoid receptor: Recognition of multiple receptor forms in vitro and distinct localization of cytoplasmic and nuclear receptors. Mol. Endocrinol **90:** 1427–1436.
14. CEKAN, S. Z. 1987. Biases in the assays of steroids and their binding proteins. J. Steroid Biochem. **27:** 95–98.
15. DIBATTISTA, J. A., J. MARTELL-PELLETIER, J.-M. CLOUTIER & J.-P. PELLETIER. 1991. Modulation of glucocorticoid receptor expression in human articular chondrocytes by cAMP and prostaglandins. J. Rheumatol. S27, **18:** 102–105.
16. FALUS, A., E. WALCZ & J. SMOLEN. 1991. Effectiveness of interleukin-1 and interleukin-6 on the corticosteroid binding of peripheral blood mononuclear cells. Clin. Exp. Rheumatol. **9:** 5.
17. STEINER, G., G. WITZMANN, A. STUDNICKA-BENKE, E. HÖFLER, G. PARTSCH & J. SMOLEN. 1992. Cytokines in sera and synovial fluids from patients wtih inflammatory arthritides. Clin. Rheumatol. **11:** 141.
18. SAWADA, T., S. HIROHATA, T. INOUE & K. ITO. 1991. Correlation between rheumatoid factor and IL-6 activity in synovial fluids from patients with rheumatoid arthritis. Clin. Exp. Rheumatol. **9:** 363–368.
19. HOLTMANN, H., C. BRAKEBUSH, M. KÖNIG, R. WINZEN, K. RESCH & D. WALLACH. 1991. Mechanisms controlling the level of receptors for tumor necrosis factor. Agents and Actions **32:** 106–108.
20. BOMSZTYK, K., J. W. ROONEY, T. IWASAKI, N. A. RACHIE, S. K. DOWER & C. H. SIBLEY. 1991. Evidence that interleukin-1 and phorbol esters activate NF-kB by different pathways: Role of protein kinase C. Cell Regulation **2:** 329–337.

DISCUSSION OF THE PAPER

P. HEINRICH (*Klinikum der RWTH Aachen, Institut für Biochemie, Aachen, Germany*): You have observed the increase in gp80 after dexamethasone treatment on iodinated IL-6 binding. Have you an idea what mechanism might be involved?

A. FALUS: Well, actually, that was a binding assay only, and just a phenomenological approach. So, in my opinion, the amount of the 80kD might have been increased, but I have never checked it myself at the mRNA level.

HEINRICH: There are at least two laboratories (J. Content's and ours) who have done this. We measured increased mRNA levels. And it could also be a matter of stabilization. I think that glucocorticoids are known to stabilize mRNA.

FALUS: Yes, in addition to the IL-6 binding test findings, earlier we checked for upregulation of gp130 by Northern blot analysis of mRNA. I think that I showed this slide once a couple of years ago, but I was not able to confirm these results later.

G. FEY (*University of Erlangen-Nürnberg, Erlangen, Germany*): I have a question about the same aspect. The strong increase in gp80 and also the increase in gp130 you observe in HepG2 and HepG3—which is actually affecting the sensitivity of the cell?

FALUS: I have no idea.

FEY: May I ask you please to clarify that. So Peter [Heinrich] says he sees increased gp80 after corticosteroids in human HEPG2 cells. And you say that sometimes you saw it and sometimes you did not, but you clearly see an increased level in IL-6 binding in binding studies. Has anybody done ^{35}S-methionine continuous labeling or pulse chase and subsequently the immunoprecipitation to measure the half-life of these proteins? And you say that there is an effect on the half-life of the mRNA. And if I compare the two sets of data I would expect an even stronger effect on the half-life of the protein.

HEINRICH: I did not say that we measured the stability of mRNA after dex treatment in our case, but we could show an increase in functional protein, for instance.

FEY: But, if the increase of the mRNA as shown by Northern blot is small. . . .

HEINRICH: There is quite a nice increase; it is three- to fivefold.

FEY: The increase in IL-6 binding was more than that?

FALUS: May I make one point? You might have misunderstood me. I thought that we have found the binding increase very well, but we found that upregulation of gp130 expression was not always reproducible. But the binding activity was reproducibly increased, particularly in Hep3B cells.

FEY: How much? Threefold? Fivefold? Tenfold?

FALUS: Five- or sixfold. That was a very strong effect. But I have no idea about the molecular background.

HEINRICH: The gp130 mRNA increases after IL-6 in the presence of dex?

FALUS: Yes.

HEINRICH: This has also been shown by several laboratories.

FEY: So the consensus will be that there is no need to look at the stability of the protein? It could all be explained by the effect of glucocorticoids on the message for the receptor components?

HEINRICH: I would still do the experiment.

FEY: I would like to see the ^{35}S-methionine protein labeling, the immunoprecipitation, pulse chase, and the half-life measurements of the protein.

A. LANGE (*Institute of Immunology and Experimental Therapy, Wrocław, Poland*): This is quite a simple question, which may be of clinical relevance. You have found that the number of receptors has been increased after glucocorticoid treatment, and then there is a concurrent lower affinity of these receptors. Could you explain the effect in terms of the acute phase proteins in the *in vitro* system?

FALUS: Well, I'm afraid not. I would like to quote Dr. Akira who answered all the time that this is too difficult a question to answer, so I have no idea. But we have found that logically and philosophically it is very hard to understand how it is possible that the Kd value is so strongly reduced, there is no change at the mRNA level, and yet we found more binding sites. So it might be that due to activation of the cell some immunogenic epitopes will be much more reliable, and therefore, we found at the beginning such a sharp staining positivity, and we have found a few more binding sites but with less binding capacity. I have no idea how to explain it.

HEINRICH: I am not a specialist on glucocorticoid receptors, but, to my knowledge, there are heat-shock proteins (hsp90) involved in binding. Could involvement of such proteins explain why you get an increase in binding sites?

FALUS: There is an easy explanation. I have a slide which I keep that shows that there is an inhibitory element which belongs to the hsp90 family. That could be simultaneously increased availability of one epitope, but I still have no idea why the Kd value has dropped. I was very, very upset about that Scatchard that we found.

Regulation of Interleukin-6 Gene Expression by Steroids[a]

ANURADHA RAY, DONG-HONG ZHANG, MARK D. SIEGEL,
AND PRABIR RAY

Department of Internal Medicine, Pulmonary and Critical Care Section
Yale University School of Medicine
New Haven, Connecticut 06520

The neuroendocrine and immune systems are now known to be intimately linked. Cytokines such as interleukin-1 (IL-1)[1,2] and IL-6[3] can directly cause increased systemic adrenocorticotrophic hormone (ACTH) levels via release of corticotropin releasing factor (CRF) from the hypothalamus. The ensuing increased levels of circulating endogenous glucocorticoids control important immune functions under the control of the hypothalamic-pituitary-adrenal axis. IL-6, which can itself be produced by the folliculostelate cells of the anterior pituitary, has been reported to directly stimulate the release of anterior pituitary hormones ACTH, prolactin, growth hormone and luteinizing hormone.[4,5]

Glucocorticoids act through multiple mechanisms on multiple target cells to elicit their pleiotropic effects. The therapeutic potential of glucocorticoids in asthma and a number of inflammatory conditions has long been recognized. For a family of compounds with such profound effects on the immune system, it is surprising that so little is known about the mechanisms by which glucocorticoids exert their antiinflammatory activities. It is now believed that the anti-inflammatory effects of glucocorticoids result, to a great extent, from their ability to inhibit the cellular release of inflammatory mediators and cytokines.

Regulation of gene transcription by steroid hormones, including glucocorticoids, is mediated by intracellular receptors.[6,7] Steroid hormone receptors belong to a complex superfamily of ligand-binding transcription factors. Members of this superfamily include the glucocorticoid receptor (GR), the mineralocorticoid receptor (MR), the estrogen receptor (ER) and the thyroid hormone receptor (TR). These receptors may be found in both the cytosolic and nuclear fractions of a tissue homogenate. Immunocytochemical studies with monoclonal antibodies against the various receptors indicate that most steroid hormone receptors, such as the estrogen receptor and the progesterone receptor, are nuclear even in the absence of hormone.[8,9] GR and MR appear to be exceptions to this general rule. In the absence of hormone, these latter receptors appear largely cytoplasmic and concentrate in the nucleus only after hormone addition.[10,11]

Actions of Glucocorticoids on the Immune System

One of the major targets of the antiinflammatory actions of glucocorticoids is cytokine production by cells of the monocyte/macrophage lineage and T lymphocytes.

---

[a] This work was supported by a grant from NIH (AI31137) and a Special Fellowship from The Leukemia Society of America (A.R.).

Glucocorticoids inhibit cytokine production to keep a heightened immune response to an antigen in check, thereby preventing uncontrolled proliferation of cells of the immune system. Cytokines whose expression is repressed by glucocorticoids include IL-1, IL-2, IL-5, IL-6, IL-8, TNF-α and interferon-γ. These effects of glucocorticoids, among others, form the basis for their therapeutic use.

MECHANISM OF REPRESSION OF GENE EXPRESSION BY STEROID RECEPTORS-nGREs

Steroid receptors can interfere with transcriptional activation of genes via different mechanisms. Most genes that are negatively regulated by glucocorticoids lack consensus glucocorticoid response elements (GRE) in their regulatory regions.[12] In the case of the human glycoprotein α-subunit gene,[13] bovine prolactin gene,[14] the rat pro-opiomelanocortin gene,[15] and the IL-6 gene,[16] binding of GR to sequences overlapping with the binding sites for positive transcription factor was noted. These negative GREs (nGREs), however, have limited sequence similarity. The binding of intact GR to the IL-6 promoter is weak, similar to the weak binding of the receptor to the prolactin and the proliferin promoters. In the case of the proliferin gene, the concentration of the steroid receptor and nonsteroid factors was found to dictate the final outcome: activation vs. repression. To explain these findings, the term "composite GRE" was coined. The composite GRE in the proliferin promoter has a binding site for the receptor adjacent to and overlapping with an AP1 binding site. Thus, while induction of the proliferin gene by the AP-1 complex (fos/jun heterodimer) was repressed by a combination of dexamethasone (dex) and GR, induction by the jun/jun or jun/fra heterodimer was actually augmented by the receptor.[17]

DIRECT PHYSICAL ASSOCIATION BETWEEN STEROID RECEPTORS AND POSITIVE TRANSCRIPTION FACTORS

Although both the collagenase gene and the proliferin gene are induced by AP-1, there are differences in the mechanisms by which GR interferes with the transactivation functions of AP-1 in the two promoters. In the case of the collagenase gene, inhibition occurs through direct interaction with AP-1, independent of any DNA-binding by GR.[18-20] With the proliferin gene, repression by GR appears to involve both binding of the receptor across the composite GRE sequence in the proliferin promoter and protein-protein interaction between GR and AP-1.[17] Utilizing a variety of techniques, we performed DNA-binding studies of GR to the IL-6 promoter which indicated that GR binds weakly to IL-6 promoter sequences.[16,21] We therefore investigated alternate mechanisms of IL-6 gene repression by glucocorticoids such as protein-protein interactions between the steroid receptor and activators of IL-6 gene expression.

REPRESSION OF IL-6 GENE EXPRESSION BY GLUCOCORTICOIDS INVOLVES PROTEINS OTHER THAN AP-1

Our earlier studies on activation of the IL-6 promoter by multiple stimuli indicated that 225 bp of IL-6 5'-flanking sequences linked to the CAT gene (pIC225), is sufficient for conferring response to IL-1 and additional agents.[16,21–23] The region between −145 and −158 of the promoter was implicated in the responsiveness to cytokines such as IL-1 and TNF by us and others. This region was also identified as the binding site for nuclear factor IL-6 (NF-IL6). Another overlapping AP-1-like sequence was also found to be responsive to phorbol esters and protein kinase A agonists in functional experiments. An IL-6 promoter construct pIC110 that contained 110 bp of IL-6 5′-flanking sequence including the NF-κB site between −64 and −73 was unresponsive to IL-1 and additional stimuli.[15,22,23] In view of the implication of the role of this NF-κB site in the induction of the IL-6 gene by TNF and phorbol esters,[24,25] we mutated each of the above-mentioned response elements and explored the IL-1 inducibility of the mutated promoters. Mutation at the AP-1-like site did not reduce the responsiveness of the promoter to IL-1 in HeLa cells. The construct pmMRE IIb225 mutated at the NF-IL6 site had greatly diminished responsiveness to IL-1 in HeLa cells, while pmNF-κB225 harboring a mutation at the NF-κB site completely lost IL-1 responsiveness.

To further investigate if the activation of pIC225 depends on the presence of both the NF-IL6 (also called multiple cytokine- and second messenger-responsive enhancer sequence II or MRE II) and the NF-κB sites, we performed a similar experiment in undifferentiated F9 embryonal carcinoma cells which lack NF-IL6, NF-κB and AP-1-like activities. The F9 cells were cotransfected with pIC225 and expression vectors for various transcription factors either singly or in combinations. The effect of overexpression of these transcription factors on IL-6 promoter activity was assayed. In F9 cells, no pIC225 expression was detected with any of the singly co-transfected expression vectors. Only a combination of CMVNF-IL6 and pRSV65 (expression vectors for human NF-IL6 and the p65 subunit of NF-κB respectively) yielded a 10-fold increase in CAT expression over basal expression.[26] Interestingly, co-expression of p49, the processed product of p100, similar to p50 of NF-κB, completely inhibited the increased CAT expression obtained by a combination of pRSV65 and CMVNF-IL6.[26] Other combinations of expression vectors had no effect on CAT expression.[26] These results indicate that these two subunits of NF-κB differ in their abilities to modulate IL-6 gene expression in combination with NF-IL6.

Based on the results of our mutational analyses, it appeared unlikely that the transcription factor AP-1 would be a target for repression of IL-6 gene expression by GR since the AP-1-like sequence in the IL-6 promoter did not appear to contribute to its activation in F9 cells and to at least IL-1 in HeLa cells. Repression of IL-6 gene expression could not be explained by the weak binding of GR to IL-6 promoter sequences alone since such weak interactions did not seem adequate to exclude the positive factors from their binding sites.

IS NF-κB A TARGET FOR REPRESSION BY GR?

Given that the NF-κB site in the IL-6 promoter was clearly important for its activation, and since NF-κB is involved in the activation of multiple inflammation-associated genes, we reasoned that it might be a target for repression by GR, at least in the context of IL-6-promoter activity.

In cotransfection experiments in F9 cells, activation of the IL-6 promoter by a combination of NF-IL6 and the p65 subunit of NF-κB was significantly reduced by GR in the presence of dexamethasone.[26] Furthermore, in electrophoretic mobility shift experiments, a deletion derivative of GR, GRΔS, devoid of its steroid binding domain, greatly diminished the ability of p65 to bind to the IL-6-κB sequence.[26]

DIRECT PHYSICAL ASSOCIATION BETWEEN GR AND p65

To investigate the possibility that the antagonism between GR and p65 might be due to direct association, we tested whether the proteins in solution could be chemically cross-linked. We also examined whether p49 and the leucine zipper and basic amino acid domain of NF-IL6 (ΔNF-IL6) could interact with GRΔS. For these experiments, p49, ΔNF-IL6 and p65 were synthesized in reticulocyte lysates in the presence of [^{35}S]methionine. Due to the similar molecular sizes of P65 and GRΔS, which did not allow resolution of the bands present in the same lane, GRΔS was synthesized in the presence of an amino acid mixture containing unlabeled methionine. The receptor construct GRΔS retained i) the two zinc-fingers, which are required for its repressor function on the IL-6 promoter[16,21] and the AP-1 site[17-20] and ii) the adjacent putative amphipathic helix that has been proposed to be involved in protein-protein interactions. Unlabeled GRΔS was incubated with either of the radio-labeled proteins p65, p49 or ΔNF-IL6 and the mixtures were treated with the cross-linking agent dithio-*bis* (succinimidyl propionate) (DSP). The reactions were immunoprecipitated with receptor-specific antibody, the immune complexes were reduced (to reverse the cross-links) and the labeled proteins were subjected to SDS-PAGE (FIG. 1).

Under these conditions, only labeled p65 was co-precipitated, and neither of the other two proteins could be detected (FIG. 1). The fuzzy band on the top migrating above p65 are from non-specific interactions with inefficiently reversed cross-linked proteins as has been previously observed by others.[17] The experiment was next repeated using control antiserum in parallel with the specific antisera. Non-immune serum did not coimmunoprecipitatie p65 under similar conditions.[26] In additional experiments we have also demonstrated association between GR and p65 in intact cells.[26] The oligomeric composition of the interacting proteins has not been addressed in our experiments.

p65 Represses GR-mediated Activation

The experiments discussed above suggested that GR can interact with p65 to inhibit its activity. In the event of such an interaction, it seemed conceivable that p65 will inhibit the the ability of GR to activate transcription. Wild-type GR is a potent hormone-dependent activator of the murine mammary tumor virus (MTV) long terminal repeat (LTR) in HeLa cells. Cotransfection of pRSV65 inhibited the GR-dependent activation of pMTV-CAT.[26] This inhibition was p65-specific and not due to cross-competition for common transcription factors between the promoters RSV and MTV, since cotransfection with pRSV49 had no effect on *trans*activation of the MTV promoter by GR and Dex.[26]

Our studies have identified a novel target for GR which is the p65 subunit of NF-κB. A possible explanation for our failure to detect an interaction between GR and NF-IL-6, as reported by Nishio *et al.*,[27] is that the complex was unstable under our assay conditions.

NEGATIVE REGULATION OF IL-6 GENE EXPRESSION BY 17β-ESTRADIOL

The secretion of interleukin-6 from freshly explanted endometrial stromal cells, in response to cytokines such as IL-1 and tumor necrosis factor (TNF) and interferon-

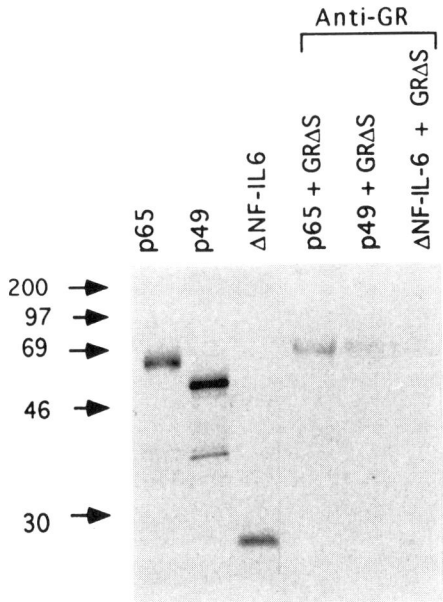

FIGURE 1. Cross-linking of *in vitro* synthesized p65 and GRΔS. GRΔS comprised amino acids 1-596 of human GR. p65, p49 and truncated NF-IL6 (ΔNF-IL-6 contained amino acids 111-276 of murine NF-IL6) were prepared *in vitro* using TNT rabbit reticulocyte lysates (Promega) in the presence of [^{35}S]labeled-methionine. Unlabeled GRΔS was synthesized similarly using a complete amino acid mixture containing unlabeled methionine. The labeled translation products (2 μl) are shown in the left three lanes and represent a 6 hour exposure. 10 μl samples of the labeled translation mixtures were incubated with 10 μl of a mixture containing unlabeled GRΔS. The reaction mixtures were then subjected to chemical cross-linking with DSP and the cross-linked products were immunoprecipitated with an anti-GR antibody raised against rat GR. The immunoprecipitates were washed extensively before cross-links were reduced by boiling in 2 × SDS-PAGE sample buffer containing 10% β-mercaptoethanol. The products were resolved on a 15% SDS-polyacrylamide and the gel was subjected to fluorography and autoradiography. The lanes showing the immunoprecipitated products represent a 2 day exposure.

γ, can be inhibited by estradiol-17β (E2).[28] Based on inhibition of IL-6 production by estrogens in bone-derived cells and osteoblastic cells,[29] and the promotion of osteoclast formation by IL-6,[30] it has been suggested that uninhibited production of IL-6 in an estrogen-depleted state may contribute to postmenopausal osteoporosis in women.

Inhibition of IL-6 gene expression by estrogens is the only physiologically relevant example of repression of gene expression by estrogens. It was intriguing to investigate the mechanism by which this is achieved in light of the fact that the IL-6 promoter lacks consensus estrogen response elements (EREs).

In transient transfection experiments, IL-1-induced activation of the IL-6 promoter was efficiently inhibited by wt ER.[31] However, estrogen receptors carrying mutations within or overlapping with the DNA-binding domain did not repress IL-6 promoter activity.[31] Furthermore, activation of the IL-6 promoter, elicited by a combination of NF-IL6 and the p65 subunit of NF-κB was inhibited by the wt receptor but not by a receptor containing a mutation in its DNA-binding domain. The repression of the IL-6 promoter by a combination of ER and E2, unlike activation of EREs by the same combination, did not appear to be mediated via high-affinity binding of the receptor to the promoter.[31] In functional experiments, the transactivator function of ER was totally inhibited by overexpression of p65 and to a lesser extent by that of NF-IL6. These results indicate that ER may repress expression in the absence of high-affinity DNA-binding.

FUNCTIONAL ANTAGONISM BETWEEN STEROID RECEPTORS AND NF-κB?

What is the biological significance of the reciprocal functional antagonism between steroid receptors and the p65 subunit of NF-κB? NF-κB is an inducible transcription factor which participates in the induction of numerous cellular and viral genes.[32] The target genes of NF-κB include the cytokine genes and other inflammation-associated genes.[32] The transcriptionally active complex of classical NF-κB is composed of two subunits p65 and p50.[33,34] It is not surprising that the p65 subunit of NF-κB is a target for repression by steroids given that independent transactivation potential of p65 is now well established. Recently, the potential role of individual subunits of NF-κB in regulation of gene expression was examined by introducing anti-sense oligonucleotides complementary p50 and p65 into embryonic stem cells.[35] Antisense oligonucleotides to p65 alone caused profound inhibition of cell adhesion.[35] It was suggested that p65 has important functions in resting cells and cannot exist solely complexed with the cytoplasmic inhibitor IκB.[35] p65 has been recently mapped to 11q13, a site involved in several types of tumor-associated abnormalities including breast cancer.[36]

A MODEL FOR SYNERGISM AND ANTAGONISM BETWEEN STEROID RECEPTORS AND POSITIVE TRANSCRIPTION FACTORS

It appears that steroid receptors can synergize with positive transcription factors to activate gene expression typically when the cognate consensus binding sites for both are present in the promoter of the particular gene. For example, in certain host cells, GR and OTF-1 synergize to activate promoters containing an octamer site in close proximity to the GRE.[15,37,38] Similarly, GR and NF-IL6 can synergistically activate the expression of the α_1-acid glycoprotein gene which contains the binding sites for both transcription factors.[27] However, OTF-1 can also be the target for negative regulation by GR via direct protein-protein interactions, in the absence of a GRE in the promoter of the target gene.[39] Similarly, NF-IL6/p65 may be the target for negative regulation by steroids, in the absence of high-affinity binding sites for steroid receptors in the promoters of genes such as the IL-6 gene.[26,31]

According to the simple model in FIGURE 2, negative regulation by steroid receptors might occur when the receptor binds to a site overlapping with the binding site of the positive factor such that the net outcome of the interaction would be just the reverse of what occurs in a synergistic interaction between the factors leading to activation of the promoter. Since most often the binding of the steroid receptor to these "nGRE" sites is weak, the positive factor binding to the adjacent site may help to tether the receptor to DNA at the cost of its transactivation function. This model might explain glucocorticoid repression of the gene for the α-subunit gene of the glycoprotein hormone.[13] In the case of the nGRE characterized in the mouse proliferin

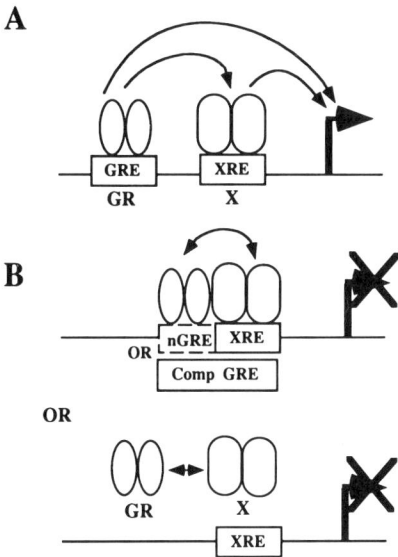

FIGURE 2. Model for (A) activation and (B) repression of gene transcription by the liganded glucocorticoid receptor (GR). A: Activation by GR is induced by binding of GR to consensus glucocorticoid response elements (GRE) and the simultaneous binding of the positive factor X to the cognate response element (XRE). Activation may result from simultaneous interaction of the two proteins with the basal transcription apparatus which may also involve direct association between the proteins GR and X. B: Repression may result from binding of the repressor (GR) an the activator (X) to nonoverlapping or overlapping DNA sequences. In this scheme, protein-protein interactions between the bound transcription factors would affect the activation function of X without compromising its DNA-binding. The nGRE might be similar to the ones identified in the human glycoprotein α-subunit gene, the bovine prolactin gene or the IL-6 gene (across the NF-IL6 binding site) or may be a composite GRE such as the one described in the mouse proliferin promoter. In the case of the proliferin composite GRE receptor activity is determined by the ratio of different non-receptor factors. Repression by GR may also result from interaction between GR and X such that the activator X is prevented from binding DNA. This model might explain transcriptional interference between i) GR and AP-1 in inhibition of the collagenase gene and ii) GR and p65 in GR-mediated inhibition of the IL-6 gene.

promoter, the net outcome in the presence of glucocorticoids appears to depend on the concentration of the nonreceptor factors. In the presence of excess Jun, which would lead to formation of Jun homodimers, interaction of GR with the nGRE and the simultaneous interaction of Jun with the AP-1 site would actually enhance the activation mediated by Jun alone, as proposed by Yamamoto and his colleagues.[17] However, the binding of the receptor to the same nGRE sequence together with binding of the Jun:Fos heterodimer to the AP-1 site would lead to inhibition of expression from the AP-1 site.[17] It is important to realize that the composite GRE does not respond to glucocorticoids alone. The expression of the collagenase gene is also dependent on an AP-1 site in the promoter. However, although glucocorticoids also downmodulate expression of the collagenase gene, the receptor in this case does not bind to the promoter. In this case, transcriptional interference between AP-1 and

GR has been proposed to involve nonproductive heterodimeric complexes between GR and Fos/Jun.

In the case of the IL-6 gene, we propose that the interaction between the p65 subunit of NF-κB and GR is similar to the collagenase situation involving interference without binding of the receptor to the NF-κB site (FIG. 2B). If the interaction between GR and NF-IL6, as proposed by Nishio *et al.*, can occur on DNA, inhibition would result by a mechanism somewhat similar to the AP-1/GR interaction on the composite GRE in the proliferin promoter. Therefore, in summary, the repression of the IL-6 gene by steroids may involve a combinatorial mechanism involving both receptor-interacting and non-interacting sites.

REFERENCES

1. NAITOH, Y., J. FUKATA, T. TOMINAGA, S. TAMAI, K. MORI & H. IMURA. 1988. Biophys. Res. Commun. **155:** 1459–1463.
2. RIVIER, C., W. VALE & M. BROWN. 1989. Endocrinology **125:** 3096–3102.
3. GWOSDOW, A., M. KUMAR & H. BODE. 1990. Am. J. Physiol. **258:** E65–E70.
4. SPANGELO, B. L., A. M. JUDD, P. C. ISAKSON & R. M. MACLEOD. 1989. Endocrinology **125:** 575–577.
5. VANKELECOM, H., P. CARMELIET, J. VAN DAMME, A. BILLIAU & D. DENEF. 1989. Neuroendocrinology **49:** 102–106.
6. EVANS, R. M. 1988. Science **240:** 889–895.
7. LUCAS, P. C. & D. K. GRANNER. 1992. Am. Rev. Biochem. **61:** 1131–1173.
8. KING, W. J. & G. L. GREENE. 1984. Nature (Lond.) **307:** 745–749.
9. PERROT-APPLANAT, M., F. LOGEAT, M. T. GROYER-PICARD & E. MILGROM. 1985. Endocrinology **116:** 1473–1484.
10. FUXE, K., A. C. WIKSTROM, S. OKRET, L. F. AGNATI, A. HARFSTRAND, Z. Y. YU, L. GRANHOLM, M. ZOLI, W. VALE & J. A. GUSTAFSSON. 1985. Endocrinology **117:** 1803–1812.
11. LOMBES, M., N. FARMAN, M. E. OBLIN, E. E. BAULIEU, J. P. BONVALET, B. F. ERLANGER & J. M. GASC. 1990. Proc. Natl. Acad. Sci. USA **87:** 1086–1088.
12. BEATO, M. 1989. Cell **56:** 335–344.
13. AKERBLOM, I. E., P. E. SLATER, M. BEATO, J. D. BAXTER & P. L. MELLON. 1988. Science **241:** 341–343.
14. SAKAI, D., D. D. HELMS, S. HELMS, J. CARLSTEDT-DUKE, J. A. GUSTAFSSON, F. M. ROTTMAN & K. R. YAMAMOTO. 1988. Genes Dev. **2:** 1144–1154.
15. SCHULE, R., M. MULLER, C. KALTSCMIDT & R. RENKAWITZ. 1988. Science **242:** 1418–1420.
16. RAY, A., K. S. LAFORGE & P. B. SEHGAL. 1990. Mol. Cell. Biol. **10:** 5736–5746.
17. DIAMOND, M. I., J. N. MINER, S. K. YOSHINAGA & K. R. YAMAMOTO. 1990. Science **249:** 1266–1272.
18. JONAT, C., H. J. RAHMSDORF, K.-K. PARK, A. C. B. CATO, S. GEBEL, H. PONTA & P. HERRLICH. 1990. Cell **62:** 1189–1204.
19. SCHULE, R., P. RANGARAJAN, S. KLIEWER, L. J. RANSONE, J. BOLADO, N. YANG, I. M. VERMA & R. M. EVANS. 1990. Cell **62:** 1217–1226.
20. YANG-YEN, H.-F. Y., J. C. CHAMBARD, Y.-L. SUN, T. SMEAL, T. J. SCHMIDT, J. DROUIN & M. KARIN. 1990. Cell **62:** 1205–1215.
21. RAY, A., K. S. LAFORGE & P. B. SEHGAL. 1991. Proc. Natl. Acad. Sci. USA **88:** 7086–7090.
22. RAY, A., S. B. TATTER, L. T. MAY & P. B. SEHGAL. 1988. Proc. Natl. Acad. Sci. USA **85:** 6701–6705.
23. RAY, A., P. SASSONE-CORSI & P. B. SEHGAL. 1989. Mol. Cell. Biol. **9:** 5537–5547.
24. LIEBERMANN, T. A. & D. BALTIMORE. 1990. Mol. Cell. Biol. **10:** 2327–2334.
25. ZHANG, Y., J.-X. LIN & J. VILCEK. 1990. Mol. Cell. Biol. **10:** 3818–3823.
26. RAY, A. & K. E. PREFONTAINE. 1994. Proc. Natl. Acad. Sci. USA **91:** 752–756.

27. NISHIO, Y., H. ISSHIKI, T. KISHIMOTO & S. AKIRA. 1993. Mol. Cell. Biol. **13:** 1854–1862.
28. TABIBZADEH, S. S., U. SANTHANAM, P. B. SEHGAL & L. T. MAY. 1989. J. Immunol. **142:** 3134–3139.
29. GIRASOLE, G., R. L. JILKA, G. PASSERI, S. BOSWELL, G. BODER, D. C. WILLIAMS & S. C. MANOLAGAS. 1992. J. Clin. Invest. **89:** 883–891.
30. JILKA, R. L., G. HANGOC, G. GIRASOLE, G. PASSERI, D. C. WILLIAMS, J. S. ABRAMS, B. BOYCE, H. BROXMEYER & S. C. MANOLAGAS. 1992. Science **257:** 88–91.
31. RAY, A., K. E. PREFONTAINE & P. RAY. 1994. J. Biol. Chem. **269:** 12940–12946.
32. BAEUERLE, P. A. & D. BALTIMORE. 1991. Transcription. P. Cohen & J. G. Foulkes, Eds. 409–432. Amsterdam: Elsevier/North Holland Biomedical Press.
33. BAEUERLE, P. A. & D. BALTIMORE. 1989. Genes Dev. **3:** 1689–1698.
34. KAWAKAMI, K., C. SCHEIDERIET & R. G. ROEDER. 1988. Proc. Natl. Acad. Sci. USA **85:** 4700–4704.
35. NARAYANAN, R., K. A. HIGGINS, J. R. PEREZ, T. A. COLEMAN & C. A. ROSEN. 1993. Mol. Cell. Biol. **13:** 3802–3810.
36. MATHEW, S., V. V. V. S. MURTY, R. DALLA-FAVERA & R. S. K. CHAGANTI. 1993. Oncogene **8:** 191–193.
37. WIELAND, S., U. DOBBELING & S. RUSCONI. 1991. EMBO J. **10:** 2513–2521.
38. BRUGGEMEIER, U., M. KALFF, S. FRANKE, C. SCHEIDEREIT & M. BEATO. 1991. Cell **64:** 565–572.
39. KUTOH, E., P.-E. STROMSTEDT & L. POELLINGER. 1992. Mol. Cell. Biol. **12:** 4960–4969.

DISCUSSION OF THE PAPER

H. BAUMANN (*Roswell Park Cancer Institute, Buffalo, NY*): In your experiments you use an expression vector with the CAT reporter gene construct, which has a very low basal level. In essence, what one sees is actually prevention of IL-1 stimulation, or can you rule out in another experiment an active suppression by glucocorticoid receptors, such as by using a slightly higher expression vector which does not need stimulation to prove the point of the inhibition by glucocorticoid?

A. RAY: What you are asking perhaps relates to the binding of the receptor to the basal elements. I might add again that the binding affinity to any of these sites is extremely weak, and if we do activate the promoter with IL-1 then without adding the ligand dexamethasone we do not see any inhibition, which shows that it is ligand dependent. We do see that over and above the basal level whatever activation we can get can be actually brought down to low basal levels, so we feel that it may be that the binding to the basal promoter element is relevant. We have not so far addressed this in our studies.

BAUMANN: So, that is only because your treatment period is probably 24h. It is a very long time considering the action of the glucocorticoids.

RAY: We have also done shorter time points. The results we have shown were over long periods of time, but it also happens when you treat for shorter periods.

G. FEY (*University of Erlangen-Nürnberg, Erlangen, Germany*): Could you explain once more, please, your last interpretation where you tried to explain what you have observed in the IL-6 gene following the models of Yamamoto and Miner with the composite GRE and Michael Karin's collegenase model? And you said that you might have a combination of both. What does that mean?

RAY: We feel that in the sense that we do not see any binding, at least by footprinting studies or DNA sequence-binding immunoprecipitation studies as well as by gel-shift experiments. We have not seen any binding of the receptor to the NF-κB site.

FEY: So, that would be more like the collagenase model.

RAY: Exactly. However, we have seen repeatedly binding across the MRE region which has the NF-IL-6 site. And we have not been able to demonstrate any interaction between NF-IL-6 and GR. Dr. Kishimoto and his colleagues have shown an interaction between the two proteins, and if that is the case, then we believe that this might occur through a mechanism similar to the proliferin gene.

FEY: Well, Dr. Kishimoto's data are co-transfections with expression constructs for both. They have not actually shown direct interaction between both proteins.

RAY: That is in the case of the α_1-acid glycoprotein gene, right? But there is GRE present.

FEY: Yes, but they have not done co-precipitations.

RAY: I thought they had.

FEY: No. I think that your data point more in the direction of collagenase. Let me ask you something about estrogen, the repression by estrogen. Probably I did not get the point, but do you have evidence that you have these protein-protein interactions for the estrogen receptor as for the glucocorticoid receptor?

RAY: Yes, we have. But we have not really worked out all the details. We are working on it.

FEY: And for the androgen receptor? Because there are also examples of repression by androgens.

RAY: No, I have no evidence for that.

FEY: And the repression mechanism that you observe for estrogen is also interaction with p65?

RAY: Yes.

G. CILIBERTO: Do you think that the repression is due to inhibition of nuclear localization of the complex? Do you think that the mechanism might be inhibition of the nuclear translocation of p65?

RAY: Well, if it is, that would be very interesting, because, again, it does not seem to occur with other members. I showed you with p49. As you know, both of these proteins exist in the native state as multi-subunit complexes. We do not know whether GR interacts with p65 in the cytoplasm.

HEINRICH: What happens if you also co-transfect the p50 and the inhibitor?

RAY: We are now doing that experiment.

Interleukin-11 in Respiratory Inflammation

O. EINARSSON,[a] G. P. GEBA,[a] Z. ZHOU,[a] M. L. LANDRY,[b]
R. A. PANETTIERI, JR.,[c] D. TRISTRAM,[b] R. WELLIVER,[d]
A. METINKO,[a] AND J. A. ELIAS[a,e]

[a]*Section of Pulmonary and Critical Care Medicine*
Department of Internal Medicine
Yale University School of Medicine
333 Cedar Street, 105 LCI
New Haven, Connecticut 06520-8057

[b]*Department of Laboratory Medicine*
Yale University School of Medicine
333 Cedar Street
New Haven, Connecticut 06520

[c]*Pulmonary and Critical Care Division*
University of Pennsylvania Medical Center
8004 East Gates
3400 Spruce Street
Philadelphia, Pennsylvania 19104-4283

[d]*Division of Infectious Diseases*
State University of New York at Buffalo
219 Bryant Street
Buffalo, New York 14222

INTRODUCTION

It was not long ago that asthma was considered largely in terms of abnormal airway smooth muscle contractility. The well known clinical observation that steroids are an effective treatment for the majority of patients with asthma and more recent studies using bronchoalveolar lavage (BAL) and bronchial biopsy have, however, prompted a re-evaluation of this concept and a renewed appreciation of the role of inflammation in this disorder.[1,2] As a result, asthma is now felt to be a chronic inflammatory disorder involving a variety of cells, including mast cells, T lymphocytes (particularly Th$_2$ cells), macrophages, granulocytes, platelets, basophils and epithelial cells.[1-4] They have also demonstrated that the cell-cell interactions that occur in the asthmatic inflammatory response are extremely complex and that a variety of mediators including histamine, prostaglandins, and cytokines may play important roles in this inflammatory process.[5-8] Dysregulated interleukin-6 (IL-6) production has also been well documented in antigen-induced asthma and airway inflammation.[5,7] However, the role that IL-6 plays in asthma and the importance in asthma of other IL-6-type cytokines such as interleukin-11 (IL-11) have not been adequately investigated.

---

[e] Address correspondence and reprint requests to Jack A. Elias, M.D.; Tel: (203) 785-4163.

IL-11 is a newly appreciated pleotropic cytokine that was originally discovered as a cross-reacting cytokine in an IL-6 bioassay.[9] Early studies of this molecule focused on its roles in hematopoiesis, its ability to stimulate the acute phase response and its ability to inhibit adipocyte differentiation. There are, however, a number of features of IL-11 that make it a particularly intriguing cytokine for students of asthmatic inflammation. First, IL-11 is unusual among cytokines in that it is a highly cationic molecule (pI ≥ 11). Cationic molecules like eosinophil major basic protein (pI 10.9) are felt to play an important role in asthma since they induce bronchospasm and airway hyperresponsiveness *in vivo*.[10] Secondly, IL-11 is known to be a T cell–dependent stimulator of B cell immunoglobulin production[11] and activated T cells are felt to play an important role in the pathogenesis of asthma.[3,12] Lastly, IL-11 is a member of the IL-6-type cytokine family and members of this family, in particular leukemia inhibitory factor (LIF), have the ability to induce cholinergic neuronal differentiation and stimulate tachykinin production.[13] Cholinergic hyperactivity and increased tachykinin production could contribute to the airways hyperresponsiveness and bronchospasm characteristic of the asthmatic diathesis.[14,15] As a result of these properties, we speculated that IL-11 might play an important role in the inflammation and physiology of the asthmatic airway. To test this hypothesis we characterized the ability of lung stromal cells (fibroblasts, epithelial-like cells and smooth muscle cells) to produce IL-11, investigated whether IL-11 was detectable in complex human biologic fluids and determined whether IL-11 had definable effects on the physiology of the mouse airway. Our studies demonstrate that a variety of stromal cells have the ability to produce IL-11 and that they do so in response to inflammatory cytokines and after infection with respiratory viruses. They also demonstrate that IL-11 can be found in the nasal secretions from children with upper respiratory tract infections and that aspiration of IL-11 into the mouse airway results in a state of airways hyperresponsiveness to methacholine.

MATERIALS AND METHODS

Cells and Cell Culture

CCL-202 human lung fibroblasts and A549 transformed alveolar epithelial-like cells were obtained from the American Type Culture Collection (ATCC, Rockville, MD). 9HTE transformed bronchial epithelial-like cells were obtained courtesy of Drs. D. Gruenert (University of CA at San Francisco) and J. Fine (Norwalk Hospital, Norwalk, CT). Human airway smooth muscle cells were prepared from surgical specimens and characterized using techniques previously described by our laboratories.[16] Each cell type was grown to confluence in nutritionally complete medium supplemented with 10% fetal calf serum. Once confluent they were washed and incubated in the presence and absence of mediator(s) and/or virus. When cytokines or histamine were employed the cells were incubated with the stimulant(s) throughout the incubation period. When viruses were employed the cells were incubated with virus at a multiplicity of infection (M.O.I.) of 3 for 90 minutes, washed and then incubated in complete medium. At the end of the incubation period, supernatant IL-11 levels and steady state IL-11 mRNA levels were quantitated as described below.

Quantification of IL-11

The IL-11 levels in supernatants from unstimulated and stimulated cells were evaluated by ELISA as previously described.[17] Monoclonal antibody 11h3/19.6.1 was used as the capture antibody and the monoclonal antibody 11h3/15.6.1 was used as the detection antibody. Both antibodies were gifts of Dr. Edward Alderman (Genetics Institute, Cambridge, MA).

mRNA Isolation and Analysis

Total cellular RNA was extracted from cell monolayers using the acid-guanadinium-thiocyanate-phenol-chloroform extraction protocol previously described.[17] The RNA was then size fractionated by electrophoresis through agarose-formaldehyde gels, transferred to nylon membranes and hybridized with ^{32}P-labeled cDNA probes. Clone pHuIL-11/PMT, a 1,250 bp IL-11 cDNA, was a gift of Dr. Paul Schendel (Genetics Institute). It was labeled via nick translation and its binding assessed after washing under conditions of high stringency. The adequacy of gel loading was assessed via ethidium-bromide staining or by hybridizing with cDNA encoding control genes.

Nasal Aspirate IL-11 Levels

Studies were undertaken to determine if IL-11 could be detected in the nasal secretions from children with upper respiratory tract infections. To accomplish this nasal aspirates were obtained from children presenting to Yale-New Haven Hospital with a clinical picture compatible with respiratory syncytial virus (RSV) infection. Nasal aspirates were also obtained from non-infected floor mates and children with a variety of other disorders. In all cases, 0.5–1.0 ml of sterile normal saline was instilled into the nasal cavity and then aspirated. The IL-11 in these aspirates was evaluated by ELISA as described above after appropriate samples were removed for viral culture and/or RSV antigen detection. The correlations between IL-11 levels and clinical characteristics were undertaken after a retrospective chart analysis.

Characterization of the Effects of IL-11 on Mouse Airway Physiology

Studies were undertaken to determine whether IL-11 could alter airway physiology *in vivo*. To accomplish this mice were lightly anesthetized and allowed to aspirate rhIL-11 (10 μg/animal) or vehicle control into their lungs. Twenty-four to 48 hours later airways resistance was evaluated using the techniques of Martin *et al*.[18] Pulmonary resistance was calculated using the method of Amdur and Mead.[19] Methacholine sensitivity was also assessed. This was done using techniques as previously described by our laboratories[20] and expressed as the PC_{100}, the dose of methacholine (μg/ml) required to increase airways resistance by 100%.

RESULTS

Lung Cell IL-11 Production

To begin to understand the role(s) that IL-11 plays in pulmonary biology, studies were undertaken to characterize the cells in the lung that have the ability to produce this cytokine. Since previous studies have demonstrated that stromal cells can produce IL-11 under appropriate circumstances,[9] lung fibroblasts, A549 cells, 9HTE cells and airway smooth muscle cells were the focus of these studies. Their responses to cytokines, histamine, viruses and other infectious agents were evaluated.

Cytokine Regulation of IL-11

Under basal culture conditions the levels of IL-11 produced by all 4 cell populations were near or below the limits of detection with our ELISA (50–100 pg/ml). In contrast, recombinant interleukin-1-α (rIL-1-α) and transforming growth factor-β_1 (TGF-β_1) were effective stimulators of IL-11 production by all 4 cell populations. In all cases, the effects were dose-dependent with peak stimulation being noted with concentrations of rIL-1-α ≥ 2.5 ng/ml and concentrations of TGF-β_1 ≥ 10 ng/ml. The elaboration of IL-11 in response to these cytokines was also time-dependent, being noticeable after within 4 hours and quite prominent after 24–48 hours of incubation. These stimulatory effects of rIL-1-α and TGF-β_1 were, at least partially, pretranslationally mediated since they were associated with comparable alterations in IL-11 mRNA accumulation. They were not generalizable, however, to all inflammatory cytokines since rIL-7, rIL-10 and rIL-4 at comparable concentrations did not have similar effects. A representative example of the stimulatory effects of rIL-1-α and TGF-β_1 on human airway smooth muscle cell IL-11 production can be seen in TABLE 1.

Since target tissues *in vivo* are likely to be exposed to multiple cytokines simultaneously, studies were undertaken to determine whether IL-1, TGF-β_1 and IL-4 interacted in the regulation of IL-11 production. In studies performed with CCL-202 lung fibroblasts, A549 epithelial-like cells and airway smooth muscle cells, a remarkable interaction of IL-1 and TGF-β_1 was appreciated. In all cases, the IL-11 production and mRNA accumulation of cells incubated with rIL-1-α plus TGF-β_1 in combination, was significantly greater than the sum of the levels produced by cells incubated with these cytokines individually. These interactions were synergistic in nature as demonstrated by isobolographic analysis. They were also at least partially specific for IL-1 and TGF-β_1 since IL-4 did not interact with rIL-1-α or TGF-β_1 in a similar fashion. In fact, in CCL-202 human lung fibroblasts, IL-4 inhibited rIL-1-induced and TGF-β_1-induced IL-11 protein production and mRNA accumulation in a dose- and time-dependent fashion (TABLE 2), suggesting that IL-4 may serve to dampen IL-11 production *in vivo*.

Histamine Regulation of IL-11

To determine if IL-11 plays a role in histamine-mediated biologic events, studies were undertaken to determine whether CCL-202 human lung fibroblasts produced

TABLE 1. Cytokine Stimulation of Human Airway Smooth Muscle IL-11

Incubation Conditions[a]	IL-11[b]
Unstimulated	0.13
IL-1	10.29
TGF-β_1	13.65
IL-1 + TGF-β_1	106.30

[a] Human airway smooth muscle cells were incubated for 48 hours in the presence and absence of rIL-1-α (2.5 ng/ml) and/or TGF-β_1 (10 ng/ml) as noted.

[b] IL-11-ng/ml; values represent mean of duplicates that were within 10% of one another.

TABLE 2. IL-4 Regulation of Human Lung Fibroblast IL-11

Incubation Conditions[a]	IL-11[b]
Unstimulated	N.D.
IL-1	2.11
TGF-β	6.53
IL-4	N.D.
IL-1 + IL-4	0.51
TGF-β + IL-4	1.13

[a] Fibroblasts were incubated for 24 hours with rIL-1-α (2.5 ng/nl), TGF-β_1 (10 ng/ml) and/or rIL-4 (10 ng/ml) as noted.

[b] IL-11 production; ng/10^6 cells. Values represent means of duplicate assays that were within 10% of one another. N.D. = None detected.

IL-11 in response to this mediator. Unstimulated fibroblasts did not produce significant amounts of IL-11. Histamine was a weak stimulator of fibroblast IL-11 production but only at high concentrations (≥ 20 μM). When fibroblasts were incubated with histamine and TGF-β_1 in combination a remarkable interaction was noted. Under these conditions fibroblasts produced levels of IL-11 that were significantly greater than the levels produced by cells stimulated with these mediators individually. This interaction was dose- and time-dependent. It could be appreciated within 4 hours and was more prominent after 24 hours of fibroblast-TGF-β_1-histamine incubation. The highest levels of IL-11 were noted in supernatants from fibroblasts incubated with 10 ng/ml of TGF-β_1 and doses of histamine ≥ 20 μM. However, doses of histamine as low as 0.2 μM and TGF-β_1 as low as 0.1 ng/ml interacted in a significant fashion to augment IL-11 production. This interaction was synergistic in nature as demonstrated by isobolographic analysis. It was also at least partially pretranslationally mediated since TGF-β_1 and histamine-induced alterations in IL-11 protein production were associated with comparable alterations in IL-11 mRNA accumulation. Interestingly, serotonin and tumor necrosis factor, at similar concentrations, did not interact in a similar fashion with TGF-β_1 and histamine, respectively.

Many of the effects of histamine are mediated by membrane histamine receptors. Thus, studies were undertaken to determine whether H_1 and/or H_2 histamine receptors were responsible for the synergistic interaction of histamine and TGF-β_1 noted in these studies. This was accomplished by determining whether H_1 and/or H_2 receptor antagonists abrogated this synergistic interaction and whether H_1 receptor and/or H_2 receptor agonists could replace histamine in this interactive process. Cimetidine (10^{-5}–10^{-6} M), a selective H_2 blocker[21] did not significantly alter the stimulatory effects of histamine, alone or in combination, with TGF-β_1. In contrast, the H_1 blockers pyrilamine (10^{-6} M) and diphenhydramine (10^{-5} M) were effective antagonists of these effects. In accord with these findings, 2-methylhistamine, a preferential H_1 receptor agonist, interacted with TGF-β_1 to synergistically augment fibroblast IL-11 production while 4-methylhistamine, a preferential H_2 agonist[21] did not share these properties (TABLE 3). These studies demonstrate that the synergistic stimulation of fibroblast IL-11 production caused by histamine and TGF-β_1 is largely dependent upon H_1 versus H_2 histamine receptor activation.

Viral Stimulation of IL-11

Studies were undertaken to determine if respiratory viruses stimulated fibroblast and epithelial-like cell IL-11 production. These studies were accomplished by infecting

TABLE 3. Histamine Analog Stimulation of IL-11

Fibroblast Incubation Conditions[a]	IL-11[b]
Unstimulated	0.12
2-methylhistamine	0.13
4-methylhistamine	0.10
TGF-β_1	3.87
TGF-β_1 + 2-methylhistamine	18.83
TGF-β_1 + 4-methylhistamine	4.1

[a] CCL-202 human lung fibroblasts were incubated for 24 hours in the presence of media alone (unstimulated) or TGF-β_1 (10 ng/ml), 2-methylhistamine (20 μM) and 4-methylhistamine (20 μM) as noted.

[b] IL-11 production; ng/10^6 cells. Values represent means of duplicates that were within 10% of one another.

cell monolayers with virus and characterizing IL-11 production at intervals thereafter. RSV (Long strain), parainfluenza virus type 3 and rhinovirus 14 were potent stimulators of A549 cell and CCL-202 lung fibroblast IL-11 production (TABLE 4) and mRNA accumulation. In contrast, herpes simplex virus Type 2 did not effectively stimulate and cytomegalovirus and adenovirus only weakly stimulated stromal IL-11 production despite documentable cell infection (TABLE 4). In addition, pneumococcus, staphylococcus and myobacterium avium intracellulare (provided courtesy of Dr. Keith Joiner, Yale University School of Medicine) also did not stimulate A549 cell or CCL-202 lung fibroblast IL-11 elaboration (TABLE 4).

IL-11 in Airway Fluids

To determine if the ability of specific viruses to stimulate IL-11 production *in vitro* was relevant to the *in vivo* state, studies were undertaken to determine if IL-11 could

TABLE 4. Stimulation of A549 Cell IL-11 Production by Infectious Agents

Experiment No.	Incubation Conditions[a]	IL-11[b]
1	Unstimulated	0.55
	RSV	3.93
	Rhino	6.39
	Parainfluenza 3	3.18
	HSV-2	0.61
	Adeno	0.89
	CMV	0.85
2	Unstimulated	0.21
	RSV	6.28
	Pneumococcus	0.29
	Staphylococcus	0.10
	Streptococcus	0.15

[a] A549 cells were either uninfected (unstimulated) or incubated with RSV (Long strain), Rhinovirus 14 (Rhino), Parainfluenza virus type 3, Herpes Simplex Virus type 2 (HSV-2), or cytomegalovirus (CMV), at a M.O.I. = 3 as noted.

[b] IL-11 ng/10^6 cells. Values represent means of duplicates that were within 10% of one another.

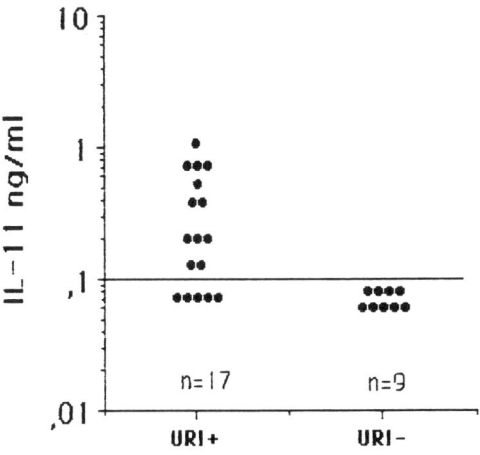

FIGURE 1. Demonstration of the IL-11 levels in nasal aspirates from children with clinical upper respiratory tract infections (U.R.I.+) and asymptomatic controls (U.R.I.−).

be detected in the airway secretions from patients with upper respiratory tract infections. To accomplish this we prospectively measured the IL-11 levels in nasal samples sent to the Virology Laboratory at Yale-New Haven Hospital for RSV isolation and/ or antigen detection during the 1993–1994 RSV season. The IL-11 levels in secretions from children with upper respiratory tract symptomatology were compared to the levels from children whose nasal aspirates were done for surveillance purposes or for other reasons. As can be seen in FIGURE 1, the IL-11 levels in the nasal aspirates from all of the children who did not have upper respiratory tract symptomatology were at or below the limits of detectability of our assay. In contrast, although some children with upper respiratory tract symptomatology had levels of IL-11 that were at or below the limits of detectability of this assay, the majority had elevated levels, many of which were easily detectable in the ng per ml range (FIG. 1). Similar differences were seen when the IL-11 levels of RSV positive (by antigen determination and/or culture) symptomatic patients were compared to those from RSV negative asymptomatic children. Interestingly, higher levels of IL-11 were detected in the secretions from children with reactive airway disease (children that were clinically found to be wheezing) than in children who did not manifest bronchospasm. These studies clearly demonstrate that, in contrast to controls, IL-11 can be detected in the nasal secretions from children with upper respiratory tract infections, particularly those due to RSV, and that the presence of IL-11 in these respiratory secretions correlates with the presence of bronchospasm in these children.

Effect of IL-11 on Airways Hyperresponsiveness in Vivo

The demonstration that viruses stimulate IL-11 production *in vitro* and the observation that IL-11 is present in the respiratory secretions of patients with respiratory viral infections led us to hypothesize that IL-11 plays an important role in the physiologic abnormalities (such as the airways hyperresponsiveness) seen in viral airways disorders. To test this hypothesis we determined whether IL-11 altered the airway physiology of BALB/c mice. In these experiments mouse lungs were airway challenged with rIL-11 (10 μg) or vehicle control and airways resistance and methacholine sensitivity

TABLE 5. Effect of IL-11 on Airways Hyperresponsiveness *in Vivo*

Treatment[a]	Log PC$_{100}$[b]
IL-11	0.49 ± 0.2
Vehicle Control	2.5 ± 0.25

[a] 10–12 week old female BALB/c mice aspirated rIL-11 (10 μg/animal) or vehicle control into their lungs and their methacholine sensitivity was measured 48 hours later.

[b] PC$_{100}$ = provocative challenge 100 = dose of methacholine (μg/ml) required to double airways resistance.

were evaluated 48 hours later. The baseline airways resistance of rIL-11 treated animals was not significantly different than the resistance of animals treated identically with vehicle control. IL-11 did, however, cause a marked increase in methacholine sensitivity with mice that received rIL-11 achieving a 100% increase in airways resistance at an approximately 100-fold lower dose of methacholine than the animals that received the vehicle control (TABLE 5). These studies clearly demonstrate that rIL-11 induces a state of airways hyperresponsiveness to methacholine *in vivo*.

DISCUSSION

To begin to understand the role that IL-11 plays in pulmonary biology and homeostasis, studies were undertaken to characterize the lung stromal cells that produce IL-11, to determine if IL-11 could be found in respiratory secretions and to characterize the effects of IL-11 on airway physiology. These studies demonstrate that a variety of stromal cells including smooth muscle cells, fibroblasts and alveolar and tracheobronchial epithelial-like cells produce IL-11 and that they do so in response to inflammatory cytokines, histamine and specific viruses. They also demonstrate that dysregulated IL-11 production can be detected in the airways of children with viral upper respiratory tract infections and that IL-11 is a potent stimulator of airways hyperresponsiveness *in vivo*.

The importance of an individual mediator within the complex cytokine networks regulating biologic homeostasis can often be deduced from an understanding of the stimuli that induce its production. Our studies demonstrate that IL-1, TGF-β_1 and histamine stimulate lung stromal cell IL-11 production while IL-4 inhibits IL-1 and TGF-β_1-stimulated IL-11 production by human lung fibroblasts. As a result of these studies, a complex network of interacting mediators (illustrated schematically in FIG. 2) appears to be involved in the regulation of the production of this important cyto-

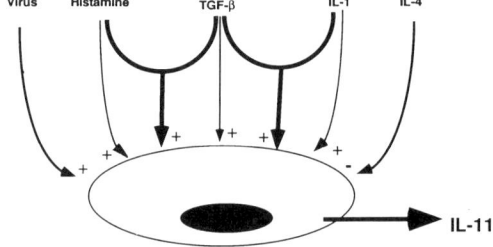

FIGURE 2. Schematic illustration of mediators and agents regulating stromal cell IL-11 production. Synergistic interactions are indicated by thick black arrows.

kine. These observations raise the possibility that some of the biologic effects attributed to IL-1, TGF-β_1 and/or histamine are mediated by IL-11. Alternatively, IL-11 might be an autocrine/paracrine inhibitor of IL-1-, TGF-β_1- and/or histamine-induced biologic effects. These findings also raise the possibility that IL-11 induction by histamine and inflammatory cytokines may contribute to the pathogenesis of chronic pulmonary inflammation, particularly the inflammation that frequently follows acute allergic phenomena, mast cell activation and histamine release.

Respiratory viruses are a major source of morbidity and mortality. This is clearly illustrated in asthma where viral infection is known to frequently cause disease exacerbation.[22,23] Epidemiologic studies have shown that the type of respiratory pathogen that causes an illness is an important determinant of its ability to induce an asthmatic exacerbation. RSV, parainfluenza virus and rhinovirus are the most likely to provoke asthma.[22,23] In contrast, CMV, HSV-2, adenovirus and bacterial and myobacterial infections are not associated with an increased incidence of asthmatic exacerbation.[22,23] Our studies demonstrate that RSV, parainfluenza type 3 and rhinovirus are major stimulators of IL-11 production, that CMV and adenovirus only weakly stimulate IL-11 production and that HSV-2, gram positive bacteria and mycobacteria do not stimulate stromal cell production of this cytokine. Thus, there is an impressive correlation between the ability of an infectious agent to stimulate lung stromal cell IL-11 production *in vitro* and the ability of this agent to cause an asthmatic exacerbations *in vivo*. This observation, our demonstration that IL-11 is detectable in the respiratory secretions of children with upper respiratory tract infections and our demonstration that IL-11 induces airways hyperresponsiveness, led us to speculate that IL-11 plays an important role in virus-induced asthmatic exacerbations. Underlying this speculation is the hypothesis that the ability of a virus to cause an asthmatic exacerbation is somehow related to its ability to induce IL-11 production and that the ability of IL-11 to induce airways hyperresponsiveness is directly involved in the pathogenesis of virally induced asthma. There are at least three ways that IL-11 could contribute to asthmatic exacerbations. First, the effects of IL-11 on T cells and B cells could contribute to the mononuclear cell infiltrate that is characteristic of this disorder. Second, IL-11 might also mediate the wheezing and bronchospasm that are frequently experienced by virally infected patients via its cationic nature (its pI is ≥ 11) since cationic molecules such as eosinophil major basic protein (pI 10.9) are important inducers of airways hyperreactivity.[10] Lastly, IL-11, IL-6, LIF, ciliary neurotropic factor and oncostatin M have recently been grouped together as the IL-6-type cytokines based on their overlapping spectra of biologic activity and commonality of subunit usage in their receptor complexes. One of the fascinating properties of some of these cytokines is their ability to stimulate neurons to take on a cholinergic phenotype and increase their production of tachykinins.[13] The induction of a cholinergic phenotype and stimulation of tachykinin production could further contribute to and exacerbate the asthmatic state.

A cardinal feature of asthma is the exaggerated bronchospastic response of the asthmatic to antigen and non-specific agents such as methacholine, histamine and cold air.[24] Although airways hyperresponsiveness and resulting bronchospasm was formerly thought to be the primary problem of the asthmatic airway, inflammation with the release of mediators from inflammatory cells is now thought to be the cause of this physiologic abnormality.[24] Consequently, bronchial hyperresponsiveness is now widely recognized as an index of airway inflammation[24] with the acknowledgment that there is a complex relationship between airways hyperresponsiveness and the inflammatory process. Despite the importance of airways hyperresponsiveness in asthma, the inflammatory events that mediate airways hyperresponsiveness are poorly understood. The limited information that is available suggests that, under appropriate circumstances, a variety of cytokines including IL-1,[25] TNF,[26] IL-5,[27] and IL-2[28] can contribute to asthmatic physiology. Our studies add to this body of data by demonstrating that IL-11 has the ability to induce airways hyperresponsiveness *in vivo* and by implicating IL-11 in the pathogenesis of viral asthmatic exacerbations.

In contrast to most inflammatory responses, asthmatic inflammation and bronchial hyperreactivity are often life-long processes. The mechanism(s) of this chronicity, however, is poorly understood. Persistent and/or latent viral infection, the persistence of sensitizing antigen, diminished alveolar macrophage suppressive influences, fibrosis-induced physiologic alterations, exaggerated steroid metabolism, local tissue T cell memory, and local neuronal alterations in the asthmatic airway have all been proposed as mechanisms for this chronicity. Evidence supporting or disproving these proposals, however, has not been forthcoming. Our studies demonstrate that lung stromal cells have the ability to produce IL-11. As such, they are in agreement with a large body of data demonstrating that stromal cells such as fibroblasts and epithelial cells have potent immune effector capabilities that can contribute to disease chronicity by amplifying and maintaining local tissue inflammation.[29–31] The ability of IL-11 to regulate the function of T and B lymphocytes[17] and possibly local neurons,[13] suggests that stromal cell-derived IL-11 production may play a role in the chronicity of the asthmatic inflammatory response.

In summary, our studies demonstrate that a variety of stromal cells in the human lung have the ability to produce IL-11 and that they do so in response to inflammatory cytokines, histamine, and specific respiratory viruses. They also demonstrate that there is a correlation between the ability of an infectious agent to stimulate stromal cell IL-11 production *in vitro* and the ability of this agent to cause asthmatic exacerbations *in vivo*. Finally, they demonstrate that dysregulated IL-11 can be detected in patients with upper respiratory tract infections and that IL-11 can induce airways hyperresponsiveness *in vivo*. As a result of these studies it is reasonable to conclude that IL-11 may be an important mediator in the pathogenesis of asthma and other chronic inflammatory disorders of the airway, particularly those that are virally induced.

REFERENCES

1. HOLGATE, S. T., J. R. WILSON & P. H. HOWARTH. 1991. New insights into airway inflammation by endobronchial biopsy. Am. Rev. Resp. Dis. **145:** S2–S6.
2. KAY, A. B. 1991. Asthma and inflammation. J. Allergy. Clin. Immunol. **87:** 893–910.
3. CORRIGAN, C. J. & A. B. KAY. 1992. T cells and eosinophils in the pathogenesis of asthma. Imunol. Today **13:** 501–507.
4. LEFF, A. R., K. J. HAMANN & C. D. WEGNER. 1991. Inflammation and cell-cell interactions in airway hyperresponsiveness. Am. J. Physiol. **260** (Lung Cell. Mol. Physiol. 4): L189–L206.
5. BROIDE, D. H., M. LOTZ, D. A. COBURN, E. C. FEDERMAN & S. I. WASSERMAN. 1992. Cytokines in symptomatic asthma airways. J. Allergy Clin. Immunol. **89:** 958–967.
6. CASALE, T. B., D. WOOD, H. B. RICHERSON, S. TRAPP, W. J. METZGER, D. ZAVALA & G. W. HUNNINGHAKE. 1987. Elevated bronchoalveolar lavage fluid histamine levels in allergic asthmatics are associated with methacholine bronchial hyperresponsiveness. J. Clin. Invest. **79:** 1197–1203.
7. GOSSET, P., A. TSICOPOULOS, B. WALLAERT, C. VANNIMENUS, M. JOSEPH, A. B. TONNEL & A. CAPRON. 1991. Increased secretion of TNF alpha and IL-6 by alveolar macrophages consecutive to the development of the late asthmatic reaction. J. Allergy Clin. Immunol. **88:** 561–571.
8. LIU, M. C., W. C. HUBBARD, D. PROUD, B. A. STEALEY, S. J. GALLI, A. KAGEY-SOBOTKA, E. R. BLEECKER & L. M. LICHTENSTEIN. 1991. Immediate and late inflammatory re-

sponses to ragweed antigen challenge of the peripheral airways in allergic asthmatics. Am. Rev. Resp. Dis. **144:** 51–58.
9. PAUL, S. R., F. BENNETT, J. A. CALVETTI, K. KELLEHER, C. R. WOOD, R. M. O'HARA JR., A. C. LEARY, B. SIBLEY, S. C. CLARK, D. A. WILLIAMS & Y-C. YANG. 1990. Molecular cloning of a cDNA encoding interleukin-11, a stromal cell-derived lymphopoietic cytokine. Proc. Natl. Acad. Sci. USA **87:** 7512–7516.
10. GUNDEL, R. H., L. G. LETTS & G. J. GLEICH. 1991. Human eosinophil major basic protein induces airway constriction and airway hyperresponsiveness in primates. J. Clin. Invest. **87:** 1470–1473.
11. YIN, T., P. SCHENDEL & Y-C. YANG. 1992. Enhancement of *in vitro* and *in vivo* antigen-specific antibody responses by interleukin-11. J. Exp. Med. **175:** 211–216.
12. ROBINSON, D. S., Q. HAMID, S. YING, A. TSICOPOULOS, J. BARKANS, A. M. BENTLEY, C. CORRIGAN, S. R. DURHAM & A. B. KAY. 1992. Predominant T_{H2}-like bronchoalveolar T-lymphocyte population in atopic asthma. N. Engl. J. Med. **326:** 298–304.
13. PATTERSON, P. & H. NAWA. 1993. Neuronal differentiation factors/cytokines and synaptic plasticity. Cell **72** (Suppl.): 123–137.
14. NADEL, J. A. 1992. Regulation of neurogenic inflammation by neutral endopeptidase. Am. Rev. Resp. Dis. **145:** S48–S52.
15. IHRE, E. & K. LARSSON. 1990. Airways responses to ipratropium bromide do not vary with time in asthmatic subjects. Studies of interindividual and intraindividual variation of bronchodilatation and protection against histamine-induced bronchoconstriction. Chest **97:** 46–51.
16. PANETTIERI, R. A., R. K. MURRAY, L. R. DEPALO, T. A. YADISH & M. I. KOTLIKOFF. 1989. A human airway smooth muscle cell line that retains physiological responsiveness. Am. J. Physiol. **259:** C329.
17. ELIAS, J. A., T. ZHENG, N. L. WHITING, T. K. TROW, W. W. MERRILL, R. ZITNIK, P. RAY & E. M. ALDERMAN. 1994. Interleukin-1 and transforming growth factor-β regulation of fibroblast-derived interleukin-11. J. Immunol. **152:** 2421–2429.
18. MARTIN, T., N. GERARD, S. GALLI & J. DRAZEN. 1988. Pulmonary responses to bronchoconstrictor agonists in the mouse. J. Appl. Physiol. **64**(6): 2318–2323.
19. AMDUR, M. O. & J. MEAD. 1958. Mechanics of respiration in unanesthetized guinea pigs. Am. J. Physiol. **192:** 364–368.
20. GEBA, G. P., C. D. WEGNER, W. N. WOLYNIEC & W. P. ASKENASE. Cell mediated asthma: Airway hyperresponsiveness is mediated by Thy 1 + CD45RA + antigen specific lymphocytes. Submitted.
21. CAVANAH, D. K. & T. B. CASALE. 1993. Histamine. *In* The Mast Cell in Health and Disease (Lung Biology, Health and Disease Series). M. Kaliner & D. Metcalfe, Eds. Vol. **62:** 321. New York: Marcel Dekker.
22. PATTEMORE, P. K., S. L. JOHNSTON & P. G. BARDIN. 1992. Viruses as precipitants of asthma symptoms. I. Epidemiology. Clin. Exp. Allergy **22:** 325–336.
23. BJORNSDOTTIR, U. S. & W. W. BUSSE. 1992. Respiratory infections and asthma. Clin. Allergy **76:** 895–915.
24. PUERINGER, R. J. & G. W. HUNNINGHAKE. 1992. Inflammation and airway reactivity in asthma. Am. J. Med. **92:** (6A)32–38.
25. WATSON, M. L., D. SMITH, A. D. BOURNE, R. C. THOMPSON & J. WESTWICK. 1993. Cytokines contribute to airway dysfunction in antigen-challenged guinea pigs: Inhibition of airway hyperreactivity, pulmonary eosinophil accumulation, and tumor necrosis factor generation by pretreatment with an interleukin-1 receptor antagonist. Am. J. Resp. Cell Mol. Biol. **8:** 365–369.
26. KIPS, J. C., J. TAVERNIER & R. A. PAUWELS. 1992. Tumor necrosis factor causes bronchial hyperresponsiveness in rats. Am. Rev. Resp. Dis. **145:** 332–336.
27. VAN OOSTERHOUT, A. J., A. R. LADENIUS, H. F. SAVELKOUL, I. VAN ARK, K. C. DELSMAN & F. P. NIJKAMP. 1993. Effect of anti-IL-5 and IL-5 on airway hyperreactivity and eosinophils in guinea pigs. Am. Rev. Resp. Dis. **147:** 548–552.
28. PRETOLANI, M. & B. VARGAFTIG. 1993. From lung hypersensitivity to bronchial hyperreactivity. Biochem. Pharmacol. **45:** 791–800.
29. ELIAS, J. A., R. J. ZITNIK & P. RAY. 1992. Fibroblast immune-effector function. *In* Pulmonary Fibroblast Heterogeneity. R. Phipps, Ed., 295–322. Boca Raton, FL: CRC Press.

30. ELIAS, J. A. & M. M REYNOLDS. 1990. IL-1 and TNF synergistically stimulate lung fibroblast IL-1α production. Am. J. Resp. Cell Mol. Biol. **3:** 13–20.
31. MARINI, M., E. VITTORI, J. HOLLEMBORG & S. MATTOLI. 1992. Expression of the potent inflammatory cytokines, GM-CSF, IL-6 and IL-8 in bronchial epithelial cells of patients with asthma. J. Allergy Clin. Immunol. **89:** 1001–1009.

DISCUSSION OF THE PAPER

G. FEY (*University of Erlangen-Nürnberg, Erlangen, Germany*): It is clear from your data that the eosinophils do not produce the IL-11 themselves. Is it a *trans* effect on stromal fibroblasts?

J. A. ELIAS: In our experiments we did not see IL-11 that was passively transferred with the MBP. I cannot, however, tell you that eosinophils do not make IL-11. The studies that we performed were not designed to test this question. In these studies we simply looked at the ability of purified MBP to stimulate stromal cell IL-11 production and found that MBP interacted in a synergistic fashion with IL-1 and TGF-β, in the induction of IL-11.

FEY: Does MBP, being a basic protein, have DNA binding activity?

ELIAS: I am not aware of MBP having DNA binding activity.

M. KOPF (*Max-Planck-Institut für Immunobiologie, Freiburg, Germany*): You mentioned that IL-4 reduces the stimulatory effects of IL-1 and TGFβ on IL-11 expression.

ELIAS: In our studies, IL-4 inhibited cytokine-stimulated IL-11 production by lung fibroblasts.

KOPF: And what effect did it have on IL-6 expression?

ELIAS: We have not looked extensively at the effect of IL-4 on IL-6 production in this system.

H. BAUMANN (*Roswell Park Cancer Institute, Buffalo, NY*): In the TGF-β knockout mice, is the expression of IL-11 in the lung or in lung cells reduced? This would confirm some functional role of TGF-β.

ELIAS: We have not had the opportunity to look at IL-11 expression in TGF-β knockout mice to see whether the levels of IL-11 are altered. An extension of what you are saying is the possibility that IL-11 may mediate some of the effects of TGF-β. We have looked at this in a number of systems, but it is too soon to discuss these studies at the present time.

UNIDENTIFIED SPEAKER: You have nicely shown the production of IL-11 in the lung, but I have not seen evidence of the binding of IL-11 to lung cells. Do you have any information about the expression of the IL-11 receptor in the lung?

ELIAS: No, I do not. I suspect, however, that gp130, a component of IL-11 receptor complex, is ubiquitously expressed in the lung. We need to know more about the composition of the IL-11 receptor to analyze this question much further. Keep in mind, however, that it is possible that IL-11 can have effects in the lung that are mediated by its cationic nature and not by receptor binding. We have not yet been able to differentiate the contribution that receptor binding and charge make to the processes we describe.

P. C. HEINRICH (*Klinikum der RWTH Aachen, Institut für Biochemie, Aachen, Germany*): Does histamine release TGF-β? How do you explain the synergistic effect on IL-11 production of histamine and TGF-β?

ELIAS: That is an issue that we are actively investigating. I can tell you that the ability of histamine and TGF-β to synergistically stimulate IL-11 is blocked by agents that antagonize calmodulin and chelate intracellular calcium. This suggests that a calcium/calmodulin-dependent pathway is involved in this synergistic interaction. This is compatible with our finding that this interaction is mediated by H1 versus H2 histamine receptors, since the former are known to regulate the levels of intracellular calcium. We have also recently used confocal microscopy with calcium dyes to assess the levels of calcium in human lung fibroblasts in the presence and absence of histamine and TGF-β_1. These studies demonstrated that histamine causes a modest biphasic increase in calcium content and that TGF-β_1 did not significantly alter intracellular calcium content. Interestingly, the majority of cells stimulated with histamine and TGF-β_1 in combination demonstrated an impressive oscillating calcium signal, suggesting that the synergy caused by these agents may, in some way, be related to this qualitatively different pattern of calcium fluxuation. We have no evidence that histamine releases TGF-β_1.

HEINRICH: But A. Falus is showing a direct effect of histamine on acute phase protein induction.

A. FALUS (*National Institute of Rheumatology and Physiotherapy, Budapest, Hungary*): One possible explanation for your question is that histamine is not only inducing acute phase but is also inducing IL-1. We have recently shown that histamine can very actively upregulate IL-6 in all cell types. So it might be a local effect of histamine on IL-1 and thus it can be an indirect effect on IL-11. What do you think?

ELIAS: We have not looked at the effects of histamine on IL-1 production.

Do Post-transcriptional Mechanisms Participate in Induction of C-reactive Protein and Serum Amyloid A by IL-6 and IL-1?[a]

IRVING KUSHNER, SHUN-LIN JIANG, DONGXIAO ZHANG, GERARD LOZANSKI, AND DAVID SAMOLS

Department of Medicine
at MetroHealth Medical Center
Cleveland, Ohio 44109-1998
and
Department of Biochemistry
Case Western Reserve University School of Medicine
Cleveland, Ohio 44106

The two major human acute phase proteins are C-reactive protein (CRP) and serum amyloid A (SAA). Both display rapid and marked increases in concentration following inflammatory stimuli, levels several thousand–fold greater than baseline being achieved in some severely inflamed individuals as a result of increased synthesis in hepatocytes. In addition, the genes encoding these proteins are similar in their response to cytokines. Both are induced by interleukin-6 (IL-6) in most model systems studied,[1-5] and addition of IL-1 to IL-6 has been shown to have a synergistic effect on each protein.[2,4-6] Studies in our laboratory have shown that both genes required the combination of IL-6 and IL-1 to achieve maximal response in Hep 3B cells while IL-6 alone was sufficient in NPLC/PRF/5 cells.

Previous studies have clearly indicated that transcription plays a major role in induction of both CRP and SAA.[7-9] In addition, however, the possibility of post-transcriptional regulation has been raised for both proteins. Studies of the effects of IL-6 and IL-1 on CRP induction,[5] employing CRP-CAT constructs transfected into Hep 3B cells, showed the major inducer of these constructs to be IL-6; the IL-1 effect was found to be exerted at the level of sequences downstream to the TATA box, including the first 15 nucleotides of the 5' untranslated region (UTR). The authors concluded that the effect of IL-1 must be exerted at a post-transcriptional level, probably at the level of translation.

Two studies have been interpreted as indicating that post-transcriptional mechanisms play a significant role in SAA induction. In the first of these, increase in SAA mRNA accumulation was somewhat greater than increase in transcription following LPS administration to mice and transcription was found to decrease while the rate of mRNA accumulation was increasing, suggesting to the authors that mRNA stabilization might be participating in SAA induction.[10] In a second study,[11] the murine liver-derived cell line BNL was incubated with conditioned medium (CM) from a mouse macrophage cell line. While SAA3 mRNA rose substantially, no effect on transcription could be shown, suggesting participation of post-transcriptional mechanisms. It is of interest that this cell line did not express SAA1 and SAA2, the major

---

[a] This work was supported by NIH grant number AG 02467.

murine acute phase reactants. The current studies were therefore undertaken to further explore the possible participation of post-transcriptional mechanisms in induction of human CRP and SAA by IL-6 and IL-1 in Hep 3B cells.

C-REACTIVE PROTEIN

In studies of CRP regulation, we investigated the effects of IL-6 and IL-1β on both the endogenous CRP gene and on CRP-CAT constructs in Hep 3B cells. We addressed two issues in kinetic studies of the endogenous gene: 1) Does IL-1β enhance CRP transcription in the presence of IL-6? 2) Does magnitude of increase in CRP message level quantitatively reflect increases in transcription, and does production of CRP protein parallel message levels?

To answer these questions, Hep 3B cells were exposed to cytokines for 72 hours; medium was changed and cytokines replaced every 24 hours. The kinetics of CRP mRNA accumulation were determined by Northern blotting, while changes in transcription rate were determined by nuclear run-on assays in aliquots of the same cells (FIG. 1). IL-1β alone had no effect on mRNA levels while IL-6 caused about a 50-fold increase in CRP mRNA by 24 h, which thereafter decreased by 48 and 72 h despite readdition of cytokines after 24 h and 48 h. The combination of IL-6 and IL-1β caused an increase in mRNA abundance about 6-fold greater than that seen with IL-6 alone. Nuclear run-on studies showed that IL-6 alone increased transcription by about 40-fold over baseline values. Addition of IL-1β to IL-6 substantially enhanced transcription by about 3.5-fold more. We concluded, in answer to the first question posed above, that IL-1β clearly had a transcription effect on the endogenous CRP gene in the presence of IL-6.

We further investigated level of regulation by comparing magnitudes of increase in mRNA levels and transcription, and by comparing CRP protein production with mRNA levels. Magnitudes of increase of mRNA and transcription rates induced by these cytokines were roughly comparable, given the limitations of the method. Similarly, secretion of CRP protein during each 24 h period roughly paralleled mRNA

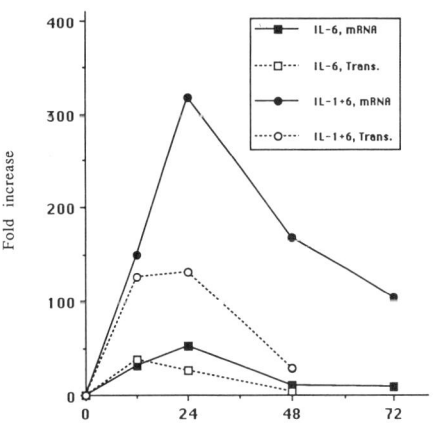

FIGURE 1. Kinetics of change in transcription (trans) and mRNA accumulation (mRNA) of CRP in Hep 3B cells during 72 h of incubation with either IL-6 (200 U/ml) or the combination of IL-6 (200 U/ml) and IL-1β (400 U/ml). Points are plotted as fold increase over baseline values set equal to 1.

levels. These findings do not provide support for post-transcriptional regulation of CRP, although they do not, of course, rule it out.

The transcriptional role of IL-1β in CRP induction was confirmed by transient transfection studies. To determine if the effect of IL-1β was mediated by the 5' UTR of the CRP gene, as reported,[5] cells were transfected with CRP-CAT constructs differing in the length of the 5' UTR ($-157/+104$, $-157/+15$ and $-157/+3$). Results were the same for all three constructs: IL-1β had a minimal effect, IL-6 alone a moderate effect and the combination of IL-6 and IL-1β a marked effect on CAT expression in every case. These studies indicated that the effects of both IL-6 and IL-1β are exerted at the transcriptional level and that the upstream 157 bases of the CRP promoter contain elements necessary for both IL-6 induction and the synergistic effect of IL-1β on transcription.

SERUM AMYLOID A

Substantially different results were found when kinetic studies of the SAA gene, comparable to those described above for CRP, were carried out. In initial studies we determined the effect of CM from LPS-stimulated monocytes on mRNA levels and transcription of a number of acute phase genes. Two patterns of response were found. For α_1-protease inhibitor and α-fibrinogen, increases in mRNA abundance and transcription were comparable and paralleled one another, resembling the findings for CRP described above. In contrast, SAA, factor B and C3 all showed increases in mRNA abundance 10-fold or more greater than increases in transcriptional and mRNA peaks were attained substantially later than were peaks in transcription. For SAA, mRNA increase was about 20-fold greater than increase in transcription. However, interpretation of these data are difficult for several reasons. 1) Very low baseline values for either transcription rate or mRNA can lead to substantial errors when magnitudes of increase are calculated. 2) Several-fold errors in nuclear run-on are not unexpected, and 3) True steady states may not be achieved since transcription rates, mRNA levels, and mRNA degradation rates may all be changing during the course of the experiment.

To avoid some of these problems we sought help from Dr. Isaac Greber, Professor of Mechanical and Aerospace Engineering at Case Western Reserve University. Since our data provided relative, rather than absolute values for mRNA levels and transcription rates, Dr. Greber developed a method of mathematical analysis, in which Northern blot and nuclear run-on values were referred to an assumed constant—the abundance ratio—representing the average mRNA level from all measurements divided by total transcription over the entire course of the study. The abundance ratio was not known, but alternative possible values could be assigned to it. This approach avoids a major pitfall in interpretation of our data since it relies on estimation of *mean* rather than initial mRNA levels and *total* rather than initial transcription rates. This analysis indicated that the rate of SAA mRNA degradation fell sharply following CM addition for all possible values of the abundance ratio, supporting a post-transcriptional effect of CM on SAA expression.

We then pursued the precise roles of IL-6 and IL-1β In this process, in similar kinetic studies. Both IL-1β and IL-6 alone induced little SAA expression, but their combination was markedly synergistic. The kinetics of SAA induction differed considerably from those of CRP. The combination of IL-6 + IL-1β caused about a 23-fold increase in transcription, which then declined somewhat, but persisted at a lesser level for the duration of the experiment. Throughout the remainder of the 72 hours of incubation, however, mRNA levels continued to rise, ultimately achieving levels more than 1100-fold greater than base. The massive difference between increases in SAA mRNA accumulation and transcription induced by IL-6 + IL-1β suggests participation of post-transcriptional mechanisms. In contrast to CRP, the marked lag between transcription peak and mRNA peak suggests that SAA mRNA is relatively stable.

In addition, like several other groups,[6,12–14] we found the mean size of SAA mRNA to decrease following its initial detection. It is of interest that SAA mRNA displayed considerable heterogeneity in size during this period, suggesting simultaneous synthesis of new, larger, presumably polyadenylated molecules and an increasing pool of aged, and therefore shortened molecules. Studies of SAA protein secreted by these cells indicated that SAA secretion was closely parallel to mRNA levels for each 24 h time period, failing to provide support for SAA regulation at the translational level.

mRNA HALF LIFE ESTIMATION

We attempted to determine half lives of both CRP and SAA mRNA following 24 hours of pre-incubation with the combination of IL-6 + IL-1β. Cells were then washed and medium replaced with fresh medium lacking cytokines. Under these conditions CRP transcription fell to minimally detectable levels and CRP mRNA fell with a half disappearance time of about 2-½ hours. In view of the relatively small amount of CRP transcription occurring at this time, it is likely that this value does not differ very much from the actual half-life of CRP mRNA. Further, the close temporal proximity of the peaks of transcription and mRNA accumulation in kinetic studies also suggested that endogenous CRP mRNA is relatively unstable.

Different results were obtained for SAA. Substantial on-going transcription was seen following cytokine withdrawal, in the range of 20–40% of that existing following the period of pre-incubation. Under these conditions the half disappearance time of SAA mRNA was about 8-½ hours; this value represents the maximal possible half-life. Actinomycin studies were not helpful in determining SAA mRNA half life; essentially no decrease in SAA mRNA was seen over a 24-hour period, as reported by others.[6,11] One possible explanation for this finding is that SAA mRNA degradation requires transcription of a gene whose product is required for that process.

OVERVIEW

It is enlightening to directly compare our findings in kinetic studies of CRP and SAA in Hep 3B cells (FIG. 2). Although the patterns of increase in serum concentrations of these two proteins are equally dramatic and closely parallel one another following inflammatory stimuli, the kinetics of CRP and SAA mRNA accumulation and transcription in response to IL-6 + IL-1β were found to differ strikingly in several ways. 1) The transcriptional response of CRP was much more transient than that of SAA. 2) The magnitude of the CRP transcriptional response appeared to be considerably greater than that of the SAA transcriptional response and may itself account for the entire CRP mRNA increase. 3) In contrast, the SAA mRNA response was many times greater than the transcriptional response, suggesting participation of post-transcriptional mechanisms. 4) The delayed SAA mRNA peak suggests that SAA mRNA is relatively stable compared to CRP mRNA.

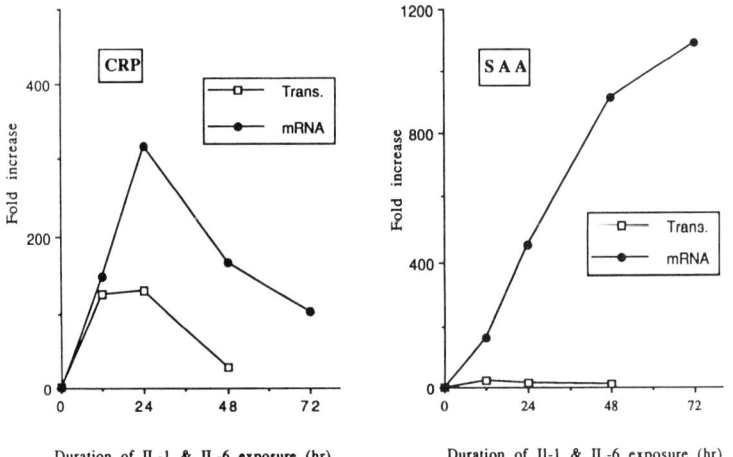

FIGURE 2. Kinetics of change in transcription (trans) and mRNA accumulation (mRNA) of CRP and SAA in Hep 3B cells during 72 h of incubation with the combination of IL-6 and IL-1β. Points are plotted as fold increase over baseline values set equal to 1. Note that maximal SAA transcription after 12 h of incubation was 23-fold greater than baseline.

Taken together, these data suggest that the comparable induction of CRP and SAA by IL-6 and IL-1 may be achieved by substantially different molecular mechanisms.

REFERENCES

1. GANAPATHI, M. K., L. T. MAY, D. SCHULTZ, A. BRABENEC, J. WEINSTEIN, P. B. SEHGAL & I. KUSHNER. 1988. Role of interleukin-6 in regulating synthesis of C-reactive protein and serum amyloid A in human hepatoma cell lines. Biochem. Biophys. Res. Commun. **157:** 271–277.
2. GANAPATHI, M. K., D. SCHULTZ, A. MACKIEWICA, D. SAMOLS, S. I. HU, A. BRABENEC, S. S. MACINTYRE & I. KUSHNER. 1988. Heterogeneous nature of the acute phase response. Differential regulation of human serum amyloid A, C-reactive protein, and other acute phase proteins by cytokines in Hep 3B cells. J. Immunol. **141:** 564–569.
3. CASTELL, J. V., M. J. GOMEZ-LECHON, M. DAVID, T. HIRANO, T. KISHIMOTO & P. C. HEINRICH. 1988. Recombinant human interleukin-6 (IL-6/BSF-2/HSF) regulates the synthesis of acute phase proteins in human hepatocytes. FEBS Lett. **232:** 347–350.
4. WOO, P., J. SIPE, C. A. DINARELLO & H. R. COLTEN. 1987. Structure of a human serum amyloid A gene and modulation of its expression in transfected L cells. J. Biol. Chem. **262:** 15790–15795.
5. GANTER, U., R. ARCONE, C. TONIATTI, G. MORRONE & G. CILIBERTO. 1990. Dual control of C-reactive protein gene expression by interleukin-1 and interleukin-6. EMBO J. **8:** 3773–3779.
6. STEEL, D. M., J. T. ROGERS, M. C. DEBEER, F. C. DEBEER & A. S. WHITEHEAD. 1993. Biosynthesis of human acute phase serum amyloid A protein (A-SAA) in vitro: The roles of mRNA accumulation, poly(A) tail shortening and translational efficiency. Biochem. J. **291:** 701–707.
7. MORRONE, G., G. CILIBERTO, S. OLIVIERO, R. ARCONE, L. DENTE, J. CONTENT & R.

CORTESE. 1988. Recombinant interleukin 6 regulates the transcriptional activation of a set of human acute phase genes. J. Biol. Chem. **263:** 12554–12558.
8. GOLDBERGER, G., D. H. BING, J. D. SIPE, M. RITS & H. R. COLTEN. 1987. Transcriptional regulation of genes encoding the acute-phase proteins CRP, SAA, and C3. J. Immunol. **138:** 3967–3971.
9. BETTS, J. C., J. K. CHESHIRE, S. AKIRA, T. KISHIMOTO & P. WOO. 1993. The role of NF-kB and NF-IL6 transactivating factors in the synergistic activation of human serum amyloid A gene expression by interleukin-1 and interleukin-6. J. Biol. Chem. **268:** 25624–24631.
10. LOWELL, C. A., R. S. STEARMAN & J. F. MORROW. 1986. Transcriptional regulation of serum amyloid A gene expression. J. Biol. Chem. **261:** 8453–8461.
11. RIENHOFF, H. Y. J. & M. GROUDINE. 1988. Regulation of amyloid A gene expression in cultured cells. Mol. Cell. Biol. **8:** 3710–3716.
12. DOWTON, S. B., C. N. PETERS & J. J. JESTUS. 1991. Regulation of serum amyloid A gene expression in Syrian hamsters by cytokines. Inflammation **15:** 391–397.
13. BRISSETTE, L., I. YOUNG, S. NARINDRAWORASAK, R. KISILEVSKY & R. DEELEY. 1989. Differential induction of the serum amyloid A gene family in response to an inflammatory agent and to amyloid-enhancing factor. J. Biol. Chem. **264:** 19327–19332.
14. SELLAR G. C., M. C. DEBEER, J. M. LELIAS, P. W. SNYDER, L. T. GLICKMAN, P. J. FELSBURG & A. S. WHITEHEAD. 1991. Dog serum amyloid A protein. J. Biol. Chem. **266:** 3505–3510.

Modified Proteins as Possible Signals in the Acute Phase Response[a]

ALEKSANDER KOJ AND AMALIA GUZDEK

Institute of Molecular Biology
Jagiellonian University
Al. Mickiewicza 3
31-120 Kraków, Poland

INTRODUCTION

Tissue damage induces macrophages and some other cells to synthesize and release numerous cytokines which are responsible for various signs of the acute phase response including a profound rearrangement of plasma protein synthesis in liver parenchymal cells.[1,2] Classification of inflammation-associated acute-phase cytokines remains controversial[3] but at least three groups of these regulatory molecules may be distinguished:

- Early and proinflammatory cytokines initiating the cascade of events: tumor necrosis factor (TNF-α), interleukin-1 (IL-1),[4,5] interferon-γ (IFN-γ),[6–8] interleukin-8 (IL-8) and related chemotactic factors.[9] They usually appear first in the site of tissue damage and elicit limited response in the immune system and in liver (except IL-8 which is induced by TNF and IL-1 and has no effect on liver parenchymal cells although it can be produced there).[10,11]
- Cytokines belonging to interleukin-6 (IL-6) family: IL-6, leukemia inhibitory factor (LIF), interleukin-11 (IL-11), oncostatin M (OSM) and ciliary neutrophic factor (CNTF) are held responsible for the main features of acute phase response in a variety of tissues, including liver.[12–16]
- Antiinflammatory cytokines down-regulating the acute-phase response: interleukin-10 (IL-10), interleukin-4 (IL-4) and interleukin-13 (IL-13).[17–24]

This classification is certainly oversimplified since some cytokines play various roles depending on the stage of inflammation (*e.g.* IFN-γ or IL-6). Moreover, there are known other important cytokines involved in the modulation of acute phase response, such as transforming growth factor-β,[25–28] hepatocyte growth factor,[29–31] and several hemopoietic regulators.[32] The acute phase response is further modified by hormones, mainly by glucocorticoids and insulin.[12,31,16]

The sequence of events during induced synthesis of acute phase cytokines is still disputed but it appears that TNF and IL-1 are produced earlier than IL-6[32,33] and directly stimulate IL-6 synthesis in model experiments. Bacterial endotoxin (LPS) is regarded as the most potent inducer of acute phase cytokines, whereas corticosteroids inhibit induction[4,13,35] (see also papers by A. Ray, and by A. C. Allison, this volume). On the other hand, taxol, a complex diterpene which stabilizes microtubules and exhibits anti-cancer activity, stimulates macrophages similarly to endotoxin.[36] Production of IL-6 and other cytokines *in vitro* is also stimulated by some viruses and synthetic polynucleotides, by second messenger agonists, and even by serum.[37]

---

[a] This study was supported by the State Committee for Scientific Research, Warsaw, Poland (KBN grant 2238/4/91).

However, the primary signals eliciting synthesis of acute phase cytokines in aseptic tissue necrosis, such as myocardial infarction, remain unidentified. Among candidates to function as "alarm molecules" are free radicals, prostaglandins and modified proteins recognized as foreign materials. The reaction is certainly complex and involves activation of the complement system, accumulation of leukocytes, stimulation of cyclooxygenase-lipooxygenase pathways and generation of free radicals.[38] Free radicals may directly affect cytokine-producing cells or modify proteins in the extracellular fluids. Proteins modified by these radicals, or by leukocyte proteinases, will be taken up by "scavenger-type" or specific receptors present on macrophages, fibroblasts or endothelial cells, and by an unknown mechanism switch on the synthesis of acute phase cytokines.

Proteinase-inhibitor complexes or proteolytically modified inhibitors from the serpin family represent such candidates for initiating signals. Perlmutter and co-workers[39] demonstrated that α_1-antitrypsin elastase complexes mediate increased expression of the antitrypsin gene not only in monocytes and macrophages but also in human HepG2 cells. However, Kurdowska and Travis[40] and Koj et al.[41] found that HepG2 cells could be stimulated to produce several acute phase proteins only indirectly by conditioned media from human lung fibroblasts which were exposed to modified serpins or serpin-proteinase complexes.

Fibrinogen is another plasma protein damaged by proteinases during acute inflammation. In 1985 Princen et al.[42] reported that several fibrinogen degradation products (FDPs) increase levels of plasma fibrinogen in vivo, while in the primary cultures of rat hepatocytes only peptide E was active. Moshage et al.[43] found that induction of fibrinogen synthesis in cultured rat hepatocytes by fragment D was possible only if liver parenchymal cells were co-cultured with macrophages, thus confirming an earlier suggestion of Ritchie and co-workers[44] on the indirect pathway of fibrinogen biosynthesis.

C-reactive protein (CRP) belongs to the most spectacular acute phase proteins in human sera.[2] Robey and co-workers[45] observed that proteolysis of human CRP produces peptides with potent immunomodulating activity, and Thomassen et al.[46] confirmed activation of human monocytes and alveolar macrophages by a synthetic peptide derived from CRP. Even native CRP added to cultured human macrophages can stimulate synthesis and release of TNFα, IL-1 and IL-6[47] by inducing the expression of corresponding cytokine genes.[48]

Elevated concentrations of glucose in the blood and body fluids occurring in diabetes lead to non-enzymatic glycosylation (glycation) of ϵ-amino group of lysine residue in proteins resulting in the formation of advanced glycosylation end products (AGEs). Glycated proteins are bound to specific receptors and taken up by macrophages, the removal process being associated with production and secretion of acute phase cytokines, such as TNF-α and IL-1.[49,50]

The purpose of the experiments described here was to determine the effects of proteolytically modified human plasma proteins: fibrinogen degradation products (FDPs), papain-cleaved α_1-antitrypsin (API*) and glycated human serum albumin (AGE-HSA) on synthesis and release of IL-1 and IL-6 by cultured human blood monocytes and alveolar macrophages. Moreover, the influence of taxol and foreign materials stimulating macrophage phagocytosis (silica particles) was evaluated. The preliminary report of these experiments has already been published.[51]

MATERIALS AND METHODS

Materials

All the materials were prepared using pyrogen-free water, and during experimental procedure precautions were undertaken to avoid contamination with endotoxin.

Fibrinogen fragments were prepared by Dr. E. Korzus (Department of Biochemistry, University of Georgia, Athens, GA, USA) essentially as described by Dang et al.[52] with the following modification. Human fibrinogen was solubilized to concentration 5 mg/ml in 50 mM Tris/HCl, 150 mM NaCl and 5 mM $CaCl_2$. Human plasmin (Boehrniger, Mannheim) was added (0.05 units per 10 mg of fibrinogen) and the mixture was incubated at 37°C for 14 h. The digestion was ended by adding ε-aminocaproic acid (final conc. 0.1 M) and PMSF (final conc. 1 mM). The digest was chromatographed on a column of DEAE-cellulose (Sigma) in 10 mM Na-bicarbonate-carbonate buffer pH 8.9, and fibrinogen fragments eluted with NaCl gradient. Purity of fragments was tested on SDS-PAGE slab gel electrophoresis in 7.5% polyacrylamide: fragment D gave a single band (above 94 kD), whereas fragment E (ca 52 kD) contained small amounts of peptide D. Samples were extensively dialyzed against water and lyophilized. Just before the experiment they were dissolved in RPMI containing 2% fetal calf serum (FCS) and filter sterilized (Millipore, 0.22 μm) before addition to macrophage culture.

Human $α_1$-proteinase inhibitor (API) was isolated from human plasma by Dr. J. Potempa (Institute of Molecular Biology, Jagiellonian University) and subjected to limited cleavage by papain as described by Johnson and Travis.[53] The modified inhibitor (API*) was separated from proteinase by MonoQ fast protein liquid chromatography, concentrated on Amicon P10 membrane, dialyzed against PBS, aliquoted and frozen at −20°C. Just before addition to macrophage culture a sample of API* was thawed, diluted to appropriate concentration with RPMI containing 2% FCS and filter-sterilized.

Glycated human serum albumin (AGE-HSA) was obtained by incubation of FPLC-purified HSA (Sigma, Deisenhofen, Germany) in sterile conditions for 14 days in PBS with 150 mM glucose.

Endotoxin (lipolysaccharide from *E. coli* 026-86, Sigma, Germany) was dissolved in sterile PBS to obtain the concentration of 1 mg/ml.

Polymyxin B sulfate (PMB, Fluka, Germany) was dissolved in PBS to the concentration of 2 mg/ml and filter-sterilized.

Silica particles (quartz dust, 20–200 μm, Johannesburg, kindly by Prof. W. Ptak, Department of Immunology, Jagiellonian University School of Medicine) were sterilized by heating for 3 h at 200°C and then suspended in sterile PBS to obtain 10% suspension (w/w). After shaking in an Eppendorf tube and sedimentation for 60 sec to remove coarse particles 10 μl of the suspension was added per 1 ml of macrophage culture.

Taxol (Paclitaxel, NSC 125973-L) was kindly provided by Dr. V. L. Narayanan (Drug Synthesis and Chemistry Branch, National Cancer Institute, Bethesda, MD). It was dissolved in DMSO to obtain 10 mM stock solution kept at −20°C and just before the experiment was suitably diluted in RPMI containing 2% FCS.

Monospecific antisera to rat plasma proteins were prepared by immunization of rabbits with purified antigens as described previously.[54]

Culture and Stimulation of Macrophages

Mononuclear cells were prepared from 50 ml of fresh human blood from a healthy donor by centrifugation with Mono-Poly resolving medium (ICN Biomedicals, Meckenheim, Germany)[55] and seeded in 6-well cluster plates (Nunclon, Kamstrup, Denmark) in RPMI containing 5% fetal calf serum (initial density of approximately 3 × 10^6 cells per 35-mm diameter well). After 2 h at 37°C in 5% CO_2 the non-adherent cells were removed by washing the wells (2 × 1 ml) with serum-free RPMI and the remaining cells were cultured overnight in RPMI containing 8% FCS. Then the media were replaced with RPMI containing 2% FCS and the tested factors added at indicated concentrations. After further culture for 24 h the media were collected, centrifuged for 3 min at 14 000 × g and kept at +4°C until used for the determination of cytokines.

Human lung macrophages were obtained by fiberoptic bronchoscopy of patients examined for diagnostic purposes following the guidelines of the American Thoracic Society.[56] Bronchoscopy and lung lavage were carried out by Dr. K. Sladek at the Pulmonological Clinic (Head: Prof. E. Niżankowska, Jagiellonian University School of Medicine). The cells were collected in sterile PBS, centrifuged, suspended in RPMI containing 8% FCS and seeded in 6-well cluster plates; subsequent procedure was as described for blood mononuclear cells.

Assay of IL-1 and IL-6

The contents of acute phase cytokines in the macrophage media was carried out either directly with specific kits, or by bioassays with rat hepatoma H-35 cells. These cells upon stimulation produce 2 classes of acute phase proteins; class 1 includes α_1-acid glycoprotein (AGP) and C3 component of the complement (CC3) and is induced by IL-1/TNF and IL-6/IL-11/LIF/OSM, whereas class 2 includes fibrinogen (FBG) and α_2-macroglobulin (A2M) and is induced by cytokines from IL-6 family alone (IL-1 or TNF even inhibit the response).[31]

For the bioassay hepatoma cells were grown in Dulbecco's modified Eagle's medium (DMEM) containing 5% FCS in 6-well cluster plates to the stage of subconfluent monolayer. Then the medium was changed to 0.9 ml of serum-free DMEM containing 1 μM dexamethasone and 0.3 ml of the tested macrophage media added. To evaluate cell response to cytokines human recombinant IL-6 (20 ng/ml) or IL-6 and IL-1 (100 units/ml) were added to certain wells (positive control). After 24 h of culture with macrophage supernatants the media were collected, dialyzed, concentrated by lyophilization and selected proteins were determined by rocket immunoelectrophoresis.[54]

Direct measurements of IL-6 concentrations in macrophage media were carried out with ELISA immunoassay (Predicta kit, Genzyme, Cambridge, MA, USA) according to supplier's instructions. IL-1α was measured with RIA Kit (Genzyme, Cambridge, MA, USA) and IL-1β with immunoenzymetric assay IL-1β-EASIA (Medgenix, Fleurus, Belgium).

RESULTS AND DISCUSSION

As expected, endotoxin stimulated synthesis of IL-1 and IL-6 by human blood-derived or lung macrophages and this effect was considerably reduced by polymyxin B (TABLE 1). Production of acute phase cytokines could be also induced by papain-inactivated α_1-proteinase inhibitor (API*) (TABLE 1) in agreement with the report of Kurdowska & Travis[40] who observed a similar effect with human fibroblasts stimulated with antichymotrypsin-cathepsin G complexes. Native inhibitor, at the final concentration of 0.5 mg/ml media, also slightly stimulated macrophages and this may be explained by progressive modification of API by endogenous macrophage proteinases during tissue culture.

Vlassara et al.[49] reported that non-enzymatically glycosylated serum albumin and tissue matrix proteins stimulate macrophages to produce IL-1 and TNF. In the present experiments we found that advanced glycosylation products of human serum albumin (AGE-HSA) can also induce synthesis of IL-6 (TABLE 1).

TABLE 1. Cytokine Synthesis in Human Alveolar Macrophages Stimulated by Endotoxin, Taxol and Some Modified Proteins

Macrophage Culture	IL-6 (ng/ml)	IL-1α (ng/ml)	IL-1β (ng/ml)
Control	0.03 ± 0.01	≤0.04	0.04
LPS	3.52 ± 0.9	0.75 ± 0.32	0.66 ± 0.07
LPS + PMB	0.28 ± 0.19	0.41	0.11
API*	2.76	N.D.	N.D.
API* + PMB	2.04	N.D.	N.D.
FDPs	1.53 ± 0.23	0.36	0.61 ± 0.05
FDPs + PMB	1.35 ± 0.41	0.23	0.32
FDPs + Taxol	1.63	N.D.	0.39
AGE-HSA	0.10 ± 0.02	0.14 ± 0.07	N.D.
Silica	0.18 ± 0.02	0.83 ± 0.41	0.90

Cytokines were measured by immunoassays in the media of macrophages cultured for 2 days and then exposed for 24 h to LPS (500 ng/ml), polymyxin B (PMB, 10 μg/ml), papain-inactivated antitrypsin (API*, 200 μg/ml), fibrinogen degradation products D or E (FDPs, 200 μg/ml), taxol (10 μM), glycated human serum albumin (AGE-HSA, 300 μg/ml) or silica particles (100 μg/ml). Means of 3–7 estimations, ± S.D. whenever calculated. N.D.—not determined.

Human alveolar macrophages obtained by fiberoptic bronchoscopy are significantly stimulated, as shown by production of cytokines eliciting synthesis of acute phase proteins in rat hepatoma cells (data not shown). However, this synthesis of cytokines was always considerably reduced after at least one day of culture *in vitro*, but could be again enhanced by adding to the media fibrinogen fragments D or E (FIGS. 1 and 2). The stimulation was dose-dependent in the range of 100–500 μg

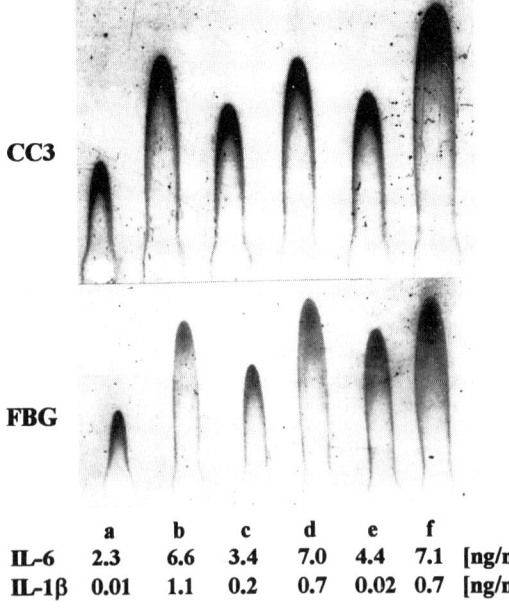

FIGURE 1. Comparison of cytokine immunoassay and bioassay with rat H-35 cells using 2 indicator proteins: C3 complement (CC3) and fibrinogen (FBG). Hepatoma cells were cultured with supernatants from non-stimulated human lung macrophages (control, well a), macrophages exposed to fibrinogen degradation product E (200 μg/ml, well b), macrophages exposed this product in the presence of polymyxin B (10 μg/ml, well c), or in the presence of 10 μM taxol (well d), macrophages exposed to fragment D (200 μg/ml, well e), and macrophages exposed to LPS (500 ng/ml). Direct measurements of IL-6 and IL-1 in the tested macrophage supernatants are reported below the photographs of the rockets.

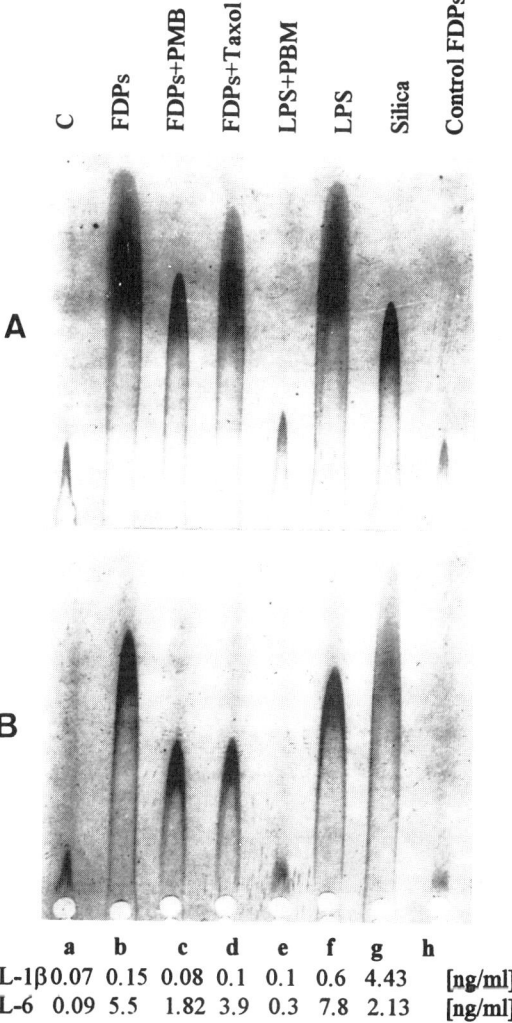

FIGURE 2. Bioassay of acute phase cytokines with rat H-35 cells using the same indicator proteins: fibrinogen (A) and C3 complement (B). The cells were cultured with: (a) control supernatants of non-stimulated human lung macrophages, (b) macrophages exposed to fibrinogen degradation product E (150 μg/ml), (c) macrophages exposed to this product in the presence of polymyxin B (10 μg/ml), (d) in the presence of 10 μM taxol, (e) macrophages exposed to LPS (500 ng/ml) and polymyxin B (10 μg/ml), (f) macrophages exposed to LPS alone (500 ng/ml), (g) macrophages exposed to silica (100 μg/ml). Well (h) media from H-35 cells cultured without macrophage supernatant but with FDPs added directly to hepatoma culture (100 μg/ml). Direct measurements of IL-6 and IL-1 in the tested macrophage supernatants are reported below the photographs of rockets.

	a	b	c	d	e	f	g	h	
IL-1β	0.07	0.15	0.08	0.1	0.1	0.6	4.43		[ng/ml]
IL-6	0.09	5.5	1.82	3.9	0.3	7.8	2.13		[ng/ml]

FDPs/ml of culture medium. Addition of polymyxin B to fibrinogen degradation products reduced to a variable extent the production of IL-1 and IL-6, whereas addition of taxol augmented synthesis of IL-6 but decreased of IL-1. The mean results of cytokine bioassays with H-35 cells are summarized in FIGURE 3.

In general, there was agreement between the direct assay of cytokines by immunological techniques and bioassay in hepatoma cells: as shown in FIGURE 1 IL-6–dependent synthesis of FBG (class 2 acute phase proteins) was more augmented by taxol than synthesis of CC3 (class 1 acute phase proteins, requiring the mixture of IL-6 and IL-1). Similar results were obtained with murine peritoneal macrophages stimulated by fragment E of human fibrinogen: taxol enhanced production of IL-6 but

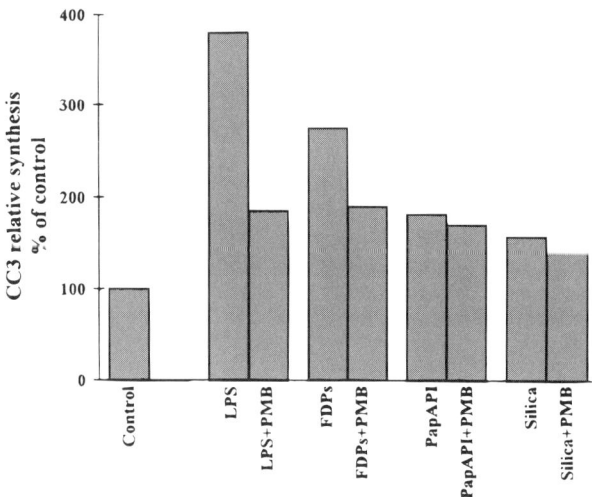

FIGURE 3. Synthesis of C3 complement (CC3) by H-35 cells cultured in the presence of media from human alveolar macrophages exposed to LPS (0.5 μg/ml), FDPs (0.2 mg/ml), papain-modified API (0.3 mg/ml) or silica (10 μg/ml). Polymyxin B (PMB), whereas present, was added to the concentration of 10 μg/ml. The results are means of at least 3 independent experiments.

not of IL-1, as judged by induced synthesis of fibrinogen and C3 complement in rat H-35 cells (Guzdek and Koj, unpublished observations). Taxol is known to induce the expression of endotoxin-responsive genes,[36] but at the same time it may inhibit IL-1 production induced by colchicine.[57] Cellular microtubule network, involved in cell differentiation, phagocytosis and secretion, appears to be important for the induced synthesis of cytokines. Our results obtained with taxol are in agreement with the observations by Manie and co-workers[57] on selective induction of acute phase cytokines by microtubule-modifying agents.

The effect taxol clearly depends on the functional state of macrophages since in some experiments addition of taxol slightly reduced synthesis of both IL-6 and IL-1 (FIG. 2). On the other hand, polymyxin almost abrogated the effect of endodoxin but only marginally affected synthesis of cytokines, and this suggests that the action of modified proteins cannot be explained by contamination with LPS (FIG. 2). In agreement with the results reported by other authors,[58] endotoxin-free silica particles were usually a potent stimulant of cytokine synthesis (FIG. 2 and TABLE 1). These particles elicit in macrophages phagocytosis and respiratory burst. The mechanism of action of modified proteins is unknown but the available evidence suggests that they are bound by the cell-surface receptors of macrophages and can also stimulate phagocytosis, and subsequently synthesis of cytokines.

The major problem in the interpretation of results with modified proteins is related to ubiquitous presence of endotoxin. The effects of polymyxin B observed in our experiments with fibrinogen-derived peptides, modified α_1-antitrypsin or glycated albumin suggest that these preparations were not endotoxin-free. Therefore, it cannot be firmly concluded that modified proteins are the primary signals eliciting the acute phase response, but it is likely that they act as co-stimulators of macrophages primed by trace amounts of endotoxin, or by other factors present in the culture media. The relevance of these observations to the *in vivo* effects requires further studies.

ACKNOWLEDGMENTS

We are grateful to Dr. E. Korzus (Department of Biochemistry, University of Georgia, Athens, GA) for providing purified fibrinogen degradation products, to Dr. J. Potempa for modified API, and to Ms. K. Stalinska, and Ms. M. Weigt-Wadas for technical assistance.

REFERENCES

1. KOJ, A. 1989. The role of interleukin-6 as the hepatocyte stimulating factor in the network of inflammatory cytokines. Ann. N. Y. Acad. Sci. **557:** 1–8.
2. KUSHNER, I. & A. MACKIEWICZ. 1993. The acute phase response: An overview. *In* Acute Phase Proteins, Molecular Biology, Biochemistry and Clinical Applications. A. Mackiewicz, I. Kushner & H. Baumann, Eds. Vol. 1: 3–19. Boca Raton, Ann Arbor, London, Tokyo: CRC Press.
3. NATHAN, C. & M. SPORN. 1991. Cytokines in context. J. Cell Biol. **113:** 981–986.
4. BEUTLER, B., N. KROCHIN, I. W. MILSARK, C. LUEDKE & A. CERAMI. 1986. Control of cachectin (tumor necrosis factor) synthesis: Mechanisms of endotoxin resistance. Science **232:** 977–980.
5. DINARELLO, C. 1991. Interleukin-1 and interleukin-1 antagonist. Blood **77:** 1627–1652.
6. BANCROFT, G. J., R. D. SCHREIBER, G. C. BOSMA, M. J. BOSMA & E. R. UNANUE. 1987. A T-cell-independent mechanism of macrophage activation by interferon-γ. J. Immunol. **139:** 1104–1107.
7. LUEDKE, C. E. & A. CERAMI. 1990. Interferon-γ overcomes glucocorticoid suppression of cachectin/tumor necrosis factor biosynthesis by murine macrophages. J. Clin. Invest. **86:** 1234–1240.
8. SANCEAU, J., J. WIJDENES, M. REVEL & J. WIETZERBIN. 191. IL-6 and IL-6 receptor modulation by IFN-γ and tumor necrosis factor-α in human monocytic cell line (THP-1). Priming effect of IFN-γ. J. Immunol. **147:** 2630–2637.
9. BAGGIOLINI, M. & I. CLARK-LEWIS. 1992. Interleukin-8, a chemotactic and inflammatory cytokine. FEBS Lett. **307:** 97–101.
10. THORNTON, A. J., R. M. STRIETER, I. LINDLEY, M. BAGGIOLINI & S. L. KUNKEL. 1990. Cytokine-induced gene expression of a neutrophil chemotactic factor/IL-8 in human hepatocytes. J. Immunol. **144:** 2609–2613.
11. KASAHARA, K., R. M. STRIETER, T. J. STANDIFORD & S. L. KUNKEL. 1993. Interleukin-4 differentially regulates tumor necrosis factor-α gene expression by human T lymphocytes and monocytes. Pathobiology **61:** 57–66.
12. HEINRICH, P. C., J. W. CASTELL & T. ANDUS. 1990. Interleukin-6 and the acute phase response. Biochem. J. **265:** 621–636.
13. SEHGAL, P. B. 1990. Interleukin-6: Regulator of plasma protein gene expression in hepatic and nonhepatic tissues. Mol. Biol. Med. **7:** 117–130.
14. BAUMANN, H. & P. SCHENDEL. 1991. Interleukin-11 regulates the hepatic expression of the same plasma protein genes as interleukin-6. J. Biol. Chem. **266:** 20424–20427.
15. SCHOOLTINK, H., T. STOYAN, E. ROEB, P. C. HEINRICH & S. ROSE-JOHN. 1992. Ciliary neurotrophic factor induces acute-phase protein expression in hepatocytes. FEBS Lett. **314:** 280–284.
16. BAUMANN, H. & J. GAULDIE. 1994. The acute phase response. Immunol. Today. **15:** 74–80.
17. OSWALD, I. P., R. T. GAZZINELLI, A. SHER & S. L. JAMES. 1992. IL-10 synergizes with

IL-4 and transforming growth factor-β to inhibit macrophage cytotoxic activity. J. Immunol. **148**: 3578–3582.
18. MOORE, K. W., A. O'GARRA, R. DEWAAL MALEFYT, P. VIEIRA & T. R. MOSMANN. 1993. Interleukin-10. Annu. Rev. Immunol. **11**: 165–190.
19. STANDIFORD, T. J., T. LINDSTEN, C. B. THOMPSON, R. M. STRIETER & S. L. KUNKEL. 1992. Interleukin-4 differently regulates tumor necrosis factor-a gene expression by human T lymphocytes and monocytes. Pathobiology **60**: 100–107.
20. MORI, N., F. SHIRAKAWA, S. MURAKAMI, S. ODA & S. ETO. 1993. Inhibitory effect of interleukin-4 on production of interleukin-6 by adult T-cell leukemia cells. Cancer Res. **53**: 4643–4647.
21. LOYER, P., G. ILYIN, Z. A. RAZZAK, J. BANCHEREAU, J. F. DEZIER, J. P. CAMPION, C. GUGUEN-GUILLOUZO & A. GUILLOUZO. 1993. Interleukin-4 inhibits the production of some acute-phase proteins by human hepatocytes in primary culture. FEBS Lett. **336**: 215–220.
22. MINTY, A., P. CHALON, J. M. DEROCQ, X. DUMONT, J. C. GUILLEMOT, M. KAGHAD, C. LABIT, P. LAPLATOIS, P. LIAUZUN, B. MILOUX, C. MINTY, P. CASELLAS, G. LOISON, J. LUPKER, D. SHIRE, P. FERRARA & D. CAPUT. 1993. Interleukin-13 is a new human lymphokine regulating inflammatory and immune responses. Nature **362**: 248–250.
23. DOHERTY, T. M., R. KASTELEIN, S. MENON, S. ANDRADE & R. L. COFFMAN. 1993. Modulation of murine macrophage function by IL-13. J. Immunol. **151**: 7151–7160.
24. ZURAWSKI, G. & J. E. DE VRIES. 1994. Interleukin 13, an interleukin 4-like cytokine that acts on monocytes and B cells, but not on T cells. Immunol. Today **15**: 19–26.
25. SPORN, M. B. & A. ROBERTS. 1990. TGFβ: Problems and prospects. Cell Regulation **1**: 875–882.
26. KULKARNI, A. B. & S. KARLSSON. 1993. Transforming growth factor-β_1 knockout mice. A mutation in one cytokine gene causes a dramatic inflammatory disease. Am. J. Pathol. **143**: 3–9.
27. MAUVIEL, A., Y. Q. CHEN, W. DONG, C. H. EVANS & J. UITTO. 1993. Transcriptional interactions of transforming growth factor-β with proinflammatory cytokines. Current Biol. **3**: 822–831.
28. CAMPOS, S. P., Y. WANG, A. KOJ & H. BAUMANN. 1993. Divergent transforming growth factor-β effects on IL-6 regulation of acute phase plasma proteins in rat hepatoma cells. J. Immunol. **151**: 7128–7137.
29. ROSEN, E. M., R. J. ZITNIK, J. A. ELIAS, M. M. BHARGAVA, J. WINES & I. D. GOLDBERG. 1993. The interaction of HGF-SF with other cytokines in tumor invasion and angiogenesis. In Hepatocyte Growth Factor-Scatter Factor (HGF-SF) and the C-Met Receptor. I. D. Goldberg & E. M. Rosen, Eds. Vol. 1: 301–310. Basel, Switzerland: Birkhauser Verlag.
30. KOJ, A., E. KORZUS, H. BAUMANN, T. NAKAMURA & J. TRAVIS. 1993. Regulation of synthesis of some proteinase inhibitors in human hepatoma cells HepG2 by cytokines, hepatocyte growth factor and retinoic acid. Biol. Chem. Hoppe-Seyler **374**: 193–201.
31. KOJ, A., J. GAULDIE & H. BAUMANN. 1993. Biological perspectives of cytokine and hormone networks. In Acute Phase Proteins. Molecular Biology, Biochemistry and Clinical Applications. A. Mackiewicz, I. Kushner & H. Baumann, Eds. Vol. 1: 275–287. Boca Raton, Ann Arbor, London and Tokyo: CRC Press.
32. BAIGRIE, R. J., P. M. LAMONT, M. DALLMAN & P. J. MORRIS. 1991. The release of interleukin-1β (IL-1) precedes that of interleukin-6 (IL-6) in patients undergoing major surgery. Lymphokine Cytokine Res. **10**: 253–256.
33. ULICH, T. R., K. GUO, D. REMICK, J. DEL CASTILLO & S. YIN. 1991. Endotoxin-induced cytokine gene expression in vivo. J. Immunol. **146**: 2316–1323.
34. PARANT, M., C. LE CONTEL, F. PARANT & L. CHEDID. 1991. Influence of endogenous glucocorticoid on endotoxin-induced production of circulating TNFα. Lymphokine Cytokine Res. **10**: 265–271.
35. AMANO, Y., S. W. LEE & A. C. ALLISON. 1993. Inhibition by glucocorticoids of the formation of interleukin-1-α, interleukin-1β and interleukin-6: Mediation by decreased messenger RNA stability. Molec. Pharmacology **43**: 176–182.
36. MANTHEY, C. L., M. E. BRANDES, P. Y. PERERA & S. N. VOGEL. 1992. Taxol increases

steady-state levels of lipopolysaccharide genes and protein-tyrosine phosphorylation in murine macrophages. J. Immunol. **149:** 2459–2465.
37. RAY, A., S. B. TATTER, U. SANTHANAM, D. C. HELFGOTT, L. T. MAY & P. B. SEHGAL. 1989. Regulation of expression of interleukin-6: Molecular and clinical studies. Ann. N. Y. Acad. Sci. **557:** 353–362.
38. ENTMAN, M. L., L. MICHAEL, R. D. ROSSEN, W. J. DREYER, D. C. ANDERSON, A. A. TAYLOR & C. W. SMITH. 1991. Inflammation in the course of early myocardial ischemia. FASEB J. **5:** 2529–2537.
39. PERLMUTTER, D. H., G. I. GLOVER, M. RIVETNA, C. S. SCHASTEEN & R. J. FALLON. 1990. Identification of a serpin-enzyme complex receptor on human hepatoma cells and human monocytes. Proc. Natl. Acad. Sci. USA **87:** 3753–3757.
40. KURDOWSKA, A. & J. TRAVIS. 1990. Acute phase protein stimulation by α-1-antichymotrypsin-cathepsin G complex. J. Biol. Chem. **265:** 21023–21026.
41. KOJ, A., H. ROKITA, T. KORDULA, A. KURDOWSKA & J. TRAVIS. 1991. Role of cytokines and growth factors in the induced synthesis of proteinase inhibitors belonging to acute phase proteins. Biomed. Biochim. Acta **50:** 421–425.
42. PRINCEN, H. M. G., H. J. MOSHAGE, J. J. EMEIS, H. J. W. DE HAARD, W. NIEUWENHUIZEN & S. H. YAP. 1985. Fibrinogen fragments X, Y, D and E increase levels of plasma fibrinogen and liver mRNAs coding for fibrinogen polypeptide in rats. Thromb. Hemostasis **53:** 212–215.
43. MOSHAGE, H. J., H. M. G. PRINCEN, J. VAN PELT, H. M. J. ROELOFS, W. NIEUWENHUIZEN & S. H. YAP. 1990. Differential effects of endotoxin and fibrinogen degradation products (FDPS) on liver synthesis of fibrinogen and albumin: Evidence for the involvement of a novel cytokine in the stimulation of fibrinogen synthesis induced by FDPS. Int. J. Biochem. **22:** 1393–1400.
44. RITCHIE, D. G., B. A. LEVY, M. A. ADAMS & G. M. FULLER. 1982. Regulation of fibrinogen synthesis by plasmin-derived fragment of fibrinogen and fibrin: An indirect pathway. Proc. Natl. Acad. Sci. USA **79:** 1530–1534.
45. ROBEY, F. A., K. OHURA, S. FUTAKI, N. FUJI, H. YAJIMA, N. GOLDMAN, K. D. JONES & S. WAHL. 1987. Proteolysis of human C-reactive protein produces peptides with potent immunomodulating activity. J. Biol. Chem. **262:** 7053–7057.
46. THOMASSEN, M. J., D. P. MEEKER, S. D. DEODHAR, H. P. WIEDEMANN & B. BARNA. 1993. Activation of human monocytes and alveolar macrophages by a synthetic peptide of C-reactive protein. J. Immunother. **13:** 1–6.
47. BALLOU, S. P. & G. LOZANSKI. 1992. Induction of inflammatory cytokine release from cultured human monocytes by C-reactive protein. Cytokine, **4:** 361–368.
48. GALVE-DE ROCHEMONTAIX, B., K. WIKTOROWICZ, I. KUSHNER & J. M. DAYER. 1993. C-reactive protein increases production of IL-1α, IL-1β and TNFα, and expression of mRNA by human alveolar macrophages. J Leukoc. Biol. **53:** 439–445.
49. VLASSARA, H., M. BROWNLEE, K. R. MANOGUE, C. A. DINARELLO & A. PASAGIAN. 1988. Cachectin/TNF and IL-1 induced by glucose-modified proteins: Role in normal tissue remodelling. Science **240:** 1546–1548.
50. GUZDEK, A. & K. STALINSKA. 1992. Glycated proteins as inducers of acute phase cytokines. Folia Histochem. Cytobiol. **30:** 167–170.
51. KOJ, A., A. GUZDEK, J. POTEMPA, E. KORZUS & J. TRAVIS. 1994. Origin of circulating acute phase cytokines: modified proteins may trigger IL-6 production by macrophages. Preliminary report. J. Physiol. Pharmacol. **45:** 69–80.
52. DANG, C. V., W. R. BELL, D. KAISER & A. WONG. 1985. Disorganization of cultured vascular endothelial cell monolayers by fibrinogen fragment D. Science **227:** 1487–1490.
53. JOHNSON, D. & J. TRAVIS. 1977. Inactivation of human α-1-proteinase inhibitor by thiol proteinases. Biochem. J. **163:** 639–641.
54. KOJ, A., J. GAULDIE, E. REGOECZI, D. N. SAUDER & G. SWEENEY. 1984. The acute phase response of cultured rat hepatocytes. Biochem. J. **224:** 505–514.
55. NEEDHAM, P. L. 1986. The separation of human blood using mono-poly resolving medium. J. Immunol. Meth. **99:** 283–284.
56. AMERICAN THORACIC SOCIETY GUIDELINES. 1985. Summary and recommendation of a

workshop on the investigational use of fiberoscopic bronchoscopy and bronchoalveolar lavage in asthmatics. Am. Rev. Resp. Dis. **132:** 180–182.
57. MANIE, S., A. SCHMID-ALLIANA, J. KUBAR, B. FERRUA & B. ROSSI. 1993. Disruption of microtubule network in human monocytes induces expression of interleukin-1 but not that of interleukin-6 nor tumor necrosis factor-α. J. Biol. Chem. **268:** 13675–13681.
58. EUGUI, E. M., B. DELUSTRO, S. ROUHAFZA, M. ILNICKA, S. W. LEE, R. WILHELM & A. C. ALLISON. 1994. Some antioxidants inhibit, in a coordinate fashion, the production of tumor necrosis factor-α, IL-1β, and IL-6 by human peripheral blood mononuclear cells. Inter. Immunology **6:** 409–422.

DISCUSSION OF THE PAPER

G. FEY (*University of Erlangen-Nürnberg, Erlangen, Germany*): I would like to ask whether the effect of taxol on IL-1 is on new protein synthesis? Or is it on release of presynthesized protein?

A. KOJ: So far we have measured only IL-1 that has been released to the medium. But taxol affected both IL-1α and IL-1β. The difference is considerable. I do not think that it would be explained by interfering with release, but until the mRNA level is measured, I cannot answer your question. It is crucial whether it is a release or a *de novo* synthesis.

FEY: So you can exclude the possibility that it is a stimulation of a processing enzyme for IL-1, which would be very interesting.

KOJ: We do not know, but you are absolutely right. There are probably many more side effects of taxol which have not yet been recognized. And it will be very interesting to find out whether it interferes with cleaving enzyme.

H. BAUMANN (*Roswell Park Cancer Institute, Buffalo, NY*): You place the major role for initiating the acute phase to the activation of macrophage. So, recognition of strange material like modified proteins is important. Now, our favorite model in acute phase is actually tissue damage. It means exposing cells to a very high level of a compound at the site of injury. Does that reflect the high concentration of activated resident macrophages which then, in turn, will activate the cascade sufficiently to support the acute phase? Or do you now need to maintain a high level of modified protein to support the system?

KOJ: I think that it is a very good point that you raised. We presented macrophages with a single dose of modified proteins. It just happened that we are using this macrophage model, but the same may be valid for any other cell that is capable of producing cytokines. So, perhaps an even better model would be fibroblasts which would not respond to endotoxin. I would agree that the macrophages are not the only source of cytokines in full-scale acute phase response. Other cells should be taken into account, including fibroblast and endothelial cells.

P. C. HEINRICH (*Klinikum der RWTH Aachen, Institut für Biochemie, Aachen, Germany*): Alex, I have problems with your CRP experiments, which you referred to. Actually, if you need to increase CRP it is really negligible. There are extremely low levels in plasma, so how can this lead to stimulations of cytokines?

KOJ: I showed this on purpose, because this may be a sort of vicious circle. Usually we refer to acute phase proteins as positive because they help to restore homeostasis. This may be the case where CRP acts in a bad manner. It stimulates synthesis of cytokines, which would then cause the acute phase response to be self-perpetuating. It stimulates synthesis of cytokines and more cytokines and more CRP and so on until something else goes into play. I hope that it might be another cytokine: cytokine 4, 10 or 13; but actually not only cytokines are involved in regulation of acute phase response. This is a cytokine meeting, so it concentrates on cytokines, but we have to be aware that there are many other factors which influence acute phase response. But you raised a very good question about what happens if this perpetuation of acute phase goes on. We then see prolonged inflammatory reaction or prolonged disease.

HEINRICH: And how about this endocytosis business? Is there any clue how endocytosis triggers cytokine release?

KOJ: Well, there is no direct proof about endocytosis as such, but probably by coupling with a respiratory burst. I cannot give a straightforward answer to whether a respiratory burst is a side effect or is necessary for production of cytokines. Maybe somebody else knows the answer.

I. KUSHNER (*Case Western Reserve University, Cleveland, OH*): Years ago, decades ago, I used to give talks about acute phase response and I used to say "inflammatory stimuli," and then I said to myself: "What are inflammatory stimuli?" And I happened to be working on a chapter with one of Tony Allison's students at the time, Phil Davis, who was an expert on inflammation. And he said "tissue injury." So that little sentence found its way into the first NYAS title that Pravin Sehgal showed earlier today. But I am a rheumatologist, and we see lots of people with gout who have spectacular CRP and SAA elevation and wonderful acute phase response. And for the life of me I could not see that urate crystals in the synovial fluid caused tissue injury, and in fact the people who are studying the effect of urate crystals have been looking at that themselves. What they found is in fact one of the first things that you said, Alex: the ingestion of urate crystals by macrophages leads to the release of the inflammatory mediators. And there are numbers of studies showing that opsonic uptake by macrophages can start the whole process of production of inflammatory mediators. What keeps them going, that's another story.

P. SEHGAL (*New York Medical College, Valhalla*): With Dr. May's permission, I think that you need to remember or recognize that CRP or a fragment of CRP can bind IL-6 and at least a working hypothesis in our corner of the world is that CRP can itself shut down IL-6 biological activity. And I think that we will hear a lot more about it in the next day or two.

Interleukin-6 Chaperones in Blood[a]

LESTER T. MAY,[b] MACKEVIN I. NDUBUISI, KIRIT PATEL, AND
DORYS GARCÍA

Department of Microbiology and Immunology
Basic Science Building
New York Medical College
Valhalla, New York 10595

Numerous studies investigating interleukin-6 (IL-6) expression *in vitro* have revealed that this multifunctional cytokine can be synthesized and secreted by many different cell-types. Endothelial cells lining the vasculature[1,2] as well as the underlying vascular smooth muscle cells[3] can produce copious amounts of IL-6 when appropriately stimulated. In the blood, monocytes[4,5] as well as B-cells[6] can also secrete significant amounts of IL-6. In every tissue that has been studied cells producing IL-6 have been found, including fibroblasts,[5] endometrial stromal cells,[7] normal keratinocytes,[8] pancreatic islet cells,[9] osteoclasts,[10] astrocytes and virtually every type of tissue macrophage.[11,12] In fact only normal human T-cells seem to distinguish themselves by their inability or, at best, poor facility to express IL-6.[13] Paradoxically it was a T-cell line from which IL-6 was cloned as a B-cell differentiation factor (Bcdf), and on this basis it was originally suggested that Bcdf is a T-cell replacement factor.[14] Now it is clear that IL-6 can be produced in virtually every tissue in the body and the range of cell-type-specific inducers is extensive and includes IL-1α, IL-1β, TNF-α, lymphotoxin, interferons, IL-2, IL-4, IL-11, all types of viruses (single or double-stranded RNA or DNA), bacterial products (Gram negative or positive-derived) lipopolysaccharide (LPS) and muramyl dipeptides and virtually every recognized second messenger agonist[12] IL-6 promoter dissections have revealed multiple response elements consistent with what has been seen in whole cell expression of IL-6.[15]

In 1992 we demonstrated that IL-6 is a normally circulating plasma protein.[16] Despite all of the intriguing cell-specific regulation of IL-6 gene expression, it became clear that there was always a significant level of IL-6 in blood ($\geq$10 nanograms/ml). However, this circulating IL-6 was completely camouflaged from the routine IL-6 bioassay, the B9 cell-growth-factor assay. Furthermore, this endogenous IL-6 found in serum or plasma was essentially transparent to all of the customary enzyme-linked immunosorbent assay (ELISA). Thus, we could identify as much as 5 μg/ml of IL-6 (confirmed by amino acid analysis) in serum or plasma that scored less than 200 picograms/ml in a commercially available ELISA and less than 50 picograms/ml by B9 cell growth factor assay.[16] Normal individuals, without any overt clinical symptoms suggestive of infection, scored undetectable levels of IL-6 in any assay (limits of detection ranged from 5–50 picograms/ml contingent on the assay used) when the actual mass numbers revealed more than 10 nanograms/ml. Current attempts to elucidate the physiological role of IL-6, to pharmacologically exploit known IL-6 biological activities (*e.g.*, its thrombopoietic activities), or even to inhibit potentially pathophysiological responses to inappropriately presented IL-6 must consider IL-6 already pres-

---

[a] Supported by a Research Grant-in-Aid from the American Heart Association, New York State Affiliate (92-363GS).

[b] Address correspondence to Dr. L. T. May; Tel: 914-993-4181; Fax: 914-993-4825.

ent in the systemic circulation. The following studies reveal some counterintuitive results that have profound implications concerning our lack of understanding of IL-6 physiology. IL-6 is found in normal human blood at levels sufficient to elicit the entire spectrum of known IL-6 effects, but remains inert. Does this circulating IL-6 act as a reservoir that can be activated or regulated? The current studies that attempt to answer this question are of general importance as they relate to all circulating cytokines or hormones.

THE MASKING OF HUMAN IL-6

The first indication that natural human IL-6 was not being measured accurately by all currently used assay systems was our finding that IL-6 secreted from human fibroblasts was predominantly multimeric and that this highly ordered IL-6 had an extremely low specific activity in the B9 cell growth factor assay and almost no IL-6 ELISA reactivity in an ELISA that was sensitive to *E. coli*-derived recombinant human IL-6 (rIL-6) at between 1–10 picograms/ml.[17] These oligomeric forms of natural human IL-6 were not attributable to the artifactual intercystine bridges frequently encountered with rIL-6. Instead this ability of IL-6 to form oligomers was found to be directly related to the degree of post-translational modifications that occur in human IL-6 synthesized in eucaryotic cells, but not in bacterial cells engineered to express human IL-6. Both increasing phosphorylation and glycosylation of IL-6 were shown to result in an increasingly higher ordered structure.[17] On gel filtration chromatography the monomeric forms of IL-6 were measured accurately by the same assays (B9 and ELISA) that were not able to determine oligomeric IL-6 amounts quantitatively indicating that the formation of quaternary structure for human IL-6 alters some immunological and biological properties. Conversely, the ability of human IL-6 to stimulate hepatocytes *in vitro* remains unaffected by differences in quaternary structure.[17]

Despite the hundreds of investigations concerned with IL-6 levels in blood which conclude that IL-6 concentrations exceed 100 picograms/ml in serum only after a response to some injury or infection we have *never* failed to isolate from serum or plasma less than 10 nanograms/ml. In all cases that were determined on patients with infection, especially those that are intercurrent with some other body trauma, we can measure amounts in excess of 100 nanograms/ml of IL-6 and have found levels as high as 5 μg/ml.[16] These numbers are only a lower estimate since they represent yields of amino acids released during an automated Edman degradation. Thus, for each purification of IL-6 from serum or plasma we can, at once, confirm the identity from an amino-terminal sequence as well as concomitantly establish amounts of IL-6 from the amounts of amino acids released during the Edman degradation. Two significant points concerning the recognition of the IL-6 found in blood are: 1) the ability to, at least, qualitatively recognize the endogenous IL-6 in circulation rested on a monoclonal antibody (4IL6) that, in comparison with other monoclonal antibodies (mAbs) to human IL-6, only poorly recognized rIL-6 and 2) the fact that essentially all of the IL-6 that was detected in blood and ultimately purified existed in a high molecular weight complexes.

The initial development of mAbs to human IL-6 revolved around routine screening and characterization of those Abs. Our major interest was to identify those mAbs with the highest affinity, as compared by dissociation constants for rIL-6, and binding to epitopes that did not cross-react or compete with each other. Using mAbs to IL-6 that fulfilled such criteria has led to the development of extremely sensitive IL-6 sandwich ELISAs that can recognize as little as 1 picogram/ml of rIL-6. This provided us with both a bioassay (B9 cell growth factor assay) and antigen/immunological assays (via different sandwich ELISAs) which, in theory, could offer two distinct and sensitive measures for IL-6 concentrations that are two to three orders of magnitude below the half-maximal concentrations for IL-6 biological activities. However, we discovered that a less sensitive IL-6 bioassay based on IL-6 hepatocyte stimulating activity (HSF; stimulation of Hep 3B cells to synthesize α_1-antichymotrypsin) as well as an IL-6 ELISA that used as its capture mAb 4IL6, which was relatively insensitive to rIL-6, could now recognize IL-6 in serum or plasma that was seemingly transparent to the assays more sensitive to rIL-6. We began to characterize this apparent IL-6 biological activity and immunoreactivity. The first step characterized the sieving properties of both serum and plasma IL-6 through gel filtration chromatography.[16] Normal serum or plasma showed no detectable IL-6, at any associated molecular mass by the customary IL-6 assays. However, we could detect small amounts of HSF activity, as well as IL-6 immunoreactivity by our 4IL6/5IL6 sandwich ELISA in fractions that were marked between 150–500 kD. Only in patients who were demonstrably septic did we detect any low molecular weight IL-6 that was representative of a monomeric form of endogenous IL-6 (*i.e.*, in fractions marked between 14–30 kD) through the customary IL-6 assays. In the same serum or plasma sample gel chromatography fractionations we detected no IL-6 in the higher molecular weight-associated fractions using the traditional assay systems. In contrast, switching to the HSF assay and 4IL6/5IL6 ELISA systems demonstrated that the bulk of the IL-6 was associated with the higher molecular fractions. Affinity purification of IL-6 from these different molecular weight fractions confirmed the qualitative picture established by the HSF activity and 4IL6/5IL6 ELISA immunoreactivity by Western blot analysis that essentially all of the IL-6 was in fractions marked between 150–500 kD.

The immunoaffinity purification of the IL-6 from these high molecular weight fractions also provided us with a clue as to why this endogenous IL-6 was transparent to so many IL-6 assays. By freeze-drying aliquots of the IL-6 immunoaffinity chromatography-generated fractions we were able to sufficiently concentrate the various proteins to run them on an SDS-PAGE and stain the protein bands with Coomasie Blue. Aside from the multiple forms of IL-6 (ranging in size from 15–30 kD) we were able to detect additional protein bands that we identified by direct amino-terminal amino acid sequencing. Each affinity-purified fraction that contained IL-6 also contained C-reactive protein (CRP), fragments of complement factors C3 (C3c) and C4 (γ-chain of C4b). More recently we have also verified that a soluble form of the IL-6R (sIL-6R) is also present in association with the IL-6 in these high molecular weight fractions. There also appears to be a soluble form of gp130 (sgp130) that has been shown to be directly involved in the signal transduction of IL-6 (18) after IL-6 binds to the IL-6R, which then associates with the membrane-bound form of gp130.

Although we have not rigorously established that these IL-6-associated proteins are directly responsible for the camouflaging of circulating, high molecular weight IL-6, we are beginning to elucidate the effects of these various normal plasma protein components on IL-6 recognition, *in vitro*. Thus far we can state that these plasma proteins do interact with IL-6 or with one or another component of this high molecular weight complex. We are currently developing assays to uncover the stoichiometric relationships among the various plasma components that we have identified in these high molecular weight IL-6-associated complexes. It is interesting that as the CRP levels increase in plasma or serum there is an increasing problem in quantitatively measuring actual circulating IL-6 levels. Since IL-6 is considered the most important cytokine affecting the dramatic increases in CRP production by hepatocytes,[19] the possibility that CRP, in turn, is somehow involved in regulating IL-6 presentation in the systemic circulation could constitute a feedback loop for even extremely elevated levels of IL-6.

ANTIBODIES CHAPERONE CIRCULATING IL-6

The use of passive immunization on experimental animals with neutralizing or blocking Abs has been a powerful approach in attempts to evaluate the contribution(s) of various cytokines to their relevant array of biological effects. Recent data from this laboratory as well as others indicate that this approach is profoundly faulted.[20,21] Rather than simply inhibiting the biological effect of the cytokine in question, administration of "neutralizing" mAb actually serves to prolong the effect. TABLE 1 illustrates how preinjection or coinjection of rat anti-murine IL-6 mAb (20F3) before or with the addition recombinant murine IL-6 i.p. into CD2F1 mice serves to maintain this administered IL-6 in the circulation. More importantly, the antibody does not neutralize the response to the injected IL-6 (Experimental groups 4 and 6), as the fibrinogen levels are elevated beyond what is found in mice injected with a similar amount of IL-6 (Exp. group 2) or IL-6 and irrelevant mAb (Exp. groups 3 and 5). The same experiments were repeated using human rIL-6 with murine anti-human IL-6 mAb (5IL6) in order to avoid any potential contribution of endogenously produced IL-6[21] that may have been induced by the antigen/antibody complex. In this way we were able to verify that only the injected human IL-6 was circulating in the mice blood by assaying the serology of any IL-6 activity. The results we obtained with the administered human IL-6 into mice were identical to what we obtained for the murine IL-6. Basically, the addition of mAb prolonged the amount of time that the administered IL-6 remained in circulation and the effect of this prolonged circulation of this (human IL-6)/anti-human IL-6 antibody) complex was not inhibitory to the IL-6 effects of increasing fibrinogen concentration in plasma. In fact the fibrinogen levels were significantly above those where IL-6 was administered without antibody (regardless of whether murine or human IL-6 was used). This paradoxical effect of so-called neutralizing antibody actually enhancing the effect intended to be inhibited was stud-

TABLE 1. Serum IL-6 and Fibrinogen Levels in Mice Coinjected with rMuIL-6 and anti-MuIL-6 mAb(Antigen and mAb Mixed Prior to Injection)

Experimental Group	IL-6	mAb	IL-6 (B9 U/ml)		Fibrinogen (mg/dl)
			2 hours	18–20 hours	18–20 hours
1.	Saline		9		186 ± 25
2.	MuIL-6		529	9	336 ± 52
3.	MuIL-6	GL113(coinj)	579	44	284 ± 6
4.	MuIL-6	20F3(coinj)	633,013	135,150	404 ± 44
5.	MuIL-6	GL113(pre)	302	9	373 ± 31
6.	MuIL-6	20F3(pre)	729,977	61,008	356 ± 23
7.	HuIL-6	5IL6	8,377	14,644	496 ± 65
8.	HuIL-6		979	170	237 ± 81

rMuIL-6 2 µg/mouse i.p.; mAb 20F3 or GL113 100 µg/mouse coinjected (premixed) with rMuIL-6 (coinj). For preincubation, 20F3 or GL113 600 µg/mouse was administered i.p. prior to MuIL-6 (pre). rHuIL-6 1.25 µg/mouse; mAb 20F3 100 µg/mouse. mAb and rHuIL-6 premixed prior to injection i.p.

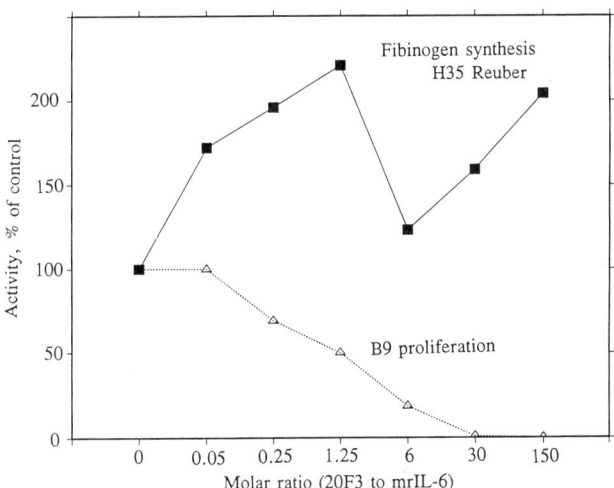

FIGURE 1. Stimulation of fibrinogen synthesis and secretion by H35 Reuber hepatoma cells in response to mouse-serum-derived IL-6. In the experiment recombinant baculovirus-vector-derived MuIL-6 ("rmIL-6") was used as the assay standard; concentrations are expressed in nanograms/ml.

ied *in vitro*. FIGURE 1 illustrates how the addition of increasing molar ratios of mAb 20F3 to recombinant murine IL-6 does neutralize the effects of IL-6 on B9 cell growth activity. However, IL-6 effect on hepatocytes is not so clearcut. In fact, we have reproducibly found that under the same conditions in which IL-6 B9 cell growth activity is completely inhibited there is an approximately 2-fold increase in IL-6-stimulated fibrinogen synthesis from rat hepatocytes (H35 Reuber cells). This enhancement effect on fibrinogen synthesis is even more pronounced when we use *in vivo*-derived IL-6/IL-6 mAb complexes and further add polyclonal antibody to murine IL-6 (see Fig. 6 of ref. 21). These observations suggest that anti-IL-6 Ab is able to alter the presentation of IL-6 to specific target tissues such that it may neutralize one effect while enhancing another.

In baboons the preinjection of mAb to human IL-6 (5IL6) two hours prior to the administration of an LPS bolus also results in the prolonged circulation of LPS-induced baboon IL-6.[21] Virtually all of the IL-6 found in circulation that had been induced by LPS is then found in an IL-6/anti-IL-6 antibody complex. Without addressing any of the normally circulating IL-6 in baboon blood that is, as in humans, difficult to recognize or measure, it was observed that these complexes also led to an enhancement in the actual amounts or concentrations of IL-6 that continued to increase even eight hours after the LPS injection. In contrast, the administration of the same amount of LPS without prior passive immunization with anti-IL-6 Ab led to a much smaller and far more transient rise in measurable IL-6 levels (for both B9 cell-growth-factor activity as well as IL-6 ELISA reactivity). The salient point in the mouse and baboon studies is that anti-IL-6 antibodies act as carriers helping to create a reservoir of circulating IL-6, which is both biologically active and retained in the systemic circulation. This ability to chaperone proteins, especially cytokines in the bloodstream, is currently being investigated for naturally occurring soluble forms of cytokine receptors as well as endogenous auto-antibodies to certain cytokines.[22,23] As in our studies the initial perception of these chaperoning molecules was suggested by their ability to inhibit biological activities *in vitro*. However, on re-examination the *in vivo* effects indicated an enhancement of biological effects as well as an ability to maintain this readily available reservoir of circulating cytokines.

The combination of multifunctional systemic molecules like IL-6 being chaperoned and camouflaged from the usual assay systems presents some interesting conundrums: 1) If the omnipresence of IL-6 is maintained, what type of regulation is involved in either preventing or stimulating the biological effects associated with IL-6 *in vitro*? 2) Can the presumed dysregulated gene expression of certain cytokines (including IL-6) that has been invoked for a number of pathological conditions now be accounted for by inappropriate regulation at the level of presentation of pre-existing molecules? 3) Is the reservoir of circulating IL-6 usable? 4) Does the formation of these IL-6 complexes preclude the potential use of any administered IL-6? At this time we cannot answer any of these questions completely. Without more complete answers to these questions the physiological or pathophysiological role and potential pharmacological applications may never be realized. The last section partially answers some of these questions through analyses of a particular type of patient whose unusual circumstances offer clues to the questions posed above.

SUSTAINED HIGH LEVELS OF INTERLEUKIN-6 FOLLOWING IMMUNOTHERAPY

In an attempt to study alterations of IL-6 levels in individuals that are administered rIL-6 a totally unexpected observation occurred. Armed with our traditional IL-6 sandwich ELISAs (7IL6/5IL6, IG61/5IL6), B9 cell-growth-factor assay as well as an additional IL-6 sandwich ELISA (4IL6/5IL6) that has, relative to the other IL-6 ELISAs, mediocre sensitivity to rIL-6, but an ability to at least qualitatively recognize IL-6 found in blood[16,24] we identified a class of patients that had a chronically high level of circulating IL-6 (>100 nanograms/ml). The existence of this IL-6 was only recognized by the 4IL6/5IL6 ELISA and the level of IL-6 was unaffected by any rIL-6 administration. Each of these individuals had received prior treatment for advanced malignancies. All of these patients with high IL-6 concentrations in their blood had been involved in an active immunotherapy regimen. Each of these patients had advanced melanoma and were treated with an anti-idiotypic antibody MK2-23 (raised to the high molecular weight melanoma-associated antigen) that had been conjugated to keyhole limpet hemocyanin (KLH) and administered with the adjuvant Bacillus Calmette Guerin (BCG). Plasma and serum samples taken concomitantly had essentially no B9 cell-growth-factor activity. For the other patients involved in this Phase I study that had no prior history with active immunotherapy there were small, but significant increases in B9 cell growth factor activity after subcutaneous injection that was equally reflected in the rIL-6-sensitive ELISAs (7IL6/5IL6). The rise in IL-6 levels, in these patients, was measured at no more than 100 picograms/ml. Most importantly, this IL-6 activity and immunoreactivity was all found at a molecular weight consistent with it being an uncomplexed monomer or dimer using a gel chromatography fractionation format.

Gel chromatography fractionation of the plasma samples with high 4IL6/5IL6 immunoreactivity revealed that all of the IL-6 immunoreactivity was found in a 200 kD complex. The initial 4IL6/5IL6 ELISA estimates of IL-6 levels of 600 nanograms/ml were found to be underestimates. Importantly, these complexes do have hepatocyte stimulating activity as identified by either fibrinogen or α_1-antichymotrypsin induction on Hep 3B cells. Analyses of serum proteins from a number of these patients registering high IL-6 levels has confirmed elevated levels of C-reactive protein (CRP) suggesting an ongoing acute phase response and indicating that the circulating IL-6 in these IL-6 complexes is active with respect to *in vivo* hepatocyte stimulation. Fortuitously each of the melanoma patients that had been involved in the immunotherapy program had plasma samples withdrawn and stored at $-80°C$. Thus, we were able to study the effects of immunotherapy on IL-6 levels from these archived plasma samples, which in some individuals occurred over a three year period. It became evident that during the course of treatment IL-6 levels continued to go up and never returned to basal levels found at the start of the immunotherapy. These high levels of IL-6 persisted for many months after treatment had been terminated, and when rIL-6 injections began there was no effect on IL-6 levels as measured in any of our assay systems (4IL6/5IL6 and 7IL6/5IL6 ELISAs as well as B9 cell-growth-factor assay). Affinity purification of these high molecular weight IL-6–associated complexes derived from the gel chromatography fractionation always found significant amounts of CRP, complement factor fragment C3c, a soluble form of the IL-6 receptor as well as the multiple isoforms of IL-6 whose heterogeneity (15–31 kD) made it impossible to distinguish endogenous from any of the administered rIL-6. All of this is consistent with our initial finding of these high molecular weight IL-6-associated complexes.[16]

The most dramatic observation in this study[24] is that patients receiving the same form of immunotherapy invariably sustain long-term IL-6–associated complexes in the systemic circulation, which contain very high concentrations of IL-6 (>600 nanograms/ml) associated with the soluble form of the IL-6 receptor, CRP and C3c. These IL-6–associated complexes may be a widespread consequence of aggressive immunization regimens in man. The fate of administered rIL-6 is unclear, but appears to become associated with the 200 kD IL-6 complex in patients that have received aggressive immunotherapy. Similar injections into patients who had not been involved in any immunotherapy had a 20–40 kD protein appear in their blood that had B9 cell-growth-factor activity and 7IL6/5IL6 immunoreactivity within 30 minutes after subcutaneous injection of rIL-6. The fact that these high molecular weight IL-6–associated complexes retain hepatocyte stimulating activity *in vitro* and apparent hepatocyte effect *in vivo* suggests that these complexes can be regulated as IL-6–associated complexes found in much lower concentrations, still containing sufficient IL-6 (>10 nanograms/ml) to induce all of the hepatocyte effects.

SUMMARY

There is increasing evidence that many, perhaps all, cytokines have a soluble form of their receptor in the systemic circulation at all times. There is also evidence that endogenous antibodies to some cytokines, including IL-6,[22] are also found in blood. Initially these findings were evaluated *in vitro*, and associated with inhibiting the respective effects of those cytokines. However, it is now becoming clear that the *in vivo* effects are paradoxically the reverse of what is seen *in vitro*. As we have explained here for IL-6 it is evident that many or all of these molecules that bind and/or associate with IL-6 maintain this molecule in the systemic circulation and constitute a reservoir of masked, but potentially active IL-6. The mode of regulation of the biological activity of these IL-6–associated complexes remains unknown, but needs to be uncovered in order to pharmacologically exploit many of the potentially beneficial effects or to prevent any potential pathological effects.

ACKNOWLEDGMENTS

We thank Mr. Giacomo Vinces and Dr. Damenjeet Chaubey for excellent technical help. We would also thank Dr. Pravin B. Sehgal for his continuous intellectual and spiritual support.

REFERENCES

1. MAY, L. T., G. TORCIA, F. COZZOLINO, A. RAY, S. B. TATTER, U. SANTHANAM, P. B. SEHGAL & D. STERN. 1989. Interleukin-6 gene expression in human endothelial cells: RNA start sites, multiple IL-6 proteins and inhibition of proliferation. Biochem. Biophys. Res. Commun. **159:** 991–998.
2. JIRIK, F. R., T. J. PODOR, T. HIRANO, T. KISHIMOTO, D. J. LOSKUTOFF, D. A. CARSON & M. LOTZ. 1989. Bacterial LPS and inflammatory mediators augment IL-6 secretion by human endothelial cells. J. Immunol. **142:** 144–147.
3. LOPPNOW, H. & P. LIBBY. 1990. Proliferating or interleukin-1-activated human vascular smooth muscle cells secrete copious interleukin-6. J. Clin. Invest. **85:** 731–738.
4. TOSATO, G., K. B. SEAMON, N. D. GOLDMAN, P. B. SEHGAL, L. T. MAY, G. C. WASHINGTON, K. E. JONES & S. E. PIKE. 1988. Monocyte-derived human B-cell growth factor identified as interferon-β_2 (BSF-2, IL-6). Science **239:** 502–504.
5. MAY, L. T., J. GHRAYEB, U. SANTHANAM, S. B. TATTER, Z. STHOEGER, D. C. HELFGOTT, N. CHIORAZZI, G. GRIENINGER & P. B. SEHGAL. 1988. Synthesis and secretion of multiple forms of "β_2-interferon/B-cell differentiation factor BSF-2/hepatocyte stimulating factor" by human fibroblasts and monocytes. J. Biol. Chem. **263:** 7760–7766.
6. SMELAND, E. B., H. K. BLOMHOFF, S. FUNDERUD, M. R. SHALABY & T. ESPEVIK. 1989. Interleukin-4 induces selective production of interleukin-6 from normal human B lymphocytes. J. Exp. Med. **170:** 1463–1468.
7. TABIBZADEH, S. S., U. SANTHANAM, P. B. SEHGAL & L. T. MAY. 1989. Cytokine-induced production of IFN-β_2/IL-6 by freshly explanted human endometrial stromal cells: Modulation by estradiol-17β. J. Immunol. **142:** 3134–3139.
8. KUPPER, T. S., K. MIN, P. B. SEHGAL, H. MIZUTANI, N. BIRCHALL, A. RAY & L. T. MAY. 1989. Production of IL-6 by keratinocytes: Implications for epidermal inflammation and immunity. **557:** 454–465.
9. CAMPBELL, I. L., A. CUTRI, A. WILSON & L. C. HARRISON. 1989. Evidence for IL-6 production by and effects on the pancreatic β-islet cells. J. Immunol. **143:** 1188–1191.
10. GIRASOLE, G., R. L. JILKA, G. PASSERI, S. BOSWELL, G. BODER, D. C. WILLIAMS & S. C. MANOLAGAS. 1992. 17β-estradiol inhibits interleukin-6 production by bone marrow-derived stromal cells and osteoblasts in vitro: A potential mechanism for the antiosteoporotic effect of estrogens. J. Clin. Invest. **89:** 883–891.
11. WESSELINGH, S. L., N. M. GOUGH, J. J. FINLAY-JONES & P. J. MCDONALD. 1990. Detection of cytokine mRNA in astrocyte cultures using polymerase chain reaction. Lymph. Res. **9:** 177–185.
12. HEINRICH, P. C., J. V. CASTELL & T. ANDUS. 1990. IL-6 and the acute phase response. Biochem. J. **265:** 621–636.
13. VILLIGER, P. M., M. T. CRONIN, T. AMENOMORI, W. WACHSMAN & M. LOTZ. 1991. IL-6 production by human T-lymphocytes. J. Immunol. **146:** 550–559.
14. HIRANO, T., K. YASUKAWA, H. HARADA, T. TAGA, Y. WATANABE, T. MATSUDA, S. KASHIWAMURA, K. NAKAJIMA, K. KOYAMA, A. IWAMATSU, S. TSUNASAWA, F. SAKIYAMA, H. MATSUI, Y. TAKAHARA, T. TANIGUCHI & T. KISHIMOTO. 1986. Complementary DNA for a novel human interleukin (BSF-2) that induce B lymphocytes to produce immunoglobulins. Nature **324:** 73–76.
15. RAY, A., P. SASSONE-CORSI & P. B. SEHGAL. 1989. A multiple cytokine- and second messenger-responsive element in the enhancer of the human interleukin-6 gene: Similarities with c-fos gene regulation. Molec. Cell. Biol. **9:** 5537–5547.
16. MAY, L. T., H. VIGUET, J. S. KENNEY, N. IDA, A. C. ALLISON & P. B. SEHGAL. 1992. High levels of "complexed" IL-6 in human blood. J. Biol. Chem. **267:** 19698–19704.

17. MAY, L. T., U. SANTHANAM & P. B. SEHGAL. 1991. On the multimeric nature of natural human interleukin-6. J. Biol. Chem. **266:** 9950–9955.
18. HIBI, M., M. MURAKAMI, M. SAITO, T. HIRANO, T. TAGA & T. KISHIMOTO. 1990. Molecular cloning and expression of an IL-6 signal transducer, gp130. Cell **63:** 1149–1157.
19. MAJELLO, B., R. ARCONE, C. TONIATTI & G. CILIBERTO. 1990. Constitutive and IL-6-induced nuclear factors that interact with human C-reactive protein promoter. EMBO J. **9:** 457–465.
20. FINKELMAN, F. D., K. B. MADDEN, S. C. MORRIS, J. M. HOLMES, I. M. KATONA & C. R. MALISZEWSKI. 1993. Anticytokine antibodies as carrier proteins: Prolongation of in vivo effects of exogenous cytokines by injection of cytokine-anti-cytokine antibody complexes. J. Immunol. **151:** 1235–1244.
21. MAY, L. T., R. NETA, L. L. MOLDAWER, J. S. KENNEY, K. PATEL & P. B. SEHGAL. 1993. Antibodies chaperone circulating IL-6: Paradoxical effects of anti-IL-6 "neutralizing" antibodies in vivo. J. Immunol. **151:** 3225–3236.
22. HANSEN, M. B., M. SVENSON, M. DIAMANT & K. BENDTZEN. 1993. High-affinity IgG autoantibodies to IL-6 in sera of normal individuals are competitive inhibitors of IL-6 in vitro. Cytokine **5:** 72–80.
23. SVENSON, M., M. BAGGE-HANSEN & K. BENDTZEN. 1990. Distribution and characterization of autoantibodies to interleukin-1α in normal human sera. Scand. J. Immunol. **32:** 695–701.
24. MAY, L. T., K. PATEL, D. GARCÍA, M. NDIBUISI, S. FERRONE, A. MITTELMAN, A. MACKIEWICZ & P. B. SEHGAL. 1994. Sustained high levels of circulating chaperoned IL-6 following active cancer immunotherapy. Blood. In press.

DISCUSSION OF THE PAPER

G. FEY (*University of Erlangen-Nürnberg, Erlangen, Germany*): Do you have any idea of the mechanism of binding to the C3 and C4 fragments? Is that a reversible mechanism? Can IL-6 be released from its chaperone?

L. T. MAY: Yes. We are looking at that right now *in vitro*. But these are very sticky proteins, as you know. The only thing that I am convinced about is that IL-6 sticks better than, say, immunoglobulins and other molecules that we were working with *in vitro*.

FEY: But it is not a covalent bond through the sialylester of C3 or C4?

MAY: Obviously not, because we can show individual peptides on a denaturing gel.

L. NETA (*Armed Forces Radiobiology Research Institute, Bethesda, MD*): I do not know if I will confuse Heinz (Baumann) or clarify. But at least I should mention that the fibrinogen levels were measured *in vivo*, and you do not usually achieve more than three- to fourfold increase of those levels in plasma.

MAY: I do not think that he was talking about *in vivo* levels. I think that he was thinking about my H-35 assay.

NETA: I'm sorry, in this case it will not fly.

Development of Human IL-6 Receptor Antagonists

JUST P. J. BRAKENHOFF,[a] FLORIS D. DE HON,
AND LUCIEN A. AARDEN

*Central Laboratory of the Netherlands Red Cross Blood Transfusion
Service and Laboratory for Experimental and Clinical Immunology
University of Amsterdam
1066 CX Amsterdam, The Netherlands*

INTRODUCTION

IL-6 is a glycoprotein of 185 amino acids. It was first described in 1980 as a co-product with unknown function of interferon-β production by fibroblasts. In the following years IL-6 turned out to be an extremely pleiotropic cytokine. The biological activities of IL-6 include the stimulation of: Ig production by B cells, B and T cell growth, differentiation of T cells and macrophages, acute phase protein production by hepatocytes, multilineage hematopoiesis, osteoclast formation, maturation of megakaryocytes, and platelet production. IL-6 also affects the central nervous system: IL-6 is an endogenous pyrogen and can induce ACTH production by the pituitary, finally resulting in increased glucocorticoid levels in the circulation. Many of these activities are exerted in synergy with other cytokines like IL-1α/β, TNF-α, IL-3 etc. (reviewed in refs. 1, 2). IL6 is structurally related to, and shares many activities with leukemia inhibitory factor (LIF), oncostatin M (OSM), ciliary neurotrophic factor (CNTF), and IL-11 because they all use a common signal transducer (gp130) in their receptor complex[3,4] (see below). Recent experiments with IL-6 knock-out mice suggest that despite this redundancy in gp130-activators, IL-6 is crucial to an optimal acute phase response after tissue damage and infection with gram-positive (but not gram-negative) bacteria, and for an optimal immune response to viruses and bacteria.[5] IL-6 also turned out to be essential for mucosal IgA production[6] and to play a role in bone metabolism.[7]

MECHANISM OF ACTION OF IL-6

IL-6 exerts its activity through triggering of a transmembrane receptor that is present on all target cells. Currently, the only known specific step in the IL6 signaling cascade is the binding of IL-6 to a low affinity "α"—chain of 80 kD (CD126). The complex of IL6 and α-chain subsequently binds with high affinity to the (non-specific) signal transducing "β" chain, gp130 (also: IL 6Rβ, CD130[1]). Both chains belong to the class I family of the cytokine receptor superfamily.[8] Association of the IL6/α-chain complex leads to homodimerization and tyrosine phosphorylation of gp130 and signal transduction.[9] The stoichiometry of the active receptor complex is not en-

---

[a] Author to whom correspondence should be addressed at Central Laboratory of the Netherlands Red Cross Blood Transfusion Service, Plesmanlaan 125, 1066 CX Amsterdam or P.O. Box 9190, 1006 AD Amsterdam; Fax: (20) 512 3170.

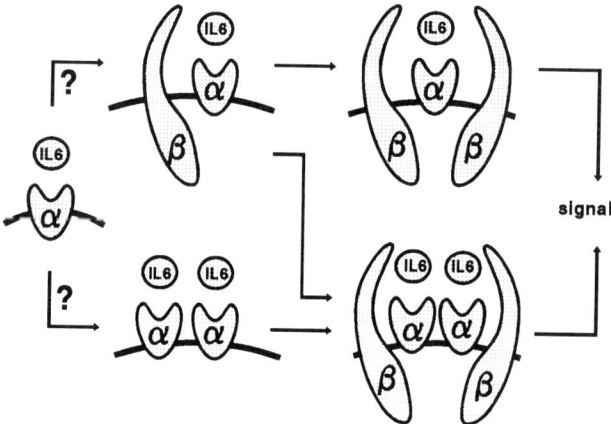

FIGURE 1. Models of IL-6 receptor interaction

tirely clear. Very recently, Ward *et al.* have found by studying complex formation of IL-6 with the soluble extracellular domains of α- and β chain that the active receptor complex may consist of two molecules of each IL6, α- and β chain[10] (see FIG. 1). The activation of gp130 by IL-6 results in the activation of various signal-transduction pathways which can also be triggered by other cytokines.[4,11] IL-6 induces tyrosine phosphorylation of the tyrosine kinases Jak1, Jak2, and Tyk2.[12,13] These in turn may tyrosine phosphorylate transcription factors Signal transducer and activator of transcription (Stat) 1α and Stat3/APRF (acute-phase response factor).[12,14,15] Other proteins that become tyrosine phosphorylated in response to IL-6 are Hck, phosphotyrosine phosphatase-1D (PTP1D, Syp or SH-PTP2), phospholipase C-gamma (PLCgamma), the 110 kD catalytic subunit of PI-3 kinase, pp120 src-substrate, proteins involved in the ras signal-transduction pathway, including Shc, Grb2, Raf-1, Mapk1 and 2, and pp90[rsk] (ribosomal S6 kinase) and a protein called p72[sak] (Stat-associated 72-kD tyrosine kinase).[16-20]

ROLE OF IL-6 IN DISEASE

In healthy individuals no or only very low levels of IL-6 (<10 pg/ml) are detectable in the circulation. In many different diseases however, IL-6 levels are increased and have been postulated to play a causative role in the pathogenesis (for reviews see refs. 2 and 21–23. Examples are multiple myeloma, AIDS lymphoma, polyclonal B cell activation as observed in AIDS, rheumatoid arthritis, cardiac myxoma and Castleman's disease, mesangial proliferative glomerulonephritis, psoriasis, cancer-associated cachexia, postmenopausal osteoporosis, sepsis, alcohol cirrhosis, and diseases of the central nervous system like Alzheimer.[7,24–30] Clearcut evidence for a causative role of IL-6 in the pathogenesis of some of these diseases has come from phase I/II clinical trials with IL-6–neutralizing monoclonal antibodies.[24,31–33] Administration of anti-IL-6 mAb to patients with multiple myeloma and AIDS lymphoma resulted in a temporary blockade of tumor cell growth in some of the patients.[24,31] Anti-IL-6 also reversed fever, acute phase reaction, night sweats, bone destruction, and cachexia.[24,31] Treatment of a patient with Castleman's disease with anti-IL-6 reduced acute phase protein levels, fever, anemia, thrombocytosis, and hypergammaglobulinemia.[32] Improvement of disease parameters was also observed[33] in patients with rheumatoid arthritis. However, inhibition of IL-6 activity with these mAbs has its limitations: firstly, in some patients a human anti-mouse antibody response is observed; and secondly, owing to complex formation with the mAb, the half-life of IL-6 in the circulation is prolonged, leading to accumulation of IL-6.[26,34] Leakage of IL-6 from such a depot might explain in part why the tumor cells in myeloma and AIDS patients escape anti-IL-6 therapy.

DEVELOPMENT AND CHARACTERIZATION OF IL-6 RECEPTOR ANTAGONISTS

In view of the deleterious effects of IL-6 in diseases, and of the limited efficacy of anti-IL-6 mAb, the development of additional IL-6 inhibitors seems desirable. IL-6 receptor antagonists may offer an alternative strategy. Targeting of the α-chain of the receptor guarantees specific inhibition of IL-6 activities. A further advantage of such molecules may be that besides the membrane-bound receptor, they also neutralize the soluble form of IL-6Rα. The soluble extracellular domain of IL-6Rα is biologically active and increases the sensitivity of cells for IL-6.[35] Moderately increased levels of IL-6Rα have been found in patients with HIV infection and multiple myeloma and suggested to enhance the effects of IL-6.[36,37]

STRUCTURE-FUNCTION ANALYSIS OF HUMAN IL-6: SEPARATE REGIONS OF IL-6 ARE IMPORTANT FOR α- AND (α-CHAIN DEPENDENT) β-CHAIN INTERACTION

IL-6 belongs to the long chain family of cytokines with a similar antiparallel four α-helical bundle core structure as growth hormone, G-CSF and LIF, of which the crystal structures have been determined.[38-40] Based on these crystal-structures a 3D-model of IL-6 has been constructed.[41] A greatly simplified version of this model is shown in FIGURE 2. By using mutagenesis approaches and epitope mapping of neutralizing mAb, we and others have identified regions of human IL-6 important for receptor interaction. Residues important for interaction with IL-6Rα are located in the A- and D-helix and in the loop between helices A and B (reviewed in refs. 41 and 42). Collectively we call this region site I or the α-site. Three regions have currently been identified that are important for β-chain interaction. Mutations in these regions abolish binding of the IL-6/IL-6Rα complex to gp130 in assays with soluble receptor components. By using neutralizing mAb we identified a region comprising residues Gln153-His165 (site II, or β_1).[42] A second site consisting of residues Lys42-Ala57 (region 2A) was identified by Ehlers et al. by studying human/mouse chimeras of IL-6.[41] This is here referred to as the β_2 site. Savino et al. identified a third region formed by residues Gly32 and Tyr36, here provisionally called β_3.[43] The position of α- and β-sites is indicated in FIGURE 2.

IL-6 MUTANTS WITH SUBSTITUTIONS IN SINGLE β-SITES ARE PARTIAL ANTAGONISTS OF WILD TYPE (wt) IL-6

We hypothesized that variants of IL-6 with the α-site intact, but with substitutions in β-sites may be receptor antagonists of wtIL-6, by virtue of their capability to

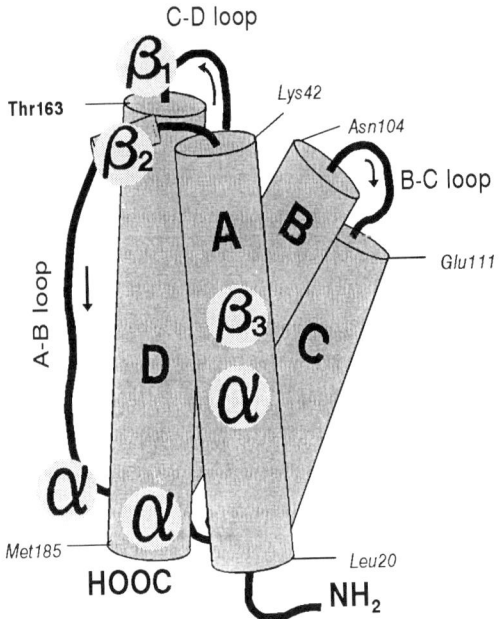

FIGURE 2. Simple version of the putative tertiary structure of IL-6. This figure is adapted from Brakenhoff *et al.*[42] Shown are the helices A–D with connecting loops and a small α-helix in the A–B loop. α's indicate the regions important for IL-6Rα interaction. β1–3 indicate the regions important for (α-chain dependent) gp130 interaction and are further described in the text.

compete for α-chain binding. Indeed we have now identified two IL-6.β_1 mutant proteins (IL-6.Q160/T163P and IL-6.W158R/T163P) capable of antagonizing wtIL-6 activity on HepG2 (hepatoma) and CESS (EBV-transformed B) cells.[42,45] The IL-6.β_2 mutant protein described above (Lys42-Ala57 of human IL-6 replaced with the corresponding residues of mouse IL-6) showed a strongly reduced activity in a variety of bioassays, but displayed no antagonistic activity.[41] The IL-6.β_3 protein showed partial antagonism on Hep3B (hepatoma) cells.[43] Interestingly however, IL-6.β_1 and IL-6.β_2 mutants which were (almost completely) inactive on HepG2 and CESS cells, were still active (with a ~1000-fold reduced activity compared to wtIL-6) on XG-1 (myeloma) and TF-1 (erythroleukemia) cells.[41,44]

IL-6.$\beta_{1,2}$ MUTANT PROTEINS ARE INACTIVE ON AND ANTAGONIZE wtIL-6 ACTIVITY ON HUMAN MYELOMA CELLS

When we combined β_1 with the β_2 mutations in one mutant protein (IL-6.$\beta_{1,2}$, IL-6.Q160E/T163P, β_2), the resulting protein was completely devoid of activity on XG-1 and TF-1 cells, and could partially antagonize wtIL-6 activity on these cells.[44] By introducing two further substitutions the affinity of the IL-6.$\beta_{1,2}$ for IL-6Rα, was ~5-fold increased. The resulting mutant protein (IL-6.$\beta_{1,2}$/F171L and S177R) could completely antagonize wtIL-6–induced proliferation of XG-1 and TF-1 cells, but not the activity of OSM, LIF, and GM-CSF on TF-1 cells.[44]

SUMMARY AND CONCLUSIONS

We have shown that through mutagenesis of IL-6 it is possible to separate receptor binding from signal transduction of the cytokine. Mutations in residues important for signal transduction via gp130 result in IL-6 variants that can competitively inhibit wtIL-6 activity *in vitro*. The differential effects of these signaling deficient mutants on various cell lines of human origin suggest that receptor composition and/or signal transduction pathways may vary between cells of different origin. The observations that three sites have been identified which are important for gp130 interaction raises the question what the role of each region is in the stepwise formation of the active IL-6 receptor complex. The overall tertiary conformation of the β-site mutants is intact, as judged from their binding characteristics to conformation specific mAbs and IL-6Rα. As can be deduced from FIGURE 1, β-site mutations may therefore affect a direct interaction with gp130, dimerization of IL-6, or maybe a conformational change in IL-6Rα, important for gp130 interaction. A future challenge will therefore be to determine the function of each of the β-sites in IL-6 receptor interaction.

ACKNOWLEDGMENTS

This work could not have been accomplished without the contribution of many collaborators. First of all we would like to thank Hanny Klaasse Bos, Saskia Ebeling, Margreet Hart, Els de Groot, Edwin ten Boekel, and Menno van der Hoorn. Special thanks also to Marc Ehlers and Stefan Rose-John. Furthermore we would like to acknowledge Rob Kastelein, Fernando Bazan, John Wijdenes, Peter Heinrich, Tetsuya Taga, Tadamitsu Kishimoto, Kioyshi Yasukawa, Yoshiyuki Ohsugi, Bernard Klein, Armen Shanafelt, Claude Clement, Jean Herrman, Veronique Fontaine, and Jean Content who all one way or another contributed to this work.

REFERENCES

1. KISHIMOTO, T., S. AKIRA & T. TAGA. 1992. Science **258**: 593–597.
2. AKIRA, S., T. TAGA & T. KISHIMOTO. 1993. Adv. Immunol. **54**: 1–78.
3. BAZAN, J. F. 1991. Neuron **7**: 197–208.
4. KISHIMOTO, T., T. TAGA & S. AKIRA. 1994. Cell **76**: 253–262.
5. KOPF, M., H. BAUMANN, G. FREER, M. FREUDENBERG, M. LAMERS, T. KISHIMOTO, R. ZINKERNAGEL, H. BLUETHMANN & G. KÖHLER. 1994. Nature **368**: 339–342.
6. RAMSAY, A. J., A. J. HUSBAND, I. A. RAMSHAW, S. BAO, K. I. MATTHAEI, G. KÖHLER & M. KOPF. 1994. Science **264**: 561–563.
7. POLI, V., R. BALENA, E. FATTORI, A. MARKATOS, M. YAMAMOTO, H. TANAKA, G. CILIBERTO, G. A. RODAN & F. COSTANTINI. 1994. EMBO J **13**: 1189–1196.
8. BAZAN, J. F. 1990. Proc. Natl. Acad. Sci. USA **87**: 6934–6938.
9. MURAKAMI, M., M. HIBI, N. NAKAGAWA, T. NAKAGAWA, K. YASUKAWA, K. YAMANISHI, T. TAGA & T. KISHIMOTO. 1993. Science **260**: 1808–1810.
10. WARD, L. D., G. J. HOWLETT, G. DISCOLO, K. YASUKAWA, A. HAMMACHER, R. L. MORITZ & R. J. SIMPSON. 1994. J. Biol. Chem. **269**: 23286–23289.
11. HIRANO, T., T. MATSUDA & K. NAKAJIMA. 1994. Stem Cells **12**: 262–277.
12. LÜTTICKEN, C., U. M. WEGENKA, J. YUAN, J. BUSCHMANN, C. SCHINDLER, A. ZIEMIECKI, A. G. HARPUR, A. F. WILKS, K. YASUKAWA, T. TAGA, T. KISHIMOTO, G. BARBIERI, S. PELLEGRINI, M. SENDTNER, P. C. HEINRICH & F. HORN. 1994. Science **263**: 89–92.
13. STAHL, N., T. G. BOULTON, T. FARRUGGELLA, N. Y. IP, S. DAVIS, B. A. WITTHUHN, F. W. QUELLE, O. SILVENNOINEN, G. BARBIERI, S. PELLEGRINI, J. N. IHLE & G. D. YANCOPOULOS. 1994. Science **263**: 92–95.

14. ZHONG, Z., Z. WEN & J. E. DARNELL, JR. 1994. Science **264:** 95–98.
15. AKIRA, S., Y. NISHIO, M. INOUE, X.-J. WANG, S. WEI, T. MATSUSAKA, K. YOSHIDA, T. SUDO, M. NARUTO & T. KISHIMOTO. 1994. Cell **77:** 63–71.
16. ERNST, M., D. P. GEARING & A. R. DUNN. 1994. EMBO J. **13:** 1574–1584.
17. BOLTON, T. G., N. STAHL & G. D. YANCOPOULOS. 1994. J. Biol. Chem. **269:** 11648–11655.
18. YIN, T. & Y.-C. YANG. 1994. J. Biol. Chem. **269:** 3731–3738.
19. DAEIPOUR, M., G. KUMAR, M. C. AMARAL & A. E. NEL. 1993. J. Immunol. **150:** 4743–4753.
20. MATSUDA, T. & T. HIRANO. 1994. Blood **83:** 3457–3461.
21. HIRANO, T., S. AKIRA, T. TAGA & T. KISHIMOTO. 1990. Immunol. Today **11:** 443–449.
22. BAUER, J. & F. HERRMANN. 1991. Ann. Hematol. **62:** 203–210.
23. HIRANO, T. 1992. Clin. Immunol. Immunopathol. **62:** S60–S65.
24. EMILIE, D., J. WIJDENES, C. GISSELBRECHT, B. JAROUSSE, E. BILLAUD, J.-Y. BLAY, J. GABARRE, J.-P. GAILLARD, J. BROCHIER, M. RAPHAEL, F. BOUE & P. GALANAUD. 1994. Blood **84:** 2472–2479.
25. STRASSMANN, G., M. FONG, J. S. KENNEY & C. O. JACOB. 1992. J. Clin. Invest. **89:** 1681–1684.
26. HEREMANS, H., C. DILLEN, W. PUT, J. VAN DAMME & A. BILLIAU. 1992. Eur. J. Immunol. **22:** 2395–2401.
27. VAN DER POLL, T., M. LEVI, C. E. HACK, H. TEN CATE, S. J. H. VAN DEVENTER, A. J. M. EERENBERG, E. R. DE GROOT, J. JANSEN, H. GALLATI, H. R. BÜLLER, J. W. TEN CATE & L. A. AARDEN. 1994. J. Exp. Med. **179:** 1253–1259.
28. DEVIERE, J., J. CONTENT, C. DENYS, P. VANDENBUSSCHE, L. SCHANDENE, J. WYBRAN & E. DUPONT. 1989. Clin. Exp. Immunol. **77:** 221–225.
29. CAMPBELL, I. L., C. R. ABRAHAM, E. MASLIAH, P. KEMPER, J. D. INGLIS, M. B. A. OLDSTONE & L. MUCKE. 1993. Proc. Natl. Acad. Sci. USA **90:** 10061–10065.
30. VANDENABEELE, P. & W. FIERS. 1991. Immunol. Today **12:** 217–219.
31. KLEIN, B., J. WIJDENES, X. G. ZHANG, M. JOURDAN, J. M. BOIRON, J. BROCHIER, J. LIAUTARD, M. MERLIN, C. CLEMENT, B. MOREL-FOURNIER, Z. Y. LU, P. MANNONI, J. SANY & R. BATAILLE. 1991. Blood **78:** 1198–1204.
32. BECK, J. T., H. SU-MING, J. WIJDENES, R. BATAILLE, B. KLEIN, D. VESOLE, K. HAYDEN, S. JAGANNATH & B. BARLOGIE. 1994. N. Engl. J. Med. **330:** 602–605.
33. WENDLING, D., E. RACADOT & J. WIJDENES. 1993. J. Rheumatol. **20:** 259–262.
34. LU, Z. Y., J. BROCHIER, J. WIJDENES, H. BRAILLY, R. BATAILLE & B. KLEIN. 1992. Eur. J. Immunol. **22:** 2819–2824.
35. TAGA, T., M. HIBI, Y. HIRATA, K. YAMASAKI, K. YASUKAWA, T. MATSUDA, T. HIRANO & T. KISHIMOTO. 1989. Cell **58:** 573–581.
36. HONDA, M., S. YAMAMOTO, M. CHENG, K. YASUKAWA, H. SUZUKI, T. SAITO, Y. OSUGI, T. TOKUNAGA & T. KISHIMOTO. 1992. J. Immunol. **148:** 2175–2180.
37. GAILLARD, J.-P., R. BATAILLE, H. BRAILLY, C. ZUBER, K. YASUKAWA, M. ATTAL, N. MARUO, T. TAGA, T. KISHIMOTO & B. KLEIN. 1993. Eur. J. Immunol. **23:** 820–824.
38. SPRANG, S. R. & J. F. BAZAN. 1993. Current Opinion in Structural Biology **3:** 815–827.
39. HILL, C. P., T. D. OSSLUND & D. EISENBERG. 1993. Proc. Natl. Acad. Sci. USA **90:** 5167–5171.
40. ROBINSON, R. C., L. M. GREY, D. STAUNTON, H. VANKELECOM, A. B. VERNALLIS, J.-F. MOREAU, D. I. STUART, J. K. HEATH & E. Y. JONES. 1994. Cell **77:** 1101–1116.
41. EHLERS, M., J. GRÖTZINGER, F. D. DE HON, J. MÜLLBERG, J. P. J. BRAKENHOFF, J. LIU, A. WOLLMER & S. ROSE-JOHN. 1994. J. Immunol. **153:** 1744–1753.
42. BRAKENHOFF, J. P. J., F. D. DE HON, V. FONTAINE, E. TEN BOEKEL, H. SCHOOLTINK, S. ROSE-JOHN, P. C. HEINRICH, J. CONTENT & L. A. AARDEN. 1994. J. Biol. Chem. **269:** 86–93.
43. SAVINO, R., A. LAHM, A. L. SALVATI, L. CIAPPONI, E. SPORENO, S. ALTAMURA, G. PAONESSA, C. TONIATTI & G. CILIBERTO. 1994. EMBO J. **13:** 1357–1367.
44. DE HON, F. D., M. EHLERS, S. ROSE-JOHN, S. B. EBELING, H. KLAASSE BOS, L. A. AARDEN & J. P. J. BRAKENHOFF. 1994. J. Exp. Med. **180:** 2395–2400.
45. DE HON, F. D., E. TEN BOCKEL, J. HERRMAN, C. CLEMENT, M. EHLERS, T. TAGA, K, YASUKAWA, Y. OHSUGI, T. KISHIMOTO, S. ROSE-JOHN, J. WIDENES, R. KASTELEIN, L. A. AARDEN & J. P. J. BRAKENHOFF. 1995. Cytokine. In press.

DISCUSSION OF THE PAPER

P. Sehgal (*New York Medical College, Valhalla*): So, what is screwed up in B9 cells?

L. A. Aarden: That is a good question. Until now we have not been able to develop an antagonist for B9 cells. Of course, B9 cells are peculiar in the sense that they are 100-fold more sensitive to IL-6 than the primary cells that you isolate from primary organs or blood. And what this means, I do not know. I have no idea what is different in B9 cells from the other cells.

G. Ciliberto (*Istituto di Ricerche di Biologia Moleculare P. Angletti, Rome Italy*): I would like to comment on that point. I think that there is nothing wrong with B9. Simply, there is a difference between human and mouse because we have mutants which are equivalent biologically on human cells and they are not active at all on mouse cells. They are not active as antagonist, so they are fully active not only on B9 cells, but also on H-35 cells. Heinz Baumann has tested them, so I think that there is a difference in receptor system or between signaling in human and mouse which nobody has ever investigated carefully.

Aarden: I agree. We have also tested these mutants on T 1165 cells, which are a plasmacytoma cell line and which are 200-fold less sensitive than B9 and also there they are active.

Sehgal: Perhaps I need a little clarification here. When we worked with human IL-6 coming from human plasma or serum we had a tremendous problem getting that registered on B9 cells. But whenever we work with murine IL-6 coming from mouse plasma we have never had a problem making that register on B9 cells. So I think that the point that there is something different between the human and mouse IL-6 working on B9 cells is a point well taken.

Aarden: Well there is a main difference that everyone should know. I got a lot of complaints from people working with B9 that become independent; it was my fault, of course, and I had to work on that. It turns out that if people grow B9 cells on murine recombinant IL-6 they tend to become independent very quickly and that we could repeat, and then we went after what was going on. It turns out that murine IL-6 is consumed rapidly by B9 cells. Human IL-6 is not consumed by B9 cells. So if you take 10 pg of human IL-6 and you grow a full bottle of cells, the IL-6 is still there. If you take mouse IL-6 it is gone within 2 days, and you need to add 1000 pg to keep them growing until you have the full bottle. So that is a large difference between these two.

M. Revel (*Weizmann Institute of Science, Rehovot, Isreal*): You said that you have an antagonist. What are the prospects of treating myeloma with it?

Aarden: I'm not so sure that these antagonists are going to be used for the treatment of patients. I think it is more a pointer to what regions of IL-6 are involved in receptor binding, and I'm not sure whether these antagonists are then any better than neutralizing monoclonal antibodies; so I think it is more a lead to what regions are involved in receptor binding and how we could develop a low molecular weight antagonist.

H. Baumann (*Roswell Park Cancer Institute, Buffalo, NY*): In the poster session a hexameric structure for the receptor was proposed. In your design you are still looking at a single α subunit present. Would that really change your design strategy now?

Aarden: No, but if indeed there is a hexameric structure, two IL-6, two gp80, two gp130, you could imagine that we have to be aware that IL-6–IL-6 interaction might also be a target. Until now we have not found that.

The Molecular Design of Human IL-6 Receptor Antagonists[a]

A. LAHM, R. SAVINO, A. L. SALVATI, A. CABIBBO,
L. CIAPPONI, A. DEMARTIS, C. TONIATTI, G. PAONESSA,
S. ALTAMURA, AND G. CILIBERTO

Istituto di Ricerche di Biologia Molecolare P. Angeletti (IRBM)
Via Pontina km 30,600
00040 Pomezia (Rome), Italy

INTRODUCTION

Physiologically, interleukin-6 (IL-6) acts as a growth and differentiation factor on various cell types and plays a major role in the induction of acute phase gene expression in hepatocytes.[1] Overproduction of IL-6 is associated with the development of several diseases, like multiple myeloma, post-menopausal osteoporosis, and chronic autoimmune diseases, and is therefore believed to be involved in their pathogenesis.[2,3] This hypothesis is strongly supported by evidence that administering IL-6 neutralizing monoclonal antibodies in human clinical studies and animal models of diseases produces therapeutic effects.[4-6] The development of potent and selective IL-6 receptor antagonists is thus considered of potentially high therapeutic value.

Activation of intracellular pathways by IL-6 depends on its sequential interaction with two transmembrane glycoproteins, IL-6Rα and gp130, which together constitute the high affinity IL-6 receptor.[7] After the initial specific binding of IL-6 to IL-6Rα, the IL-6/IL-6Rα complex associates with gp130.[8] This latter molecule undergoes a ligand-dependent homodimerization, which is followed by the activation of intracellular tyrosine kinases of the Jak family and phosphorylation of Stat transcription factors.[9] While the intracytoplasmic domain of IL-6Rα does not carry information relevant to signal transduction, the extracytoplasmic domain shows a peculiar biological property when expressed in soluble form: it behaves as an IL-6 agonist due to its ability to form IL-6/IL-6Rα complexes which bind and activate gp130.[10] The receptor complex assembled by IL-6 is believed to be structurally related to that of a great number of cytokines, including growth hormone (GH).[11] The similarity is thought to be even more pronounced for the group of cytokines that include leukemia inhibitory factor (LIF), ciliary neurotrophic factor (CNTF), interleukin 11 (IL-11) and oncostatin M (OM), which all require gp130 as the signal-transducing subunit.[12] Strong support to there being structural similarities in the receptor complexes assembled by these cytokines is provided by the following evidence: 1) the growing number of cytokine structures already determined confirm predictions of a common topology, an antiparallel four α-helix bundle[13]; 2) the existence of a significant sequence homology in the extracellular domain of the corresponding receptors has led to the identification of a region of about 200 amino acids, called the cytokine binding domain (CBD), which is predicted to fold into two consecutive "barrel-like" subdomains of seven β-strands, very similar to immunoglobulin constant domains[14]; 3) all these cytokines trigger the sequential assembly of either homo- or heterodimeric receptor complexes.[15]

---

[a] This work was supported in part by EEC grant BRIDGE BIOT-CT91-0260 to G. C.

The recently determined x-ray structure of the complex between hGH and CBDs of its homodimeric receptor (hGHbp) provides a first detailed insight into the mode of interaction established by this class of molecules.[16] GH serves as a bridging ligand between two receptor molecules, and three interacting surfaces can be identified in the assembled receptor complex: a binding site on GH for its first receptor (Site 1); a second binding site on GH for its second receptor (Site 2) and an interface between the two receptors. The structural and functional information deriving from the study of the GH complex can therefore be used as a template for the construction of 3D models of the interaction between other helical cytokines and their corresponding homo- or heterodimeric receptors. These models could help to identify the residues which constitute Site 1 and Site 2 in the cytokine of interest and also those located at the interface between the two receptors. Their mutagenesis may be used to confirm the validity of the model and also lead to its further improvement. At the same time, some targeted mutations could result in the generation of receptor antagonists. We have applied this process to IL-6 and obtained different classes of receptor antagonists.

EXPERIMENTAL PROCEDURES

Molecular Modeling

Construction of the model of IL-6 has already been described.[17] Modeling of the IL-6Rα and gp130 CBDs initiated by manually aligning their amino acids sequence against the corresponding part of the hGHbp. This initial alignment was then inscribed into the structural scaffold provided by the x-ray structure of the hGH-h(GHbp)$_2$ complex.[16] The packing of side-chains within the hydrophobic core of the two subdomains was optimized; the subsequent remodeling of the loop regions (including insertions and deletions) produced the final receptor models, with the relative orientation of the two CBDs, apart for minor adjustments, kept practically identical to the one present in the hGH-h(GHbp)$_2$ structure.[16] A model of the interaction between IL-6 and the CBDs of IL-6Rα and gp130 was obtained as described.[17] All modeling was performed using either the WHATIF[18] or INSIGHT[19] molecular modeling software. Structures for hGH-(hGHbp)$_2$, the Tenascin and Ig-constant domains were taken from the PDB protein structure database[20] (entries 2HHR, 1TEN and 1FDL, respectively).

IL-6 and IL-6Rα Mutagenesis and Expression of Recombinant Proteins

IL-6 mutagenesis was performed as described.[17] Expression of IL-6 mutant proteins was performed as described, either intracytoplasmically in the *E. coli* BL21 (DE3) LysE strain[21] or as secretion product in the periplasmic space of the same *E. coli* strain.[17]

For the production of soluble human IL-6Rα (shIL-6Rα) in COS-7 cells, the cDNA coding for a truncated form (aa. 1-324) of hIL-6Rα, with an additional C-terminal stretch of six-histidines, was generated by PCR and inserted into pcDNAI (Invitrogen), thus generating the COS expression vector pc6FRH. This last plasmid was used as a template to derive, by using PCR methods, a series of pc6FRH constructs encoding histidine-tagged mutant forms of shIL-6Rα (Mut-1/Mut-8).

For the generation of Baculovirus recombinant transfer vectors, the cDNAs coding for wild-type and Mut-4 shIL-6Rα were introduced into the pBlueBacIII (Invitrogen) plasmid. Expression of proteins in HighFive™ insect cells using recombinant Baculovirus was performed as described.[22] Purification of receptors using metal affinity chromatography was achieved using standard protocols.[23]

In Vitro *Receptor Binding Assays and Immunoprecipitations*

In vitro receptor binding assays for IL-6 mutant proteins were performed as described.[17] Immunoprecipitations experiments with anti human IL-6Rα monoclonal antibody I6R1/9G.11 were performed as described.[23]

Biological Assays

The stimulation of transcription of the IL-6 inducible C-reactive protein (CRP) gene promoter transfected in hepatoma cells was measured as described.[24] To measure DNA binding activity of transcription factor APRF/STAT3,[25] whole-cell[26] or nuclear[27] extracts from HepG2 hepatoma cell were prepared, with the addition of 5 mM of NaF phosphatase inhibitor to all buffers used for extract preparation. APRF/STAT3 activation was then monitored by gel retardation as described.[27]

RESULTS

Molecular Modeling

The process of sequential receptor dimerization first observed for GH is believed to apply to most helical cytokines, including IL-6.[13] It is therefore plausible that the overall architecture of the hGH-h(GHbp)$_2$ complex may serve as a three-dimensional template for the IL-6/IL-6Rα/gp130 complex. We previously generated a 3D model of human IL-6 starting from a multiple sequence alignment with G-CSF and the recently determined x-ray 3D structure of bovine G-CSF.[17] This model predicts residues 12 to 184 of IL-6 as forming a 4-helix bundle as in the case of GH (FIG. 1).

The aminoacid sequences of human IL-6Rα and gp130 CBDs can be aligned with that of hGHbp taking advantage of conserved residues such as the four cysteines predicted to form disulfide bridges, prolines in the interdomain linker, and the WSXWS motif.[14] A three-dimensional model for CBDs of both receptor chains was constructed by inscribing their aligned sequences onto the structural scaffold of hGH-(hGHbp)$_2$ complex (see experimental procedures). Deletions and insertions occur predominantly outside the β-strands (FIG. 2) and the relative orientation of the two subdomains is predicted to be identical to hGHbp. The latter can be deduced from the absence of insertions or deletions in between subdomains 1 and 2 and the conservation of a PXPP motif at the beginning of subdomain 2 (FIG. 2). In conclusion, since both IL-6Rα and gp130 CBDs are predicted to have a β-strand composition and subdomain orientation identical to GHbp, we combined their 3D models with that of IL-6[17] and oriented the three molecules as in the hGH-h(GHbp)$_2$ complex.[16] The resulting model of the IL-6 in the context of its hetero-dimeric receptor is shown in FIGURE 3.

The model predicts that in IL-6 the contact surface for the IL-6Rα (Site 1) is composed of residues that form the long loop connecting helices A and B (AB loop) and of exposed residues in the carboxy-terminal end of helix D. On the other side of

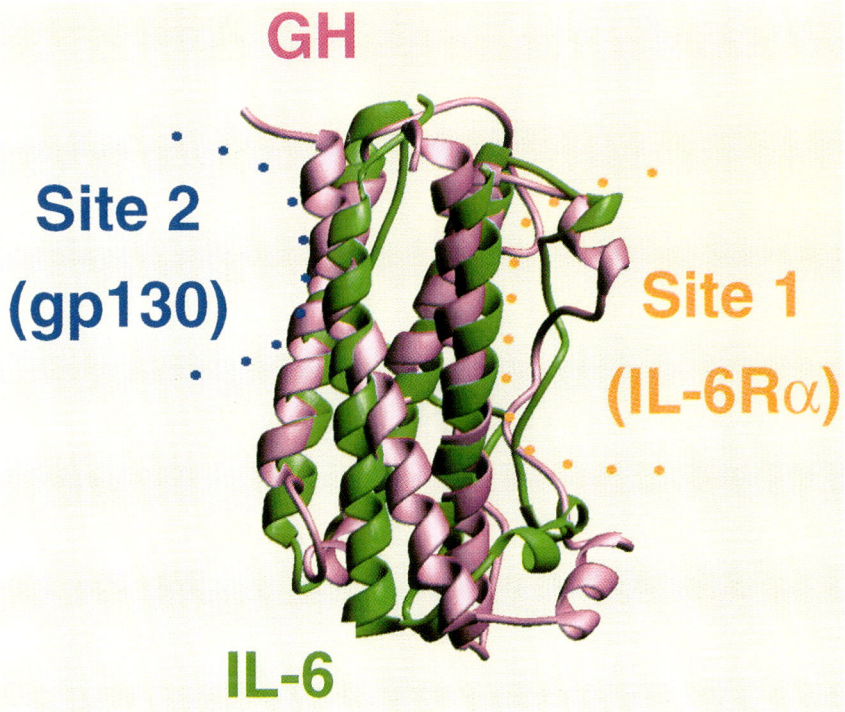

FIGURE 1. Superposition of the IL-6 model (green) onto hGH (magenta). The overall very similar topology of the two molecules suggests that, in analogy to hGH, two distinct patches on the surface of the IL-6 molecule are involved in the interaction with the receptors: Site 1 (orange), including residues from helix D and the AB loop, should specifically recognize the IL-6Rα and, on the opposite site of the molecule, gp130 should make contact with Site 2 (blue) formed by residues from helices A and C. (Figure was drawn using the RIBBONS software.[41])

the cytokine, it should be the exposed residues in helices A and C of IL-6 that are responsible for interaction with gp130 (Site 2): their mutagenesis should give rise to variants with unimpaired IL-6Rα binding but decreased biological activity (FIG. 3). The model also predicts, in analogy with GH, that IL-6Rα residues in the E2 strand and AB2 loop of the CBD are involved in the heterodimerization with gp130. Variants of the IL-6Rα mutated at these positions should accordingly still bind IL-6 but no longer interact with gp130 and consequently lose their agonistic activity (FIG. 3). Both types of mutants are expected to behave as IL-6 antagonists.

Mutagenesis of IL-6 Residues in Helices A and C

The hIL-6 residues identified as possible candidates for making contact with gp130 (27, 28, 31 and 35 on helix A and 118, 121 and 125 on helix C) were mutated by PCR, at the cDNA level, either singly or in combination. Mutant proteins were

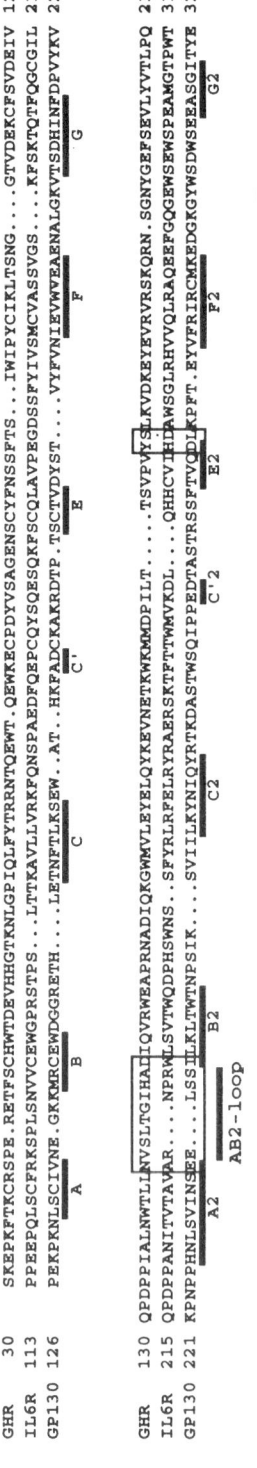

FIGURE 2. Alignment of the IL-6Rα and gp130 CBDs with the extracellular domain of hGHbp according to our model. Regions from the hGH-(hGHbp)₂ complex structure implicated as participating in receptor dimerization (AB2 loop and E2 strand) are indicated by black boxes. Black lines below the alignment mark the presence of the seven β-strands within the two subdomains.

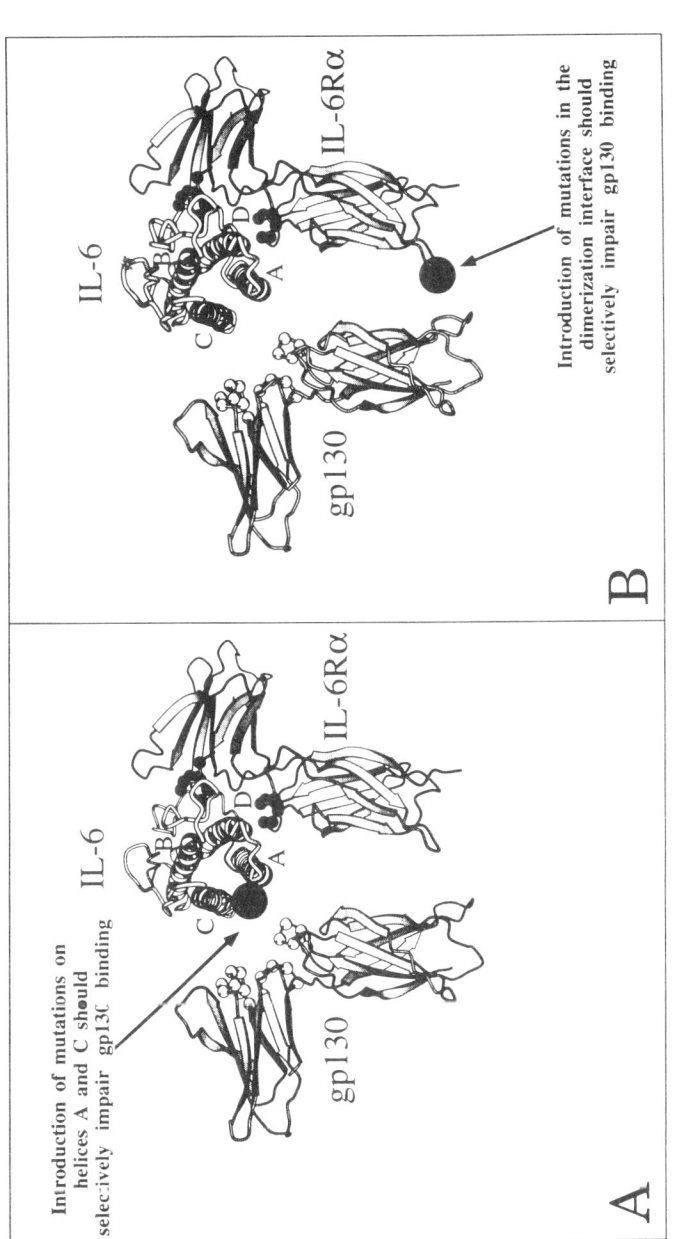

FIGURE 3. Schematic MOLSCRIPT[42] representations of the model describing the complex between IL-6 and the CBDs of the IL-6Rα and gp130. For demonstration purposes, gp130 has been slightly removed from its actual position to pronounce the predicted effect of mutations at Site 2 of IL-6 (**A**) and within the dimerization interface (strand E2 and AB2 loop) of the IL-6Rα (**B**), both of which should prevent the recruitment of gp130 and thus impair complex assembly. Loop regions of the two receptors involved in interaction with the cytokine are indicated by *small filled circles* (IL-6Rα) or *open circles* (gp130), *big circles* mark the sites where mutations were introduced.

TABLE 1. Biological Activity and Receptor Binding of IL-6 Mutants

Mutations				Biological Activity		Receptor Binding (% of wt)
Helix A		Helix C		EC_{50} ng/ml	Maximal Activity (% of wt)	
Y31	G35	S118	V121	0.8 ± 0.2	100	100
D				2.1 ± 0.2	105 ± 15	111 ± 19
	R			0.8 ± 0.1	100 ± 20	NT[a]
	L			1.1 ± 0.1	100 ± 15	NT
D	Y			18 ± 4	53 ± 5	73 ± 17
D	F			40 ± 9	51 ± 7	84 ± 9
			D	1.4 ± 0.5	100 ± 5	78 ± 2
		R		1.2 ± 0.2	100 ± 9	81 ± 18
		L	D	2.2 ± 0.2	100 ± 4	92 ± 34
		R	D	22.8 ± 3.3	66 ± 6	66 ± 5
D	F	L		57 ± 9.7	58 ± 7	20 ± 2
D	F	R		14.7 ± 3.1	63 ± 7	66 ± 2
D	F	R	D[b]	>4000	0	97 ± 15
D	F	L	D	>4000	0	69 ± 18

Biological activity is measured as activation the IL-6 inducible CRP gene promoter transfected in human Hep 3B hepatoma cells.[24] The EC_{50} is the concentration of each mutant which gives 50% of the wt IL-6 maximal stimulation, and is determined by dose-response curves as described.[17] The first lane in the table shows the wt IL-6 sequence in positions 31, 35, 118 and 121. For each mutant, where no change is indicated the wild-type residue is present.

[a] NT, not tested.
[b] This mutant will be referred in the text as DFRD.

expressed in *E. coli*: their *in vitro* binding to IL-6Rα was determined by ELISA and their biological activity verified on human hepatoma cells. The most significant results are presented in TABLE 1. Only mutants with specific double substitutions of residues 31 and 35 on helix A (upper part of TABLE 1) or of residues 118 and 121 on helix C (middle part of TABLE 1) displayed strongly reduced bioactivity while maintaining, as expected, normal binding to IL-6Rα. When mutations at these residues were combined, as in the quadruple mutant DFRD, no residual bioactivity could be detected, while affinity for IL-6Rα was unchanged. From these results we can conclude that residues 31/35 in helix A and 118/121 in helix C, from which our model predicts as forming a continuous patch on the IL-6 surface (FIG. 4), all participate in triggering signaling events in IL-6–stimulated cells, probably through direct interaction with gp130. Indeed, we have previously shown that amino acid substitutions in the same area selectively decreased the ability of IL-6 to interact *in vitro* with gp130.[17]

One of the mutants which showed complete loss of activity, namely DFRD, was tested for its capacity to antagonize wt IL-6 on human hepatoma HepG2 cells. Two assays were used, stimulation of transcription from a transfected IL-6-dependent promoter[24] and fast activation of DNA binding activity for transcription factor APRF/Stat3.[25] In the first case a dose-dependent inhibition curve was obtained with full inhibition at a 2000-fold mutant vs. wild-type IL-6 molar excess (FIG. 5A). In the second, a 1000-fold molar excess of DFRD was able to fully block APRF activation as assessed by electrophoretic mobility shift assay (EMSA) with an APRF binding site (FIG. 5B). Interestingly, antagonism is highly specific, as DFRD was unable to inhibit the bioactivity of the related cytokine OM (FIG. 5B).

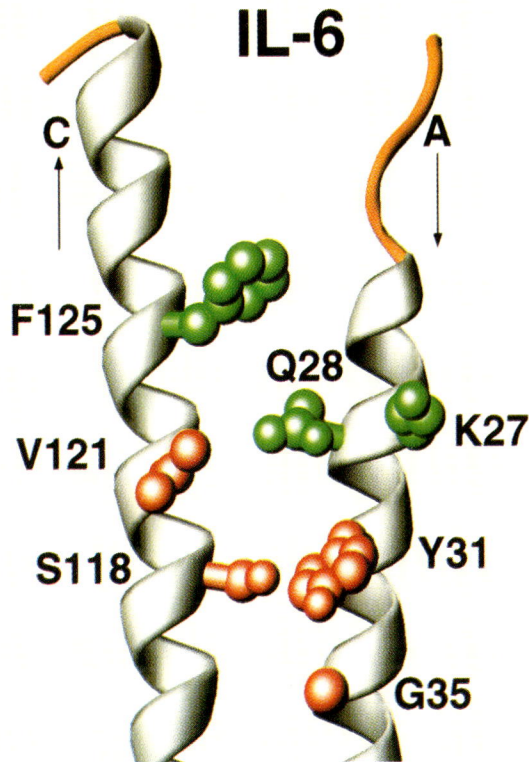

FIGURE 4. Residues on IL-6 helices A and C that were initially predicted to interact with gp130 at Site 2 are shown. Whereas mutations at positions 27, 28 and 125 (green) did not affect the biological activity, the combined mutation of residues 31, 35, 118 and 121 (red) generated the IL-6 DFRD variant that behaves as specific IL-6 antagonist. Specific interactions between IL-6 and gp130 should therefore center around the continuous patch formed by these four residues.

Generation of IL-6 Superantagonist by Mutagenesis of Helix D

As described above, the model also predicts that IL-6 residues from two regions that are spatially close to each other, the AB loop and the carboxy-terminal part of helix D, should constitute the contact surface with the IL-6Rα. The involvement of the latter part of the IL-6 molecule in IL-6Rα binding has indeed been demonstrated by site directed mutagenesis.[28,29] The model further predicted that by increasing the affinity of an antagonist for IL-6Rα, its effectiveness as inhibitor at low concentrations should also increase. In a previous study we generated an IL-6 variant with the single substitution S176R, showing a 3-fold increased affinity for IL-6Rα.[29] Recently, we also identified in the same region the substitutions Q175I and Q183A, which, when combined with the mutation S176R in the triple mutant IL-6 IRA, cause a 4.5-fold increase in receptor binding (A. Cabibbo et al., submitted). These three substitutions in the D helix were inserted in the context of the mutant DFRD, thus generating the mutant IL-6 DFRDIRA. Like DFRD, the IL-6 DFRDIRA variant showed no bioactivity, but its receptor-binding activity increased approximately 4-fold as compared to wt IL-6 and DFRD (data not shown). This experimental result confirms a total independence of Sites 1 and 2 in receptor interaction. Furthermore, when tested for antagonism on HepG2 cells, DFRDIRA proved to be a more effective IL-6 inhibitor than the parent mutant, because it reaches full inhibition at a 250-fold molar excess, as compared with the 2000-fold molar excess of DFRD required to achieve the same effects (FIG. 6).

Mutagenesis of the Presumptive IL-6Rα/gp130 Interface

To generate an IL-6Rα variant impaired in the interaction with gp130, a double substitution of residues H280 and D281 on strand E2 was introduced (Mut-1, TABLE 2), in positions that correspond to hGHbp residues Y200 and S201 known to be involved in homodimer formation.[16] In the second region implicated in receptor dimerization, the AB2 loop, we decided to mutate N230 either separately (Mut-2)

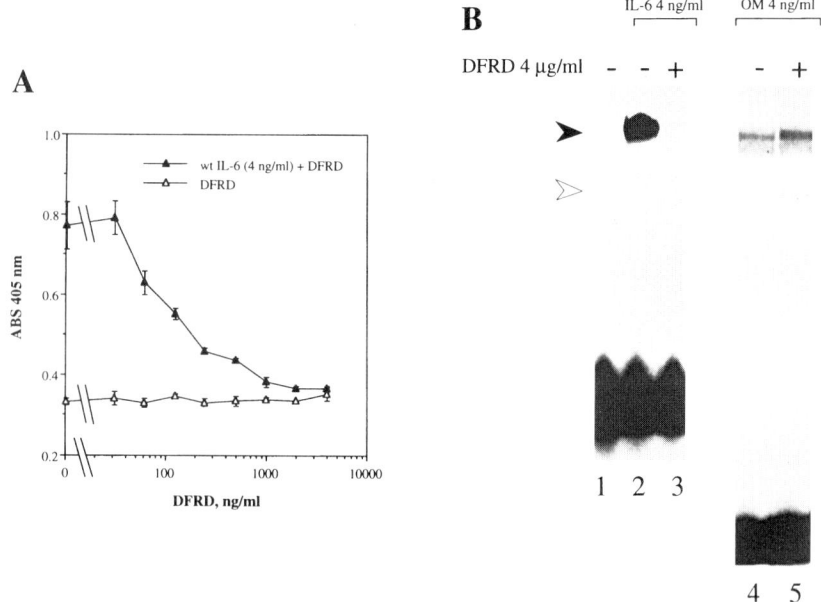

FIGURE 5. Mutant DFRD antagonizes wt IL-6 activity on human HepG2 hepatoma cells. **A:** Human HepG2 cells were transfected with the IL-6–inducible CRP gene promoter fused to a reporter gene[24] and incubated with increasing amounts of DFRD in the presence *(filled symbols)* or in the absence *(open symbols)* of 4 ng/ml of wt IL-6. The transcriptional activity from the CRP gene promoter was quantified as described.[24] **B:** HepG2 cells were incubated (15 min) with no cytokine (lane 1), with 4 ng/ml of wt IL-6 (lanes 2 and 3) or of OM (lanes 4 and 5) in the absence or in the presence of 4 μg/ml of mutant DFRD, as indicated. Whole cell extracts[26] and EMSAs[27] were performed as described. DFRD inhibits APRF activation *(closed arrowhead)* by IL-6, but not by OM. The *open arrowhead* indicates the position of an unspecific signal.

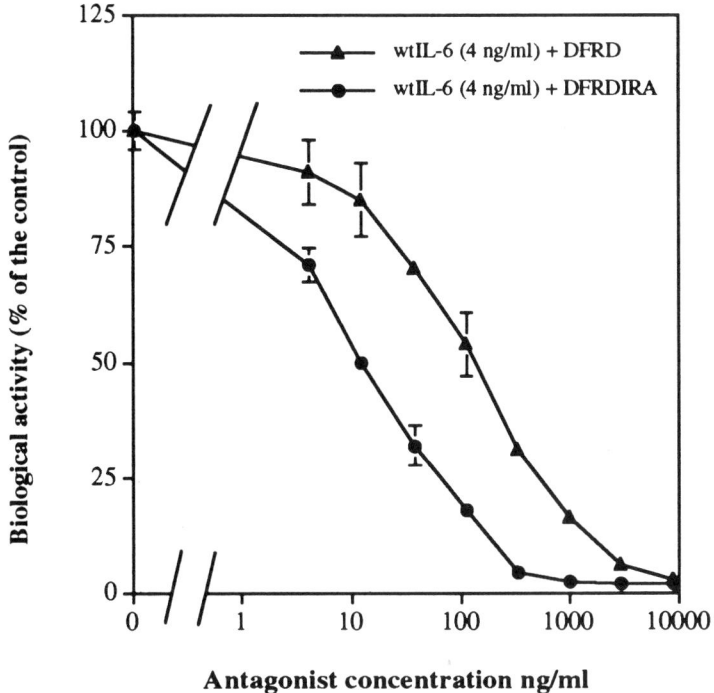

FIGURE 6. IL-6 DFRDIRA is a more effective antagonist than DFRD. Human HepG2 cells were transfected as in FIGURE 5 and induced with 4 ng/ml of wt IL-6 in the presence of increasing concentrations of IL-6 DFRD or IL-6 DFRDIRA, as indicated. The transcriptional activity from the CRP gene promoter was quantified as described[24] and expressed as a percentage of the transcriptional efficiency in cells incubated with 4 ng/ml of wt IL-6 only, after subtraction of the background signal given by transfected control (non-induced) cells.

or in combination with A228 (Mut-3) and, combining Mut-1 and Mut-3, we also constructed a mutant that carried all four substitutions (Mut-4, TABLE 2). In a more drastic approach to prove the involvement of the AB2 loop in receptor dimerization, the loop was substituted with corresponding or similar segments of structurally related molecules (Mut-5, Mut-6, Mut-7). In a first variant (Mut-5), the predicted AB2 loop of shIL-6Rα was substituted with that of hGHbp (TABLE 2). Two shorter AB2 loop variants (Mut-6 and Mut-7) carried the equivalent regions of the tenth domain of Tenascin[30] and of an immunoglobulin constant domain,[31] respectively (TABLE 2). Finally, substitution of a loop region from a structurally unrelated molecule produced an even longer version of the AB2 loop (Mut-8) that, with the introduction of two prolines at appropriate positions, should become conformationally locked (TABLE 2).

All these mutants were generated in the context of a cDNA encoding a truncated form of human IL-6Rα (shIL-6Rα)[23] with an artificial termination codon introduced at aa. position 324 and a C-terminal stretch of six histidine residues immediately upstream of it. Wild type and mutant soluble IL-6 receptors were produced in transiently transfected COS-7 cells. To normalize their expression level we performed immunoprecipitations with a non-neutralizing anti-hIL-6Rα monoclonal antibody.

The expression level of the various mutants was comparable to that of the wild type with the exception of Mut-5, Mut-6 and Mut-7 which were constantly produced in lower amounts (TABLE 2), suggesting that the mutations introduced might affect either stability or the secretion of the protein.

We next determined the affinity of the various shIL-6Rα variants for IL-6 using a recently developed technique which exploits C-terminal histidine tagging.[23] The results obtained with the various IL-6Rα variants are summarized in TABLE 2: point mutations in the E2 strand and AB2 loop did not significantly affect binding affinity; on the contrary, all variants in which the complete AB2 loop had been substituted (Mut-5 to Mut-8), displayed a strongly decreased ability to interact with the cytokine. Since the mutants with the weakest affinity for IL-6 also showed the lowest level of expression (Mut-5, Mut-6 and Mut-7), it is conceivable that major changes in the AB2 loop sequence cause severe and unpredicted conformational changes which alter the IL-6 binding site and/or protein stability. We therefore selected the mutants that show an IL-6 binding affinity in the same order of magnitude as the wild-type and assessed their binding to soluble gp130 (sgp130) by coimmunoprecipitation in the presence of IL-6. The results are shown in TABLE 2. As expected, substitutions at the beginning of the putative E2 strand (Mut-1) strongly reduced the association of the IL-6/sIL-6Rα complex with sgp130 molecules. However, also the single and double substitution mutants in the AB2 loop, Mut-2 and Mut-3, showed a decreased interaction with sgp130 (TABLE 2). Intriguingly, the quadruple mutant Mut-4 displayed the lowest ability to coimmunoprecipitate ^{35}S-sgp130, thus suggesting an additive effect of the mutations located in different regions of the receptor.

These results indicated Mut-4 as the receptor mutant whose binding to gp130 is most heavily affected, without decreasing affinity for IL-6. In order to study the biological properties of Mut-4, its production and that of wt soluble receptor was scaled up using the Baculovirus expression system. Both His-tagged proteins were produced at high levels and purified from the supernatant of infected insect cells by

TABLE 2. Amino Acid Sequence, Expression Level, Affinity for hIL-6 and Ability to Associate with gp130 of shIL-6Rα Mutants

| Mutant | Amino Acid Sequence | | % Expression[a] | % IL-6 Binding[a] | % gp130 Association[a] |
	AB-2 Loop Mutations	E-2 Strand Mutations			
Mut-1	wild-type sequence	I_{279} SV A_{282}	100	70	10
Mut-2	T_{225} AVARDPRW L_{234}	Wild-type sequence	100	100	30
Mut-3	T_{225} AVDRDPRW L_{234}	Wild-type sequence	100	100	30
Mut-4	T_{225} AVDRDPRW L_{234}	I_{279} SV A_{282}	100	90	5
Mut-5	T_{225} LNVSLTGIHAD L_{234}	Wild-type sequence	1	<1	N.D.
Mut-6	V_{224} KDVTDTT L_{234}	Wild-type sequence	20	<1	N.D.
Mut-7	V_{224} HPASN L_{234}	Wild-type sequence	10	<1	N.D.
Mut-8	T_{225} WDPTKGEPM L_{234}	Wild-type sequence	100	10	N.D.
Wt	T_{225} AVARNPRW L_{234}	I_{279} HD A_{282}	100	100	100

The substitutions introduced in the predicted AB-2 loop and E-2 strand are indicated. The sequence of the wild-type IL-6Rα is shown for comparison. To monitor the expression level of receptor variants, tranfected COS-7 cells were metabolically labeled with ^{35}S-methionine and the conditioned medium was immunoprecipitated with anti hIL-6Rα mAb 16R1/9G.11. Immunoprecipitates were resolved by SDS/PAGE analysis and ^{35}S-labeled receptors were quantified by densitometric scanning of the gel using Phosphorimager software (Molecular Dynamics). The affinity of each receptor mutant for IL-6 was determined by cold-ligand competition assay as described.[20] The ability of COS-produced shIL-6Rα variants to co-immunoprecipitate ^{35}S-labeled sgp130 in the presence of hIL-6 was monitored in experiments performed as described.[17,20] Immunoreactive complexes were electrophoresed on SDS/polyacrylamide gel and immunoprecipitated ^{35}S-sgp130 was quantified by densitometric analysis of the gel.

[a] Relative to wt.

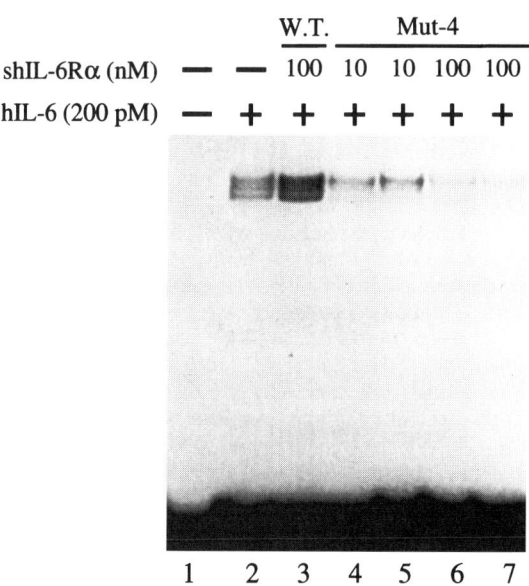

FIGURE 7. Mutant shIL-6Rα Mut-4 inhibits IL-6 dependent APRF activation in cultured hepatoma cells. HepG2 cells were incubated (15 min) with IL-6 alone (lane 2) or in combination with either 100 nM wild-type shIL-6Rα (lane 3) or increasing concentrations of mutant Mut-4 (lanes 3–7). In a control experiment (lane 1), no IL-6 was added to the medium. Nuclear extracts were prepared and induction of APRF/STAT3 DNA binding activity was monitored as described.[27]

metal-affinity chromatography. Their biological activity was tested on human hepatoma HepG2 cells using the APRF activation assay.[27] Human HepG2 cells were stimulated with 200 pM hIL-6, together with either wild-type or mutant receptors. As shown in FIGURE 7, while shIL-6Rα potentiated APRF induction by IL-6 (FIG. 7, lane 3), we observed that Mut-4 not only showed no sign of agonistic activity, but rather inhibited the cytokine activity in a concentration-dependent fashion (FIG. 7, lanes 4–7). Interestingly, the effect is specific for IL-6 since no inhibition of OM-dependent APRF induction was observed (not shown).

DISCUSSION

In this paper we present the construction of a three-dimensional model of the interaction between IL-6 and its two receptor chains, based on the known structure of the hGH-h(GHbp)$_2$ complex, and demonstrate how this model is used to selectively introduce mutations in either IL-6 or the IL-6Rα in order to modify their biological properties.

The results of the analysis of IL-6 mutants clearly show that it is possible to fully dissociate IL-6Rα binding from signal transduction through mutagenesis of the surface area predicted to interact with gp130 (Site 2). However, several residues had to be mutagenized either alone or in combination in order to identify a patch of four amino acids (31/35/118/121) fundamental for signal transduction. Interestingly, individual substitutions of these residues were not able to significantly affect the biological activity which was completely abolished only when mutating all of them together. In conclusion our data confirm that our three-dimensional model is valid, and allow us to position Site 2 of IL-6 approximately in the same spatial location as in GH.

Although our molecular model has identified the exposed residues in helix A and C as contact points with gp130, it does not explain the recent results reported by Brakenoff and colleagues.[32] These authors, using a different approach, have obtained a partial IL-6 antagonist by substituting residues 159 and 162, predicted to be located at the beginning of helix D and thus far from our proposed Site 2. Although this would indicate that our model is incomplete, it might denote the existence of a second binding site for gp130 on IL-6 (Site 3), which is perfectly in line with the observation that the last step in IL-6 receptor assembly is homodimerization of the gp130 chain.[33] It is therefore possible that Site 2 and Site 3 mutants are inactive because they cannot bind two gp130 molecules simultaneously. Additional mutagenesis of IL-6 and the determination of the receptor complex stoichiometry *in vitro* will be necessary to further clarify this point.

The mutagenesis we performed on IL-6Rα, demonstrates that it is possible to dissociate IL-6 binding from signal transduction. In fact, while the soluble form of the receptor is a potentiator of the cytokine activity, the variant Mut-4 is not only devoid of enhancing function, but acts as a dominant negative modulator of IL-6. These results provide greater insight into the mechanisms of interaction between helical cytokines and their receptors. The involvement of residues in the E2 strand and AB2 loop in the receptor-receptor interface had until now been demonstrated at structural and functional level only for the homodimerizing GHbp.[16,34] Our data in addition demonstrate the involvement of these same regions also in the stabilization of a heterodimeric (IL-6Rα/gp130) receptor complex, similar to those assembled by several other cytokines like IL-3, IL-4, IL-5 or GM-CSF.[15]

We observed that mutations in the E2 strand and in the AB2 loop individually weaken binding to gp130. Combining these mutations causes a further decrease, but does not totally abolish this interaction, and this is in line with the Mut-4 being only a partial antagonist. There are several possible explanations to this finding. First, we did not test all the possible substitutions at positions 280 and 281 and did not mutagenize all the residues of the AB2 loop. Thus, it cannot be excluded that a more systematic approach could lead to a full antagonist like the one recently discovered for hGHbp.[34] In this latter case, however, one must consider that since the receptor is a homodimer, the observed mutation is going to simultaneously affect interactions formed by both receptor chains.[16,34] Finally, as discussed above for IL-6, the possible existence of another binding surface for a second gp130 molecule cannot be excluded for IL-6Rα either. Future efforts will hence be directed towards further mutagenizing shIL-6Rα, in order to completely abolish binding to gp130 without disturbing protein folding. In multiple myeloma, IL-6 has been shown to act as an autocrine as well as a paracrine growth factor[35,36] and to cause the development of plasmacytoma and myeloma kidney in transgenic mice.[37,38] Generating potent IL-6 antagonists has thus been anticipated as a possible therapeutic strategy. This task is made particularly difficult both by the high degree of sensitivity of myeloma cells to IL-6[39] and by the high level of this cytokine produced by the majority of patients.[40] An appropriate solution to this problem is to produce selective and potent IL-6 antagonists. Preliminary results obtained in our laboratory have indicated that the IL-6 mutant DFRD is able to fully inhibit the growth of the IL-6 dependent human myeloma cell line XG-1, and that this effect is even more pronounced by using the "superantagonist" DFRDIRA.

Generating cytokine antagonists is of paramount importance in view of their potential applications in the therapy of cancer, inflammatory and autoimmune diseases. The work presented in this paper demonstrates that detailed knowledge of the 3D structure of the cytokine-receptors complex (information not available in the case of IL-6) is not an absolute prerequisite for the generation of a full antagonist when structural information is available from homologous systems, hence allowing the problem to be addressed by molecular modeling.

ACKNOWLEDGMENTS

We thank J. Clench for critical reading of the manuscript, Yves M. Cully for artwork and I. Bagni for excellent secretarial assistance.

[**Note Added in Proof:** A related work describing the isolation of a polypeptide inhibitor of hIL-6 using the phage-display technique has recently been published.[43]]

REFERENCES

1. VAN SNICK, J. 1990. Annu. Rev. Immunol. **8:** 253–278.
2. AKIRA, S., T. TAGA & T. KISHIMOTO. 1993. Adv. Immunol. **54:** 1–78.
3. POLI, V., R. BALENA, E. FATTORI, A. MARKATOS, M. YAMAMOTO, H. TANAKA, G. CILIBERTO, G. A. RODAN & F. COSTANTINI. 1994. EMBO J. **13:** 1189–1196.
4. KLEIN, B., J. WIJDENES, X-G. ZHANG, M. JOURDAN, J-M. BOIRON, J. BROCHIER, J. LIAUTARD, M. MERLIN, C. CLEMENT, B. MOREL-FOURNIER, Z-Y. LU, P. MANNONI, J. SANY & R. BATAILLE. 1991. Blood **78:** 1198–1204.
5. JILKA, R. L., G. HANGOC, G. GIRASOLE, G. PASSERI, D. C. WILLIAMS, J. S. ABRAMS, B. BOYCE, H. BROXMEYER & S. C. MANOLAGAS. 1992. Science **257:** 88–91.
6. BECK, J. T., S-M HSU, J. WIJDENES, R. BATAILLE, B. KLEIN, D. VESOLE, K. HAYDEN, S. JAGANNATH & B. BARLOGIE. 1994. New Engl. J. Med. **330:** 602–605.
7. KISHIMOTO, T., S. AKIRA & T. TAGA. 1992. Science **258:** 593–597.
8. HIBI, M., M. MURAKAMI, M. SAITO, T. HIRANO & T. KISHIMOTO. 1990. Cell **63:** 1149–1157.
9. KISHIMOTO, T., T. TAGA & S. AKIRA. 1994. Cell **76:** 253–262.
10. ROSE-JOHN, S. & P. C. HEINDRICH. 1994. Biochem. J. **300:** 281–290.
11. WELLS, J. A. 1994. Curr. Opin. Cell Biol. **6:** 163–173.
12. STAHL, N. & G. D. YANCOPOULOS. 1993. Cell **74:** 587–590.
13. SPRANG, S. R. & J. FERNANDO BAZAN. 1993. Curr. Opin. Struct. Biol. **3:** 815–827.
14. BAZAN, J. F. 1990. Proc. Natl. Acad. Sci. USA **87:** 6934–6939.
15. SATO, N. & A. MYAJIMA. 1994. Curr. Opin. Cell Biol. **6:** 174–179.
16. DE VOS, A. M., M. ULTSCH & A. A. KOSSIAKOFF. 1992. Science **255:** 306–312.
17. SAVINO, R., A. LAHM, A. L. SALVATI, L. CIAPPONI, E. SPORENO, S. ALTAMURA, G. PAONESSA, C. TONIATTI & G. CILIBERTO. 1994. EMBO J. **13:** 1357–1367.
18. VRIEND, G. 1990. J. Mol. Graph. **8:** 52–56.
19. DAYRINGER, H. E., A. TRAMONTANO, S. R. SPRANG & R. J. FLETTERICK. 1986. J. Mol. Graphics **4:** 82–87.
20. BERNSTEIN, F. C., T. F. KOETZLE, G. J. B. WILIAMS, E. F. MEYER, JR., M. D. BRICE, J. R. RODGERS & O. KENNARD. 1977. J. Mol. Biol. **112:** 535–542.
21. ARCONE, R., P. PUCCI, F. ZAPPACOSTA, V. FONTAINE, A. MALORNI, G. MARINO & G. CILIBERTO. 1991. Eur. J. Biochem. **198:** 541–547.

22. O'REILLY, D. R., L. K. MILLER & V. A. LUCKOW, EDS. 1992. Baculovirus expression vectors, a laboratory manual. New York: W. H. Freeman and Company.
23. SPORENO, E., G. PAONESSA, A. L. SALVATI, R. GRAZIANI, P. DELMASTRO, G. CILIBERTO & C. TONIATTI. 1994. J. Biol. Chem. **269:** 10991–10995.
24. GREGORY, B., R. SAVINO & G. CILIBERTO. 1994. J. Immunol. Methods **170:** 47–56.
25. ZHONG, Z., Z. WEN & J. E. DARNELL, JR. 1994. Science **264:** 95–98.
26. ZIMARINO, V. & C. WU. 1994. Science **327:** 727–730.
27. WEGENKA, U. M., J. BUSCHMANN, C. LUTTICKEN, P. C. HEINRICH & F. HORN. 1993. Mol. Cell. Biol. **13:** 276–288.
28. LEEBEK, F. W. G., K. KARIYA, M. SCHWABE & D. M. FOWLKES. 1992. J. Biol. Chem. **267:** 14832–14838.
29. SAVINO, R., A. LAHM, M. GIORGIO, A. CABIBBO, A. TRAMONTANO & G. CILIBERTO. Proc. Natl. Acad. Sci. USA **90:** 4067–4071.
30. LEAHY, D. J., W. A. HENDRICKSON, I. AUKHIL & H. P. ERICKSON. 1992. Science **258:** 987–991.
31. FISCHMANN, T. O., G. A. BENTLEY, T. N. BHAT, G. BOULOT, R. A. MARIUZZA, S. E. V. PHILIPPS, D. TELLO & R.J. POLJAK. 1991. J. Biol. Chem. **266:** 12915–12923.
32. BRAKENOFF, J. P. J., M. HART, E. R. DE GROOT, F. DI PADOVA & L. A. AARDEN. 1990. J. Immunol. **145:** 561–568.
33. MURAKAMI, M., M. HIBI, N. NAKAGAWA, T. NAKAGAWA, K. YASUKAWA, K. YAMANISHI, T. TAGA & T. KISHIMOTO. 1993. Science **269:** 1808–1810.
34. DUQUESNOY, P., M. L. SOBRIER, B. DURIEZ, F. DASNOT, C. R. BUCHANAN, M. O. SAVAGE, M. A. PREECE, C. T. CRAESCU, Y. BLOQUIT, M. GOOSSENS & S. AMSELEM. 1994. EMBO J. **13:** 1386–1395.
35. KAWANO, M., T. HIRANO, T. MATSUDA, T. TAGA, Y. HORII, K. IWATO, H. ASAOKU, B. TANG, O. TANABE, H. TANAKA, A. KURAMOTO & T. KISHIMOTO. 1988. Nature **332:** 83–85.
36. KLEIN, B., X-G ZHANG, M. JOURDAN, J. CONTENT, F. HOUSSIAU, L. A. AARDEN, M. PIECHACZYC & R. BATAILLE. 1989. Blood **73:** 517–526.34.
37. SUEMATSU, S., T. MATSUDA, A. KATSUYUKI, S. AKIRA, N. NAKANO, S. OHNO, J. MIYAZAKI, K. YAMAMURA, T. HIRANO & T. KISHIMOTO. 1989. Proc. Natl. Acad. Sci. USA **86:** 7547–7551.
38. FATTORI, E., C. DELLA ROCCA, P. COSTA, M. GIORGIO, B. DENTE, L. POZZI & G. CILIBERTO. 1994. Blood **83:** 2570–2579.
39. JOURDAN, M., X-G XUE, M. PORTIER, J-M BOIRON, R. BATAILLE & B. KLEIN. 1991. J. Immunol. **147:** 4402–4407.
40. LU, Z-Y, H. BRAILLY, J-F ROSSI, J. WIJDENES, R. BATAILLE & B. KLEIN. 1993. Cytokine **5:** 578–582.
41. CARSON, M. 1987. J. Mol. Graphics **5:** 103–106.
42. KRAULIS, P. J. 1991. J. Appl. Crystallog. **24:** 946–950.
43. MARTIN, F., C. TONIATTI, A. L. SALVATI, S. VENTURINI, G. CILIBERTO, R. CORTESE & M. SOLLAZZO. 1994. EMBO J. **73:** 5303–5309.

DISCUSSION OF THE PAPER

P. SEHGAL (*New York Medical College, Valhalla*): Do you have any pharmacokinetic data with the IL-6 and IL-6 receptor mutants in animal situations? Because from everything I have heard there is an aspect that would bother me a lot, and that is that these molecules *in vivo* instead of inhibiting will act as carriers and will increase the half-life by 1000-fold; instead of the 1000-fold inhibition that you see in culture you will get a 10- to 100-fold increase *in vivo* in biological activity. And that is something that we have become acutely cautious about.

G. CILIBERTO: We are aware of that; however, we do not have any pharmacokinetic data with our antagonists. I think that the only way we could know something about their possible function will be to finally have a molecule that has inhibitory activity on murine cells and then test it on transgenic animals. This would be the right way to use transgenic animals, for example, IL-6 transgenic animals that suffer from IL-6–dependent pathology. At this point we cannot have a direct proof of their *in vivo* effect.

SEHGAL: What is the point of testing them in transgenic animals? That was going to be my second question. What are the human disease states that you would seriously consider the use of such antagonists in? What are the clinical situations today that you can identify where you would in serious fashion consider the use of such antagonists?

CILIBETO: The only one is multiple myeloma.

SEHGAL: I would not consider this very seriously, because from the data that I am aware of the moment you stop the antagonist, in that case the neutralizing antibody, the myeloma comes right back up.

CILIBERTO: The antibody I agree with you is not a good way of treating multiple myeloma because it gives stabilization of IL-6 and gives increased production, but the ability of cells taken from myeloma patients treated with antibody to respond to monoclonal antibodies *in vitro* is maintained, so that in this case the treatment with antibody does not select IL-6-resistant cells; that is proven by the Montpelier group.

SEHGAL: That point is well taken, but I am still struggling with the question: In which clinical disease state would you actually consider using an IL-6 antagonist?

CILIBERTO: We believe that myeloma can be a good target. Together with that, the availability of a good antagonist that also works on mouse cells and its testing in particular animal models will give the final answer about the role of IL-6 in particular diseases; also for chronic immunological diseases this would be very important to know.

M. REVEL (*Weizmann Institute of Science, Rehovot, Israel*): It is beautiful work. I wanted to ask you about the peptide library you described that you have found or sequences that resemble a piece of the IL-6 receptor. But among the other phages that you got did you have many peptides which were equivalent to the IL-6 receptor? Can you give us some statistics?

CILIBERTO: Actually, most of the clones that were selected had the sequence in the loops that resembled parts of the receptor. However, the minibody protein by itself is rather sticky, so we discarded many of the selected variants because they were giving us other problems in the ELISA assay. So we end up only with this, but actually the selected sequence in most of the cases looks like receptor loops.

R. G. HAWLEY (*Sunnybrook Health Science Centre, Toronto, Ont., Canada*): Did you say that you tested your IL-6 antagonist on B-9 cells? And does it inhibit as an antagonist?

CILIBERTO: Unfortunately, it is an agonist on B-9 cells.

HAWLEY: So the model system in the transgenic mice will be one that is making human IL-6.

CILIBERTO: They are making human IL-6. But, of course, what we are trying to do now is to put additional mutations into proteins in order to get something that is not species-specific, but also is an antagonist on rodent cells.

Alanine-scanning Mutagenesis of Human Interleukin-11: Identification of Regions Important for Biological Activity

MARTA CZUPRYN, FRANN BENNETT, JENNIFER DUBE,
KATHY GRANT, HUBERT SCOBLE,
HEMCHAND SOOKDEO, AND JOHN M. McCOY[a]

Genetics Institute Inc.
87 Cambridge Park Drive
Cambridge, Massachusetts 02140

INTRODUCTION

Interleukin-11 (IL-11) was originally identified as a factor produced by a bone marrow–derived stromal cell line which could stimulate the proliferation of IL-6-dependent plasmacytoma cells.[1] However, it is now recognized that the biological activity of interleukin-11 is not limited to the B-cell lineage; the molecule is a truly multi-functional cytokine[2-4] with effects on the proliferation and differentiation of early pluripotent stem cells, the proliferation of megakaryocyte,[5] erythroid[6] and myeloid[7] progenitors, induction of the acute-phase response in hepatocytes,[8] and on the inhibition of pre-adipocyte differentiation.[9] Although some of the elements of the IL-11 receptor complex remain unknown, one component is thought to be gp130,[10] placing IL-11 into the sub-class of cytokines which use this molecule for signal transduction. Members of this sub-class include interleukin-6 (IL-6), leukemia inhibitory factor (LIF), oncostatin M (OSM) and ciliary neurotrophic factor (CNTF). Together with IL-11 these molecules are collectively referred to as the IL-6-type cytokines.[11]

Although the three dimensional structure of a representative of the IL-6-type cytokine sub-class remains to be determined experimentally, it has been proposed based on physical studies, computer modeling and mutagenesis experiments that they possess a distinctive four-helix bundle tertiary fold.[12-14] This fold,[15,16] comprising four packed α-helices interconnected by loop regions of varying length and stabilized by the presence of disulfide bonds, has been observed experimentally in the tertiary structures of a number of other cytokines, including growth hormone (GH), interleukin-2 (IL-2), interleukin-4 (IL-4), granulocyte colony stimulating factor (G-CSF), and granulocyte-macrophage colony stimulating factor (GM-CSF). Furthermore, the regions of human growth hormone that interact with its homodimeric receptor were revealed unambiguously by x-ray crystallography of the growth hormone/receptor complex.[17] The primary receptor binding site of human growth hormone (site I) includes surface residues of helix D, residues at the C-terminal end of helix A and residues in the long loop connecting helices A and B, including one of the two segments of mini-helix present in this loop. The secondary receptor binding site (site II) comprises surface residues at the N-terminus of helix A, residues in helix C, and residues in the loop

---

[a] Author to whom all correspondence should be addressed.

between helices B and C. This detailed structural data has provided a paradigm for the proposed receptor binding sites of other cytokines.[14,18]

To date there has been little information available on the structure/function relationships of human IL-11 (hIL-11). Recently, however, a four-helix bundle fold was proposed for the molecule[19] based on a number of lines of evidence including; the high helicity of the molecule revealed by circular dichroism measurements, computer predictions of secondary structure, the locations of intron/exon boundaries in the IL-11 gene, and limited proteolysis experiments showing degradation predominantly in proposed inter-helical regions. In agreement with the model and proposed receptor binding regions selective chemical modification experiments implicated methionine 58 (thought to lie in a mini-helix within the AB loop) and lysine 98 (located at the N-terminus of a putative helix C) in the biological activity of hIL-11. Moreover C-terminal deletion studies suggested that this region of IL-11 was important both for the stability and biological activity of the molecule. To provide additional support for this structural hypothesis, and to complement ongoing multi-dimensional NMR structural studies, the structure/function relationships of hIL-11 were probed in the present study using alanine-scanning mutagenesis. We present evidence for helical structure at both the N- and C-termini of hIL-11, and describe a number of mutated forms of hIL-11 with greatly diminished biological activities.

METHODS

Bacterial Strains and Plasmid Constructions

E. coli K12 strain GI724 (ATCC 55151)[20] was used for the expression work and as the host for plasmid constructions. The strain contains the bacteriophage λ repressor (cI) gene stably integrated into the chromosomal *amp*C locus. Repressor synthesis is under the transcriptional control of a synthetic *Salmonella typhimurium trp* promoter integrated upstream of cI in the chromosome. GI724 is a host strain suitable for pL promoter expression vectors, pL-directed transcription being inducible in GI724 by the addition of tryptophan to the growth medium.

The expression plasmid used for synthesis of both wild-type and mutant hIL-11 was based on pTRXFUS, a vector which has been successfully used for the production of a wide range of cytokines in a soluble form in the *E. coli* cytoplasm as C-terminal thioredoxin fusion proteins.[20] pTRXFUS contains a colE1 origin of replication, a β-lactamase gene as a selectable marker and the bacteriophage λ pL promoter located upstream of the *E. coli* thioredoxin (*trx*A) gene. A short DNA sequence encoding the linker peptide "-GSGSGDDDDK-", positioned in frame at the 3'-end of *trx*A, provides a specific enterokinase site[21] at the point of fusion of thioredoxin to cytokine fusion partners. This allows for specific cleavage of the fusion protein to release the cytokine if desired. Further downstream in the vector lies a polylinker DNA sequence containing convenient restriction sites and also an *asp*A transcription terminator sequence.

The wild-type human interleukin-11 referred to in this paper is missing the first proline residue of the natural sequence (des-Pro hIL-11), and comprises 177 amino-acid residues with a calculated molecular mass of 19047 Da. The gene for wild-type hIL-11 was fused to the thioredoxin gene in pTRXFUS to generate a fusion expression vector, pTRXF-EKIL11dp-781. Alanine substitutions were introduced into hIL-11 in this vector by means of cassette mutagenesis. Before commencing the N-terminal alanine-scan a modified vector, pTRXF-EKIL11dp-781(K41E), was constructed. In

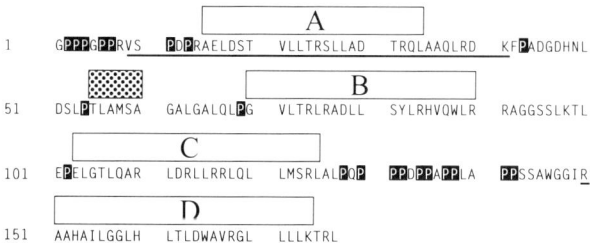

FIGURE 1. The primary sequence of human interleukin-11. Shown is the des-Pro form which lacks the amino-terminal proline residue found in the natural sequence. The open boxes labelled A, B, C and D denote the predicted locations of α-helices. The shaded box marks the location of a predicted mini-helix containing methionine 58, a residue thought to be involved in the biological activity of the molecule [19]. The distribution of proline residues in the hIL-11 sequence is indicated by black boxes. Note particularly that there are no prolines within predicted helical regions, and note also the preponderance of prolines in the C-D loop region. Underlined are the residues mutated in this study.

this plasmid a unique EcoR1 site was introduced into the hIL-11 gene at the codon encoding lysine 41, changing it to a glutamate codon (the effect of this mutation, K41E, on bioactivity is presented in the results section). The DNA lying between this new EcoR1 site and a naturally occurring unique Xho1 site in the hIL-11 gene, situated at the codon for arginine 8, was replaced with 32 separate synthetic oligonucleotide duplexes encoding mutations at every position between valine 9 and aspartate 40 (FIG. 1). Each wild-type hIL-11 codon in this section was replaced with an alanine codon, or if the wild-type residue at any position was already an alanine, it was changed to a serine. Introduction of the synthetic oligonucleotide in each case removed the EcoR1 site, reverting position 41 back to the original lysine residue. For the C-terminal alanine-scan mutagenesis a unique BamH1 site was introduced into the hIL-11 DNA sequence in pTRXF-EKIL11dp-781 at a position corresponding to glycine 148. In this case the introduction of the new restriction site was translationally silent. The DNA between the new BamH1 site and a downstream Acc1 site was replaced by 28 separate synthetic oligonucleotide duplexes encoding mutations at every position between arginine 150 and leucine 177 of hIL-11 (FIG. 1). Again each wild-type hIL-11 codon in this section was replaced with an alanine codon, or if the wild-type residue at any position was already alanine, it was changed to serine.

Production and Quantitation of Thioredoxin/hIL-11 Mutants

Conditions for the growth and induction of pTRXFUS expression plasmids in GI724 are described elsewhere.[20] Wild-type and mutant hIL-11 fusions were produced at levels of approximately 3–5% of total soluble *E. coli* cell protein at an induction temperature of 37°C. Bacterial cells expressing the various mutant genes were lysed in a French pressure cell and fractionated into soluble and insoluble fractions by centrifugation at 15,000 × g for 10 minutes. The two fractions were run on separate SDS-polyacrylamide gels[22] and stained with Coomassie blue. Following destaining, the gels were dried between sheets of cellophane and scanned on a flat-bed grey-scale scanner. The gel scans were visualized and the pixel values of individual protein bands measured using the program IMAGE from NIH. Data was first normalized for gel loading with reference to a strong *E. coli* band on the gel, and then corrected for background density. The amount of each hIL-11 mutant was then expressed as a percentage of a wild-type hIL-11 control which was included on every gel.

Biological Assay

In vitro biological activity of wild-type thioredoxin/hIL-11 and mutants was assessed in a proliferation assay performed on the murine plasmacytoma cell line T10.[1] Purification of the mutant thioredoxin/hIL-11 fusion proteins was typically unnecessary since the T10 assay could be performed successfully on crude bacterial lysates. Cleavage of the thioredoxin/hIL-11 fusion proteins with enterokinase to release free hIL-11 was also usually unnecessary, since hIL-11 fused to thioredoxin has full biological activity. Assays used serial dilutions of sterile-filtered, clarified bacterial lysates containing the mutant fusion proteins. Inhibition of the assay caused by bacterial cell components at low dilutions did not interfere with the assessment of hIL-11 activity, which was always made at much higher dilutions.

Structure Predictions

Predictions of secondary structure of hIL-11 were performed according to Chou and Fasman[23] and Garnier *et al.*[24] using the GCG computer program package. The length of α-helices was determined from helical wheel projections based on the preservation of amphipathic character.

RESULTS

C-Terminal Alanine-Scan

The thioredoxin/hIL-11 fusion gene is expressed well in *E. coli* and the fusion protein, made at about 3–5% of the cell protein at 37°C, is all soluble and fully active in bioassays. Previous mutagenesis work[19] had shown that successive deletions of blocks of four amino-acid residues from the C-terminus of hIL-11 had led immediately to a marked reduction in biological activity, and progressively to protein insolubility as evidenced by the appearance of the fusion protein in the pellet fraction of *E. coli* cell lysates. Since this result implicated residues at the C-terminus of hIL-11 in both biological activity and in protein stability, an alanine-scan was performed on this region to define the exact residues contributing to each of these effects. By analogy to growth hormone this region of hIL-11 may correspond to helix D, and constitute part of site I, the primary receptor binding site.

The length of the region chosen for the mutagenesis was based on computer predictions of secondary structure[23,24] and extended from arginine 150 to the C-terminal residue of hIL-11, leucine 177. A total of 28 mutants were made across this region, with each residue in turn being mutated to an alanine, or to a serine if alanine was already the wild-type residue. Although the mutants all accumulated to similar extents following induction as judged by gels of whole *E. coli* cell lysates, when SDS-PAGE

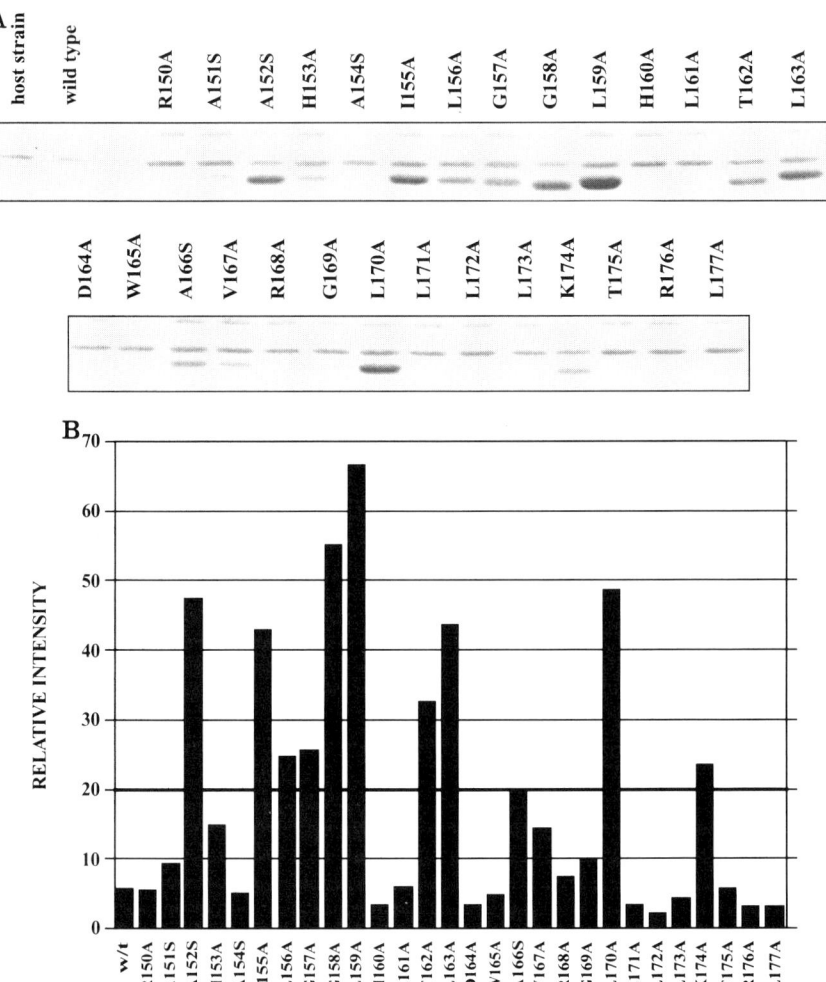

FIGURE 2. A: The insoluble cell-pellet fractions from the C-terminal alanine-scan experiment, Coomassie-blue stained SDS-PAGE gels. **B:** Quantitation of the thioredoxin/hIL-11 mutant bands in the gels shown in FIGURE 2A. Relative intensity is expressed in arbitrary units derived from the pixel values of gel scans. Values are normalized for gel loading and expression levels.

gels of the cell-pellet fractions (the inclusion body fractions) were examined (FIG. 2a) it was clear that several mutants were structurally unstable. Quantitation of the amounts of fusion protein in the insoluble fraction from gel scans (FIG. 2b) revealed that A152S, I155A, G158A, L159A, T162A, L163A, and L170A were particularly noteworthy in this respect. The spacing of these residues relative to each other along the primary structure appeared to exhibit an approximate periodicity of 3 or 4 residues, suggestive of an α-helical secondary structure. Since most of these residues possess hydrophobic side chains, they may make important contributions to the stability of the folded molecule by being buried in the interior of the molecule as the hydrophobic face of an amphipathic α-helix. Although it is possible that the instability caused by the mutations is at the level of protein folding, overall the more likely explanation is the disruption of important tertiary interactions.

To assess the effects of mutations on the biological activity of hIL-11, soluble fractions from the C-terminal alanine-scan inductions were submitted for T10 bioassay. FIGURE 3a shows the activity results, normalized for expression and gel loading

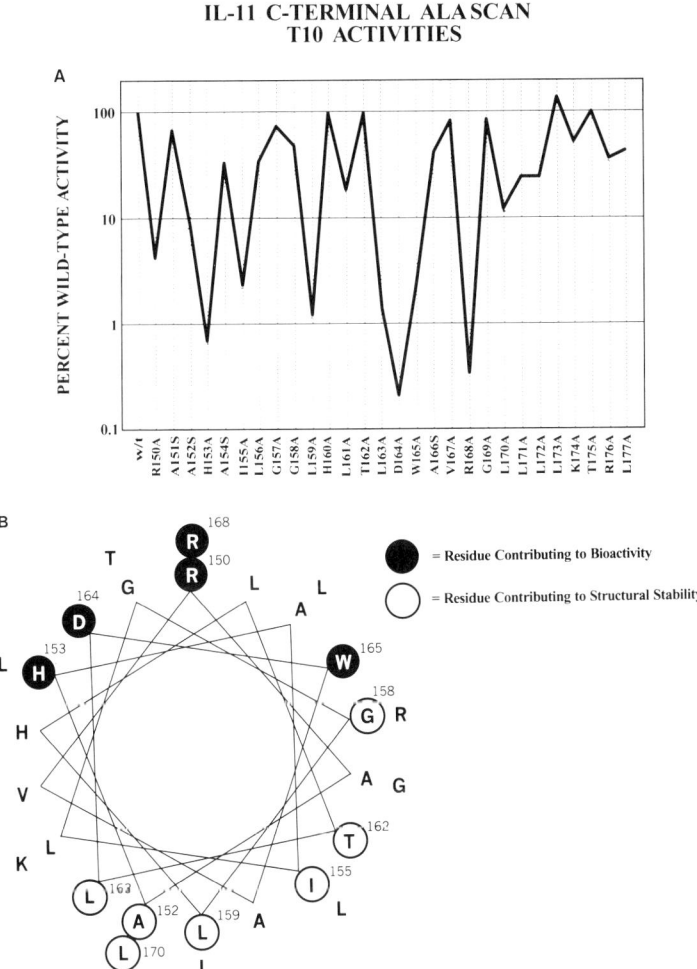

FIGURE 3. A: Activities of C-terminal alanine-scan mutants in the T10 murine plasmacytoma proliferation assay. Activities are expressed as a percentage of wild-type hIL-11. **B:** Helical wheel projection of the C-terminal hIL-11 sequence from arginine 150 to leucine 177. Residues thought to be involved in both bioactivity and structural stability are marked.

differences and presented as a percentage of wild-type activity. There were a number of mutants where the observed specific activity was below 5% of the wild-type level, notably R150A, H153A, D164A, W165A and R168A (the activities observed for I155A, L159A and L163A were also low, but for each of these mutants severe instability problems were the probable cause). Note that while D164A exhibited a large reduction in specific activity, having only 0.2% of the activity of wild-type hIL-11, none of this particular mutant appeared in the insoluble fraction (FIG. 2a), suggesting that it was correctly folded. As a further check that the effects on activity were truly specific to the mutated side-chains, and not due to a general protein folding defect, four of the mutants fusions with reduced activity (R150A, H153A, D164A and W165A) were cleaved with enterokinase and the mutant hIL-11 species purified to homogeneity. All of the purified mutants ran as monomeric species with no apparent aggregation on size exclusion columns (data not presented), and H153A and D164A both had circular dichroism spectra that were identical to wild-type hIL-11, indicating that as judged by these criteria they were correctly folded.

The effects on activity, like the effects on solubility, also appeared to show a rough periodicity. FIGURE 3b plots those residues thought to be involved in stability and those thought to be involved in bioactivity on a helical wheel. The projection clearly shows a hydrophobic face and a hydrophilic face of a putative C-terminal helix D. Strikingly, residues which the alanine-scan showed to have effects on stability all map to the hydrophobic face, and all the residues which had less than 5% activity when mutated lie on the hydrophilic face. These data provide a strong argument for the presence of amphipathic helical structure at the C-terminus of hIL-11.

N-Terminal Alanine-Scan

Based on computer predictions a second alanine-scan was performed on another region of hIL-11 thought to possess a helical secondary structure, a segment lying between the glutamate residue at position 16 an the leucine at position 34. By analogy to growth hormone this region may correspond to helix A, which contains residues contributing to both receptor binding sites I and II.

The segment chosen for mutagenesis was valine 9 to lysine 41, covering the entire predicted helix A and extending into the adjacent loop regions. The mutants were expressed and analyzed identically to the C-terminal mutants described above; however, in sharp contrast, no solubility problems were noted for any of the N-terminal mutants. FIGURE 4a shows the results of activity assays. Mutation of several amino-acid residues in putative helix A caused severe reductions in bioactivity, and as was seen with the C-terminal helix D, these N-terminal activity mutants displayed an apparent periodicity with respect to the primary sequence. Mutations showing less than 5% of wild-type activity included P13A, E16A, L17A, L22A, R25A, L28A, T31A, R32A, L34A and R39A. The two mutants L17A and R25A were each less than 0.1% as active as wild-type hIL-11. A helical wheel plot of the N-terminal region of hIL-11 is presented in FIGURE 4b. The distribution of mutations effecting activity can be interpreted as demonstrating a helical secondary structure, although not as clearly as was seen with the C-terminal alanine-scan. One face of the putative helix exhibits most of the activity mutations, with the other face being comparatively open.

At the N-terminus a clear mapping on an amphipathic helix of activity mutations on a hydrophilic face and structural mutations on a hydrophobic face could not be drawn. This contrasted with observations of the effects of mutations made at the C-terminus, and might point to a more critical involvement of hydrophobic interactions in the maintenance of structure in that region of the molecule.

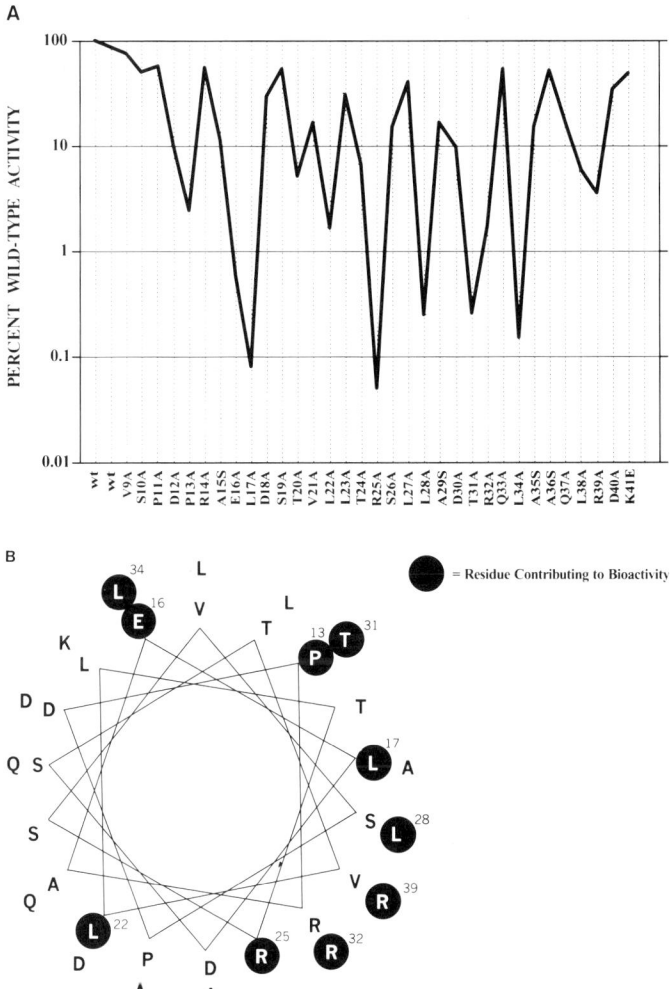

FIGURE 4. A: Activities of N-terminal alanine-scan mutants in the T10 murine plasmacytoma proliferation assay. Activities are expressed as a percentage of wild-type hIL-11. **B:** Helical wheel projection of the N-terminal hIL-11 sequence from valine 9 to lysine 41. Residues thought to be involved in bioactivity are marked.

DISCUSSION

At first glance it seems unlikely that human interleukin-11 would be be a four-helix bundle cytokine, since the molecule is rich in proline residues (12%), and a predominantly helical secondary structure might appear improbable. Furthermore, all of the known members of the four-helix bundle cytokine class possess stabilizing disulfide cross-links, whereas hIL-11 lacks cysteine residues altogether. Recently, however, the availability of purified recombinant hIL-11 has enabled the structure of the molecule to be probed by physical and biochemical techniques. Circular dichroism measurements reveal that despite its content of proline, hIL-11 is in fact highly helical (57 ± 1%, John Steckert, personal communication) and that, even though it lacks disulfide bonds, the molecule is extremely thermally stable (Tm = 90°C, Nicholas Warne, personal communication). Chemical modification experiments performed on purified hIL-11 have identified methionine 58, and either or both of lysine residues 41 and 98, as being important for biological activity. Chemical modification has also shown that the N-terminal glycine residue of hIL-11 is not involved in activity, whereas specific amino-acid deletions have suggested that residues at the C-terminus of the molecule are important not only for activity but also for stability.[19] Recently it was reported that hIL-11 transduces its signal using gp130, the shared subunit of all IL-6 type cytokine receptor complexes.[10] This places hIL-11 firmly into the family of IL-6 type cytokines, and although a representative tertiary structure has not yet been experimentally determined for this class of proteins, there are a wealth of studies which support their possession of a four-helix bundle fold. Based on a consideration of all these data a four-helix bundle model was proposed for the hIL-11 structure and some additional evidence supporting the model obtained from the results of limit proteolysis.[19] Degradation of hIL-11 in these experiments was seen mostly in potential inter-helix loop regions, and not within the proposed helices themselves. Continuing these studies, we have in this paper used alanine-scanning mutagenesis to probe those regions of hIL-11 which, according to the four-helix bundle model, may possibly contain critical elements of receptor binding sites.

In any mutagenesis approach it is difficult to separate specific efforts on protein function from the potentially deleterious effects of introduced mutations on the global fold of the protein. Such problems can be minimized, however, if the introduced changes are restricted in their scope and if the means of production of the mutated proteins does not involve an *in vitro* refolding step. For example, the true effects of particular mutations on function may be masked by protein instability caused by deletion mutations, or by mutations involving substitutions of residues with small-side chains by those with large side-chains, or by multiple mutations made simultaneously. Alanine-scanning mutagenesis (*i.e.*, the individual sequential substitution of each residue in a selected region by alanine) avoids most of these potential problems; no deletions are introduced, each mutant is a single change, and the introduced alanine side-chain is small. Alanine substitutions are particularly suitable for proteins containing large amounts of α-helix, since the alanine residue is well tolerated in helical regions.

E. coli is the organism of choice for the production of proteins when speed of analysis and high level expression are important considerations. However, heterologous proteins made in *E. coli* often require refolding, and single mutations introduced into a protein can often profoundly influence *in vitro* refolding pathways (J.M.M. unpublished observations). We chose to express hIL-11 mutants in *E. coli* as thioredoxin fusion proteins using the expression vector pTRXFUS. This system has been shown to produce many cytokines, including hIL-11, in a *soluble* and biologically active form in the *E. coli* cytoplasm,[20] which greatly facilitates structure/function studies. Since the thioredoxin/hIL-11 fusion protein is fully active, we were able to rapidly produce hIL-11 mutants in *E. coli* and analyze the effects of the mutations on biological activity. The levels of expression achieved with the system also allowed for easy purification of selected mutants in quantities sufficient to provide confirmatory evidence for their correct folding by physical methods. Additionally, since the wild-type thioredoxin/hIL-11 fusion protein was made in a soluble form, we were able to easily identify hIL-11 residues important for structural stability simply by looking for changes in

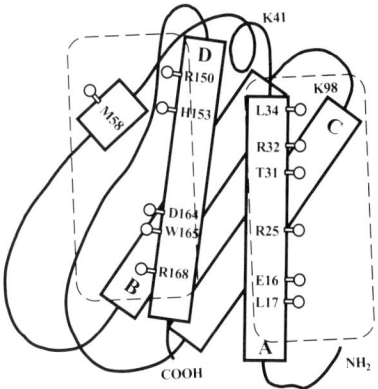

FIGURE 5. A schematic showing the proposed 4-helix bundle topology of hIL-11. Potential receptor/gp130 binding areas are indicated by dotted lines. The positions and identities of residues important for biological activity identified in this work and also in ref. 19 are indicated.

the solubility profile of each expressed mutant. This is in sharp contrast to the usual case for this type of study performed in *E. coli,* where effects like these would be masked by uncertainties regarding the efficiencies of *in vitro* refolding.

The results of the alanine-scan mutagenesis experiments performed on hIL-11 are summarized in FIGURE 5. The residues implicated in biological activity are positioned on a four-helix bundle representation of the hIL-11 structure. The hypothetical locations of receptor-binding areas are outlined in the figure, based on the known receptor-binding regions of human growth hormone.[17] Presumably binding sites for both gp130 and a hIL-11-specific receptor molecule should be present on hIL-11. Note, however, that since the hIL-11 receptor is uncharacterized, and no defined binding assay for it yet exists, we cannot distinguish between the effects of particular mutations on hIL-11 receptor binding versus effects on gp130 binding. Neither can we rule out subtle effects on conformation which may adversely influence receptor/gp130 binding at a position remote from any particular mutation.

At the C-terminus of hIL-11 residues R150, H153, D164, W165 and R168 are all involved in biological activity and can be mapped to the hydrophilic face of a putative amphipathic α-helix (FIG. 3b). In addition a number of other residues at the C-terminus of hIL-11, i.e. A152, I155, G158, L159, T162, L163, and L170, have a clear involvement in the maintenance of a stable tertiary structure, and these residues map to the opposite, hydrophobic face of the same putative amphiphatic helix, suggesting that the side-chains of these residues are buried internally in the structure and that they make important contributions to overall stability. This evidence argues persuasively that the C-terminus of hIL-11 is helical, and that this C-terminal helix constitutes a portion of the primary receptor binding site (site I). This model is in good agreement with what is observed with residues at the C-terminus of growth hormone. It should be noted also that methionine 58 of hIL-11, which had previously been shown to be involved in the biological activity of the molecule,[19] also probably contributes to site I. This would also be analogous to the situation in growth hormone, where a similar receptor-interacting region is found within the AB loop.[17]

There are precedents for structure/function relationships at the C-termini of other IL-6-type cytokines similar to those we observe in hIL-11. The C-terminal region of IL-6 itself has been shown to be important for binding to the IL-6 receptor, and in particular two arginine residues at positions 180 and 183 are thought to be essential.[13,25,26] It is also widely believed that the C-terminus of IL-6 has a helical conformation,[13,26] although it is unclear if the helix extends to the extreme C-terminus.[27] As a further example the C-terminus of oncostatin-M has similarly been proposed to be an amphiphatic helix mediating interactions with its receptor.[12]

The results of the N-terminal alanine-scan on hIL-11 are less straightforward. Numerous residues are found in this area which appear to contribute to biological activity including; P13, E16, L17, L22, R25, L28, T31, R32, L34 and R39. These residues are distributed along the primary sequence with an approximate periodicity of 3 or 4 residues, suggesting that they are in a helical secondary conformation. Like the C-terminal helix D, this putative N terminal helix A is amphiphatic, although to a lesser extent since its hydrophobic face is interrupted by the three threonine residues, T20, T24 and T31. However, when the N-terminal residues implicated in biological activity are projected onto an N-terminal helical wheel (FIG. 4b) they do not distribute neatly to a hydrophilic face as was seen for mutants at the C-terminus. Nevertheless there is a side of the putative N-terminal helix that is devoid of activity mutants which may constitute an interior "face", although this "face" is itself quite hydrophilic. No mutants were found in the N-terminal region which affected the stability of hIL-11 in the manner of certain residues at the C-terminus. The reason for this is unclear, but one could speculate that the N-terminal helix relies less on concerted hydrophobic interactions to ensure stable contacts with other elements of the hIL-11 structure, preferring instead multiple, more varied interactions. Further conformational details of the N-terminal helix await the solution of the hIL-11 tertiary structure.

It has been shown that the first 28 residues are dispensable for the biological activity of IL-6 [28]. A similar situation is probably true for hIL-11, since hIL-11 fused to thioredoxin via its N-terminus is fully active, and chemical modification of the glycine residue at the N-terminus of hIL-11 is well tolerated with no loss of activity.[19] However, the number of dispensable N-terminal residues must be smaller for hIL-11 than for IL-6, since P13A has only 2.5% of wild-type activity. Clearly for hIL-11 certain residues between P13 and K41 are involved in biological activity, and by analogy with growth hormone this region would constitute part of receptor binding site II. The C-terminal portion of helix A may also contribute some residues to site I. Recently Savino et al.[14] have developed a detailed model of the IL-6 structure based on the known structures of granulocyte colony stimulating factor and growth hormone. According to this model an N-terminal helix, helix A, was proposed to form part of a putative receptor-binding site II. The model was tested by making specific mutants and evidence was found that this region of IL-6 may indeed be part of the binding site for gp130, in particular IL-6 residues Y31 and G35. Another recent report[29] found that other residues in IL-6, specifically residues Q160 and T163 located in a region corresponding to the loop between helix C and D, may also be involved in gp130 binding. This CD loop region is interesting since the corresponding region in hIL-11 is extremely rich in prolines and bears no apparent homology to the CD loop of IL-6, despite the fact that both proteins signal through gp130.

In summary alanine-scan mutagenesis has identified a number of residues important for both the activity and structural stability of hIL-11. The C-terminus of hIL-11 is predicted to be helical (helix D) and to constitute part of the binding site (site I) of the uncharacterized hIL-11-specific receptor. Important residues contributing to receptor binding at this site may include R150, H153, D164, W165 and R168. In addition it is likely that M58 also participates in receptor binding. Residues at the extreme N-terminus of hIL-11 have been shown to be unnecessary for activity, however in a region lying between proline 13 and lysine 41 there are a number of residues which are critical in this respect, including P13, E16, L17, L22, R25, L28, T31, R32, L34 and R39. This region is predicted to be helical (helix A) and, by analogy to IL-6, some residues in this helix may constitute part of a gp130 binding site (site II) and others may be involved in site I.

SUMMARY

We have identified functionally important regions of human interleukin-11 (hIL-11) by means of alanine-scanning mutagenesis. A total of 61 mutated forms of hIL-11 were produced in *E. coli* as thioredoxin fusion proteins and tested in a murine T10 plasmacytoma proliferation assay. Mutations made at several positions proximal to the hIL-11 C-terminus caused substantial reduction in biological activity. In addition a number of other mutations in this region affected either protein folding or stability. Both effects displayed a characteristic periodicity with respect to the primary sequence which suggested that residues close to the C-terminus of hIL-11 adopt a helical conformation. Mutations made proximal to the N-terminus of hIL-11 also exhibited reduced bioactivity, although no effects on protein folding or stability were observed. The N-terminal mutations with reduced activity also mapped with a periodicity suggestive of a helical conformation. We previously have proposed a four-helix bundle topology for the hIL-11 structure based on physical studies, selective chemical modifications, positions of intron/exon boundaries, limit proteolysis experiments and site-directed mutagenesis. The alanine-scanning mutagenesis data we report here provide additional support for this model.

ACKNOWLEDGMENTS

We would like to thank Philip T. Boyle Jr., John Steckert, Nicholas Warne, and Wen Yu for their generous assistance in the execution of this work.

REFERENCES

1. PAUL, S. R., F. BENNETT, J. A. CALVETTI, K. KELLEHER, C. R. WOOD, R. M. O'HARA JR., A. C. LEARY, B. SIBLEY, S. C. CLARK, D. A. WILLIAMS & Y.-C. YANG. 1990. Proc. Natl. Acad. Sci. USA **87**: 7512–7516.
2. YANG, Y.-C. & T. YIN. 1992. BioFactors **4**: 15–21.
3. NEBEN, S. & K. TURNER. 1993. Stem Cells (Dayt) **11**(Suppl. 2). 156–62.
4. DU, X. X. & D. A. WILLIAMS. 1994. Blood **83**: 2023–2030.
5. BRUNO, E., R. BIDDELL & R. HOFFMAN. 1991. Exp. Hematol. **19**: 378–381.
6. QUESNIAUX, V.F.J., S.C. CLARK, K. TURNER & B. FAGG. 1992. Blood **80**:1218–1223.
7. KELLER, D. C., X. X. DU, E. F. SROUR, R. HOFFMAN & D. A. WILLIAMS. 1993. Blood **82**: 1428.
8. BAUMANN, H. & P. SCHENDEL. 1991. J. Biol. Chem. **266**: 20424–20427.
9. KAWASHIMA, I., J. OHSUMI, K. MITA-HONJO, K. SHIMODA-TAKANO, H. ISHIKAWA, S. SAKAKIBARA, K. MIYADAI & Y. TAKIGUCHI. 1991. FEBS Lett. **283**: 199–202.
10. YIN, T., T. TAGA, M. L.-S. TSANG, K. YASUKAWA, T. KISHIMOTO & Y.-C. YANG. 1993. J. Immunol. **151**: 2555–2561.
11. KISHIMOTO, T., T. TAGA & S. AKIRA. 1994. Cell **76**: 1–20.
12. KALLESTAD, J. C., M. SHOYAB & P. S. LINSLEY. 1991. J. Biol. Chem. **266**: 8940–8945.
13. LÜTTICKEN, A. KRÜTGEN, E. MÖLLER, P. C. HEINRICH & S. ROSE-JOHN. 1992. FEBS Lett. **282**: 265–267.
14. SAVINO, R., A. LAHM, A. L. SALVATI, L. CIAPPONI, E. SPORENO, S. ALTAMURA, G. PAONESSA, C. TONIATTI & G. CILIBERTO. 1994. EMBO J. **13**: 1357–1367.

15. Parry, D. A. D., E. Minasian & S. J. Leach. 1988. J. Molec. Recognition **1:** 107–110.
16. Bazan, J. F. 1990. Immunol. Today **11:** 350–354.
17. De Vos, A. M., M. Ultsch & A. A. Kossiakoff. 1992. Science **255:** 306–312.
18. Goodall, G. J., C. J. Bagley, M. A. Vadas & A. F. Lopez. 1993. Growth Factors **8:** 87–97.
19. Czupryn, M. J., J. M. McCoy & H. A. Scoble. 1995. J. Biol. Chem. **270:** 978–985.
20. LaVallie, E. R., E. A. DiBlasio, S. Kovacic, K. L. Grant, P. F. Schendel & J. M. McCoy. 1993. Bio/Technology **11:** 187–193.
21. LaVallie, E. R., A. Rehemtulla, L. A. Racie, E. A. DiBlasio, C. Ferenz, K. L. Grant, A. Light & J. M. McCoy. 1993. J. Biol. Chem. **268:** 23311–23317.
22. Laemmli, U. K. 1970. Nature **277:** 680–685.
23. Chou, P. Y. & G. D. Fasman. 1978. Ann. Rev. Biochem. **47:** 251–276.
24. Garnier, J., D. J. Osguthorpe & B. Robson. 1978. J. Mol. Biol. **120:** 97–120.
25. Brakenhoff, J. P., M. Hart, E. R. De Groot, F. Di Padova & L. A. Aarden. 1990. J. Immunol. **145:** 561–568.
26. Leebeek, F. W. G., K. Kariya, M. Schwabe & D. M. Fowlkes. 1992. J. Biol. Chem. **267:** 14832–14838.
27. Savino, R., A. Lahm, M. Giorgio, A. Cabibbo, A. Tramontano & G. Ciliberto. 1993. Proc. Natl. Acad. Sci. USA **90:** 4067–4071.
28. Brakenhoff, J. P., M. Hart & L. A. Aarden. 1989. J. Immunol. **143:** 1175–1182.
29. Brakenhoff, J. P. J., F. D. de Hon, V. Fontaine, E. ten Boekel, H. Schooltink, S. Rose-John, P. C. Heinrich, J. Content & L. A. Aarden. 1994. J. Biol. Chem. **269:** 86–93.

DISCUSSION OF THE PAPER

G. Ciliberto (*Istituto di Ricerche di Biologia Moleculare, Pomezia, Italy*): Do the mutants in helix A behave as antagonists?

J. McCoy: I knew you would ask that question. We have not purified them all. We purified one of the mutations, R2SA, and tested it in a T-10 assay for its ability to antagonize, and it did not.

Ciliberto: Have you also started to mutagenize helix C?

McCoy: No, we have not. We are on hold as far as mutagenesis goes because we are waiting for the structure. I think that once we have the structure we can make much more informed mutational choices.

G. Fey (*University of Erlangen-Nürnberg, Erlangen, Germany*): I was impressed by your thioredoxin expression system in which you get 20% of total cellular protein in the form of your recombinant protein. That is fairly high if it is in cytosol. Isn't it true that if you express proteins at that high level that they would precipitate out? What is the reason that IL-11 does not precipitate out? Does it not have disulfide bonds?

McCoy: I think that the reason why these proteins do show in the soluble fraction is that they are fused to a highly soluble partner. Thioredoxin acts like a covalently joined chaperone protein.

Inter-Species Chimeras of Leukemia Inhibitory Factor Define a Human Receptor Binding Site[a]

CATHERINE M. OWCZAREK,[b] MEREDITH J. LAYTON,
DONALD METCALF, ROSLYN CLARK, NICHOLAS M. GOUGH,
AND NICOS A. NICOLA

*The Cooperative Research Centre for Cellular Growth Factors and The
Walter and Eliza Hall Institute of Medical Research
PO Royal Melbourne Hospital
Melbourne, Victoria 3050, Australia*

The specific interaction of a cytokine or growth factor with its receptor is the first step in a series of complex intermolecular interactions required to ultimately transduce a biological signal. The glycoprotein leukemia inhibitory factor (LIF) was originally isolated, purified and cloned on the basis of its differentiation-inducing activity, but has since been shown to support a diverse range of physiological functions.[1] Many of the biological actions of LIF are shared by a number of other cytokines including G-CSF, oncostatin-M and interleukin-6.[2]

LIF mediates its functions by binding to a transmembrane receptor. cDNA clones have been isolated which encode a receptor that binds LIF with low affinity.[3] A high-affinity LIF receptor (LIF-R) can be generated by the interaction of the low affinity subunit (α-chain) with a second protein, gp130.[4] Both the LIF-R α-chain and gp130 are members of the recently described hemopoietic superfamily of receptors.[5] This family of receptors contain in their extracellular regions at least one copy of a hemopoietin domain, which is defined by a common secondary and tertiary structural fold, two pairs of conserved cysteines, and a Trp-Ser-X-Trp-Ser motif (where X is any amino acid) near the carboxy-terminus of the extracellular domain.

In order to define the residues involved in the interaction between LIF and its receptor we have undertaken a detailed molecular dissection of the LIF molecule. One approach that has been successfully applied to the delineation of residues involved in ligand-receptor interactions has been the generation and analysis of inter-species chimeras of the growth factor in question. LIF was an ideal candidate for mapping α-chain binding sites by this method as there were two properties specific to human LIF that we could exploit. Human LIF (hLIF) binds to the hLIF-R α-chain with low affinity, but mouse LIF (mLIF), although it is highly homologous to hLIF,[6] does not bind appreciably to this receptor.[3,7] Human LIF is biologically active on LIF responsive mouse cells, but unexpectedly it binds to the mLIF-R α-chain with an approximately 1000- to 5000-fold higher affinity than does mLIF. This unusual

---

[a] This work was supported by the National Health and Medical Research Council, Canberra; The Anti-Cancer Council of Victoria; AMRAD Corporation, Melbourne; the J. D. and L. Harris Trust Fund; the Philip Bushell Trust; the National Institute of Health, Bethesda, MD, Grant CA22556 and the Australian Government Cooperative Research Centres scheme.

[b] Author to whom correspondence should be addressed; Tel: 61-3-345-2559; Fax: 61-3-345-2616.

high-affinity binding of hLIF to the mLIF-R α-chain is primarily due to the slower rate of dissociation of hLIF, compared to mLIF, from the mLIF-R α-chain.[7] The construction and analysis of hybrid molecules composed of mLIF into which different regions of hLIF were substituted would enable us to delineate the regions of the hLIF polypeptide that confer these two properties specific to human LIF. We could determine which amino acid residues confer the first property of hLIF (binding to the hLIF-R α-chain where mLIF cannot) by evaluating the ability of a hybrid m-hLIF protein to compete with ^{125}I-hLIF for binding to the hLIF-R α-chain. The enhanced binding of hLIF to the mLIF-R α-chain would provide us with an opportunity to determine the epitopes which confer the second feature of hLIF by evaluating the ability of a m-hLIF hybrid protein to compete with ^{125}I-hLIF for binding to the mLIF-R α-chain. Furthermore, the 1000- to 5000-fold difference in the ability of mLIF and hLIF to compete with ^{125}I-hLIF for binding to the mLIF-R α-chain provides large window in which to measure the degree of hLIF-like binding in this assay.

The ligands for the hemopoietin family of receptors are predicted to have a common overall topology, although they are not related at the primary amino acid sequence level.[8] This structure, which is characterized by four anti-parallel α-helices connected by one short and two long loops, has been confirmed experimentally for a number of cytokines including granulocyte colony stimulating factor (G-CSF),[9] granulocyte-macrophage CSF (GM-CSF),[10] growth hormone (GH),[11,12] interleukin-2 (IL-2),[13,14] IL-4[15] and IL-5.[16] An x-ray crystal structure or NMR structure of LIF has not been described so we utilized published secondary and tertiary structural predictions[17] to divide the LIF sequence into a series of α-helices and connecting loops (FIG. 1). We then constructed a series of hybrid proteins where the mLIF amino acid sequence was used as a molecular framework into which specific regions of the hLIF amino acid sequence were substituted (FIG. 2) and (TABLE 1). Each hybrid protein was produced as a GST fusion protein in *E. coli*, affinity purified and separated from the GST portion by cleavage with thrombin.[18,19] After purification to homogeneity on S-Sepharose, the amount of each protein was quantified by amino acid analysis.[20] A silver-stained[21] SDS-polyacrylamide gel[22] with a selection of m-hLIF hybrid proteins

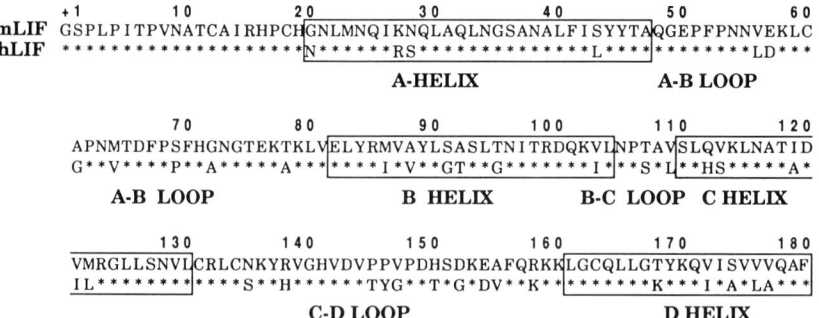

FIGURE 1. Comparison of mouse and human LIF amino acid sequences. Amino acid residues that are identical between mLIF and hLIF are indicated by asterisks and predicted α-helices A, B, C and D are surrounded by boxes. The numbering of the amino acid residues of each protein starts at +1 (serine) of the mature, native proteins; however, the thrombin cleavage results in an additional glycine residue at position −1 in recombinant mLIF, hLIF and all m-hLIF hybrids. The single-letter amino acid code is used throughout.

TABLE 1. Amino Acid Sequence Specifications for m-hLIF Hybrid Proteins

Hybrid	Amino Acid Sequence Specification
M	M1–180
H	H1–180
MH1	H1–102:M103–180
MH2	M1–102:H103–180
MH3	M1–160:H161–180
MH4	M1–109:H110–130:M131–180
MH5	M1–130:H131–160:M161–180
MH6	M1–109:H110–160:M161–180
MH27	MH5+Q112H
MH28	MH5+V113S
MH14	MH5+Q112H:V113S
MH16	M1–109:H110–153:M154–180
MH17	M1–109:H110–130:M131–153:H154–160:M161–180
MH18	MH6+H138R
MH31	MH6+T145P
MH19	MH6+Y146P
MH20	MH6+G147V
MH21	MH6+T150H
MH22	MH6+G152D
MH23	MH6+D154E
MH24	MH6+V155A
MH25	MH6+K158R
MH29	MH5+T107S
MH30	MH5+V109L
MH32	MH5+V103I
MH33	M+T107S:Q112H:V113S:A155V:R158K
MH34	MH33+H1–47
MH35	MH33+H48–81
MH36	MH33+H82–104
MH37	MH33+V103I
MH38	MH33+V56L
MH39	MH33+V109L
MH40	MH33+V56L:V103I:V109L
MH41	MH33+V56L:V103I
MH43	MH33+E57D
MH44	MH33+A61G
MH45	MH33+M64V
MH46	MH33+S69P

Sequences are designated according to the following example. M1–130:H131–160:M161–180 (MH5) denotes that residues between 1 and 130 as well as between 161 and 180 are derived from mLIF sequence and residues 131–160 are derived from hLIF sequence. Single amino substitutions are denoted as H138R, indicating that the histidine at position 138 is changed to arginine.

is shown in FIGURE 3. The high resolution of our competitive inhibition assays, and the accuracy with which we quantified the amount of protein in each preparation allowed us to determine the precise contribution of individual amino acids to ligand-receptor interactions. One of the major disadvantages in the analysis of chimeric proteins is that the overall tertiary structure may be destabilized by the amino acid substitutions involved. We tested each hybrid protein in two assays that could indicate whether the protein was correctly folded. First, mLIF and hLIF could compete simi-

HYBRID	SPECIFIC BIOLOGICAL ACTIVITY (UNITS/mg) x10^{-8}	% hLIF SCORE MEAN ± SD (mLIF-R α-CHAIN)	$\frac{ID_{50} \text{ (hybrid)}}{ID_{50} \text{ (hLIF)}}$ (hLIF-R α-CHAIN)
M	2.2	0	>10,000
H	3.8	100	1
MH1	1.4	23±2	300
MH2	1.8	86±11	2.5
MH3	0.82	7±13	1500
MH4	2.4	30±3	800
MH5	1.6	54±4	75
MH6	1.4	78±2	6
MH27	2	66±3	12
MH28	4.4	60±4	14
MH14	2.9	71±2	6
MH18	1.3	79±7	6
MH31	2.3	78±1	6
MH19	2.6	75±6	6
MH20	1.9	76±5	6
MH21	5.2	76±4	6
MH22	4.2	76±7	6
MH23	2.6	79	6
MH24	2.1	58±3	75
MH25	2.1	67±2	30
MH29	2.2	65±3	50
MH30	4.0	53±4	150
MH32	3.4	59±1	60
MH33	4.2	72±6	15
MH34	1.2	70±2	30
MH35	4.1	84±2	1.5
MH36	2.9	81±5	30
MH37	0.86	71±2	15
MH38	0.94	76±5	5
MH39	1.0	72±3	50
MH40	1.4	79±3	30
MH41	1.3	80±2	30
MH43	2.4	87±3	2.5
MH44	2.2	71±4	15
MH45	2.7	72±4	30
MH46	3.9	70±3	30

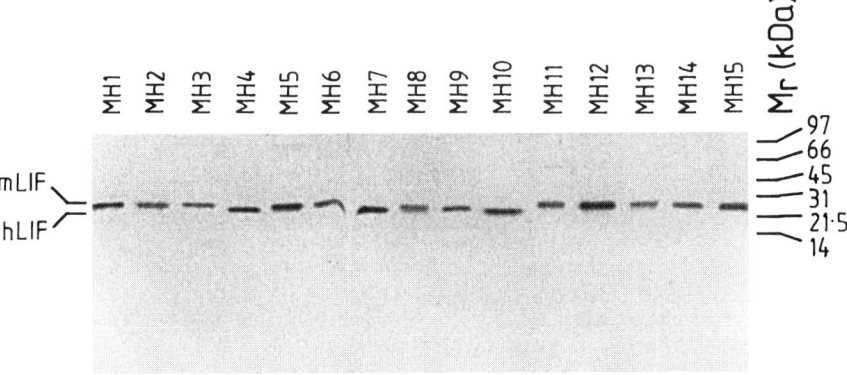

FIGURE 3. SDS polyacrylamide gel electrophoresis analysis of purified hybrid LIF proteins (MH1 to MH15). Approximately 50 ng of each protein was analyzed on a 15% polyacrylamide gel and silver-stained. The relative positions of the mouse LIF and human LIF protein bands are shown at the left of the gel. Low molecular weight (M_r) standards (BioRad) are indicated in kD. (From Owczarek et al.[25] Reproduced by permission of Oxford University Press.)

larly with ^{125}I-mLIF for binding to the mLIF-R α-chain and secondly, both mLIF and hLIF had similar abilities to induce the differentiation of mouse M1 cells into macrophages. All the chimeric molecules we constructed appeared to be folded correctly as they were essentially indistinguishable from both mLIF and hLIF in these two assays (FIG. 2).

In order to study the specific interactions between hLIF and the α-chain of its receptor, it was necessary to carry out experiments in the absence of other interacting molecules, such as the LIF-R affinity converter, gp130. As a source of the hLIF-R α-chain we expressed a plasmid encoding this protein and transfected it into a strain of COS cells that did not express detectable endogenous LIF-R or gp130. A naturally occurring, soluble form of the mLIF-R α-chain in normal mouse serum had identical binding characteristics to the membrane-bound form[23] and so was used as a source of mLIF-R α-chain.

FIGURE 2. Summary of data from biological assays and competitive binding assays of mLIF, hLIF and m-hLIF hybrid proteins. Mouse LIF sequence is represented by open boxes and human LIF sequence is represented by black boxes. The hybrid proteins are prefixed by "MH" to denote that they contain both mLIF and hLIF amino acid sequence, and their amino acid sequence specifications are listed in TABLE 1. The relative positions of the predicted α-helices, and connecting loops in the hybrid proteins can be determined by aligning the schematic representations with the diagram immediately below. The specific biological activity of each hybrid is calculated from its functional activity (ability to induce differentiation of mouse M1 myeloid leukemic cells into macrophages) per milligram of protein, as assessed by amino acid analysis. The % hLIF score is calculated from the 50% inhibitory dose (ID_{50}) for the inhibition of ^{125}I-hLIF binding to the mLIF-R α-chain by mLIF, hLIF and the m-hLIF hybrids. The ratio of the ID_{50} values for a hybrid over hLIF is calculated from the ID_{50} for the inhibition of ^{125}I-hLIF binding to the hLIF-R α-chain expressed on the surface of COS cells. Most assays were performed at least twice and the inter-assay standard deviation is shown.

The first two hybrid proteins that we constructed enabled us to quickly define which half of the hLIF molecule was involved in the unusual high-affinity interaction of hLIF with the mLIF-R α-chain. As a means of conveniently classifying each m-hLIF hybrid, we devised a means of scoring each hybrid according to how similar its activity was to hLIF. This %hLIF score was based on the concentration of mLIF, hLIF and each m-hLIF hybrid required to inhibit 50% of ^{125}I-hLIF binding to the mLIF-R α-chain (ID_{50}). The equation:

$$\% \text{ human LIF score} = \frac{\log \text{ID}_{50}(mLIF) - \log \text{ID}_{50}(hybrid)}{\log \text{ID}_{50}(mLIF) - \log \text{ID}_{50}(hLIF)} \times 100\%$$

was used to convert the ID_{50} of each hybrid into a %hLIF score. In this system, hLIF is defined as having a 100% hLIF score and mLIF as 0%. Hybrid MH1, where the amino-terminal half was composed of hLIF residues and the carboxy-terminal half was composed of mLIF residues had a %hLIF score of 23 ± 2%. This indicated that a small proportion of the residues involved in the enhanced interaction of hLIF with the mLIF-R α-chain must be located in the amino-terminal half of the hLIF polypeptide. However the reverse molecule, MH2, had a %hLIF score of 89 ± 11% (FIG. 2) implying that the carboxy-terminal half of hLIF contained the majority of these residues (FIG. 4B). Hybrid MH2 was also only 2.5-fold less efficient than hLIF at

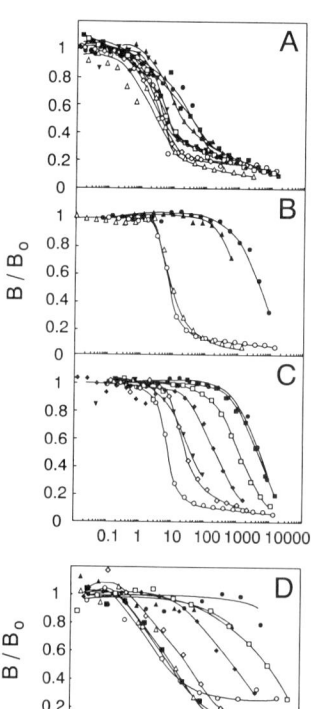

FIGURE 4. A: Competitive inhibition of ^{125}I-mLIF binding to soluble mLIF-R α-chain by mLIF, hLIF and a selection of m-hLIF hybrids. (●), mLIF; (○), hLIF; (▲), MH1; (△), MH2; (■), MH3; (□), MH4; (◆), MH5; (◇), MH6; (▼), MH14. Results for all competition assays were expressed as the number of counts bound to the receptor at a particular concentration of unlabeled competitor (B) divided by the number of counts bound to the receptor when no unlabeled competitor was present (B_0). **B:** Competitive inhibition of ^{125}I-hLIF binding to soluble mLIF-R α-chain by mLIF, hLIF and a selection of m-hLIF hybrids. (●), mLIF; (○), hLIF; (▲), MH1; (△), MH2. **C:** Competitive inhibition of ^{125}I-hLIF binding to soluble mLIF-R α-chain by mLIF, hLIF and a selection of m-hLIF hybrids. (●), mLIF; (○), hLIF; (■), MH3; (□), MH4; (◆), MH5; (◇), MH6; (▼), MH14. **D:** Competitive inhibition of ^{125}I-hLIF binding to COS cells transfected with the human LIF-R α-chain by mLIF, hLIF and a selection of m-hLIF hybrids. (●), mLIF; (○), hLIF; (▲), MH1; (△), MH2; (□), MH4; (◆), MH5; (◇), MH6; (■), MH14. (From Owczarek et al.[25] Reproduced by permission of Oxford University Press.)

FIGURE 5. Model of mLIF and hLIF binding to mouse and human LIF-R α-chains. A binding site is present on both the mLIF and hLIF ligands (a), for which there is a complementary site (A) on the mLIF-R α-chain only. A second site (b), which is present on the hLIF ligand only, and which is proposed to mediate both binding to the hLIF-R α-chain and the unusual high-affinity to the mLIF-R α-chain, interacts with a site (B) on both the mLIF-R α-chain and the hLIF-R α-chain. The site described in this study is the site on the hLIF ligand indicated by "b". (From Owczarek et al.[25] Reproduced by permission of Oxford University Press.)

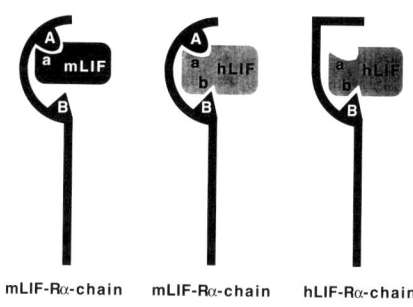

competing with ^{125}I-hLIF for binding to the hLIF-R α-chain, whilst hybrid MH1 competed only weakly (FIG. 4D).

A further series of hybrids, (MH3–MH6), in which sections of the carboxy-terminal half of the hLIF molecule were substituted into a mLIF framework were constructed (FIG. 2). Analysis of these hybrids revealed that the substitution of the predicted human D-helix did not increase the affinity of this hybrid for the mLIF-R α-chain compared to mLIF, although there were significant contributions to hLIF-like binding from the predicted C-D loop, the C-helix and also the short loop between the B and C helices (FIG. 2). The contributions from different regions appeared to be additive as combinations of these regions resulted in incremental increases in the %hLIF score (FIG. 2). These hybrids were also tested for their ability to compete with ^{125}I-hLIF for binding to the hLIF-R α-chain. Again, the competitive inhibition curves of these hybrids formed a range between the two extremes of mLIF and hLIF (FIG. 4D). Surprisingly, however, their increasing abilities to displace ^{125}I-hLIF from the hLIF-R α-chain correlated exactly with their increasing abilities to displace ^{125}I-hLIF from the mLIF-R α-chain. This unexpected observation indicated that the site that hLIF uses to bind to the hLIF-R α-chain is identical to the site that confers the unusual high-affinity binding of hLIF to the mLIF-R α-chain. An implication of this observation is that the binding of mLIF and hLIF to their isologous receptor α-chains is not through an equivalent site. However, mLIF and hLIF must share at least one receptor-binding determinant because they are also able to cross compete for binding to the mLIF-R α-chain. In the assay systems described in this study, which rely on exchange of nonconserved residues between mLIF and hLIF, this site, labeled "a" in FIGURE 5, would be undetectable. Mouse LIF is not able to bind with appreciable affinity to the hLIF-R α-chain, implying that hLIF contains a hLIF-R α-chain binding determinant that mLIF does not. Analyzing this series of m-hLIF hybrids in these two assay systems has led us to conclude that the site through which hLIF interacts with the hLIF-R α-chain, labeled "b" in FIGURE 5, is the same as that which mediates the enhanced binding of hLIF to the mLIF-R α-chain. This model is able to explain the inability of mLIF to bind to the hLIF-R α-chain as it has no site a, as well as providing a rationale for the extra interactions which cause hLIF to have a higher affinity for the mLIF-R α-chain compared to mLIF. However, it also implies that the site through which mLIF and hLIF bind to their isologous receptor α-chains has not been conserved throughout the evolution of the LIF polypeptide in different species.

Analysis of this initial series of hybrids indicated that the residues on hLIF which comprised a hLIF-R α-chain determinant were located in different regions of the primary amino sequence. Although the predominant contribution to hLIF-like activity was from residues located in the loop structure between the two carboxy-terminal α-helices, there were also significant contributions from the C-helix, the B-C loop and regions in the amino-terminus. We then proceeded to resolve the precise amino acid residues that constituted the proposed hLIF-R α-chain binding site on the hLIF molecule. A further series of hybrids was generated by site-directed mutagenesis (FIG. 2) in order to evaluate the contribution of amino acids in these regions to binding to both the hLIF-R α-chain and the enhanced binding to the mLIF-R α-chain. These hybrids were tested in both assays even though we had established that either assay could assess the contribution of the amino acid residues to hLIF-like binding. Assaying only the ability of a hybrid to displace ^{125}I-hLIF from the hLIF-R α-chain would not differentiate between a hybrid that was incorrectly folded or one that was behaving like mLIF. Because both assay systems were found to be most accurate in the middle of their range, site-directed mutants were based on a hybrid that already had an intermediate hLIF-like binding in both assays.

An example of this strategy is demonstrated in the elucidation of the critical binding residues in the predicted C-helix. Hybrids MH27 and MH28 were based on hybrid MH5, in which the C-D loop was composed of hLIF residues (53 ± 3% hLIF score),

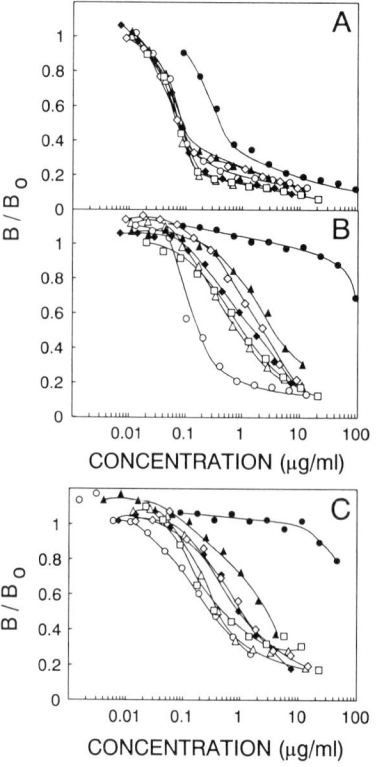

FIGURE 6. A: Competitive inhibition of ^{125}I-mLIF binding to soluble mLIF-R α-chain by (●), mLIF; (○), hLIF; (▲), MH5; (△), MH6; (◆) MH27; (◇), MH28; (□), MH14. **B:** Competitive inhibition of ^{125}I-hLIF binding to soluble mLIF-R α-chain by (●), mLIF; (○), hLIF; (▲), MH5; (△), MH6;, (◆) MH27; (◇), MH28; (□), MH14. **C:** Competitive inhibition of ^{125}I-hLIF binding to COS cells transfected with the human LIF-R α-chain by (●), mLIF; (○), hLIF; (▲), MH5; (△), MH6;, (◆) MH27; (◇), MH28; (□), MH14.

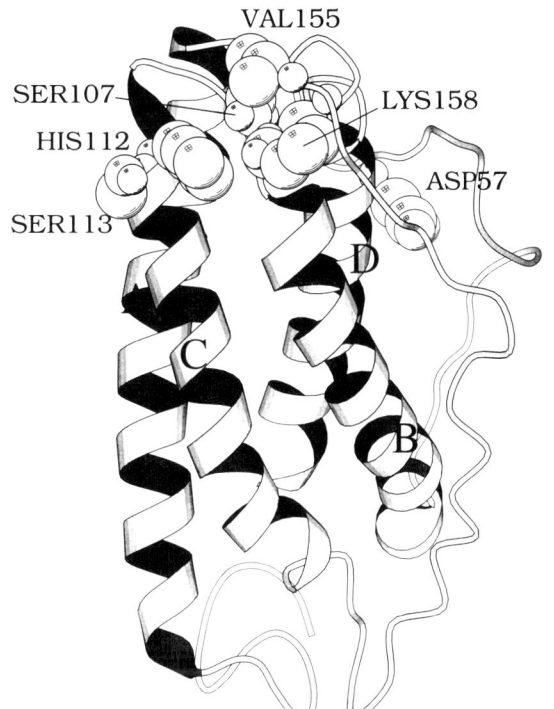

FIGURE 7. Diagram of the model of hLIF showing the polypeptide backbone. The predicted α-helices are designated A, B, C and D. Residues D57, S107, H112, S113, V155 and K158, which together make up the proposed hLIF-R α-chain binding site, are indicated. This figure was drawn using the program MOLSCRIPT[26] and is presented with the permission of D. Smith and H. Treutlein.

but also contained two additional mLIF to hLIF substitutions (Q112H and V113S respectively) in the C-helix. The presence of either hLIF amino acid substitution increased the %hLIF score, but neither alone were able to reconstitute the total contribution of the C-helix (FIG. 6B). Hybrid MH14 was also based on hybrid MH5 but had both substitutions (Q112H and V113S) and was able to increase the %hLIF score to that of hybrid MH6 in which both the C-helix and the C-D loop were made up entirely of hLIF residues (FIG. 6B). These chimeras were also tested for their ability to compete with ^{125}I-hLIF for binding to COS hLIF-R cells (FIG. 6C). Ranking this set of hybrids in the order of the concentration of each required for 50% inhibition of ^{125}I-hLIF binding to both the mLIF-R α-chain and COS hLIF-R cells again gave qualitatively the same results.

Using this systematic approach of site-directed mutagenesis we were able to identify a total of six amino acid residues in hLIF that made up the site through which it interacts with the hLIF-R α-chain. These six residues were Asp57 in the A-B loop, Ser107 in the B-C loop, His112 and Ser113 in the C-helix, and Val155 and Lys158 in the C-D loop. In order to visualize the relative positions of these residues on the hLIF molecule we utilized a three-dimensional model of hLIF which was derived by homology modeling using the known structure of a closely related cytokine, human G-CSF.[27] Translation of these six residues onto this model revealed that, although they were located in several discontinuous regions in the primary amino acid sequence, they formed a relatively contiguous cluster on the surface at one end of the predicted four α-helical bundle (FIG. 7). Hybrid proteins containing the substitutions V56L,

V103I and V109L gave equivocal results in the context of either assay so it was difficult to assign a definitive role to these in receptor binding. It is possible that they may represent additional, but minor, receptor-ligand interactions.

In order to ascertain whether these six residues on the hLIF molecule made up the entire hLIF-R α-chain binding site, and could perhaps also reconstitute the biological functions of hLIF, we constructed hybrid MH43, that was composed entirely of mLIF residues except that it had the six hLIF residues that we had determined were involved in the putative hLIF-R α-chain binding site. Hybrid MH43 had a similar specific biological activity to both mLIF and hLIF when tested for induction of differentiation of mouse M1 cells into macrophages (FIG. 8D), and competed with ^{125}I-mLIF for binding to the mLIF-R α-chain to a similar extent to both mLIF and hLIF (FIG. 8A). This indicated that substituting these six hLIF residues did not disrupt the normal secondary and tertiary structure of the polypeptide. The presence

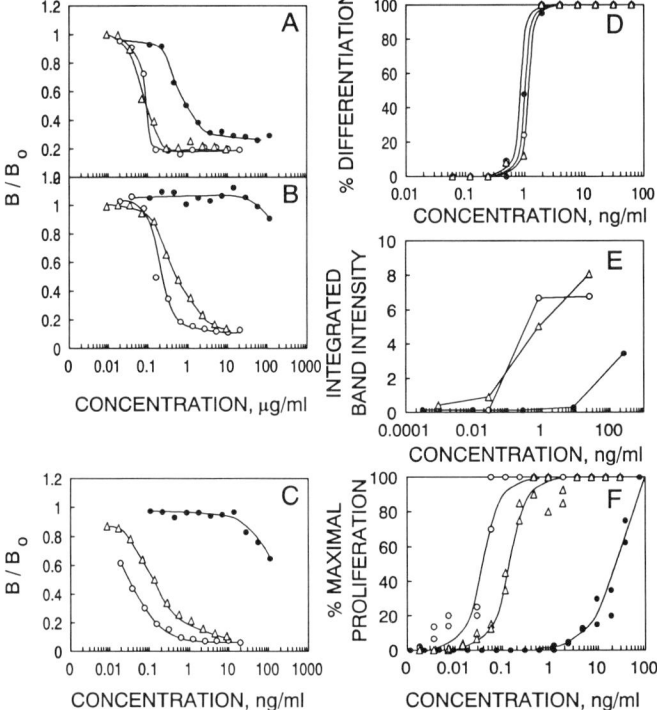

FIGURE 8. A: Competitive inhibition of ^{125}I-mLIF binding to soluble mLIF-R α-chain by (●) mLIF, (○) hLIF and (△) MH43. **B:** Competitive inhibition of ^{125}I-hLIF binding to MLIF-R α-chain by (●) mLIF, (○) hLIF and (△) MH43. **C:** Competitive inhibition of ^{125}I-hLIF binding to COS cells transfected with the hLIF-R α-chain by (●) mLIF, (○) hLIF and (△) MH43. **D:** Differentiation-inducing activity of mouse M1 cells into macrophages by (●) mLIF, (○) hLIF and (△) MH43. **E:** Detection by Western blot analysis of haptoglobin secreted by the human hepatoma cell line HepG2 in response to stimulation with (●) mLIF, (○) hLIF and (△) MH43. **F:** Proliferation of BaF/3 cells expressing the human LIF-R α-chain and mouse gp130 in response to stimulation with (●) mLIF, (○) hLIF and (△) MH43.

of these six hLIF residues on a mLIF framework resulted in a 2000-fold increase in the ability of MH43 to compete with ^{125}I-hLIF for binding to the mLIF-R α-chain compared to mLIF (FIG. 8B) giving it a %hLIF score of 87 ± 3% (FIG. 2). Hybrid MH43 was also only 2.5-fold less efficient than hLIF at competing for ^{125}I-hLIF for binding to the hLIF-R α-chain (FIG. 8C). Thus, by changing only 3% of the total amino acid residues in mLIF to the equivalent hLIF residues, to give hybrid MH43, we were able to reconstitute the binding activities that are specific to hLIF.

We also tested MH43 to see if it had gained the biological activities specific to hLIF. Because mLIF does not bind appreciably to the hLIF-R α-chain, it cannot normally activate a hLIF-R. Biological assays on human cells are therefore specific for hLIF, unlike assays on mouse cells, which respond to both mLIF and hLIF. LIF is one of a number of cytokines, including IL-6, which can induce the production of acute phase proteins in the liver. Human LIF is able to stimulate the production of haptoglobin (measured by Western analysis using an anti-haptoglobin antibody) in the human hepatoma cell line HepG2 with a 50% stimulatory dose of 150 pg/ml, while mLIF is only able to stimulate these cells at a 2000-fold higher concentration. Hybrid MH43 was able to stimulate the production of haptoglobin at a similar concentration to hLIF (FIG. 8E). BaF/3 cells are a mouse pro-B lymphocyte cell line which normally do not express either LIF receptor α-chains or gp130. LIF is able to stimulate the proliferation of BaF/3 cells that have been stably transfected with the hLIF-R α-chain and mouse gp130. Mouse LIF can stimulate proliferation of these cells, but the concentration of mLIF required is at least 600-fold higher compared to hLIF. The 50% stimulatory dose of hybrid MH43 required to induce the proliferation of the transfected BaF/3 cells was 2- to 3-fold higher than that of hLIF and 250-fold lower than that of mLIF (FIG. 8F). We have thus created a derivative of mouse LIF with biological activities that are strikingly similar to those that are elicited by human LIF.

This study has clearly defined six amino acid residues that specify the site through which hLIF interacts with the hLIF-R α-chain and thus contribute most of the binding energy required for this interaction to occur. This interaction alone does not activate the hLIF-R, so further interactions of both hLIF and the hLIF-R α-chain with human gp130 must be required for signal transduction. However, the ability of MH43 to both bind to, and activate the hLIF-R demonstrates that we have defined the majority of the residues essential for this first step in signal transduction. The most complete paradigm of a ligand-receptor interaction within the hemopoietic family of receptors is the x-ray crystallographic structure of human growth hormone (hGH) in complex with its receptor.[12] Human GH binds to one subunit of its receptor via site 1, which comprises 24 amino acid residues. A second receptor subunit subsequently interacts with both hGH and the first receptor. The site 1 hGH receptor binding site defined by mutagenesis studies[24] was much less extensive than that defined by the co-crystal structure of the hGH/hGH-R complex, indicating that not all of the contact residues in the binding surface contributed a significant amount of the actual binding energy. The six residues on hLIF that we have defined in this study are likely to constitute most of the binding energy to the hLIF-R α-chain but undoubtedly, other contact sites exist. Many analogies with hGH site 1 interactions have been made for other hemopoietic growth factors but the binding site for hLIF to the hLIF-R α-chain defined in this study appears to be somewhat different. The hGH molecule presents a helical face to the first subunit of the hGH receptor, which is presumably a relatively rigid structure, while the binding site on the hLIF molecule for the hLIF-R α-chain is largely located on flexible loop regions. This would suggest that although two molecules possess a similar tertiary structural scaffold they may not necessarily utilize the same receptor binding motifs. The role of flexibility of a molecule in intermolecular interactions has not yet been well studied as these regions are difficult to resolve in protein structures derived either by x-ray crystallography or NMR. In the model of hLIF Asp57 appears to be quite distant from the cluster of residues Ser107, His112, Ser113, Val155, and Lys158. Visualization of the actual proximity of the six residues when the crystal structure of LIF, and indeed the crystal structure of the LIF/LIF receptor complex, is solved may give some insight into whether conformational changes in the loop regions of hLIF occur on the binding of this ligand to its cognate receptor α-chain.

MATERIALS AND METHODS

All the experimental procedures used in this study are described in more detail elsewhere.[25,28]

ACKNOWLEDGMENTS

We thank D. Smith and H. Treutlein for the model of hLIF, D. Hilton for the transfected BaF/3 cell line, L. Murray and D. Hilton for advice on the HepG2 assay, S. Mifsud and L. DiRago for assistance with the M1 colony assays, R. Simpson, J. Eddes and J.-G. Zhang for assistance with the amino acid analysis, and S. Rakar for technical assistance.

[Note Added in Proof: The x-ray crystallographic structure of murine LIF has recently been solved (Robinson, R.C., L. M. Grey, D. Staunton, H. Vankelecom, A. B. Vernallis, J.-F. Moreau, D. I. Stuart, J. K. Heath, & E. Y. Jones. 1994. The crystal structure and biological function of leukemia inhibitory factor: Implications for receptor binding. Cell **77**: 1101–16). There are some differences between this structure of mLIF and the model of hLIF presented in this paper. However, the mLIF amino acid residues in the equivalent positions to the residues on hLIF that have been defined by the mutagenesis studies described in this paper as comprising the hLIF-R α-chain binding site are all exposed at the surface of the mouse LIF molecule, and form a continuous interaction surface at one end of the 4 α-helical bundle structure.]

REFERENCES

1. METCALF, D. 1991. The leukemia inhibitory factor (LIF). Int. J. Cell Cloning **9**: 95–108.
2. ROSE, T. M. & A. G. BRUCE. 1991. Oncostatin M is a member of a cytokine family that includes leukemia-inhibitory factor, granulocyte colony-stimulating factor, and interleukin 6. Proc. Natl. Acad. Sci. USA **88**: 8641–8645.
3. GEARING, D. P., C. J. THUT, T. VANDEBOS, S. D. GIMPEL, P. B. DELANEY, J. KING, V. PRICE, D. COSMAN & M. P. BECKMANN. 1991. Leukemia inhibitory factor receptor is structurally related to the IL-6 signal transducer, gp130. EMBO J. **10**: 2839–2848.
4. GEARING, D. P., M. R. COMEAU, D. J. FRIEND, S. D. GIMPEL, C. J. THUT, J. MCGOURTY, K. K. BRASHER, J. A. KING, S. GILLIS, B. MOSLEY, S. F. ZIEGLER & D. COSMAN. 1992. The IL-6 signal transducer, gp130: An oncostatin M receptor and affinity converter for the LIF receptor. Science **255**: 1434–1437.

5. COSMAN, D., S. D. LYMAN, R. L. IDZERDA, M. P. BECKMANN, L. S. PARK, R. G. GOODWIN & C. J. MARCH. 1990. A new cytokine receptor superfamily. Trends Biochem. Sci. **15:** 265–270.
6. GOUGH, N. M., D. P. GEARING, J. A. KING, T. A. WILLSON, D. J. HILTON, N. A. NICOLA & D. METCALF. 1988. Molecular cloning and expression of the human homologue of the murine gene encoding myeloid leukemia-inhibitory factor. Proc. Natl. Acad. Sci. USA **85:** 2623–2627.
7. LAYTON, M. J., P. LOCK, D. METCALF & N. A. NICOLA. 1994. Cross-species Receptor Binding Characteristics of Human and Mouse Leukemia Inhibitory Factor Suggest a Complex Binding Interaction. J. Biol. Chem. **269:** 17048–17055.
8. BAZAN, J. F. 1990. Haemopoietic receptors and helical cytokines. Immunol. Today **11:** 350–354.
9. HILL, C. P., T. D. OSSLUND & D. EISENBERG. 1993. The structure of granulocyte-colony-stimulating factor and its relationship to other growth factors. Proc. Natl. Acad. Sci. USA **90:** 5167–5171.
10. DIEDERICHS, K., T. BOONE & P. A. KARPLUS. 1991. Novel fold and putative receptor binding site of granulocyte-macrophage colony-stimulating factor. Science **254:** 1779–1782.
11. ABDEL-MEGUID, S. S., H. S. SHIEH, W. W. SMITH, H. E. DAYRINGER, B. N. VIOLAND & L. A. BENTLE. 1987. Three-dimensional structure of a genetically engineered variant of porcine growth hormone. Proc. Natl. Acad. Sci. USA **84:** 6434–6437.
12. DE VOS, A. M., M. ULTSCH & A. A. KOSSIAKOFF. 1992. Human growth hormone and extracellular domain of its receptor: Crystal structure of the complex. Science **255:** 306–312.
13. BRANDHUBER, B. J., T. BOONE, W. C. KENNEY & D. B. MCKAY. 1987. Crystals and a low resolution structure of interleukin-2. J. Biol. Chem. **262:** 12306–12308.
14. BAZAN, J. F. 1992. Unraveling the structure of IL-2. Science **257:** 410–413.
15. POWERS, R., D. S. GARRETT, C. J. MARCH, E. A. FRIEDEN, A. M. GRONENBORN & G. M. CLORE. 1992. Three-dimensional solution structure of human interleukin-4 by multidimensional heteronuclear magnetic resonance spectroscopy. Science **256:** 1673–1677.
16. MILBURN, M. V., A. M. HASSELL, M. H. LAMBERT, S. R. JORDAN, A. E. PROUDFOOT, P. GRABER & T. N. WELLS. 1993. A novel dimer configuration revealed by the crystal structure at 2.4 Å resolution of human interleukin-5. Nature **363:** 172–176.
17. BAZAN, J. F. 1991. Neuropoietic cytokines in the hematopoietic fold. Neuron **7:** 197–208.
18. SMITH, D. B. & K. S. JOHNSON. 1988. Single-step purification of polypeptides expressed in *Escherichia coli* as fusions with glutathione S-transferase. Gene **67:** 31–40.
19. GEARING, D. P., N. A. NICOLA, D. METCALF, S. FOOTE, T. A. WILLSON, N. M. GOUGH & L. WILLIAMS. 1989. Production of leukemia inhibitory factor in *Escherichia coli* by a novel procedure and its use in maintaining embryonic stem cells in culture. BioTechnology **7:** 1157–1161.
20. SIMPSON, R. J., R. L. MORITZ, E. C. NICE, B. GREGO, F. YOSHIZAKI, Y. SUGIMURA, H. C. FREEMAN & M. MURATA. 1986. Complete amino acid sequence of plastocyanin from a green alga, *Enteromorpha prolifera*. Eur. J. Biochem. **157:** 497–506.
21. BUTCHER, L. A. & J. K. TOMKINS. 1985. Anal. Biochem. **148:** 384–388.
22. LAEMMLI, U. K. 1970. Nature (London) **227:** 680–685.
23. LAYTON, M. J., B. A. CROSS, D. METCALF, L. D. WARD, R. J. SIMPSON & N. A. NICOLA. 1992. A major binding protein for leukemia inhibitory factor in normal mouse serum: Identification as a soluble form of the cellular receptor. Proc. Natl. Acad. Sci. USA **89:** 8616–8620.
24. CUNNINGHAM, B. C., P. JHURANI, P. NG & J. A. WELLS. 1989. Receptor and antibody epitopes in human growth hormone identified by homolog-scanning mutagenesis. Science **243:** 1330–1336.
25. OWCZAREK, C. M., M. J. LAYTON, D. METCALF, P. LOCK, T. A. WILLSON, N. M. GOUGH & N. A. NICOLA. 1993. Inter-species chimaeras of leukaemia inhibitory factor define a major human receptor binding determinant. EMBO J. **12:** 3487–3495.
26. KRAULIS, P. J. 1991. Molscript: A program to produce both detailed and schematic plots of protein structure. J. Appl. Cryst. **24:** 946–950.

27. D. K. SMITH, H. R. TREUTLEIN, T. MAURER, C. M. OWCZAREK, M. J. LAYTON, N. A. NICOLA & R. S. NORTON. 1994. Homology modelling and 1H NMR studies of human leukaemia inhibitory factor. FEBS Lett. **350:** 275–280.
28. LAYTON, M. J., C. M. OWCZAREK, D. METCALF, R. L. CLARK, D. K. SMITH, H. R. TREUTLEIN & N. A. NICOLA. 1994. Conversion of the biological specificity of murine to human leukemia inhibitory factor by replacing 6 amino acid residues. J. Biol. Chem. **269:** 29891–29896.

DISCUSSION OF THE PAPER

G. CILIBERTO (*Istituto Ricerche di Biologia Molecolare, Pomezia, Italy*): In your model you propose the existence of two sites in the mouse receptor for the binding to the human LIF site A and site B. Considering that the LIF receptor has two cytokine binding domains, do you know whether the two sites are located in the two different cytokine binding domains? Have you analyzed these sections of the receptor?

C. M. OWCZAREK: It is very tempting to speculate that site A or site B could be located in separate domains, and we are carrying out experiments to test this. We know from work on IL-3 common receptor, the common β chain, that only one of the hematopoietin domains is involved in receptor binding. As yet we really have no evidence to show whether it is site A or site B or both.

G. FEY (*University of Erlangen-Nürnberg, Erlangen, Germany*): Could you come back please to the last slide where you explained that mouse LIF was less efficient in stimulating acute response than human LIF. In describing this you had an explanation and I missed that. Could you say again what the explanation was?

OWCZAREK: I think that at very high concentrations mouse LIF can actually stimulate the human LIF receptor. It seems that this site A and site B hypothesis is not an all or nothing effect and that there must be some kind of residual effect when mouse LIF binds. And we have found that if you have a human LIF receptor α chain with a mouse gp130, mouse LIF can actually compete quite well. So there must be some limited species specificity with gp130 and at high concentrations of mLIF the interaction is stabilized.

H. BAUMANN (*Roswell Park Cancer Institute, Buffalo, NY*): I can actually tell you a little bit more, because we tested the mouse LIF produced by Genentech and in this particular experiment there was no difference in response between mouse and human LIF. The dose-response was the same. We have used yeast LIF, you have used bacterial LIF. We have tested Metcalf's LIF as well, which turned out to be of very low activity compared to the yeast material. I do not know whether that makes a difference. But that was our major concern too.

OWCZAREK: In the beginning we got everything turned on and then we realized that we were just overloading the system and then we titrated right down. Once we did a titration on the low end we could actually see this difference. But at first everything was stimulating everything.

BAUMANN: Yes, but I can assure you that we did a titration as well.

The Crystal Structure of Murine Leukemia Inhibitory Factor[a]

R. C. ROBINSON,[b,e] L. M. GREY,[c] D. STAUNTON,[c]
D. I. STUART,[b,d] J. K. HEATH,[c] AND E. Y. JONES[b,d]

[b]Laboratory of Molecular Biophysics
[c]CRC Growth Factor Group
[d]Oxford Centre for Molecular Sciences
Department of Biochemistry
University of Oxford
South Parks Road
Oxford OX1 3QU United Kingdom

INTRODUCTION

The history of the structural analysis of leukemia inhibitory factor (LIF) originates from the X-ray structure of porcine growth hormone[1] and the subsequent realization[2] that several other cytokines including LIF were likely to have a similar four helix bundle topology. The up-up-down-down topological arrangement of the helices is unique to these cytokines, of which several have now been demonstrated to conform to this prediction. Currently, there are nine examples of structures based on this cytokine four helix bundle topology. Five are standard four helix bundles—granulocyte macrophage colony stimulating factor (GMCSF),[3,4] interleukin 2 (IL-2)[5] and interleukin 4 (IL-4),[6–9] growth hormone,[1,10] and granulocyte colony stimulating factor (GCSF)[11]; three are dimeric molecules—macrophage colony stimulating factor (MCSF),[12] interleukin 5 (IL-5),[13] interferon γ (IFN-γ)[14,15]; and one is a five helix bundle interferon β (IFN-β).[16]

In Bazan's original analysis,[2] based on sequence comparisons, genetic organization and biological activity, LIF was grouped in a subfamily with two other cytokines: ciliary neurotrophic factor (CNTF) and oncostatin M (OSM). The significance of this classification only became apparent after the functional receptors for these molecules were identified. The biological effects of LIF are mediated by interaction ($K_d \sim 10^{-9}$ M) between the ligand and a specific LIF receptor subunit (LIF-R)[17] which is a member of the "cytokine-binding" family of receptor subunits (reviewed in refs. 18 and 19) characterized by a conserved pattern of cysteine residues and a WSXWS amino acid motif. Formation of a high affinity signaling complex ($K_d \sim 10^{-11}$ M) requires the association of the LIF/LIF-R complex with another transmembrane signal transducing molecule gp130[20,21] which itself exhibits features of the cytokine family of receptors.[22] OSM is capable of generating a biological response with the identical two receptor components LIF-R and gp130.[21,23–25] CNTF shows a more complex

---

[a] The CRC Growth Factor Group is Supported by the Cancer Research Campaign. The Oxford Centre for Molecular Sciences is supported by the SERC and MRC. EYJ is supported by a Royal Society University Research Fellowship, RCR by a MRC research studentship and LG by a CRC studentship.

[e] Author for correspondence; Tel: 0865-275397; Fax: 0865-275182.

involvement of gp130 and LIF-R in ligand-mediated signaling, utilizing a third receptor component CNTF-receptor (CNTF-R)[26,27] which acts as a specificity conferring element. Interleukin 6 (IL-6), however, which lies outside the immediate LIF subgroup, interacts with the IL-6 receptor subunit (IL-6R)[28,29] in conjunction with two molecules of gp130. Hence, LIF, OSM and CNTF are capable of binding uniquely to LIF-R as well as gp130. Such a correlation between sequence similarity and receptor binding suggests that there may be a conserved pattern of amino acids which is either directly involved in binding the LIF-R/gp130 receptor complex or responsible for maintaining a particular structural element which is important in receptor binding. The overlap in the use of receptor subunits correlates with shared biological activities between LIF and OSM,[30] CNTF[31] and IL-6.[32]

Extensive structural and functional analyses of the interaction between growth hormone and its receptor[10,33] have revealed the structural organization of the functional growth hormone ligand/receptor complex in which a single molecule of ligand is complexed to two molecules of receptor. Receptor subunit homodimerization, and consequent signaling, is brought about by the sequential interaction of two physically distinct sites on the ligand with essentially similar binding sites on each receptor subunit. The structure of the growth hormone ligand/receptor complex provides a model with which to interpret structural data for the other four helix bundle cytokine receptor complexes, in a similar way to that in which the structure of growth hormone successfully provided a model for cytokine structure. We discuss here the extension of structure/function analysis to a heterodimeric cytokine receptor system.

EXPERIMENTAL PROCEDURES

The methods of expression, purification and structure determination of LIF have been described.[34] In short, murine LIF was expressed as a fusion protein with glutathione S-transferase in *E. coli*. The fusion protein was purified on a glutathione affinity column, from which recombinant LIF was cleaved with human thrombin. This form of LIF contained one extra amino acid, glycine at the N-terminus, resulting from the engineered cleavage site in the fusion protein, and was shown to be fully active in biological assays. A final purification step of cation exchange chromatography produced material of a suitable standard for crystallization trials.

Small needle-like clusters of crystals were grown from 40% PEG 8000, 5 mM MES pH 6.0. Macroseeding reduced nucleation and allowed growth of crystals of a sufficient size for diffraction studies (0.1 × 0.1 × 1.0 mm). The crystals are of the space group $P2_12_12_1$ and a native data set to 2 Å was collected in-house using a MAR Research imaging plate and a Rigaku RU200 rotating anode X-ray generator. Multiple isomorphous replacement was the method chosen to estimate the phases. In total five heavy atom derivatives were required $K_2Pt(NO_2)_4$, $AgNO_3$, tetrakis(acetoxymercuri)·methane, mercury acetaldehyde and K_2HgI_4, probably because four out of the five derivatives share the same major site. Phase improvement by solvent flattening[35] produced an interpretable electron density map.

A putative mainchain trace in agreement with the up-up-down-down topology of growth hormone was established after electron density for 2 long loops, one of which included a short fifth helix, was identified. This trace was confirmed by the identification of electron density for the three disulfide bridges. A polyalanine model was fitted to the electron density map and, based on a tentative sequence alignment, a full model for LIF was built and refined. Further refinement and rebuilding to $2 \mid F_o \mid - \mid F_c \mid$ maps calculated with model phases at 2.0 Å resolution yielded the current model for LIF.

RESULTS

The current model of the structure of murine LIF is shown in FIGURE 1. The R value on all the data 20.0–2.0 Å including a bulk solvent correction is 18.6% with stereochemistry typified by root mean square deviations from ideal bond lengths of 0.015 Å and by root mean square deviations from ideal bond angles of 1.48°. There are no non-glycine residues in the disallowed region of the Ramachandran plot and 40 ordered waters have been added. The values of atomic temperature factors rise rapidly for the N-terminal region preceding Asn-21 in the crystal structure of LIF. The electron density continue to give a clear indication of mainchain and sidechain positions between residues Asn-9 and Asn-21, but for the region before Asn-9 the density becomes poor and the temperature factors for the mainchain atoms exceed 60 Å^2. Residues 1–8 plus the N-terminal glycine of this 181 residue form of LIF are therefore omitted from the model. Low resolution model and MIR phase combined maps do however provide some indication that the course of the N-terminal region continues away from the bulk of the molecule into a region of solvent.

A detailed description of the structure has been reported[34]; we recapitulate here the principal features. LIF is a compact molecule with overall dimensions of approximately 22 Å × 28 Å × 46 Å. As had been predicted,[2] the LIF structure conforms to the up-up-down-down four helix bundle topology common to the hematopoietic growth factors (FIG. 2). The structure thus comprises 4 main α-helices conventionally labeled A, B, C and D, linked by two long loops (AB and CD) and one short loop (BC). This topological motif may be considered in terms of two pairs of antiparallel α-helices B:C and A:D. The B and C helices (29 and 27 residues respectively), are relatively straight and pack in a classic antiparallel manner, tilted to cross approximately half way down their length. The A helix (27 residues) and the shorter D helix (23 residues with an additional 3 C-terminal residues which depart from the classic hydro-

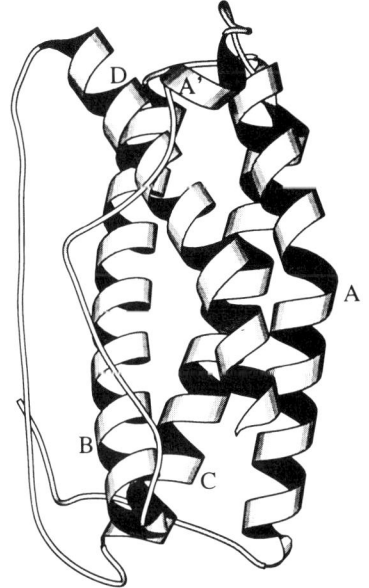

FIGURE 1. A schematic diagram of the structure of LIF. The figure was produced using the program MOLSCRIPT.[41]

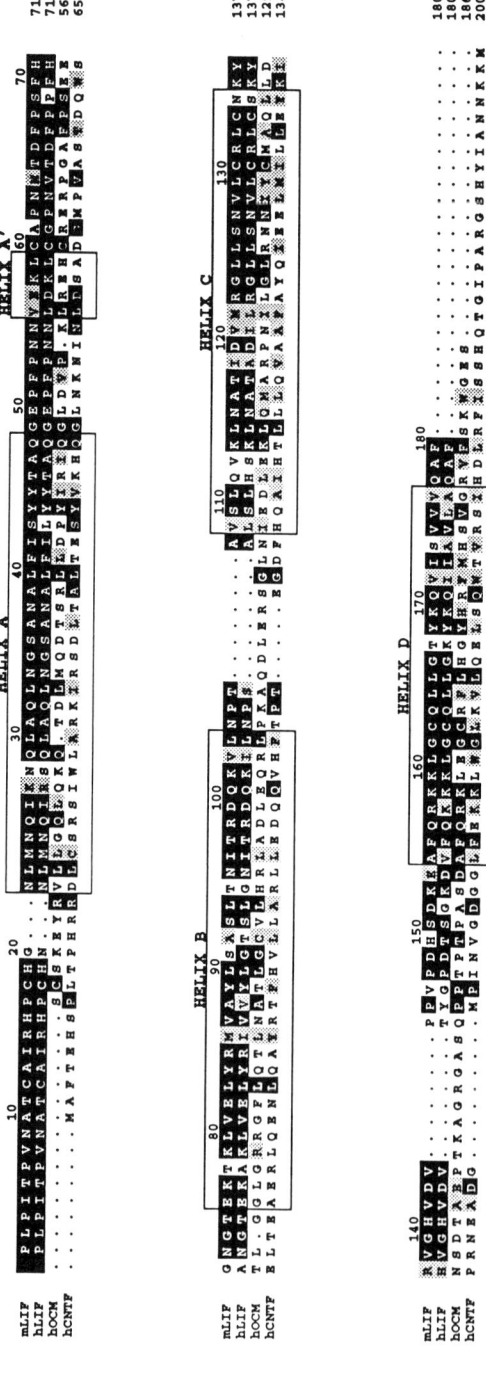

FIGURE 2. Sequence alignments for human and murine LIF, human OSM and human CNTF based on structural considerations. Conserved residues are painted black and conservative substitutions are shown in grey. Large open boxes represent the positions of the helices in murine LIF, and the residue numbers refer to the murine LIF sequence. The figure was prepared using the program ALSCRIPT—G. J. Barton, Laboratory of Biophysics, Oxford.

gen bonding pattern) exhibit pronounced kinks (most notably in helix A) which serve to maximize the region of close packed, solvent inaccessible core formed on addition of this antiparallel α-helix pair to the B:C pair to form the central four helix bundle. These kinks require breaks in the normal α-helix hydrogen bonding pattern, substitute hydrogen bonds are made to the polar sidechains of serines (Ser-36 in helix A and Ser-174 in helix D) and tightly bound water molecules (FIG. 1). The compact core is composed predominantly of hydrophobic residues contributed by the four α-helices. However, prior to helix A, between Asn-9 and Leu-22, the N-terminal region is wrapped around the molecule; the long loops AB (the first part of which contains a fifth short α-helix A') and CD are similarly tightly packed against the four helix bundle. Thus these three regions also contribute to the molecular core. The N-terminal region is pinned to the four helix bundle at the bottom of helix C by two disulfide bridges (Cys-12 to Cys-134 and Cys-18 to Cys-131). Similarly the third disulfide bridge (Cys-60 to Cys-163) tethers the first part of the AB loop to the top of helix D. This disulfide bonding pattern confirms that reported by Nicola et al.[36] The compact nature of the molecule is further emphasized on inspection of crystallographic temperature factors. These indicate no regions of high conformational mobility apart from the N-terminal region prior to Asn-21.

DISCUSSION

Structural comparisons of the LIF structure with the other long chain helical cytokines, growth hormone[10] and GCSF,[11] reveal that the lengths of the four helices and their relative positions are, to a first approximation, conserved between these three molecules—as are the conformations and positions of major portions of the long AB and CD loops. However, detailed comparisons of the structures indicate several basic points of variation. The N-terminal region in LIF, prior to helix A, follows a unique path wrapping around the base of the four helix bundle. The major variation in the four helices occurs in helix A which exhibits a distinctive kink in LIF which is thus far unique to this helical cytokine. The first part of the AB loop in all three structures contains a short helical region and the C-terminal half of this loop superimposes well between LIF and GCSF; however, this loop is markedly shorter in LIF and this is manifested in the acute angle at which the first half of the loop crosses in front of the D helix. The AB loop in LIF overlays the surface of the D helix at a point approximately one third of the way down its length rather than at its N-terminus as in growth hormone. Thus the major distinctive features of the LIF structure in comparison to GCSF and growth hormone are the N-terminal region, the kink in helix A and the position of the AB loop on crossing helix D.

FIGURE 2 includes a sequence alignment between human and murine LIF. The positions of the α-helices and the degree of residue solvent accessibility are indicated based on the murine LIF structure. The two sequences differ for 39 residues with no insertions or deletions. Of these differences none seem likely to perturb the structure greatly. The majority of the changes are at solvent exposed residues which are distributed evenly over the surface of the molecule and cannot, taken in isolation, indicate the structural basis of the species specificity which is observed for biding to human LIF-R.[34,36] The LIF structure is the first to be determined for a member of the LIF-R binding subgroup, which also includes CNTF and OSM. A revised sequence alignment[34] for LIF, OSM and CNTF, based on conservation of major structural features, is also presented in FIGURE 2. Clearly, for this level of sequence identity structural variations may occur between the molecules at several points. However, the alignment does show strong conservation of key structural residues along the lengths of all four helices, most notably in helix D, which supports the assumption of structural equivalence for residues in these regions. Given the location of the four main helices in the sequences gross comparisons may also be made with respect to the rest of the LIF structure. Thus relative to LIF the N-terminal region is truncated and the C-terminal region is extended for OSM. The AB loop in LIF and OSM is tethered by a disulfide bridge to the equivalent point on helix D. The BC loop is lengthened in OSM and, to a lesser extent, in CNTF. Several of the distinguishing features of the structure of LIF in comparison to growth hormone and GCSF are likely to be conserved in the structures of OSM and CNTF. Residue Ser-36, which mediates the kink in the A helix by hydrogen bonding back to the mainchain, is conservatively substituted to Asp in OSM and CNTF suggesting that this kink may be a common feature among these molecules. Similarly, the position at which the AB loop crosses the D helix and the N-terminal region wrapping around the A helix are fixed, at least in the case of OSM, by disulfide bonds. The nature of several exposed residues at the N-terminal end of helix D (Phe-156, Arg-158, Lys-159) is conserved. Finally, the kink in the D helix may also be a conserved feature to maximize the packing of this helix against the rest of the molecule.

Mutagenesis studies that have exploited the disparity in binding affinity of human and murine LIF for human LIF-R[34,36] have identified regions on LIF implicated in LIF-R binding. The work of Owczarek et al.[37] suggests that residues in the region of 130–160 and 103–130 are responsible for LIF-R binding. These residues (130–160) map to the CD loop and N-terminal end of the D-helix, before the point at which the AB loop crosses. The secondary region of residues (103–130) cluster around the short BC loop. The work of Robinson et al.[34] confirms the first region of interaction implicating a narrower range of residues 150–160, which map to the C-terminal end of the CD loop and the N-terminal end of the D helix. Furthermore, this study finds a LIF-R binding element within amino acids 161–180 which lie at the C-terminal end of the D helix at and beyond the region at which the AB loop crosses this helix. The data also provide indirect evidence that there is some contribution from the N-terminal half of the molecule, most probably from the AB loop. Not surprisingly some of the solvent accessible residues which are better conserved in the LIF subfamily fall into these regions of LIF-R binding specificity.

To understand this mutagenesis data in terms of the growth hormone ligand/receptor model we have overlaid the LIF structure onto that of growth hormone in the ligand/receptor complex (FIG. 3a). Receptor subunit I would be capable of interacting with region 161–180 in this arrangement, but the activity of regions 150–160 and 103–130 are not accounted for by this model. LIF-R, however, is unusual in having two "cytokine-binding" domains,[17] and we propose that the N-terminal of these domains, the one furthest from the cell membrane, can wrap around the molecule to interact with the N-terminal region of the D helix, the C-terminal end of the CD loop and the short BC loop (FIG. 3b). Such an arrangement for LIF-R binding to LIF relies heavily on the unique position at which the AB loop crosses the D helix. Firstly, this AB loop can not obscure the binding sites on this helix, and secondly, the positioning of this loop must be such as to allow LIF-R to interact with both C and N-terminal ends of the D helix. Clearly, molecules of the structure of growth hormone and GCSF, in which the AB loop crosses the N-terminal end of the D helix, would not be compatible with this model.

Receptor subunit II would hence correspond to gp130 in this model (FIG. 3), although as yet there are no data on which amino acids on LIF bind to this molecule. Mutagenesis data are however available for IL6 binding to gp130.[38] The binding arrangement appears to mimic that in the growth hormone model, where a molecule

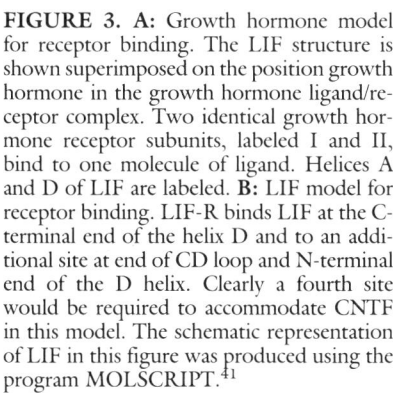
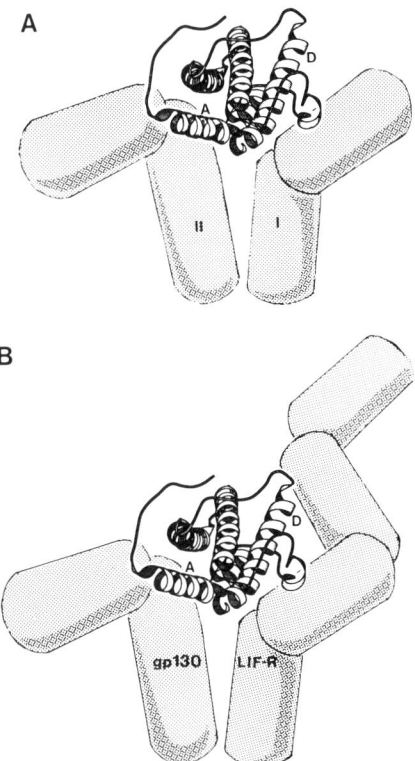

FIGURE 3. A: Growth hormone model for receptor binding. The LIF structure is shown superimposed on the position growth hormone in the growth hormone ligand/receptor complex. Two identical growth hormone receptor subunits, labeled I and II, bind to one molecule of ligand. Helices A and D of LIF are labeled. **B:** LIF model for receptor binding. LIF-R binds LIF at the C-terminal end of the helix D and to an additional site at end of CD loop and N-terminal end of the D helix. Clearly a fourth site would be required to accommodate CNTF in this model. The schematic representation of LIF in this figure was produced using the program MOLSCRIPT.[41]

of gp130 binds at both receptor sites I and II (FIG. 3). Hence, by analogy it is not unreasonable to suggest that receptor subunit II may indeed correspond to gp130 in the LIF ligand/receptor model (FIG. 3). The position of gp130 in the model is centered at the kink in the A helix, a feature likely to be conserved in OSM and CNTF, which may be important in binding this receptor component.

The IL-6-Rα binding to IL6 has also been probed by mutagenesis experiments.[39] Regions 39–96 and 134–184 on IL6, which correspond to the AB loop–B helix and to the CD loop–D helix, respectively, when mapped onto the structure of GCSF[2,11] have been shown to be involved in binding IL6-R. As the C-terminal portion of the D helix has also been shown to bind to gp130 the remaining portion of this second region, as well as the AB loop, appears to have some similarity to the regions implicated in binding the N-terminal LIF-R "cytokine-binding" domain in the LIF ligand/receptor model. It may therefore be instructive to consider LIF-R to be equivalent to a combination of gp130 and IL6-R.

CNTF binds to a third receptor subunit CNTF-R which is not accounted for by the model (FIG. 3b). Mutagenesis experiments on CNTF have identified one residue that is implicated in binding CNTF-R. This residue 63-Gln is equivalent to residue 69-Ser in LIF (FIG. 2) located in the C-terminal end of the AB loop a region not suggested, in the model (FIG. 3a), to bind to gp130 or to LIF-R.

The model (FIG. 3b) for LIF-R and gp130 binding to LIF, OSM and CNTF, clearly needs to be tested by further mutagenesis and structural studies. One anomaly, however, that still remains is a question of distance. How do molecules such as gp130 and LIF-R which have three fibronectin type III domains between the membrane and the first "cytokine binding" domain interact simultaneously with ligands that are bound to receptor subunits that have no such fibronectin domains, such as CNTF-R and IL6-R, when these molecules are attached to the cell surface? Again, further structural studies will be required to determine the geometries of these complete ligand/receptor complexes.

In conclusion we have determined the structure of LIF to 2.0 Å, a result which also has implications for the structures of CNTF and OSM. This structure, when combined with mutagenesis data, allows a proposal to be made of a receptor binding model, consistent with that of the growth hormone receptor/ligand complex but with additional novel features, which contributes to ideas on the signaling events at the cell membrane.

SUMMARY

We have determined the structure of murine leukemia inhibitory factor (LIF) by X-ray crystallography at 2.0 Å resolution. The current crystal structure comprises native LIF residues 9 to 180 with 40 ordered water molecules. For this model the R value (with a bulk solvent correction) is 18.6% on all data from 20.0 Å to 2.0 Å with stereochemistry typified by root mean square deviations from ideal bond lengths of 0.015 Å. The mainchain fold conforms to the four α-helix bundle topology previously observed for several members of the hematopoietic cytokine family. Of these, LIF shows closest structural homology to granulocyte colony stimulating factor and growth hormone. Sequence alignments for the functionally related molecules oncostatin M and ciliary neurotrophic factor, when mapped to the LIF structure, indicate regions of conserved structural and surface character. Analysis of published mutagenesis data implicate two regions of receptor interaction which are located in the fourth helix and the preceding loop. A model for receptor binding based on the structure of the growth hormone ligand/receptor complex requires additional, novel features to account for these data.

ACKNOWLEDGMENTS

We thank J. Pitt and S. Cole for assistance with protein production, D. Harvey for mass spectroscopy, T. Willis for protein sequencing and amino acid analysis, K. Harlos and the staff at the SRS, Daresbury and at the Photon Factory, Japan for help with X-ray data collection, and R. Bryan and R. Esnouf for computing facilities.

Atomic coordinates for murine LIF have been deposited with the Protein Data Bank, Brookhaven National Laboratory, USA. Prerelease coordinates are available from EYJ; e-mail address YVON@BIOP.OX.AC.UK.

REFERENCES

1. ABDEL-MEGUID, S. S. *et al.* 1987. Proc. Natl. Acad. Sci. USA **84**: 6434–6437.
2. BAZAN, J. F. 1991. Neuron **7**: 197–208.
3. DIEDERICHS, K. *et al.* Science **254**: 1779–1782.

4. WALTER, M. R. et al. 1992. J. Biol. Chem. **267:** 20371–20376.
5. BAZAN, J. F. & Q. B. MCKAY. 1992. Science **257:** 410–413.
6. WALTER, M. R. et al. 1992. J. Mol. Biol. **224:** 1075–1085.
7. WLODAWER, A. et al. 1992. FEBS Lett. **309:** 59–64.
8. SMITH, L. J. et al. 1992. J. Mol. Biol. **224:** 899–904.
9. POWERS, R., et al. 1993. Biochemistry **32:** 6744–6762.
10. DE VOS, A. M. et al. 1992. Science **255:** 306–312.
11. HILL, C. P. et al. 1993. Proc. Natl. Acad. Sci. USA **90:** 5167–5171.
12. PANDIT, J. et al. 1992. Science **258:** 1358–1362.
13. MILBURN, M. V. et al. 1993. Nature **336:** 172–176.
14. EALICK, S. E. et al. 1991. Science **252:** 698–702.
15. SAMUDZI, et al. 1991. J. Biol. Chem. **266:** 21791–21797.
16. SENDA, T. et al. 1992. EMBO J. **11:** 3193–3201.
17. GEARING, D. P. et al. 1991. EMBO J. **10:** 2839–2848.
18. COSMAN, D. et al. 1990. Trends Biochem. Sci. **15:** 265–270.
19. COSMAN, D. 1993. Cytokine **5:** 95–106.
20. GEARING, D. P. et al. 1992. Science **255:** 1434–1437.
21. GEARING, D. P. et al. 1992. Ciba. Found. Symp. **167:** 245–255.
22. HIBI, M. et al. 1990. Cell **63:** 1149–1157.
23. LIU, J. et al. 1992. J. Biol. Chem. **267:** 16763–16766.
24. YIN, T. et al. 1993. J. Immunol. **151:** 2555–2561.
25. TAGA, T. et al. 1992. Proc. Natl. Acad. Sci. USA **89:** 10998–11001.
26. DAVIS, S. et al. 1991. Science **253:** 59–63.
27. DAVIS, S. et al. 1993. Science **260:** 1805–1808.
28. KISHIMOTO, T. et al. 1992. Science **258:** 593–597.
29. TAGA, T. & T. KISHIMOTO. 1992. FASEB J. **6:** 3387–3396.
30. MALIK, N. et al. 1989. J. Mol. Cell Biol. **9:** 2847–2853.
31. STOCKLI, K. A. et al. 1989. Nature **342:** 920–923.
32. VAN SNICK, J. et al. 1988. Eur. J. Immunol. **18:** 193–197.
33. WELLS, J. A. & A. M. DE VOS. 1993. Annu. Rev. Biophys. Biomol. Struct. **22:** 329–351.
34. ROBINSON, R. C. et al. 1994. Cell **77:** 1101–1116.
35. WANG, B. C. 1985. Meth. Enzym. **115:** 90–111.
36. NICOLA, N. A. et al. 1993. Biochem. Biophys. Res. Commun. **190:** 20–26.
37. OWCZAREK, C. M. et al. 1993. EMBO J. **12:** 3487–3495.
38. SAVINO, R. et al. 1994. EMBO J. **13:** 1357–1367.
39. VAN DAM, M. et al. 1993. J. Mol. Biol. **268:** 15285–15290.
40. PANAYOTATOS, N. et al. 1993. J. Mol. Biol. **268:** 19000–19003.
41. KRAULIS, P. J. 1991. J. Appl. Cryst. **24:** 946–950.

DISCUSSION OF THE PAPER

G. CILIBERTO (*Istituto di Ricerche di Biologia Moleculare P. Angletti, Pomezia (Rome), Italy*): Based on the last model you proposed kinking of the LIF receptor in the second cytokine binding domain of the LIF receptor, which binds the LIF molecule in the part of the region where all the mutants were made. So, given the fact that oncostatin M also binds the LIF receptor, can you speak a little bit about the conservation of residues in the same region of oncostatin M which would allow binding to LIF receptor in the same way?

R. ROBINSON: There are a number of residues which are conserved between LIF, oncostatin M and CNTF, the majority of which lie at the c-terminal end of the CD loop and N-terminal end of D helix—the region we have proposed to bind to this "second" binding domain of the LIF receptor.

CILIBERTO: I see. So you can basically predict that in, say, the IL-6 where you have different residues in the same region a second gp130 molecule sits and this is the region which L. Aarden has mutagenized.

ROBINSON: We do. Mutagenesis work has been carried out on the LIF receptor whereby the two cytokine binding domains have been expressed separately. They bind to the LIF mutants in a fashion which enforces our model of receptor binding.

M. REVEL (*Weizmann Institute of Science, Rehovot, Israel*): Actually, my question is on the same topic. You know that the interferon receptor also has two binding domains, and I would like to know what the evidence is upon which you base the folding of your two sites to interact with LIF, because you could have made the opposite hypothesis—that oncostatin M interacts with one binding site and LIF with the other. So, do you have any experimental evidence to support your hypothesis?

ROBINSON: The mutagenesis which I have talked about supports the idea that the LIF receptor has two sites on LIF and the more recent data we have acquired on expressing the cytokine binding domains in the LIF-R suggests that the model is in fact correct.

REVEL: You could say that one of the two sites on LIF interacts with gp130, as you said that you did not know where to put gp130 in your model.

ROBINSON: We are proposing a three-site model. Two sites interact with LIF-R and one with gp130. There is, as yet, no evidence for the positioning of gp130 in the complex. We look forward to such data as a stern test to ideas.

Function of Hematopoietin Receptor Subunits in Hepatic Cells and Fibroblasts[a]

CHUN-FAI LAI,[b] KAREN K. MORELLA,[b] YANPING WANG,[b,c]
SATORU KUMAKI,[d] DAVID GEARING,[e] STEVEN F. ZIEGLER,[f]
DAVID J. TWEARDY,[g] SUSANA P. CAMPOS,[b,c]
AND HEINZ BAUMANN[b,h]

[b]*Department of Molecular and Cellular Biology*
Roswell Park Cancer Institute
Buffalo, New York 14263

[c]*Children's Hospital of Buffalo*
Division of Endocrinology
Buffalo, New York 14222

[d]*Immunex Corporation*
Seattle, Washington 98101

[e]*Systemix*
Palo Alto, California 94304

[f]*Darwin Molecular Corporation*
Bothell, Washington 98021

[g]*Pittsburgh Cancer Institute*
Division of Basic Research
Pittsburgh, Pennsylvania 15213

INTRODUCTION

Mammalian liver cells respond to treatments with different interleukin (IL)-6-type cytokines: IL-6, IL-11, oncostatin-M (OSM), leukemia inhibitory factor (LIF) or ciliary neurotrophic factor (CNTF), by an increase in transcription of a similar set of acute phase plasma protein (APP) genes.[1] This cytokine effect is considered to be one of the basic regulatory mechanisms that contribute to the hepatic acute phase response *in vivo*.[2] The apparent redundancy of the cytokine action has been ascribed to the facts that: i) IL-6-type cytokine receptors share a common signal-transducing subunit; ii) the receptors engage a common intracellular signal-transducing mechanism; and iii) APP genes contain in their 5'-flanking regions similar *cis*-acting DNA elements that serve as a common target of signal-transducing factors.

Receptors for the IL-6-type cytokines belong to the family of hematopoietin receptors which possess common structural motifs within their extracellular and, in a few cases, also in their intracellular domain.[3,4] The family is subdivided into several groups,

---

[a] This work was supported by NIH grants CA26122 and DK33886, ACS grant DHP-111B and grant 2709 from Women's and Children's Health Research Foundation.
[b] Author to whom correspondence should be addressed.

based on the identity of the shared signal-transducing subunits. These groups consist of: i) the receptors for IL-2, -4, -7, -9, -13, and -15 which share or are predicted to utilize IL-2Rγ; ii) the receptors for IL-3, IL-5 and granulocyte-macrophage colony stimulating factor (GM-CSF) which depend on IL-3Rβ; and iii) the IL-6-type cytokine receptors which depend on gp130.[5,6] Several of the hematopoietin receptors, including the receptor for granulocyte colony stimulating factor (G-CSF), erythropoietin (EPO), growth hormone (GH) and prolactin, function as homodimers.[7–10] Additional members, such as the receptor for thrombopoietin (c-mpl), have been identified based on sequence similarity, but their molecular mode of action remains to be defined.[11]

Although the function of most hematopoietin receptors has been associated with the control of proliferation of hematopoietic cells, the transcriptional regulation of early growth response genes and differentiated genes by several hematopoietic receptors in specific cell types has been described. Signal transduction by the ligand-occupied hematopoietin receptor is initiated by activation of receptor-bound protein tyrosine kinases (PTK) or by recruitment to and then activation of cytoplasmically located kinases. Depending upon the particular cell type in which the receptor resides, the involvement of Jak/Tyk and src-related PTKs has been identified.[12–17] A proposed immediate consequence of the kinase action is the activation by phosphorylation of cytoplasmic and nuclear transcription-controlling proteins. A particularly prominent role has been ascribed to "Signal Transducers and Activators of Transcription" (Stat proteins which bind to *cis*-acting gene sequence of cytokine and growth factor–responsive genes.[18,19] The interaction of Stat proteins with either modified *sis*-inducible element (SIE) of the *c-fos* gene[18] or the wild-type SIE-related sequence in the 3′ flanking region of the *junB* gene[20] has proven to be a highly sensitive indicator of the activity of Stat proteins. These interactions give rise to DNA-protein complexes detectable by gel mobility shift assay (GMSA) and hence termed *sis*-inducible factors (SIF).[18] Principal components of SIFs were recognized to be the SH-2 domain-dependent dimers of p91/84 (or Stat 1) and p92 (or Stat 3, or APRF).[19,21,22] Although the signal transduction of the hematopoietin receptor by the PTK-Stat pathway has been documented in numerous cell systems, the precise contribution of the Stat proteins to the transcriptional control of the target genes has yet to be delineated.[12]

Structure/function analysis of hematopoietin receptors suggest that qualitative and quantitative signaling is determined by distinct subregions of the cytoplasmic domains of the signal transducing receptor subunits. The domains directing the control of proliferation and the transcription of specific genes do not appear to coincide in all instances as observed for IL-2R,[23] GM-CSFR,[24] G-CSFR,[7,26,27] and the IL-6-type cytokine receptors.[5,27,28] Furthermore, a correlation of a specific pattern of PTK-Stat activation with a given cell response has yet to be established.

The goals of this study were: 1) to define to what extent the representative members of the hematopoietin receptors exercise similar functions in a given cell; 2) to determine whether the conserved motifs in the cytoplasmic domains of different hematopoietin receptors similarly control the expression of a specific gene element; and 3) to identify any correlation between the activation of Stat proteins and the modulation of gene expression. We have developed a test system for IL-6-type cytokine receptors using the regulation of APP gene elements in hepatoma cells and applied this system to the functional analysis of hematopoietin receptors that are not expressed in hepatic cells. The results indicate that the function of hematopoietin receptors can be reconstituted in a heterologous cell system, that the cell response is defined by the signal transducing receptor subunits, and that separate signaling mechanisms contribute to the cell regulation.

REGULATION OF SPECIFIC APP GENE ELEMENTS BY IL-6-TYPE CYTOKINE RECEPTORS

Treatment of the rat hepatoma H-35 cells (subclone T7-18-1; ref. 29), with either IL-6, IL-11, LIF, CNTF, or OSM, results in an increased expression of the representative APPs, β-fibrinogen (βFB), hemopexin (HPX), thiostatin, and haptoglobin (HP). Within 30 min of treatment, the gene transcription rates reach maximal level and are maintained at that level for hours. The magnitude of stimulation is markedly enhanced in the presence of dexamethasone for IL-6 and IL-11 but not for LIF, CNTF or OSM. All these IL-6-type cytokines, in combination with IL-1-type cytokines (IL-1α, IL-1β, TNFα, TNFβ), exert a prominent synergistic action on the type 1 APP genes, α_1-acid glycoprotein (AGP) and complement component-3 (C3).

We have identified the minimal IL-6-response elements (IL-6RE) of the βFB, HPX, and HP genes which show considerable sequence similarity to the IL-6RE of the rat α_2-macroglobulin gene and contain a core-nucleotide sequence, T/C T/C GG(G)AA(A).[30,31] The IL-6RE of the βFB gene differs, however, from those of the HP, HPX and AGP genes in that the consensus sequence is adjacent to a binding site for C/EBP, and thus, can be strongly activated by co-expressed C/EBP isoforms.[32]

These gene elements have been used to construct IL-6-regulatable reporter gene plasmids. Five copies of a 23 bp oligonucleotide representing the core segment of the IL-6RE of the HPX[30] and HP[20] genes were inserted 5′ to the enhancerless minimal SV40 promoter that controls the chloramphenicol acetyl transferase (CAT) gene. Both constructs, when transiently introduced into H-35 cells, yielded an approximate 50-fold stimulation by IL-6 but no detectable stimulation by IL-1, TNF, IFN-γ and insulin (example of HP-CAT gene regulation in FIGURE 1). The regulation via these IL-6REs was not appreciably affected by overexpressed isoforms of C/EBP,[32] NF-kB, AP-1, or glucocorticoid receptor (data not shown). These CAT reporter gene constructs were utilized to determine the activity of IL-6–type cytokine receptors and to identify the intracellular receptor domains that mediate the signaling events.

In order to unequivocally delineate the relevant signaling domains within the two signal-transducing subunits of the IL-6-type cytokine receptor, gp130 and LIFR, we needed to analyze the receptor function without potential interference from the endogenous receptor subunits, particularly, gp130. We, therefore, determined the function of the cytoplasmic domain separate from the native extracellular domain by creating chimeric receptors consisting of the extracellular domain of G-CSFR and the transmembrane and cytoplasmic domains of LIFR or gp130.[27] We selected G-CSFR because this receptor functions as a ligand-induced homodimer, independently of other hematopoietin receptor subunits.[7,26] Moreover, since G-CSFR and its ligand are not expressed by the hepatoma cells, the possibility of autocrine stimulation is eliminated.[33] The choice of G-CSFR proved to be beneficial because transient expression of full-length G-CSFR in hepatoma cells resulted in signaling events that appeared qualitatively equivalent to those observed with the endogenous IL-6R.[26,27] Since the G-CSFR transfected into hepatic cells yielded an additional example of an "IL-6–type cytokine" response, a valuable tool became available for a comparative definition of the general structural features of the cytoplasmic signaling region of functionally similar hematopoietin receptors.

Like the G-CSFR, chimeric G-CSFR-gp130 and G-CSFR-LIFR, when transfected into H-35 cells, were capable of activating the intracellular signal transduction which led to the activation of the IL-6RE-CAT gene constructs.[33] This finding indicated that the intracellular receptor domains, even in the artificial context of a G-CSFR chimera, were functional and that the experimental system was suitable for dissection of the receptor domains. By progressive carboxy terminal deletion, internal deletion

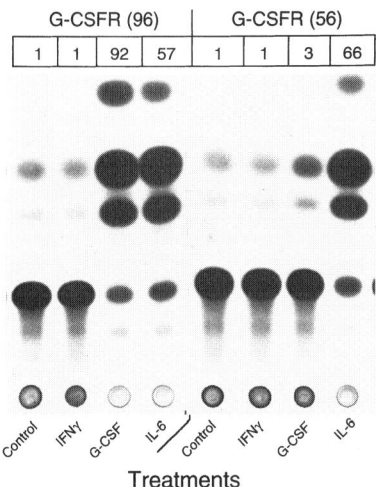

FIG 19-1

FIGURE 1. Regulation of HP IL-6RE-CAT reporter gene construct by G-CSFR in H-35 cells. Two cultures of H-35 cells in 10 cm dishes were transfected with DNA-DEAE dextran complex consisting of 15 μg pHP(5×IL-6RE)CAT [HP IL-6RE 5'-GATCCGTGGTTACTGGAACAGTA 3'] and 2.5 μg of expression vector for either G-CSFR(96) [cytoplasmic domain truncated to 96 residues; ref. 26] or G-CSFR(56) [cytoplasmic domain reduced to 56 residues and thereby deleting box 3 motif; ref. 26]. After 16 h recovery period, the transfected cultures were subdivided into 4 cultures. The subcultures were treated for 24 hours with serum-free medium containing 1 μM dexamethasone alone (=control) or in addition 100 ng/ml of murine IFN-γ (Genentech), human G-CSFR (Immunex) or human IL-6 (Genetics Institute). The cells were extracted and CAT activity determined. The values were calculated relative to the control in each series (defined as 1) and are listed above the autoradiogram. One representative enzyme reaction is shown.

and point mutation, the minimal functional domain of G-CSFR, gp130 and LIFR were assessed.[27] For each receptor, we noted that a cooperativity of separate regions were required for full function.

The minimal cytoplasmic region for IL-6RE regulation ranges from 96 amino acid residues for G-CSFR, 133 residues for gp130 to 150 residues for LIFR.[27] Although a substantial carboxy terminal part of the receptors appeared to be dispensable for signaling, those sections nevertheless were necessary to gain maximal activity of gp130 and LIFR. The minimal functional domain in all three receptors included three conserved sequence motifs: the transmembrane proximal motif termed box 1 and box 2 that have been shown to be necessary for achieving a proliferative signal by several hematopoietin receptors,[7,25,26,35–39] and the distal box 3 motif with a central tyrosine residue necessary for function.[27]

The presence of box 3 determines whether the receptor is capable of activating the IL-6RE-CAT construct. FIGURE 1 illustrates, with G-CSFR as a representative example, that when the cytoplasmic domain had been truncated from 96 residues (plus box 3) to 56 residues (minus box 3), the box 3–dependent signal which has been termed "IL-6–signal" is lost.[28] Since G-CSFR and G-CSFR–gp130 with cytoplasmic domains that contain box 1 and box 2 only were capable of stimulating proliferation in BAF cells, a separate signal derived from this region was proposed. To detect this predicted signal in our hepatic cell system, an appropriate response element was needed. Functional analysis of APP gene sequences indeed revealed that elements different from the IL-6RE were activated by receptors devoid of box 3. Two types of elements identified were: the cytokine response element (CytRE) and the hematopoietin receptor response element (HRRE). The CytRE is a 62 bp sequence representing the 5' half of the distal hormone regulatory element of the rat AGP gene[40] which, in quadruple form in CAT vectors, mediated stimulation by not only IL-6-type cytokines but also by IL-1, TNFα, insulin, hepatocyte growth factor, and interferon-γ (IFN-γ).[41,42] Since IL-6-type cytokine receptors activate Stat proteins and yield a response similar to that observed with the IFN-γ receptor,[18] we also employed for comparative purposes a CAT reporter gene construct that contained 4 tandem copies

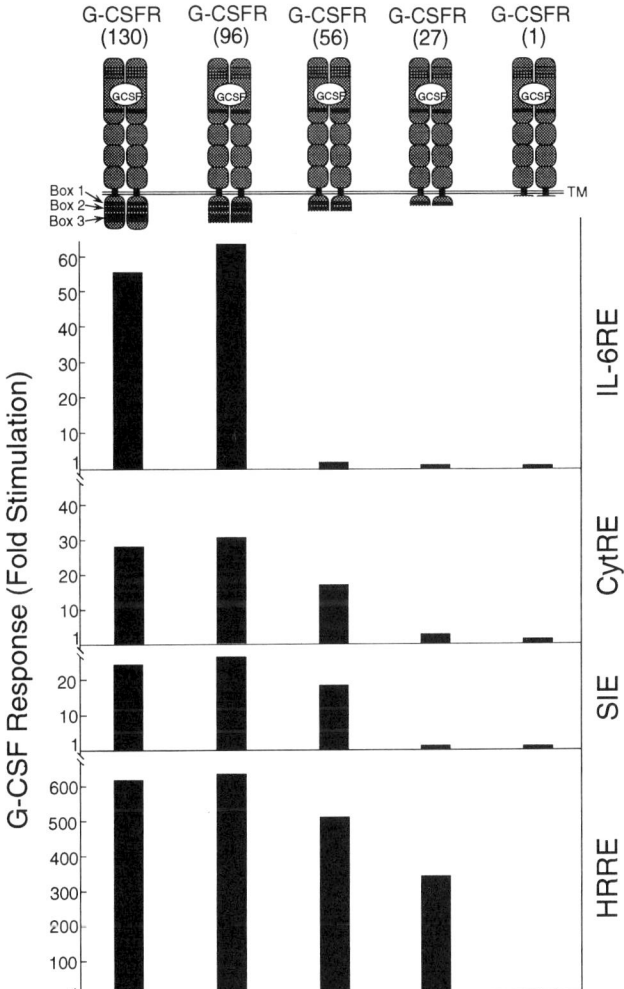

FIGURE 2. Regulatory activities of G-CSFR with progressively truncated cytoplasmic domain. H-35 cells were transfected with a pair-wise combination of CAT reporter gene constructs (10 μg) and expression vectors for the G-CSFR forms containing cytoplasmic domains of different lengths. The number of amino acid residues in the cytoplasmic domains of the receptor domains are listed schematically at the top [G-CSFR(130) represents the full-length class IV receptor.[48,49] The CAT reporter genes contain either 5 copies of rat HPX IL-6RE 5'-GATCCTGCCGGGAA-GATAGTCTGAGA-3',[30] 4 copies of the 62 bp rat AGP CytRE,[40] 4 copies of the high-affinity SIE m67,[18] or 8 copies of HRRE 5'GATCCATCCTTCTGGGAATTCTGATCA-3'.[20,43] The subcultures were treated with G-CSF and the magnitude of increase in CAT activity was determined relative to the control treatment for each transfected culture.

of the high affinity SIE.[18] HRRE represents a multimerized synthetic 27 nucleotide fragment that had been designed by modifying the consensus sequence of IL-6REs of APP genes[20,31,40] and selected for high inducibility by hematopoietin receptor signals.[43] A CAT gene construct containing 8 HRRE units was identified and utilized in this study because of its high magnitude of activation.

The four different CAT reporter gene constructs were used to probe the signaling function of the cytoplasmic domains of G-CSFR, gp130 and LIFR (FIGS. 1 and 2 show examples for G-CSFR; see also refs. 27 and 28). The data suggest that G-CSFR initiates separate signals which are distinguishable by the minimal receptor region necessary to achieve regulation of the reporter genes. The IL-6RE is regulated by the region that includes box 1 through 3, whereas CytRE and SIE similarly require the regions with only box 1 and 2, and the HRRE is dependent on box 1 region alone. The specificity for the signaling activity of the gp130 cytoplasmic domain is similar to G-CSFR.[28] The activity of LIFR proved to be somewhat different; while the G-CSFR-LIFR chimera mediated a strong IL-6 signal, a substantially weaker signal was induced by the box 1 and box 2 domain,[28] and essentially no signal was detectable with the box 1 domain alone. The failure of the box 1 domain of LIFR to regulate HRRE-CAT construct has been attributed to the fact that LIFR has a variant box 1 sequence, in that tryptophane at position 11 is replaced by tyrosine.[28] We conclude from the results of these functional analyses that IL-6-type cytokine receptors in H-35 cells mediate at least three signaling events that can be experimentally detected: 1) the "IL-6-signal" targeted to IL-6RE; 2) the "cytokine signal" targeted to CytRE and SIE; and 3) the "hematopoietin receptor signal" targeted to HRRE.

SIGNALING FUNCTION OF OTHER HEMATOPOIETIN RECEPTORS

The structural comparison of signal-transducing subunits of the various hematopoietin receptors indicate that the sequence comprising the membrane proximal cytoplasmic domain, in particular the box 1 and box 2 motifs, has been conserved.[39] Moreover, these regions are noted to be necessary for gaining a proliferative signal in hematopoietic cells as observed for c-mpl, IL-2Rβ, EPOR and GHR.[11,34,38] This structural similarity raised the question of whether these receptor domains exert functions similar to the ones defined for the IL-6–type cytokine receptors. A functional comparison seemed possible by introducing these receptors in H-35 cells and measuring the regulation of the CAT reporter constructs. The reconstitution of signaling by receptors that are not normally expressed in hepatic cells require, however, that receptors expressed in hepatoma cells are capable of recruiting the components of the signal-transduction machinery existing in the host cell. Evidently, receptors which rely on cell-type restricted signal mediators, such as receptor-interacting PTKs and/or downstream Stat protein substrates that are not present in liver cells, will appear inactive in transfected hepatoma cells.

We analyzed several members of the hematopoietin receptor family which are not found in liver. These receptors included the G-CSFR-MPL chimera[28]; IL-2R,[23,43,44] IL-7R,[45] IL-4R[46] (all of which rely on IL-2Rγ as a common subunit); and the homodimerizing EPOR.[47] GHR[43] served as an example of a hematopoietin receptor normally expressed in liver but not associated with IL-6–type cytokine receptor signaling function. Expression vectors for each receptor subunit were co-transfected into H-35 cells along with one of the four CAT reporter gene constructs. The regulation of the reporter genes by the introduced receptors were compared to that of the endogenous receptors (FIG. 3). All of the transfected receptors were able to activate HRRE-CAT

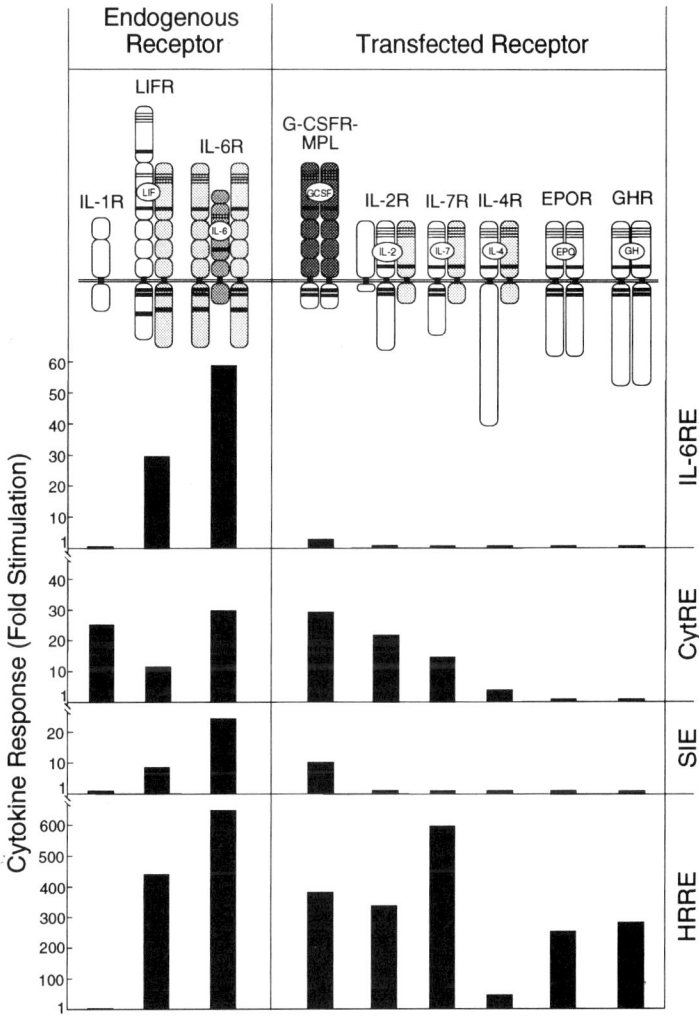

FIGURE 3. Activity of hematopoietin receptors. Using the same experimental technique as in FIGURE 2, H-35 cell cultures were transfected with expression vectors encoding either G-CSFR-mpl[11]; the three human IL-2R subunits α, β, and γ[23,43,44]; human IL 7R[45] and IL-2Rγ; human IL-4R[46] and IL-2Rγ; murine EPOR[47]; or rabbit GHR.[43] The reporter gene constructs were the same as used in FIGURE 2: pHPX(5 × IL-6RE)CAT, pAGP(4 × CytRE)CAT, p(4 × SIE)CAT, and p(8 × HRRE)CAT. Each culture was subdivided into 5, and these were treated with serum-free medium with 1 μM dexamethasone alone or containing in addition either 0.5 ng/ml human IL-1β (Immunex), 10 ng/ml human LIF (Immunex), 100 ng/ml human IL-6, G-CSF, human IL-2 (Cetus), IL-7 (Immunex), IL-4 (Immunex), EPO (Amgen), or human GH (Genentech). In separate experiments, we verified that none of the ligands for the transfected receptors was able to activate any of the CAT reporter gene constructs in H-35 cells that had not received the cognate receptor. The cytokine-induced change in CAT activity was calculated relative to the control culture in each experimental series.

expression demonstrating that the receptors are at least partially compatible with the hepatoma signal-transduction system. Unexpectedly, the pair, IL-4R/IL-2Rγ, was active at a relatively low level, even though the cytoplasmic domains of both subunits did not contain the conserved structural motif, *i.e.*, box 1 and/or box 2.[44] Remarkable receptor-specific differences in the regulation of the CAT reporter genes were observed. None of the receptors produced a significant stimulation of IL-6RE-CAT, probably due to the lack of a box 3 equivalent motif. G-CSFR-MPL was active on both CytRE and SIE, whereas the IL-2Rγ-dependent receptors could activate CytRE but not SIE. EPOR and GHR were unable to activate these CAT genes. Taken together, the analyses of hematopoietin receptors in hepatoma cells defined common and receptor-specific signaling processes.

SIF ACTIVATION AS PART OF CYTOKINE RECEPTOR ACTION

The current model of signal initiation by hematopoietin receptors proposes an activation of receptor-associated PTK or PTK kinases recruited to the receptors. These kinases include members of the Jak/Tyk family and src-related kinases. Direct or indirect targets of the kinases are Stat proteins and probably other SH2/SH3-containing signal mediating proteins.[2,21] Since a prominent role in signaling has been ascribed to Stat proteins including the SIFs (Stat 1 and Stat 3; refs. 18, 21 and 22), the question must be asked whether the regulation of gene expression by the receptor forms in our system is correlated with specific SIF activation. Previous characterization of H-35 cells[20] has indicated that all IL-6–type cytokines promote by means of their endogenous receptors an identical transient activation of SIF-A, -B and -C. Peak values were observed after a 15 to 30 min treatment followed by a rapid decline of SIF-B and -C activity, but a sustained level of SIF-A activity persisted for at least 24 h (FIG. 4, lanes 1–3). Treatment of the H-35 cells with IFN-γ primarily induced SIF-C activity which also persisted at lower levels for at least 24 h (FIG. 4, lanes 4 and 5). The regulation of SIF activity in H-35 cells follows essentially the pattern of regulation noted in HepG2 cells.[18] DNA binding activity of SIFs was readily detectable with the high affinity SIE sequence as probe, but under the same assay conditions, no binding to HP IL-6RE[20] or HRRE was observed (FIG. 4, lanes 6–10). Therefore, the detection of receptor-mediated Stat protein activation was restricted to those proteins binding to SIE.

Transient transfection of plasmid DNA into H-35 cells generally yields at best a 5% of transfection efficiency as judged by experiments in which a β-galactosidase expression vector was co-introduced, and the transfected cells were identified by staining. The low efficiency of transfection and low level expression in the total cell culture precluded a biochemical analysis of transfected cytokine receptors in H-35 cells.[27,28] Therefore, we utilized L-cells and COS-1 cells, both of which permit high level expression of transiently transfected plasmids as alternative cell systems. This switch to nonhepatic cells required that we could at least qualitatively reproduce some of the receptor function seen in H-35 cells. Our goal was to correlate receptor protein expression with SIF activation and CAT gene regulation in the *same* transfected cell culture.

Such a comparative analysis proved to be possible in L-cells but not COS-1 cells, because L-cells not only yielded relatively high level expression of receptor protein but could also regulate the same IL-6RE and HRRE CAT reporter gene constructs as seen in H-35 cells, although at a much lower magnitude of stimulation (FIG. 5). The salient features of a representative receptor analysis in L-cells are demonstrated by the cotransfection of G-CSFR(96) or G-CSFR(56) with HP-IL-6RE-CAT construct

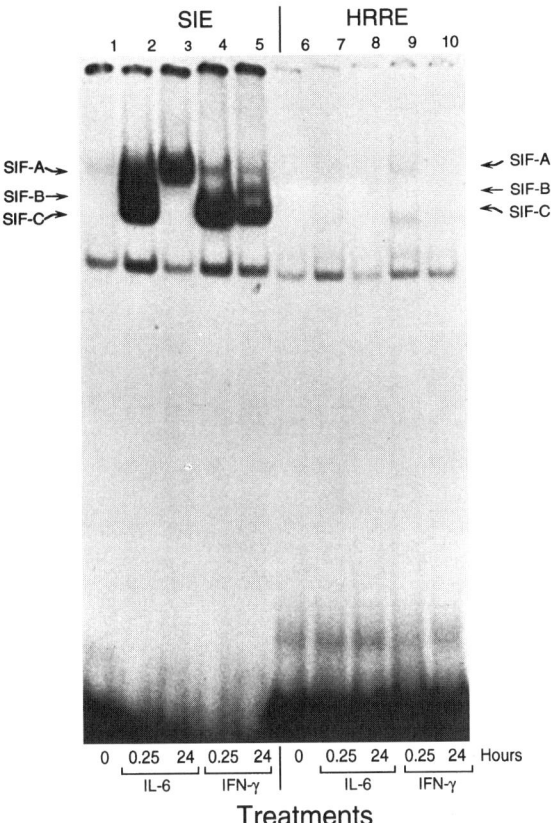

FIGURE 4. SIF activation by cytokines in H-35 cells. Five confluent cultures of H-35 cells in 10 cm dishes were maintained for 16 h in serum-free medium then treated for 15 min or 24 h with IL-6 or IFN-γ and used for extraction of nuclear proteins.[18] The duplicate aliquots of the protein extracts (10 μg) were preincubated in 20 μl reaction volume with 5 μg poly[dIdC] for 15 min on ice, and then ^{32}P-labeled SIE m67[18] or HRRE[20] was added. Incubation was continued for 15 min at room temperature, and the reaction mixture was separated onto a 4% native polyacrylamide gel in 0.5X Tris-borate-EDTA buffer. The autoradiogram after a 16 h exposure is shown. The relative positions of the SIF complexes A, B and C are indicated.

(same plasmid combination as used in H-35 cells, FIG. 1). Western blot analysis revealed that comparable levels of receptor proteins were synthesized by the cells but G-CSF induced SIF activity only in cells transfected with the box 3–containing G-CSFR(96) and not in those with the G-CSFR(56). The comparison to H-35 cells also demonstrated that L-cells had a much lower level of SIF activity than H-35 cells (on per cell basis) and that IL-6 treatment primarily induced SIF-A. The CAT gene regulation was qualitatively similar to that seen in H-35 cells in that only the box 3–containing G-CSFR(96) was effective (FIG. 5).

The test of the various G-CSFR forms with progressively truncated cytoplasmic domains for regulating the HRRE-CAT constructs in L-cells (FIG. 6) was again in

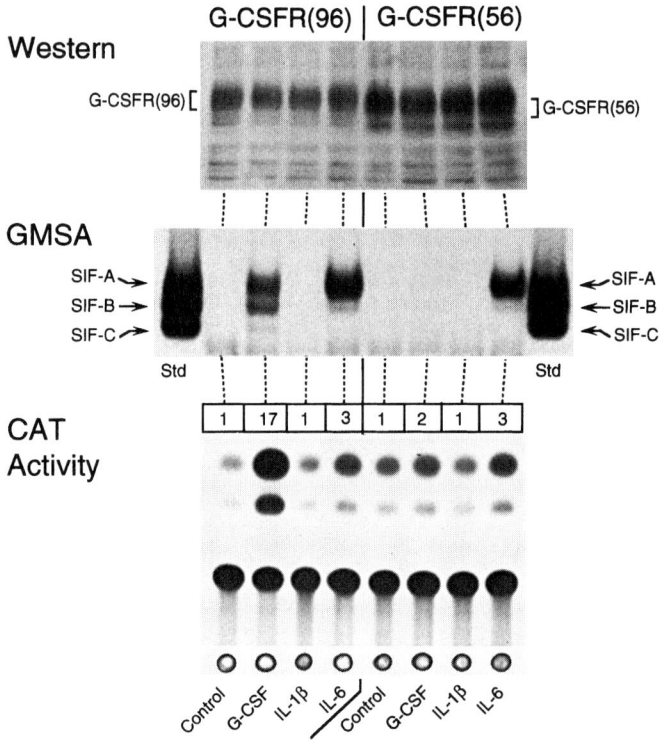

FIGURE 5. Functional analysis of G-CSFR in L-cells. Two cultures of L-cells in 15 cm dishes were transfected with 3 ml solution of DNA-DEAE-dextran mixture consisting of 10 μg pHP(5×IL-6RE)CAT and 30 μg of expression vector for either G-CSFR(96) or G-CSFR(56). After 16 h, each cell culture was released by trypsin and divided into 4 cultures in 10 cm dishes (for Western blot and GMSA) and 4 cultures in 3.5 cm dishes (for CAT activity). Twenty-four hours later, the 10 cm dishes were changed to serum-free medium, and after 16 h, cells were treated for 15 min with serum-free medium alone or containing the cytokines indicated at the bottom. The cells were scraped off the dish, and one-fourth of the cell suspension removed for *Western* blot analysis. The cells were lysed in 20 μl tris-buffered saline containing 1% NP-40 and a cocktail of protease and phosphatase inhibitors. After 20 min on ice, the lysate was centrifuged for 20 sec at 10,000 g and supernatant subjected to electrophoresis on a 5% polyacrylamide gel. Proteins were transferred onto Immobilon-P (Millipore) membrane and reacted with sheep anti-human G-CSFR[17] followed by rabbit anti-goat Ig and by alkaline phosphatase-conjugated goat anti-rabbit Ig. The pattern was visualized by 5-bromo-4-chloro-3-indoyl phosphate *p*-toluidine/*p*-nitro-blue tetrazolium chloride reaction (Bio-Rad). The remaining three-fourths of the cell suspension was centrifuged and the cell pellet resuspended in 50 μl of 20 mM Hepes pH 7.9, 300 nM NaCl, 14% glycerol and cocktail of protease and phosphatase inhibitors and processed for whole cell extraction.[18,20,43] Five μl of extract was reacted with ^{32}P-labeled SIE and subjected to GMSA as described in FIGURE 4. Nuclear extract of IL-6-treated H-35 cells served as standard *(Std)*. The 4 cultures in 3.5 cm dishes were treated for 24 h with cytokines, extracted and processed for CAT analysis. The relative change in CAT activity is indicated above the autoradiogram.

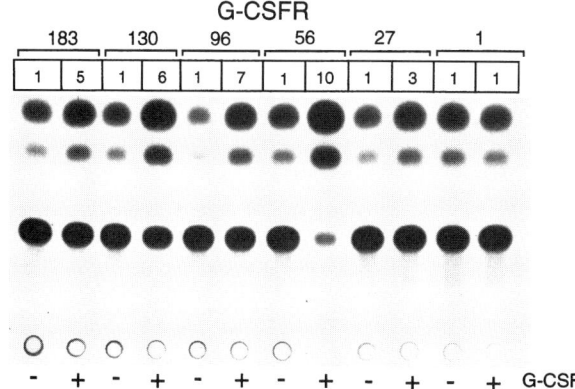

FIGURE 6. Gene regulating activity of G-CSFR with progressively truncated cytoplasmic domain in L-cells. L-cells in 10 cm dishes were transfected with DNA-DEAE dextran complex consisting of 5 μg p(8×HRRE)CAT and expression vector for either full-length G-CSFR isoform 25.1 *(183)*,[48] full-length G-CSFR isoform D7 *(130)*,[48] or truncated forms having cytoplasmic domains truncated to 96, 56, 27, and 1 residue.[26] The transfected cultures were subdivided and treated with or without G-CSFR. The relative change in CAT activity in each culture series is determined.

agreement with the results of H-35 cells. All receptor forms with the exception of G-CSFR(1) were active, even though the receptor forms with the cytoplasmic domain with less than 96 residues were not detectably inducing SIF activity (FIG. 5 and data not shown; ref. 20).

The analysis of the various hematopoietin receptors (see FIGS. 2 and 3) by the technique shown in FIGURE 5 revealed a complex pattern of cell response (summarized in TABLE 1 below). While each of the box 3–containing receptors was stimulating SIF, suggesting a correlation with IL-6RE-CAT gene regulation, a similar SIF activation was also noted for G-CSFR-MPL, EPOR, and GHR, none of which regulated the IL-6RE-CAT. No activation of SIF was observed in L-cells transfected with IL-2R, IL-4R and IL-7R, even though regulation of the HRRE-CAT construct occurred comparable to that by G-CSFR-MPL, EPOR and GHR.

The failure of detecting SIF activation with some of the receptor forms in L-cells could be conceivably attributed to the combination of: a) insufficient expression of the receptor; b) low activity of the receptors; and c) low level of STAT proteins. We, therefore, used as an additional test system COS-1 cells which have an IL-6-type cytokine specific induction kinetics and relative amounts of SIF activity comparable to H-35 cells (FIG. 7). COS-1 cells also achieve approximately 10 times higher expression levels of receptor plasmids than L-cells as determined by mRNA (Northern blot) and protein (Western blot) analyses (FIG. 8, and data not shown). In COS-1 cells, the transfected receptors, although capable of linking up to the signal transducing machinery, are unable to yield a significant regulation of cotransfected CAT reporter gene constructs (data not shown). The characterization of the G-CSFR forms in COS-1 cells (FIG. 8) yielded similar but not identical results to L-cells (FIG. 5). Major differences observed were that in COS cells, the receptors primarily activated the SIF-C form instead of SIF-A as in L-cells, and the high level of expression of G-CSFR(56) in COS-1 cells was able to induce SIF activity.

TABLE 1. Summary of the Functions Exerted by Hematopoietin Receptors in H-35, COS-1 and L-cells

	Endogenous			Transfected						
Cell Response	IL-1R, TNFR	IL-6R, IL-11R, LIFR, CNTFR, OSMR	IFN-γR	G-CSFR, G-CSFR-gp130, G-CSFR-LIFR	G-CSFR-MPL	IL-2R (α+β+γ)	IL-7R+ IL-2Rγ	IL-4R+ IL-2Rγ	EPOR	GHR
Stimulation of Gene Expression in H-35 Cells										
Il-6RE	−	+	−	+	−	−	−	−	−	−
CytRE	+	+	+	+	+	+	+	(+)	−	−
SIE	−	+	+	+	(+)	−	−	−	−	−
HRRE	−	+	(+)	+	+	+	+	(+)	+	+
Activation of Stat Proteins in COS-1 and L-Cells										
SIF	−	+	+	+	+	−	−	−	+	+

Symbols represent: −, no detectable regulation; +, regulation; (+), low level regulation (≤10% of maximal cell response).

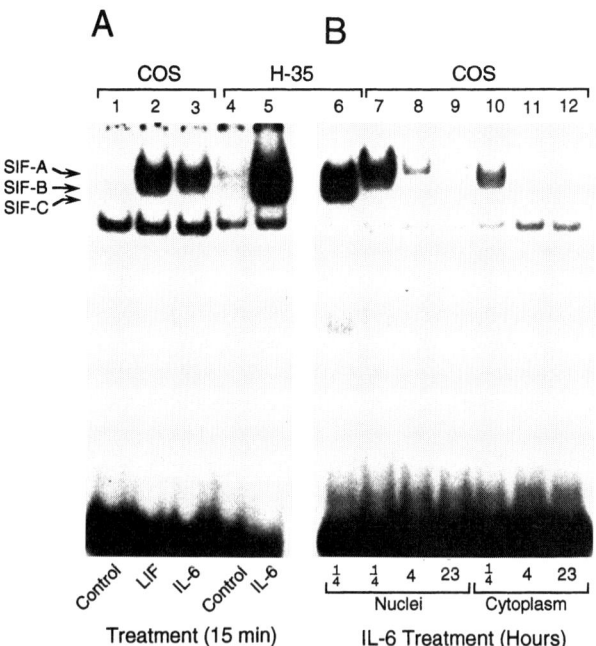

FIGURE 7. Regulation of SIF in COS-1 cells. In two separate experiments, confluent monolayers of COS-1 cells in 10 cm dishes were maintained for 16 h in serum-free medium. The cells were treated with LIF or IL-6 for 15 min (**A,** lanes 1–5) or with IL-6 for the times indicated in **B.** Whole cell extracts were prepared in **A,** or proteins extracted from nuclear and cytoplasmic fraction **B.** GMSA was carried out with ^{32}P-labeled SIE oligonucleotide as probe. Extracts of treated H-35 cells served as standard. The position of SIFA, -B and -C of H-35 cells are indicated at the left.

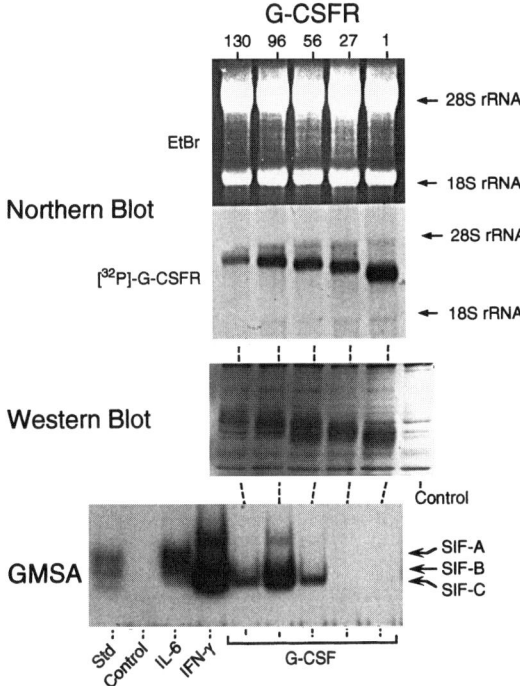

FIGURE 8. Expression and function of G-CSFR forms in COS-1 cells. COS-1 cells in 15 cm dishes were transfected with DNA-DEAE-dextran complex containing 30 μg of expression vector for the G-CSFR form indicated at the top. After a 24 h recovery period, the cells were maintained for an additional 16 h in serum-free medium. The cells were treated for 15 min with G-CSF and then collected by scraping. One half of cell suspension was used to extract total cell RNA, of which 15 μg each were subjected to Northern blot analysis. DNA separation was visualized by ethidium bromide (EtBr) staining (top panel) and to the RNA after transfer to nitrocellulose probed with ^{32}P-labeled 1 kb cDNA fragment encoding the extracellular domain of human G-CSFR. From the remaining one-half portion of the cell suspension, one quarter was processed for Western blotting and the rest for GMSA as described in FIGURE 6. In the Western blot analysis, extract of non-transfected COS 1 cells (=control) was included. To define the positions of SIF complexes, we included extracts of untransfected COS-1 cells that had been treated for 15 min with medium alone (=control) or with IL-6 or IFN-γ. Extract of IL-6-treated H-35 cells served as standard *(Std)*.

Observing that the transfected receptors in COS-1 cells were apparently not able to activate the same Stat proteins as those activated by the endogenous IL-6-type cytokine receptors or by the same transfected receptors in L-cells, the following explanations are possible: i) the production of functional receptors is in vast excess relative to the signaling kinases that are responsible for activating SIF-A, thus leading to the use of a "default system" that results in the recruitment of the kinases for SIF-C activation; ii) in COS-1 cells, the transfected receptors encounter primate signaling proteins that are structurally and/or compositionally different from those in rodent cells; and iii) the extracellular domains of human G-CSFR influence the activation process differently in primate cells compared to rodent cells. In order to address the issue of species-specific differences in SIF activation and action of G-CSFR, we compared the electrophoretic pattern of SIFs activated by endogenous hematopoietin receptors such as IL-6-type cytokine and IFN-γ receptors in H-35 and HepG2 cells and by G-CSF and IFN-γ receptors freshly isolated in human neutrophils culture with SIF patterns observed in several experimental systems including G-CSFR transfected into L-cells and COS-1 cells (FIG. 9). The results indicate that the relative mobilities of the SIF-DNA complex (SIF-A, -B and -C) were identical between the rodent cells (H-35, lanes 1 and 13) and L-cells (lanes 6 and 10), but differed from those of HepG2 cells (lanes 2 and 12) which all showed slower mobilities than the rodent counterparts. The G-CSFR induced form in neutrophils (lane 3) had a slower mobility than the LIF- or IL-6-activated SIF-A in HepG2 cells (lanes 2 and 12), suggesting that these two complexes may not be biochemically identical. G-CSFR introduced in L-cells (lane 4) activated primarily SIF-A that is electrophoretically the same as the one activated in IL-6 (lane 10) and a trace of SIF-B. In COS-1 cells, however, the transfected G-CSFR stimulated SIF-C form (lane 5) that appears to be the same as in IFN-γ–treated COS-1 (lane 8) and HepG2 cells (lane 9) but different from that in IFN-γ–treated neutrophils (lane 7). Taken together, these results indicate that there are species-, as well as cell line–specific differences in the electrophoretic mobilities of SIF-DNA complexes and in the activation pattern of SIF proteins by the same receptor form. At present, we have no molecular explanation for the drastic difference in G-CSFR action in L-cells versus COS-1 cells (lanes 4 and 5), but we assume that most of the discrepancies are caused by the receptor overexpression and cell-specific limitation for accommodating a proper signaling reaction for all receptor molecules.

Inasmuch as our transfection system did not reproduce the precise signal mechanism of endogenous receptors, a major value of the functional analyses of receptors in L-cells and COS-1 cells lies in the ability to probe the receptor domains that interact with the resident signal transduction mechanism. This is of particular interest in the case of receptors which appear to have redundantly acting motifs in their cytoplasmic domains and in which a deletion of one of these motifs does not affect CAT gene

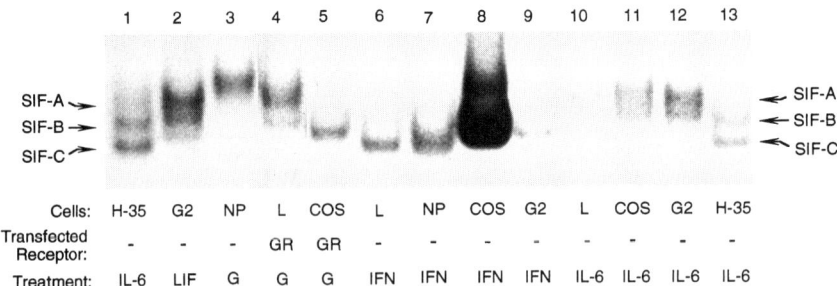

FIGURE 9. Relative mobilities of cytokine-induced SIF complexes. Whole cell extracts derived from H-35 cells, HepG2 cells (G2), primary human neutrophils (NP), L-cells (L), and COS-1 cells (COS). Also included were extracts from L-cells and COS-1 cells transfected with full-length G-CSFR (isoform D7) (GR). The treatments were all carried out for 15 min and included the cytokines IL-6, LIF, G-CSF (G) and IFN-γ (IFN). All extracts were reacted with ^{32}P-labeled SIE, and the binding reactions were analyzed on one gel. To provide an optimal presentation of the relative position of the major binding complex, a 4 h exposure of the gel for lanes 1–3 and 5–13 was used. For lane 4, a 16 h exposure was needed.

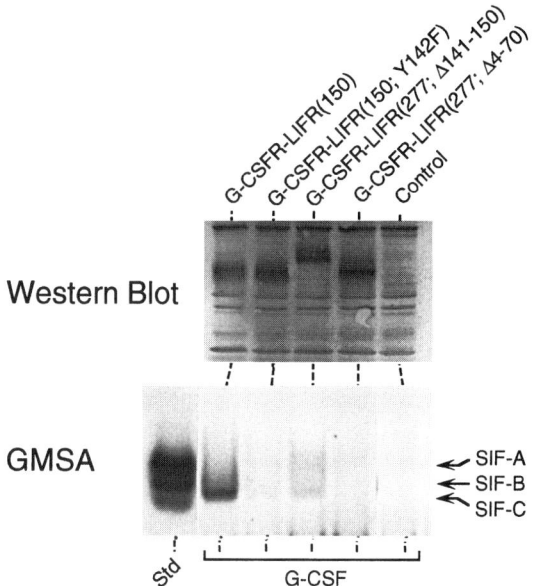

FIGURE 10. SIF-inducing activities of mutant forms of G-CSFR-LIFR chimeras. COS-1 cells in 10 cm dishes were transfected with expression vectors for the mutant G-CSFR-LIFR forms indicated at the top. Control culture represents non-transfected COS-1 cells. After stimulation for 15 min with G-CSF, the cells were divided into two parts which were processed for Western blot analysis of the G-CSFR and GMSA of SIFs as in FIGURE 8.

regulation in hepatoma cells. G-CSFR-LIFR chimera represents a prime example. By progressive carboxy terminal deletion mutation, we defined the functional relevance of box 3 at position 141 to 150 (containing the critical tyrosine residue at 142) for IL-6RE CAT gene regulation and yet observed that a deletion of this 10 residue sequence from the full-length cytoplasmic LIFR domain did not impair the IL-6 signal.[27] We have speculated that the region carboxy terminal to box 3 exerted a function redundant to box 3. Transfection of expression vectors for these chimeric receptor forms into COS-1 cells (FIG. 10) revealed that these vectors produced similar levels of the receptor protein. The minimal G-CSFR-LIFR(150) activated SIF-C, whereas the same receptor containing the mutation Y142F was ineffective. The chimeric receptor with the internal box 3 deletion ($\Delta 141-150$) displayed a detectable but much lower SIF stimulating activity than G-SFR-LIFR(150), suggesting that box 3 is indeed a major but not sole determinant of interaction with the signaling mechanism. The cooperativity of separate elements is demonstrated by the fact that box 3 motif is only active in the presence of the region containing box 1 and 2. G-CSFR-LIFR(277) with the internal deletion of residues 4 to 70 ($\Delta 4-70$) proved to be inactive in stimulating SIF (FIG. 10) and CAT reporter genes.[27]

CONCLUSION

In these studies, we attempted to define common functional properties of representative members of the hematopoietin receptor family. We devised experimental systems that allowed the identification of the structural regions in the cytoplasmic receptor domain that determine the specificity of gene regulation in rat hepatoma and the interaction with signal-transduction mechanisms in fibroblasts that lead to activation of Stat proteins. The data are summarized in TABLE 1 and indicate that regulation by hematopoietin receptors involves several signaling elements and that gene regulation cannot be strictly correlated with the activation of SIFs.

Major issues yet to be addressed are: 1) what is the identity of the signal-initiating kinases that interact with the specific cytoplasmic domains; 2) which of the kinase actions are causal to gene regulation; 3) which of the Stat- or DNA-binding proteins are mediating the activation of specific reporter gene constructs; and 4) what are the precise contributions of ubiquitous and cell-type restricted signaling components to the function of hematopoietin receptors?

ACKNOWLEDGMENTS

We thank Drs. J. N. Ihle and B. A. Witthuhn, St Jude Children's Research Hospital, Memphis, TN, for providing the expression vector for murine EPOR; Dr. W. I. Wood, Genentech, for rabbit GHR cDNA; Drs. G. G. Wong and P. Schendel, Genetics Institute, for human recombinant IL-6 and IL-11; Dr. G. Wong, Genentech for murine and human IFN-γ; and Marcia Held for secretarial assistance.

REFERENCES

1. MACKIEWICZ, A., A. KUSHNER & H. BAUMANN, Eds. 1993. Acute Phase Proteins. Molecular Biology, Biochemistry and Clinical Applications. Boca Raton, FL: CRC Press, Inc.
2. BAUMANN, H. & J. GAULDIE. 1994. Immunol. Today **15**: 74–80.
3. BAZAN, J. F. 1990. Proc. Natl. Acad. Sci. USA **87**: 6934–6938.
4. MIYAJIMA, A., T. KITAMURA, N. HARADA, T. YOKATA & K. ARAI. 1992. Ann. Rev. Immunol. **10**: 295–331.
5. MURAKAMI, M., M. HIBI, N. NAKAGAWA, T. NAKAGAWA, K. YASUKAMA, K. YAMANISHI, T. TAGA & T. KISHIMOTO. 1993. Science **260**: 1808–1810.
6. STAHL, N. & G. D. YANCOPOULOS. 1993. Cell **74**: 587–590.
7. FUKUNAGA, R., I. E. ISHIZAKA, C. X. PAN, Y. SETO & S. NAGATA. 1991. EMBO J. **10**: 2855–2865.
8. WATOWICH, S. S., A. YOSHIMURA, G. D. LONGMORE, D. J. HILTON, Y. YOSHIMURA & H. F. LODISH. 1992. Proc. Natl. Acad. Sci. USA **89**: 2140–2144.
9. DE VOS, A. M., M. ULTSCH & A. A. KOSSIAKOFF. 1992. Science **255**: 306–312.
10. ULTSCH, M. & A. M. DE VOS. 1993. J. Mol. Biol. **231**: 1133–1136.
11. VIGON, I., C. FLORINDO, S. FICHELSON, J.-L. GUENET, M. G. MATTEI, M. SOUYRI, D. COSMAN & S. GISSELBRECHT. 1993. Oncogene **8**: 2607–2615.
12. DARNELL, J. E., JR., I. M. KERR & G. R. STARK. 1994. Science **264**: 1415–1421.
13. IHLE, J. N. 1994. Trends Endocrin. Metab. **5**: 137–143.
14. WILKS, A. F. & A. G. HARPUR. 1994. BioEssays **16**: 313–320.
15. TORIGOE, T., H. U. SARAGOORI & J. C. REED. 1992. Proc. Natl. Acad. Sci. USA **89**: 2674–2678.
16. ERNST, M., D. P. GEARING & A. R. DUNN. 1994. EMBO J. **13**: 1574–1584.
17. COREY, S. J., A. L. BURKHARDT, J. B. BOLEN, R. L. GEAHEEN, L. S. TKATCH & D. J. TWEARDY. 1994. Proc. Natl. Acad. Sci. USA **91**: 4683–4687.
18. SADOWSKI, H. B., K. SHURAI, J. E. DARNELL, JR. & M. Z. GILMAN. 1993. Science **261**: 1739–1744.
19. ZHONG, Z., Z. WEN & J. E. DARNELL, JR. 1994. Science **264**: 95–98.
20. LAI, C.-F., S. IMMUENSCHUH, D. P. GEARING, S. F. ZIEGLER & H. BAUMANN. Mutation

of the box 3 motif in gp130 resulted in a concomitant loss of STAT activation and gene regulation via the interleukin-6 response element. Submitted.
21. SHUAI, K., C. M. HORVATH, L. H. TSAI-HUANG, S. QURESHI, D. COWBURN & J. E. DARNELL, JR. 1994. Cell 76: 821–828.
22. AKIRA, S., Y. NISHIO, M. IUONE, X.-J. WANG, S. WEI, T. MATSUSAKA, K. YOSHIDA, T. SUDO, M. NARUTO & T. KISHIMOTO. 1994. Cell 77: 63–71.
23. ASAO, H., T. TAKESHITA, N. ISHII, S. KUMAKI, M. NAKAMURA & K. SUGAMURA. 1993. Proc. Natl. Acad. Sci. USA 90: 4127–4131.
24. SATOR, N., K. SAKAMAKI, N. TERADA, K.-I. ARAI & A. MIYAJIMA. 1993. EMBO J. 12: 4181–4189.
25. FUKUNAGA, R., E. ISHIZAKA-IKEDA & S. NAGATA. 1993. Cell 74: 1079–1087.
26. ZIEGLER, S. F., T. A. BIRD, K. K. MORELLA, D. MOSLEY, D. GEARING & H. BAUMANN. 1993. Mol. Cell. Biol. 13: 2384–2390.
27. BAUMANN, H., A. J. SYMES, M. R. COMEAU, K. K. MORELLA, Y. WANG, D. FRIEND, S. F. ZIEGLER, J. S. FINK & D. GEARING. 1994. Mol. Cell. Biol. 14: 138–146.
28. BAUMANN, H., D. GEARING & S. F. ZIEGLER. 1994. J. Biol. Chem. 269: 16297–16304.
29. BAUMANN, H., K. R. PROWSE, S. MARINKOVIC, K.-A. WON & G. P. JAHREIS. 1989. Ann. N.Y. Acad. Sci. 557: 280–297.
30. IMMENSCHUH, S., Y. NAGAE, H. SATOH, H. BAUMANN & U. MULLER-EBERHARD. 1994. J. Biol. Chem. 269: 12654–12661.
31. HATTORI, M., L. J. ABRAHAM, W. NORTHEMANN & G. H. FEY. 1990. Proc. Natl. Acad. Sci. USA 87: 2364–2368.
32. BAUMANN, H., K. MORELLA, S. P. CAMPOS, Z. CAO & G. P. JAHREIS. 1992. J. Biol. Chem. 267: 19744–19751.
33. BAUMANN, H., K. K. MORELLA & S. P. CAMPOS. 1993. J. Biol. Chem. 268: 10495–10500.
34. COLOSI, P., K. WONG, S. R. LEONG & W. I. WOOD. 1993. J. Biol. Chem. 268: 12617–12623.
35. HATAKEYAMA, M., H. MORI, T. DOI & T. TANIGUCHI. 1989. Cell 59: 837–845.
36. D'ANDREA, A. D., A. YOSHIMURA, H. YOUSSOUFIAN, L. I. ZON, J. W. KOO & H. F. LODISH. 1991. Mol. Cell. Biol. 11: 1980–1987.
37. MIURA, O., J. L. CLEVELAND & J. N. IHLE. 1993. Mol. Cell. Biol. 13: 1788–1795.
38. QUELLE, D. E. & D. M. WOJCHOWSKI. 1991. Proc. Natl. Acad. Sci. USA 88: 4801–4805.
39. MURAKAMI, M., M. NARAZAKI, M. HIBI, H. YAWATA, K. YASUKAWA, M. HAMAGUCHI, T. TAGA & T. KISHIMOTO. 1991. Proc. Natl. Acad. Sci. USA 88: 11349–11353.
40. WON, K.-A. & H. BAUMANN. 1990. Mol. Cell. Biol. 10: 3965–3978.
41. CAMPOS, S. P., Y. WANG, A. KOJ & H. BAUMANN. 1994. Cytokine. 6: 485–492.
42. BAUMANN, H. & G. G. WONG. 1989. J. Immunol. 143: 1163–1167.
43. MORELLA, K. K., C.-F. LAI, N. KUMAKI, S. KUMAKI, Y. WANG, J. N. IHLE, J. GIRI, D. COSMAN, D. J. TWEARDY, S. P. CAMPOS & H. BAUMANN. 1995. IL-2 receptor defines a new type of signaling mechanism for hematopoietin receptors in hepatic cells and fibroblasts. J. Biol. Chem. In press.
44. ZIEGLER, S. F., K. K. MORELLA, D. ANDERSON, N. KUMAKI, W. J. LEONARD, D. COSMAN & H. BAUMANN. 1995. Eur. J. Immunol. 25: 399–404.
45. GOODWIN, R. G., D. FRIEND, S. F. ZIEGLER, R. JERZY, B. A. FALK, S. GIMPEL, D. COSMAN, S. K. DOWER, C. J. MARCH, A. E. NAMEN & L. S. PARK. 1990. Cell 60: 941–951.
46. MOSLEY, B., M. P. BECKMANN, C. J. MARCH, R. L. IDZERDA, S. D. GIMPEL, T. VAN-DENBOS, D. FRIEND, A. ALPERT, D. ANDERSON, J. JACKSON, J. M. WIGNALL, C. SMITH, G. GALLIS, J. E. SIMS, D. URDAL, M. B. WIDMER, D. COSMAN & L. S. PARK. 1989. Cell 59: 335–348.
47. WITTHUHN, B. A., F. W. QUELLE, O. SILVERNNOINEU, T. YI, B. TANG, D. MIVRA & J. N. IHLE. 1993. Cell 74: 227–236.
48. LARSEN, A., T. DAVIS, B. M. CURTIS, S. GIMPEL, J. E. SIMS, D. COSMAN, L. PARK, E. SORENSEN, C. J. MARH & C. A. SMITH. 1990. J. Exp. Med. 172: 1559–1570.
49. TWEARDY, D. J., K. ANDERSON, L. A. CANNIZZARO, R. A. STEINMAN, C. M. CROCE & K. HUEBNER. 1992. Blood 79: 1148–1154.

DISCUSSION OF THE PAPER

T. HIRANO (*Osaka University School of Medicine, Osaka, Japan*): Jak family tyrosine kinase may play an important role in activation of Stat factors, so is there any correlation between Jak kinase activation and inducibility of their SIE in your deletion experiments?

H. BAUMANN: We do not know, because we have not determined Jak activation. There are two reasons: One, transiently transfected hepatoma cells do not give us enough receptor expression for immunological detection of the receptor proteins and their associated kinases. And, two, transfection of COS or L-cells, although excellent for obtaining high levels of receptor proteins (about 100,000 to 1,000,000 binding sites per transfected cell) results in a system in which the receptors are in vast excess to the kinases. Our initial attempts to use these cells has failed to detect ligand-induced phosphorylation of receptors or kinases.

L. AARDEN (*Netherlands Red Cross Blood Transfusion Service, Amsterdam*): You saw dissociation between the Epo receptor, for example, between Stat and IL-6 receptor element activation. Is this a lack of activation or could it be a dominant negative effect? Have you looked for that possibility?

BAUMANN: EpoR and growth hormone receptors are capable of activating Stat proteins, but do not affect expression of CAT reporter gene constructs containing the IL-6REs. However, these receptors can prominently signal via the "hematopoietin receptor response element." At present, we cannot prove whether Stat activities, which are detected by the SIE probe, are indeed causal to gene regulation via the IL-6RE. Do EpoR and GHR exert a dominant negative signal? Probably not, because when EpoR or GHR-transfected cells were treated with the combination of Epo or GH and IL-6, we observed a normal IL-6 signal.

The Soluble Interleukin-6 Receptor[a]

STEFAN ROSE-JOHN,[b] MARC EHLERS,[c]
JOACHIM GRÖTZINGER, AND JÜRGEN MÜLLBERG[d]

*First Department of Internal Medicine
Section Pathophysiology,
University of Mainz
Obere Zahlbacher Str. 63
D-55101 Mainz, Germany
and
Department of Biochemistry
RWTH Aachen
Pauwelsstraße 30
D-52057 Aachen, Germany*

INTRODUCTION

The cellular receptor for interleukin-6 (IL-6) consists of at least two transmembrane proteins, an 80 kD ligand binding glycoprotein (IL-6R) and a 130 kD glycoprotein involved in signal transduction (gp130).[1-3] IL-6 first binds to the IL-6R and this complex subsequently associates with two gp130 molecules. The signal-transducing complex consists of IL-6, IL-6R, and a disulfide linked dimer of gp130.[4,5] In addition crosslinking experiments with purified IL-6 and soluble IL-6R proteins revealed complexes which from their relative electrophoretic mobility could be interpreted as dimeric IL-6 bound to dimeric IL-6R.[6] According to this view the active IL-6 receptor complex would be a hexamer of 2 molecules each of IL-6, IL-6R, and gp130.

Like other cytokine receptor proteins the two subunits of the IL-6 receptor complex are expressed at very low numbers (about 500–2000 copies per cell).[7] The expression of the IL-6R is upregulated by glucocorticoids whereas the gp 130 protein is upregulated by IL-6.[7-9]

Interestingly, soluble forms of the IL-6R and of gp130 have been detected in various body fluids of healthy donors.[10-12] Such soluble cytokine receptors have recently attracted a lot of attention since they seem to modulate the responses of the cognate cytokines.[13,14]

In the present article we focus on the mechanism of generation of soluble forms of both subunits of the IL-6 receptor complex and the state of the present knowledge of the molecular interaction between the ligand IL-6 and the two soluble receptor subunits.

---

[a] The experimental work described in this article has been supported by grants from the Deutsche Forschungsgemeinschaft, Bonn, Germany.
[b] Address correspondence to Dr. Stefan Rose-John at the First Department of Internal Medicine, Section Pathophysiology, Obere Zahlbacher Strasse 63. Johannes Gutenberg Universität, Mainz, 55101 Mainz, Germany. Tel: 49-6131-173363. E-Mail-ROSE@MZD-MZA.ZDV.UNI-MAINZ.DE.
[c] *Present address*: First Department of Internal Medicine, NMFZ, Langenbeckstrasse 63, Johannes Gutenberg Universität Mainz, 55101, Mainz, Germany.
[d] *Present address*: Immunex Corp., 51 University Street, Seattle, WA 98101, USA.

THE SOLUBLE IL-6R PROTEIN

Studying the biosynthesis of the IL-6R in transfected cells we noticed that the 80 kD membrane bound IL-6R was proteolytically cleaved and a 55 kD soluble protein was released into the supernatant (FIG. 1). Shedding of the IL-6R is dramatically increased after treatment of the IL-6R expressing cells with the phorbol ester 4β-phorbol-12-myristate-13-acetate (PMA) (FIG. 2). This activation of shedding by PMA occurs within 20–40 min and is brought about via specific activation of protein kinase C.[15,16] Primary human monocytes when treated with PMA released a soluble form of the IL-6R indicating that the soluble IL-6R found in human serum might be produced by these cells (FIG. 3).[15,16] The proteolytic cleavage site of the IL-6R has been determined to be immediately adjacent to the transmembrane domain between Gln357 and Asp358 (FIG. 4).[17] Mutational analysis of the cleavage site revealed no strict consensus sequence for a protease. It is therefore likely that not a sequence but rather a structural motif is recognized by the shedding protease.[17] Comparison with known cleavage sites of transmembrane proteins showed no similarities (TABLE 1) of the IL-6R cleavage site and those of five additional transmembrane proteins. Interestingly the shedding protease could not be inhibited by a cocktail of inhibitors of the four major classes of proteinases (serine-, acidic-, cystein-, metalloproteinases). Furthermore we could demonstrate that the cytoplasmic tail of the IL-6R protein, the phosphorylation of which is increased after treatment of cells with PMA, is not necessary for the regulation of shedding by PMA.[17] We conclude that the protease responsible for shedding of the IL-6R should be a transmembrane protein which is

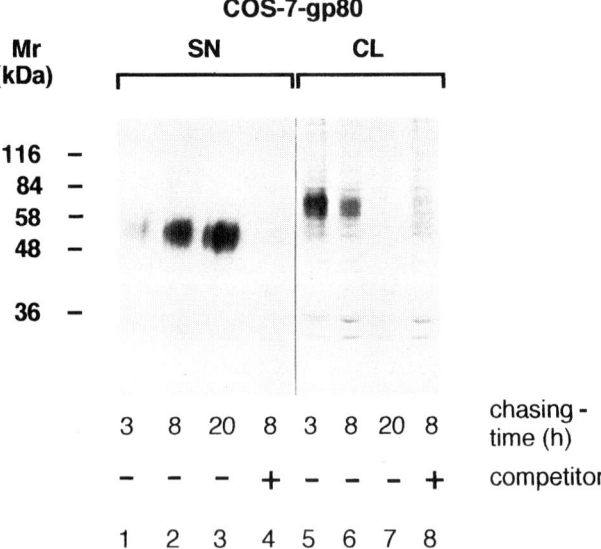

FIGURE 1. Release of a soluble form of the membrane-bound gp80 IL-6R protein by transfected COS-7 cells. 2×10^6 COS-7-gp80 cells were labeled with 50 μCi Tran[^{35}S]label in methionine/cysteine free medium for 2 h. After various times of chasing, supernatants (SN) (lanes 1–3) and cell lysates (CL) (lanes 5–7) were immunoprecipitated with a gp80 specific antiserum and analyzed by SDS-PAGE and fluorography. 1 μg of the extracellular domain of gp80 expressed in *E. coli* was added as competitor before immunoprecipitation (lanes 4, 8).

FIGURE 2. Stimulation of shedding of gp80 IL-6R by the phorbol ester 4β-phorbol-12-myristate-13-acetate (PMA). 2×10^6 COS-7-gp80 cells were labeled as described in the legend of FIGURE 1. After 1 h of chasing cells were incubated with 10^{-7} M PMA for 1 h as indicated in the figure. Cell lysates (CL) and supernatants (SN) were immunoprecipitated and analyzed by SDS-PAGE and fluorography.

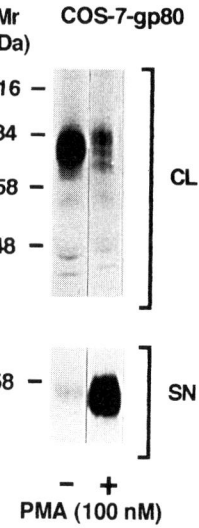

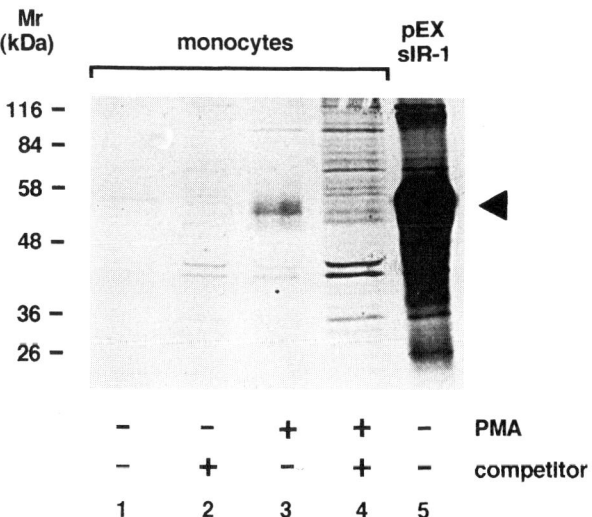

FIGURE 3. Generation of a soluble IL-6R by human peripheral blood monocytes. 10^8 primary human monocytes were labeled with 500 μCi Tran[^{35}S]label for 16 h in the absence (lanes 1, 2) or presence (lanes 3, 4) of 10^{-7} M PMA. Culture supernatants were immunoprecipitated and analyzed by SDS-PAGE and fluorography. 1 μg of the extracellular domain of gp80 expressed in E. coli was added as competitor before immunoprecipitation (lanes 2, 4). For comparison, the extracellular domain of gp80 secreted by stably transfected NIH/3T3 cells (*arrowhead*) was analyzed (lane 5).

210　　　　　　　　　　　　ANNALS NEW YORK ACADEMY OF SCIENCES

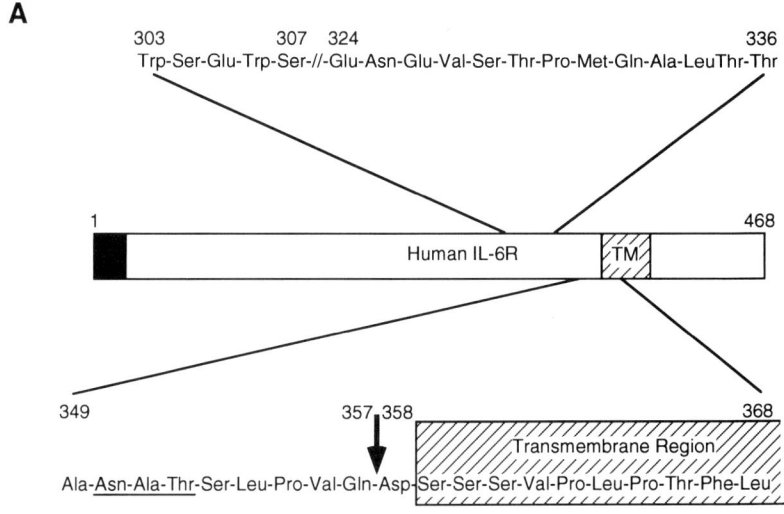

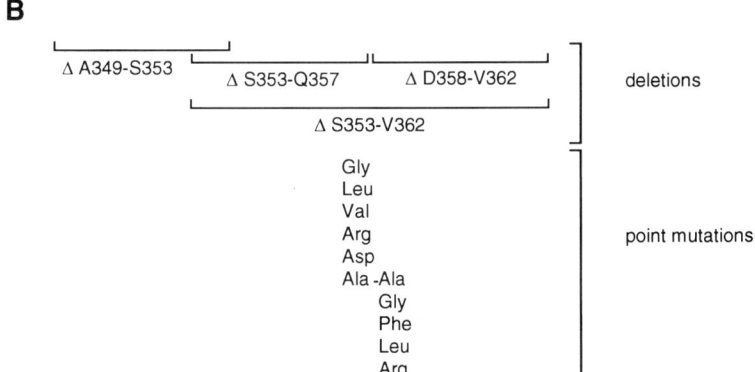

FIGURE 4. Schematic representation of the human IL-6R protein. **A:** The IL-6R protein is shown as an open bar with the signal peptide indicated by the filled and the transmembrane domain (TM) by the shaded box. Sequence elements like the WSXWS box, the recognition epitope of the anti-IL-6R antiserum and the determined cleavage site are highlighted. **B:** Deletion mutations and point mutations introduced around the cleavage site of the IL-6R.

TABLE 1. Comparison of Proteolytic Cleavage Sites of Several Membrane Proteins

IL-6R	LPVQ ⇓ DSSS
TNFR	PLAN ⇓ VTNP
EGF	WELR ⇓ HAGH
TGFα	DLLR ⇓ VVAA
AR	CGEK ⇓ SNKT
KL	PPVA ⇓ ASSR

For references see Müllberg et al.[17]

stimulated by PMA-stimulated phosphorylation at its cytoplasmic portion activating the extracellular part of the protease leading to the specific cleavage of the IL-6R protein.[17]

THE SOLUBLE FORM OF gp130

The biosynthesis of gp130 was studied in a similar fashion as in the case of the IL-6R protein.[18] In order to directly compare shedding of IL-6R and gp130, both proteins were overexpressed in the same type of cell and the release of soluble receptor forms was analyzed.[18] It turned out that also the gp130 protein is cleaved by a shedding protease to release a 100 kD soluble protein. The soluble form of the gp130 protein is recognized by three monoclonal antibodies raised against the membrane associated gp130 protein.[18] This fact together with the size of the soluble form of gp130[12,18] is an indication that the proteolytic cleavage site should be located close to the transmembrane region of the gp130 receptor protein. Interestingly, the extent to which shedding of gp130 occurs is much smaller (about 1%) when compared with the IL-6R protein (FIG. 5). Moreover, for the shedding protease responsible for the release of the soluble form of gp 130 no stimulation by PMA has been observed.[18] We conclude from these studies that shedding is not an unspecific release of all membrane proteins and that most likely two different shedding proteases are responsible for the release of soluble forms of the two IL-6 receptor subunits IL-6R and gp130.[15-18]

THE COMPLEX OF SOLUBLE IL-6R AND IL-6

The soluble IL-6R binds the ligand IL-6 with comparable affinity as the membrane-associated receptor.[6] Moreover, IL-6 bound to the soluble IL-6R generated by shed-

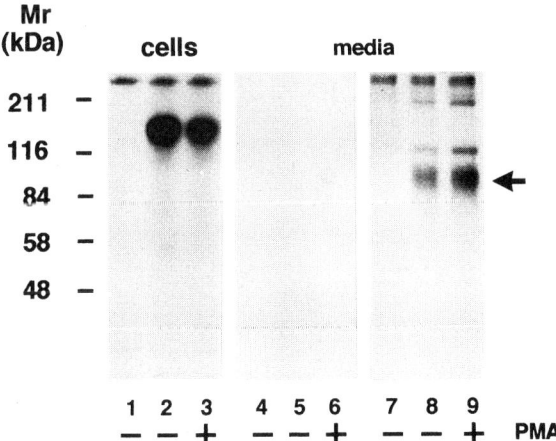

FIGURE 5. Generation of a soluble form of gp130 by limited proteolysis. MDCK-gp130 cells constitutively expressing gp130 were radioactively labeled and immunoprecipitated. Lanes 7 to 9 are identical with lanes 4 to 6 except that they were exposed ten times longer. Immunoprecipitations were performed with the gp130 specific mAb AM64. Soluble gp130 is marked by an arrow.

ding elicits an IL-6–specific signal on cells which express gp130 but not the IL-6R protein on the cell surface;[19,20] *i.e.*, which would not be able to bind IL-6 or react on IL-6. This implies that cells by releasing the soluble IL-6R protein render other cells responsive to IL-6 (*trans*-signaling). From all soluble cytokine and growth-factor receptors such an agonistic function has only been described for the IL-6R and a soluble form of the ciliary neurotrophic factor (CNTF) receptor (see ref. 14 for review).

A recently recognized example of an important physiological function of the soluble IL-6 is the regulation of the balance between osteoclasts and osteoblasts. This balance is influence by steroid hormones which act by stimulating the release of cytokines like IL-1, tumor necrosis factor (INF)-α, and IL-6.[21] The formation of osteoclasts is not stimulated by IL-6 alone but only by the combination of IL-6 and the soluble IL-6R.[22] The authors conclude that the target cells probably do not express the IL-6R protein and are dependent in their responsiveness to IL-6 on the soluble IL-6R released by other cells.[22] In line with these experiments it has been found that mice lacking endogenous IL-6 do not develop osteoporotic symptoms after ovariectomy, which in wild type animals caused a significant loss of bone matter together with an increase in bone turnover rates.[23] These experiments indicate a key role for IL-6 and the soluble IL-6R in the pathogenesis of osteoporosis.[22,23]

THE COMPLEX OF IL-6, SOLUBLE IL-6R, AND SOLUBLE gp130

It has been shown that the signal transducing complex of the IL-6 receptor system on the cell membrane consists of a disulfide linked dimer of gp130 associated with the IL-6/IL-6R complex.[4,5,24,25] Having demonstrated that soluble forms of the IL-6R and the gp130 protein are generated by shedding of the membrane-associated proteins,[15–18] we asked the question whether the soluble forms of IL-6R and gp130 together with IL-6 could form a ternary complex in solution. FIGURE 6 shows that in the presence of non-radioactively labeled IL-6 and soluble IL-6R metabolically labeled gp130 released from transfected MDCK cells by shedding could be immunoprecipitated with an antiserum directed against the soluble IL-6R.[6] These results clearly demonstrate that both soluble forms of the IL-6 receptor system associate in solution in the presence of the ligand IL-6.

These data have important implications. In the plasma of healthy donors levels of soluble IL-6R have been reported to be as high as 70 ng/ml.[11] Blood levels of soluble gp130 have been measured to be 300 ng/ml.[12] Since IL-6 concentration in healthy individuals are in the range of 1–50 pg/ml and the affinity of the soluble IL-6R is about 10^{-9} M, it can be assumed that all IL-6 in the circulation is bound to the soluble IL-6R. Furthermore there is a large depot of soluble(s) IL-6R molecules which might bind IL-6 which is synthesized after stimulation by monocytes, fibroblasts or endothelial cells.[26] The soluble form of gp130 has no detectable binding affinity for IL-6.[3,12,18] The association constant between IL-6/IL-6R and the soluble gp130 protein is not known, but the ternary complex can be detected in the serum of patients[12] and could be demonstrated to have antagonistic activity;[12] *i.e.*, the agonistically acting complex of IL-6 and IL-6R can be neutralized by the circulating soluble form of the gp130 protein.

In consequence of these findings we will have to reassess the concentrations and biological activities of IL-6 and its circulating receptor components. The accuracy of ELISAs and biological assays for IL-6 will have to be checked for the possible interference by the soluble receptor components sIL-6R or sgp130. The biological activity

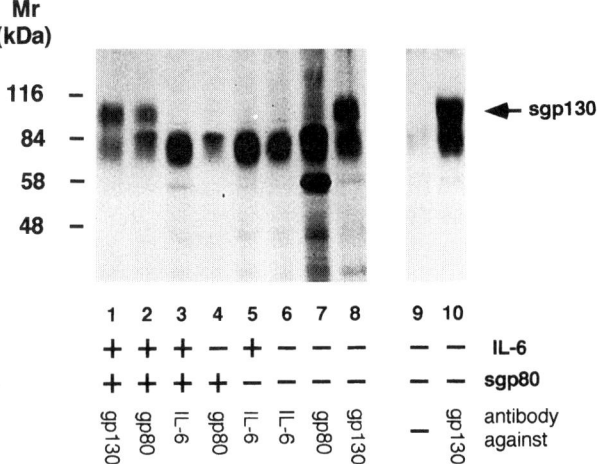

FIGURE 6. Formation of a ternary complex of IL-6, soluble IL-6R and soluble gp130. 2×10^7 MDCK-gp130 cells were labeled with 500 µCi Tran[^{35}S]label in methionine/cysteine-free medium for 2 h and subsequently chased for 16 h. To aliquots of labeled MDCK-gp130 culture medium 100 ng recombinant human IL-6 and 500 ng soluble IL-6R protein in conditioned cell culture medium were added as indicated in the figure. Immunoprecipitations were carried out using antibodies against IL-6 (polyclonal antiserum), the IL-6R (polyclonal antiserum) and gp130 (mAb AM64) as indicated in the figure.

of IL-6 can only be predicted when the concentrations of all soluble receptor components are known and the binding constants between all these components have been elucidated.

SOLUBLE FORMS OF RECEPTOR SUBUNITS OF THE IL-6–RELATED CYTOKINES LIF, CNTF, AND OSM

The IL-6 signal-transducing protein gp130 has been shown to be a component of the signaling complexes for leukemia inhibitory factor (LIF), CNTF, oncostatin M (OSM), and IL-11.[24,27] For the LIF-R protein which is the second subunit of the LIF-, OSM-, and CNTF-receptor complex, the existence of a soluble form has been demonstrated.[28] This soluble protein which is present in the serum at levels of about 1 µg/ml has been shown to exhibit antagonistic activity, i.e., the soluble receptor competes with the membrane receptor for the ligand LIF.[28]

The complex of CNTF and the CNTF-R together with gp130 and the LIF-R forms the CNTF receptor signal-transducing complex. Recently it has been demonstrated that a complex between LIF-R and CNTF/CNTF-R is formed on cells which express the LIF-R but not the gp130 protein. Such a complex presumably does not elicit a CNTF specific signal but it can be assumed that it leads to a depletion of LIF-R molecules which are not available for signaling.[29] It is not known whether the LIF-R in such a situation dimerizes. It has, however, recently been shown that in a chimeric G-CSF/LIF-R protein with an extracellular G-CSF and an intracellular LIF-R portion, the G-CSF triggered dimerization of the chimeric receptor lead to a LIF-specific signal, indicating that dimerization of the cytoplasmic domain of the LIF-R is sufficient to initiate signal transduction.[30] These results might indicate that in the presence of the CNTF/CNTF-R complex no dimerization of the LIF-R protein occurs.

A somehow similar situation has been described for the interaction of gp130 and OSM. OSM binds directly to the gp130 protein and signals via a gp130/LIF-R heterodime.[27] On the human hepatoma cell line Hep3B which has been shown to express the gp130 but not the LIF-R protein it has been demonstrated that high concentration of OSM can occupy all available gp130 proteins which in turn can not be used by IL-6 signaling.[31] On these cells OSM acts indeed as an IL-6 antagonist.

The situation that CNTF/CNTF-R complexes bind to the LIF-R or that OSM

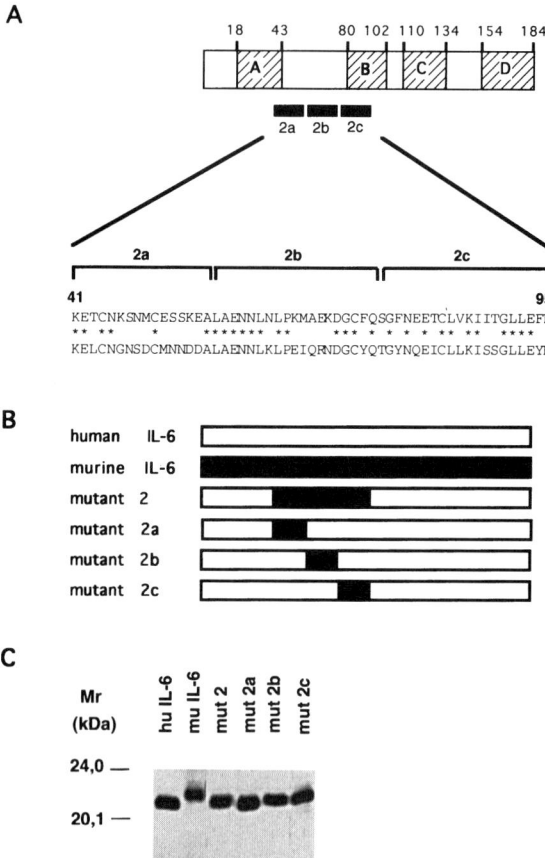

FIGURE 7. Chimeric human/murine IL-6 proteins. **A:** Representation of the human IL-6 protein with the four predicted α-helices shown as hatched boxes. Numbers indicate the predicted first and last residues of the α-helices. The amino acid sequence of the region 2 and its subdivision into the regions 2a, 2b, and 2c human (*top*) and murine (*bottom*) IL-6 is shown. **B:** Schematic representation of the human and murine IL-6 protein and chimeras thereof. **C:** The purified IL-6 variants are visualized by silverstaining after refolding, purification and SDS-PAGE.

binds directly to gp130 also applies for the soluble proteins. This immediately implies that high concentration of one cytokine of the IL-6, LIF, OSM, CNTF, IL-11 family can directly interfere with the biological activity of the other family members. Such a scenario is not likely to happen in the circulation but local concentrations of cytokines, *e.g.* in the synovia or other closed compartments can reach concentrations which make such a competition for soluble receptor components or complexes of soluble receptor components possible.

MOLECULAR DESIGN OF IL-6 RECEPTOR ANTAGONISTS

IL-6 is specifically recognized by the IL-6R and this complex associates with a dimer of gp130. It can therefore be concluded that on the surface of the IL-6 protein there should be several protein-protein interaction sites responsible for specific IL-6R and gp130 interaction. Structure-function analysis of IL-6 were used to establish the importance of the carboxy-terminus of IL-6 for binding to the IL-6R protein.[32-35]

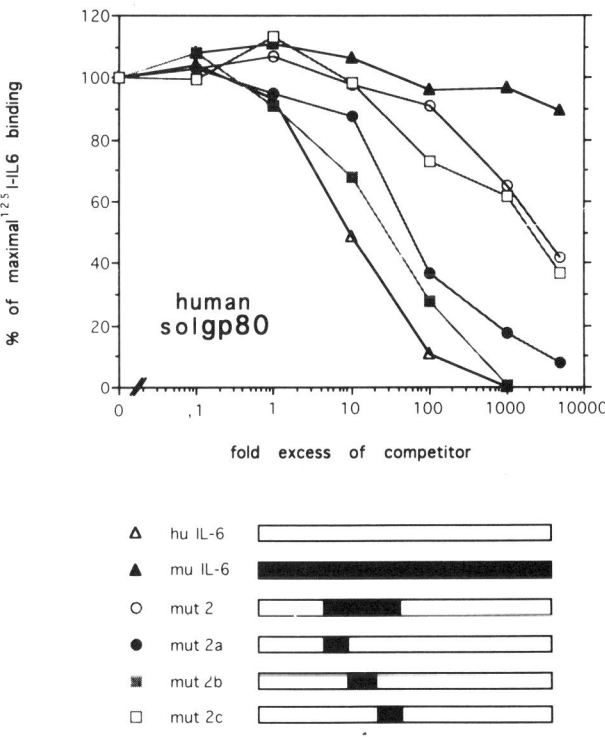

FIGURE 8. Binding of IL-6 variants to the soluble human IL-6R. Recombinant human soluble IL-6R was incubated with human ^{125}I-IL-6. Binding was competed with increasing amounts of human, murine or chimeric IL-6 proteins. The soluble IL-6R/IL-6 complexes were immunoprecipitated with a sIL-6R specific antiserum and protein A Sepharose. Radioactivity was determined by γ-counting.

In addition, the part of IL-6 comprising the long loop between the A and the B helix was implicated to be involved in the specific IL-6/IL-6R interaction.[36]

Studies with a panel of neutralizing monoclonal antibodies directed against human IL-6 resulted in the identification of two possible receptor interaction sites, called site I and site II.[37,38] It turned out that site I is identical with the C-terminus of the IL-6R whereas site II seemed to be involved in activation of gp130. Consequently, the introduction of point mutations in the region of site II which is located at the top of the D-helix of IL-6 lead to the establishment of a partial IL-6 receptor antagonist, *i.e.* a molecule which still binds to the IL-6R but can not activate gp130.[39]

Studies with human-murine chimeric IL-6 proteins identified two additional regions between helix A and helix B which turned out to be important for binding to the IL-6R (region 2C) and activation of gp130 (region 2A) (FIG. 7).[40] The specific interaction of region 2C with the IL-6R and of region 2A with gp130 was defined with the help of soluble receptor proteins[40] (FIGS. 8, 9). The exchange of region 2C with the corresponding murine sequences lead to a loss of binding to the soluble IL-6R. FIGURE 8 shows binding experiments in which the ability of the IL-6 variants to compete with human ^{125}I-IL-6 for soluble IL-6R binding is tested. The IL-6 protein with murine residues in region 2A failed to form a ternary complex between IL-6, soluble IL-6R and soluble gp130 (FIG. 9). Interestingly, in the tertiary structure

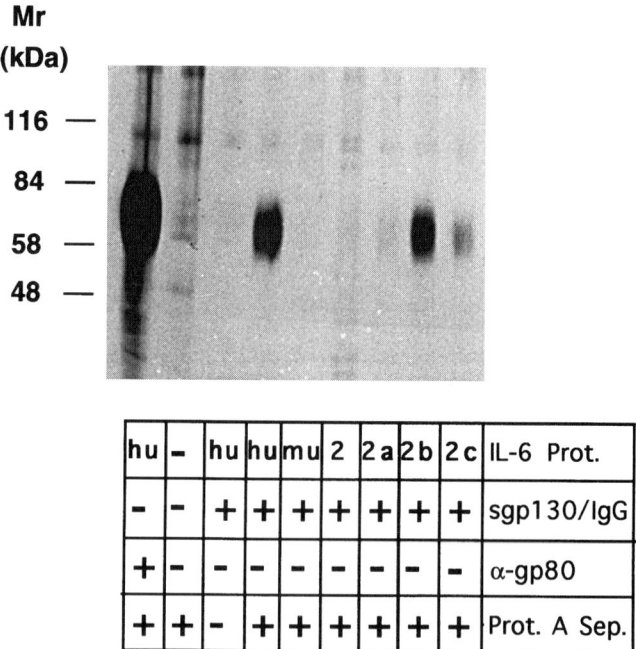

FIGURE 9. Induction of complex formation between soluble forms of IL-6R and gp130 by the IL-6 variants. Complex formation of sIL-6R, sgp130 and human, murine, or chimeric IL-6 proteins was determined using metabolically labeled [^{35}S]-sIL-6R and a fusion protein of human sgp130 and human IgG1. Complexes were precipitated with protein A Sepharose, separated by SDS-PAGE and visualized by fluorography.

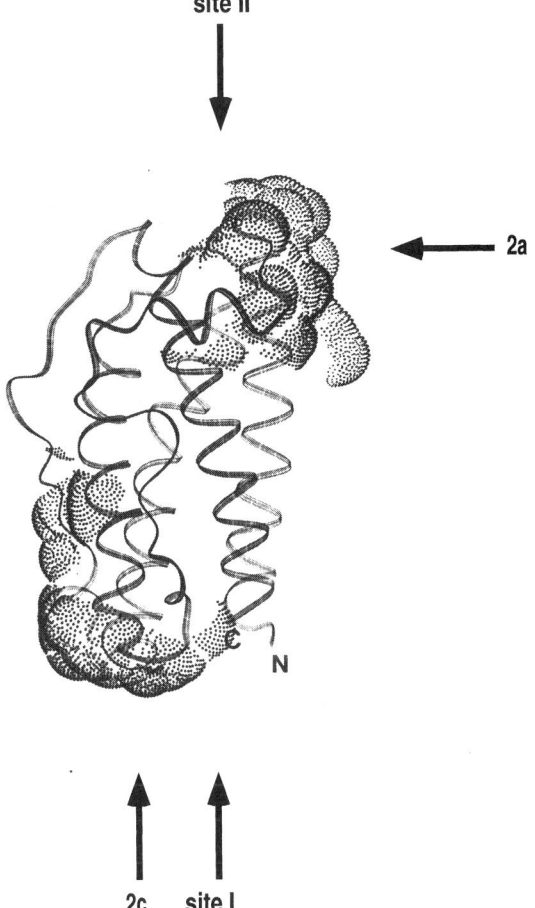

FIGURE 10. Three dimensional model of human IL-6. Ribbon representation of the human IL-6 model. Site I, site II, regions 2a and 2c (see text) are indicated by arrows. Site I and region 2c as well as site II and region 2a are in close contact. C, COOH-terminus; N, NH$_2$-terminus (corresponds to residue 17 of IL-6). The solvent-accessible surface of the regions 2a and 2c is shown in dotted surface mode.

of IL-6 which has been modeled according to the recently solved X-ray crystal structure of granulocyte colony stimulating factor,[41] region 2C which is involved in IL-6R binding is in close contact with site I whereas region 2A which activates gp130 is immediately adjacent to site II (FIG. 10). From these results we concluded that region 2C/site I and region 2A/site II form common discontinuous epitopes involved in IL-6R and gp130 interaction, respectively.[40]

In all cases when soluble IL-6 receptor proteins have been employed for structure function analysis of IL-6, the loss of ternary complex formation between IL-6, soluble IL-6R and soluble gp130 has been paralleled with a loss in biological activity of IL-6. FIGURE 11 shows an experiment in which the induction of gene expression of human haptoglobin by IL-6 variants is analyzed (comp. FIG. 9). Human IL-6 lead to full stimulation of haptoglobin gene expression whereas murine IL-6 showed no effect. Mutant 2 and the submutants 2A, 2B, and 2C were also analyzed. Mutant 2B fully stimulated haptoglobin gene expression, whereas cells treated with mutant 2C

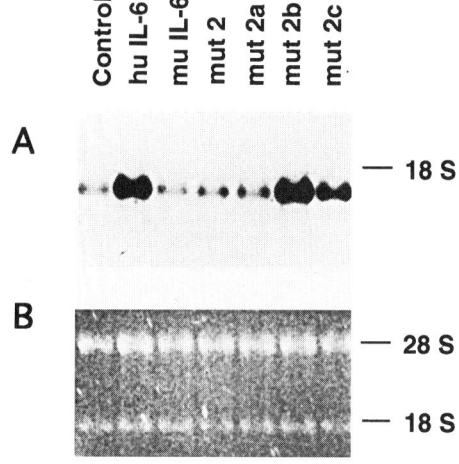

FIGURE. 11. Induction of haptoglobin gene expression in human hepatoma cells by IL-6 variants. **A:** HepG2 cells were treated for 18 h with 10 ng/ml of human, murine or chimeric IL-6 proteins. Total RNA was prepared and used for Northern blot analysis with a human ^{32}P-labeled haptoglobin cDNA as a probe. **B:** Photography of the ethidiumbromide stained RNA gel.

showed only weak gene induction. Mutant 2 and mutant 2A did not induce the expression of human haptoglobin mRNA (FIG. 11). It becomes clear from the comparison of FIGURE 9 and FIGURE 11 that complex formation between IL-6, soluble IL-6R and soluble gp130 is a good measure of the biological activity of variants of IL-6. This is also true for a number of additional structure-function studies of IL-6.[42-44] Therefore the study of the interaction between IL-6 variants and the soluble subunits of the IL-6 receptor complex is a powerful tool for the analysis of IL-6 and eventually for the rational design of human IL-6 receptor antagonists.

CONCLUSIONS

The receptor complex for the cytokine IL-6 consists of two transmembrane proteins, a ligand-binding subunit (IL-6R) and a signal-transducing protein (gp130). Both proteins are released from the cell by limited proteolysis (shedding) albeit at different efficiencies. The IL-6R is quantitatively shed after treatment of cells with the activator of protein kinase C, PMA whereas the signal-transducing subunit gp130 is only slowly released and no activation of this process by PMA is seen. The soluble IL-6R binds the ligand IL-6 with comparable affinity as the membrane-bound receptor. The complex of IL-6 and soluble IL-6R can associate in solution with the shed gp130 protein and with cell-associated gp130. Cells which only express gp130 can not be stimulated by IL-6 but by the complex of IL-6 and soluble IL-6R (*trans*-signaling). Therefore the regulated release of the soluble IL-6R protein is important to modulate the activity of the cytokine IL-6. Finally the soluble receptor subunits of the IL-6 receptor complex can be used to study the interaction of IL with the two receptor proteins. Hereby the agonistic or antagonistic potential of large numbers of IL-6 variants can be tested. This is a powerful approach for the rational design of human IL-6 receptor antagonists.

ACKNOWLEDGMENTS

The authors would like to thank U. Haßiepen and M. Robbertz for their expert help with the artwork.

[Note added in proof: After this manuscript was submitted for publication we have continued our structurfunction analysis of Interleukin-6 and have succeeded in constructing a highly effective Interleukin-6 receptor antagonist. This work is described in F. D. DeHon *et al.* 1994. J. Exp. Med. **180:** 2395–2400 and M. Ehlers *et al.* 1995. J. Biol Chem. **270:** 8158–8163.]

REFERENCES

1. YAMASAKI, K., T. TAGA, Y. HIRATA, H. YAWATA, Y. KAWANISHI, B. SEED, T. TANIGUCHI, T. HIRANO & T. KISHIMOTO. 1988. Science **241:** 825–828.
2. TAGA, T., M. HIBI, Y. HIRATA, K. YAMASAKI, T. MATSUDA, T. HIRANO & T. KISHIMOTO. 1989. Cell **58:** 573–581.
3. HIBI, M., M. MURAKAMI, M. SAITO, T. HIRANO. T. TAGA & T. KISHIMOTO. 1990. Cell **63:** 1149–1157.
4. MURAKAMI, M., M. HIBI, N. NAKAGAWA, T. NAKAGAWA, Y. YASUKAWA, K. YAMANISHI, T. TAGA & T. KISHIMOTO. 1993. Science **260:** 1808–1810.
5. DAVIS, S., T. H. ALDRICH, N. STAHL, L. PAN, T. TAGA, T. KISHIMOTO, N. Y. IP & G. D. YANCOPOULOS. 1993. Science **260:** 1805–1080.
6. STOYAN, T., U. MICHAELIS, H. SCHOOLTINK, M. VAN DAM, R. RUDOLPH, P. C. HEINRICH & S. ROSE-JOHN. 1993. Eur. J. Biochem. **216:** 239–245.
7. ROSE-JOHN, S., H. SCHOOLTINK, D. LENZ, E. HIPP, G. DUFHUES, H. SCHMITZ, X. SCHIEL, T. HIRANO, T. KISHIMOTO & P. C. HEINRICH. 1991. Eur. J. Biochem. **190:** 79–83.
8. SCHOOLTINK, H., T. STOYAN, D. LENZ, H. SCHMITZ, T. HIRANO, T. KISHIMOTO, P. C. HEINRICH & S. ROSE-JOHN. 1991. Biochem. J. **277:** 659–664.
9. SCHOOLTINK, H., H. SCHMITZ-VAN DE LEUR, P. C. HEINRICH & S. ROSE-JOHN. 1992. FEBS Lett. **297:** 263–265.
10. NOVICK, D., H. ENGELMANN, D. WALLACH & M. RUBINSTEIN. 1989. J. Exp. Med. **170:** 1409–1414.
11. HONDA, M., S. YAMAMOTO, M. CHENG, K. YASUKAWA, H. SUZUKI, T. SAITO, Y. OSUGI, T. TOKUNAGA & T. KISHIMOTO. 1992. J. Immunol. **148:** 2175–2180.
12. NARAZAKI, M., K. YASUKAWA, T. SAITO, Y. OHSUGI, H. FUKUI, Y. KOISHIHARA, G. D. YANCOPOULOS, T. TAGA & T. KISHIMOTO. 1993. Blood **82:** 1120–1126.
13. TEDER, T. F. 1991. Am. J. Respir. Cell. Mol. Biol. **5:** 305–306.
14. ROSE-JOHN, S. & P. C. HEINRICH. 1994. Biochem. J. **300:** 281–290.
15. MÜLLBERG, J., H. SCHOOLTINK, T. STOYAN, P. C. HEINRICH & S. ROSE-JOHN. 1992. Biochem. Biophys. Commun. **189:** 794–800.
16. MÜLLBERG, J., H. SCHOOLTINK, T. STOYAN, M. GÜNTHER, L. GRAEVE, G. BUSE, A. MACKIEWCIZ, P. C. HEINRICH & S. ROSE-JOHN. 1993. Eur. J. Immunol. **23:** 473–480.
17. MÜLLBERG, J., W. OBERTHÜR, F. LOTTSPEICH, E. MEHL, E. DITTRICH, L. GRAEVE, P. C. HEINRICH & S. ROSE-JOHN. 1994. J. Immunol. **152:** 4958–4968.
18. MÜLLBERG, J., E. DITTRICH, L. GRAEVE, C. GERHARTZ, K. YASUKAWA, T. TAGA, T. KISHIMOTO, P. C. HEINRICH & S. ROSE-JOHN. 1993. FEBS Lett. **332:** 174–178.
19. MACKIEWICZ, A., H. SCHOOLTINK, P. C. HEINRICH & S. ROSE-JOHN. 1992. J. Immunol. **149:** 2021–2027.
20. ROSE-JOHN, S., H. SCHOOLTINK, H. SCHMITZ-VAN DE LEUR, J. MÜLLBERG, P. C. HEINRICH & L. GRAEVE. 1993. J. Biol. Chem. **268:** 22084–22091.
21. HOROWITZ, H. C. 1993. Science **260:** 626–627.
22. TAMURA, T., N. UDAGAWA, N. TAKAHASHI, C. MIYURA, S. TANAKA, Y. YAMADA, Y. KOISHIHARA, Y. OHSUGA, K. KUMAKI, T. TAGA, T. KISHIMOTO & T. SUDA. 1993. Proc. Natl. Acad. Sci. USA **90:** 11924–11928.
23. POLI, V., R. BALENA, E. FATTORI, A. MARKATOS, M. YAMAMOTO, H. TANAKA, G. CILIBERTO, A. A. RODAN & F. COSNTANTINI. 1994. EMBO J. **13:** 1189–1196.
24. GEARING, D. P., M. R. CORMEAU, D. J. FRIEND, S. D. GIMPEL, C. T. THUT, J. MCGOURTY, K., K. BRASHER, J. A. KING, S. GILLIS, B. MOSLEY, S. F. ZIEGLER & D. COSMAN. 1992. Science **255:** 1434–1437.

25. STAHL, N. & G. D. YANCOPOULOS. 1993. Cell **74**: 587–590.
26. AKIRA, S., T. TAGA & T. KISHIMOTO. 1993. Adv. Immunol. 54: 1–78.
27. KISHIMOTO, T., . TAGA & S. AKIRA. 1994. Cell **76**: 253–262.
28. LAYTON, M. J., B. A. CROSS, D. METCALF, L. D. WARD, R. J. SIMPSON & N. A. NICOLA 1992. Proc. Natl. Acad. Sci. USA **89**: 8616–8620.
29. GEARING, D. P., S. F. ZIEGLER, M. R. COMEAU, D. FRIEND, B. THOMA, D. COSMAN, L. PARK & B. MOSLEY. 1994. Proc. Natl. Acad. Sci. USA **91**: 1119–1123.
30. BAUMANN, H., A. J. SYMES, M. R. COMEAU, K. K. MORELLA, Y. WANG, D. FRIEND, S. F. ZIEGLER, J. S. FINK & D. J. GEARING. 1994. Mol. Cell. Biol. **14**: 138–146.
31. SPORENO, E., G. PAONESSA, A. L. SALVATI, R. GRAZIANI, P. DELMASTRO, G. CILIBERTO & C. TONIATTI. 1994. J. Biol. Chem. **269**: 10991–10995.
32. KRÜTTGEN, A., S. ROSE-JOHN, C. MÖLLER, B. WROBLOWSKI, A. WOLLMER, J. MÜLLBERG, T. HIRANO, T. KISHIMOTO & P. C. HEINRICH. 1990. FEBS Lett **262**: 323–326.
33. KRÜTTGEN, A., S. ROSE-JOHN, G. DUFHUES, S. BENDER, C. LÜTTICKEN, P. FREYER & P. C. HEINRICH. 1990. FEBS Lett. **273**: 95–98.
34. LÜTTICKEN, C., A. KRÜUTTGEN, E. MÖLLER, P. C. HEINRICH & S. ROSE-JOHN. 1992. FEBS Lett. **282**: 265–267.
35. LEEBEEK, F. W. G., K. KARIYA, M. SCHWABE & D. M. FOWLKES. 1992. J. Biol. Chem. **267**: 14832–14838.
36. VAN DAM, M., J. MÜLLBERG, H. SCHOOLTINK, T. STOYAN, J. P. G. BRAKENHOFF, L. GRAEVE, P. C. HEINRICH & S. ROSE-JOHN. 1993. J. Biol. Chem. **268**: 15285–15290.
37. BRAKENHOFF, J. P. J., M. HART, E. R. DE GROOT, F. DI PADOVA & L. A. AARDEN. 1990. J. Immunol. **145**: 561–568.
38. BRAKENHOFF, J. P. J., F. D. DEHON, V. FONTAINE, M. HART, E. R. DE GROOT, J. CONTENT & L. A. AARDEN. 1992. Serono Symp. Publ. Raven Press **88**: 33–41.
39. BRAKENHOFF, J. P. J., F. D. DEHON, V. FONTAINE, E. TENBOEKEL, H. SCHOOLTINK, S. ROSE-JOHN, P. C. HEINRICH, J. CONTENT & L. A. AARDEN. 1994. J. Biol. Chem. **269**: 86–93.
40. EHLERS, M., A. GRÖTZINGER, F. D. DEHON, J. MÜLLBERG J. P. J. BRAKENHOFF, J. LIU, A. WOLLMER & S. ROSE-JOHN. 1994. J. Immunol. **153**: 1744–1753.
41. HILL, C. P., T. D. OSSLUND & D. EISENBERG. 1993. Proc. Natl. Acad. Sci. USA **90**: 5167–5171.
42. SAVINO, R., A. LAHM, A. L. SALVATI, L. CIAPPONI, E. SPORENO, S. ALTAMURA, G. POANESSA, C. TONIATTI & G. CILIBERTO. 1994. EMBO J. **13**: 1357–1367.
43. DEHON, F. D., M. EHLERS, S. ROSE-JOHN, S. EBELING, H. K. BOS, L. A. AARDEN & J. P. J. BRAKENHOFF. 1994. J. Exp. Med. **180**: 2395–2400.
44. DEHON, F. D., E. TEN BOEKEL, J. HERRMAN, C. CLEMENT, M. EHLERS, T. TAGA, K. YASUKAWA, Y. OHSUGI, T. KISHIMOTO, S. ROSE-JOHN, J. WIJDENES, R. KASTELEIN, L. A. AARDEN & J. P. J. BRAKENHOFF. 1995. Cytokine. In press.

DISCUSSION OF THE PAPER

G. CILIBERTO: (*Istituto di Ricerche di Biologia Molecolare P. Angeletti, Pomezia, (Rome), Italy*): Have you tried to block shedding by adding a large excess of peptide which contains the cleavage site?

S. ROSE-JOHN: No, we have not tried that.

CILIBERTO: Have you ever found a cell in which shedding does not take place?

ROSE-JOHN: No, we have not found such a cell. But we have been looking for one, because in the process of thinking about how to clone this protein we thought that we might find a negative cell and then try to expression clone it. So we went through at least 10–15 cell lines, and we have found none which cannot shed. Actually, we are now back to yeast and we are in the middle of experiments which look rather nice.

G. FEY (*University of Erlangen-Nürnberg, Erlangen, Germany*): I am curious about potential sequence specificity of your shedding proteases. You suggested that amino acids right outside transmembrane domain may be determining its specificity to some extent. Have you ever tried to take that sequence and insert it into another membrane? Would that lead to cleavage by the shedding proteins at that position?

ROSE-JOHN: That is in progress, but not done yet.

T. HIRANO (*Osaka University Medical School, Osaka, Japan*): Do you think that when PMA stimulation induces release of other surface molecules the same protease acts on other cell surface molecules?

ROSE-JOHN: It might very well be, we are just doing the experiment. Jürgen Müllberg, who is now at Immunex, has access to an inhibitor which apparently seems to inhibit shedding of TNF receptor. We are repeating this experiment, and it will tell us at least whether TNF receptor and IL-6 receptor are shed by the same protein. But I do not yet know.

M. REVEL (*Weizmann Institute of Science, Rehovot, Israel*): The gp130 which is shed from the cells—do you find that it has a biological activity as antagonist?

ROSE-JOHN: We have not tried that, but I think that there are data from Dr. Kishimoto's lab which suggest the antagonistic effect of soluble gp130.

REVEL: The natural gp130?

ROSE-JOHN: I think also the natural gp130.

Membrane-bound and Soluble Interleukin-6 Receptor: Studies on Structure, Regulation of Expression, and Signal Transduction[a]

PETER C. HEINRICH,[b,d] LUTZ GRAEVE,[b] STEFAN ROSE-JOHN,[b]
JENS SCHNEIDER-MERGENER,[c] ELKE DITTRICH,[b]
ANDREA ERREN,[b] CLAUDIA GERHARTZ,[b] ULRIKE
HEMMANN,[b] CLAUDIA LÜTTICKEN,[b] URSULA WEGENKA,[b]
OLIVER WEIERGRÄBER,[b] AND FRIEDEMANN HORN[b]

[b]Institut für Biochemie der RWTH Aachen
Pauwelsstraße 30
D-52057 Aachen, Germany

[c]Universitätsklinikum Charité
Humboldt-Universität zu Berlin
Institut für Medizinische Immunologie
Schumannstraße 20/21
10117 Berlin, Germany

INTERLEUKIN-6 AND ITS RECEPTOR

Interleukin-6 (IL-6), a cytokine consisting of 184 amino acids, belongs to a group of polypeptide hormones and cytokines which according to a prediction by Bazan[1] share a structure characterized by a bundle of four antiparallel α-helices. This family which also includes growth hormone, prolactin, and many cytokines—*e.g.*, granulocyte colony stimulating factor (G-CSF), erythropoietin (EPO), leukemia inhibitory factor (LIF), oncostatin (OM), and ciliary neurotrophic factor (CNTF)—has therefore been called the α-helical cytokine family. The predicted tertiary structure was confirmed by X-ray analysis of growth hormone, IL-4, and G-CSF,[2-4] and IL-6 is expected to have a similar structure. So far, however, attempts to crystallize IL-6 have failed in several laboratories.

IL-6 is produced by many different cell types, particularly after stimulation with IL-1. In monocytes, bacterial lipopolysaccharides (LPS) are important inducers of IL-6 synthesis and secretion. In turn, IL-6 acts on a wide spectrum of target cells, showing a pleiotropic spectrum of actions.[5,6] IL-6 triggers B-cells to differentiate to plasma cells and to synthesize and secrete antibodies, and is a maturation factor for T-cells. Furthermore, IL-6 has been reported to be an autocrine growth factor for

---

[a] Experiments described herein were supported by the Deutsche Forschungsgemeinschaft (Bonn) and the Fonds der Chemischen Industrie (Frankfurt).

[d] Author to whom correspondence should be addressed; Tel: +49 (241) 808-8830; Fax: +49 (241) 888-8428.

plasmacytoma and mesangial cells, and for keratinocytes. It acts on nerve cells resulting in the formation of dendrites and plays an important role in hematopoiesis and in the acute phase reaction of the liver. In response to IL-6, hepatocytes synthesize and secrete acute phase plasma proteins.[7]

IL-6 exerts its action via a cell surface receptor which consists of two subunits: the IL-6 binding protein gp80 and the signal-transducing component gp130.[8,9] Both IL-6 receptor subunits belong to the hematopoietic receptor superfamily.[10] After binding of IL-6 to gp80, the IL-6/gp80 complex interacts with gp130 which in turn dimerizes and initiates the generation of a biological signal.[11] We and others have shown that there are at least two sites in the IL-6 molecule which interact with the IL-6 receptor: one binds to gp80 while the other contacts the signal transducer gp130.[12,13]

IL-6/IL-6 RECEPTOR INTERNALIZATION

After binding to its receptor, IL-6 is rapidly internalized and degraded by rat hepatocytes and human hepatoma cells HepG2.[14,15] As we have shown previously, this internalization leads to a loss of IL-6 binding sites at the cell surface indicating that the IL-6 receptor is down-regulated by its ligand.[14] This down-regulation may play an important role in protecting the organism against overstimulation. In order to elucidate the mechanism of ligand-induced internalization and down-regulation of the IL-6 receptor, we searched for possible internalization sequences in the cytoplasmic domains of both the IL-6-binding protein gp80 and the signal transducer gp130. For this purpose, gp80 and gp130 were expressed in COS-7 cells, either alone or in combination. When gp80 was expressed alone, IL-6 was bound with low affinity ($K_D = 1 \times 10^{-8}$ M) by the transfected COS-7 cells and only a very inefficient internalization of the ligand was observed.[15] Co-expression of gp130 with gp80, however, resulted in an increased IL-6 binding affinity of $K_D = 6.3 \times 10^{-10}$ M, and 42% of initially bound IL-6 was internalized within 30 minutes. Deletion of the cytoplasmic domain of gp130 did not affect the IL-6 binding affinity but reduced the internalization efficiency by 79%. However, a gp80 lacking the complete cytoplasmic domain internalized IL-6 as efficiently as the full length protein when co-expressed with gp130.[15] These observations provide strong evidence that not the binding (gp80) but the signal transducing component (gp130) of the IL-6 receptor complex mediates the efficient uptake of IL-6. By studying gp130 mutants in which parts of the intracellular domain were deleted, a 10 amino acids region (amino acids 142-151, TQPLLDSEER) crucial for the efficient internalization of IL-6 was identified (FIG. 1). This sequence does not comprise the well-defined tyrosine-containing internalization signal described for many constitutively internalizing receptors such as the LDL, transferrin, or asialoglycoprotein receptors.[16] However, it contains a di-leucine motif, which has recently been shown to be involved in internalization and lysosomal targeting of a number of other receptors—*e.g.*, the T-cell receptor δ- and γ-chains, and the interferon-γ receptor.[17,18] Furthermore, for the transferrin receptor it has been reported that a di-leucine motif can replace the tyrosine-containing internalization sequence.[19] Murakami and co-workers described that an 61 amino acids juxtamembraneous region of gp130 is sufficient for the generation of growth signals.[20] Since it is evident from our studies that internalization is mediated by another region of gp130 we conclude that IL-6 receptor internalization is not a prerequisite for the proliferative response.

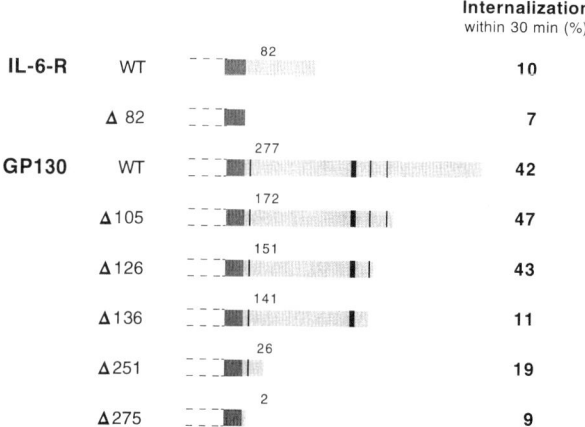

FIGURE 1. Internalization of IL-6 receptor complexes consisting of wildtype gp80 and gp130 or different deletion mutants. COS-7 cells were transiently transfected with expression vectors for gp80 alone (wildtype or 82 amino acids deletion, top two values) or for wildtype gp80 in combination with various deletion mutants of gp130. Extracellular, transmembrane, and cytoplasmic domains of the expressed proteins are schematically shown as dashes, dark grey boxes, and light grey boxes, respectively. The number of amino acids of the cytoplasmic domains is given above the grey boxes. Thick and thin bars within the cytoplasmic tail are locations of potential internalization sequences. *Thick black bar:* tyrosine containing motif; *thin black bars:* di-leucine motifs. Internalization was measured by binding 1 nM [^{125}I]-IL-6 to the transfected cells at 4°C for 2h and shifting to 37°C for 30 min. Internalized IL-6 was measured after stripping surface-bound IL-6 with a high salt/low pH wash. Internalized IL-6 is indicated at the right as percentage of initially bound IL-6. The values are means from 2–4 independent experiments.

SOLUBLE IL-6 RECEPTOR

Soluble extracellular domains of the IL-6 receptor as well as of the signal transducer gp130 have been found in human serum and urine.[21,22] We have shown in transfected COS-7 cells that the generation of the soluble IL-6 receptor from its membrane-bound form occurs by shedding (*i.e.* by limited proteolysis) and is stimulated by phorbol esters.[23] Presently, neither the tissues or cells physiologically involved in the generation of the soluble IL-6 receptor nor its target cells and functions are known. Interestingly, soluble gp80/IL-6 complexes exhibit an agonistic action on cells carrying the signal transducing subunit gp130 on their surface.[24]

As a first approach to investigate the quarternary structure of the IL-6 receptor we have expressed the extracellular domains of gp80 and gp130 in baculovirus-infected insect cells. After purification by affinity chromatography using immobilized ligand, the soluble IL-6 receptor binds IL-6 with a dissociation constant of about 0.5 nM (FIG. 2) and is biologically active when measured with hepatoma cells stably transfected with a cDNA coding for IL-6 (FIG. 3). These cells (HepG2-IL-6) which were previously established in our laboratory[24] constitutively synthesize and secrete IL-6 into the medium. By acting in an autocrine manner, the released IL-6 leads to a permanent down-regulation of IL-6 receptors. Since gp130 is still present in the HepG2-IL-6 cells, acute phase protein mRNA synthesis can be triggered by addition of soluble gp80. As shown in FIGURE 3, the mRNA levels of the acute phase protein

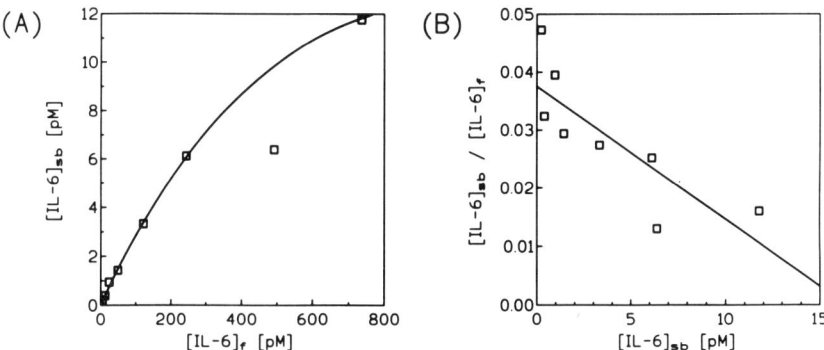

FIGURE 2. Binding of [^{125}I]-recombinant human IL-6 to soluble gp80. **A:** Soluble human gp80 was purified from conditioned media of baculovirus-infected insect cells and was incubated at a concentration of 37 pM with [^{125}I]-labeled recombinant human IL-6 at concentrations ranging from 5 to 750 pM. Complexes of IL-6 and soluble gp80 were then immunoprecipitated by the use of a polyclonal antibody to gp80 and protein A-Sepharose and analyzed by γ-counting. **B:** Scatchard transformation of the data from (**A**).

haptoglobin increased when the soluble IL-6 receptor purified from insect cells was added to HepG2-IL-6 cells.

To map regions of the IL-6 molecule involved in receptor interaction, we used iodinated soluble IL-6 receptor to probe a series of overlapping dodecapeptides bound

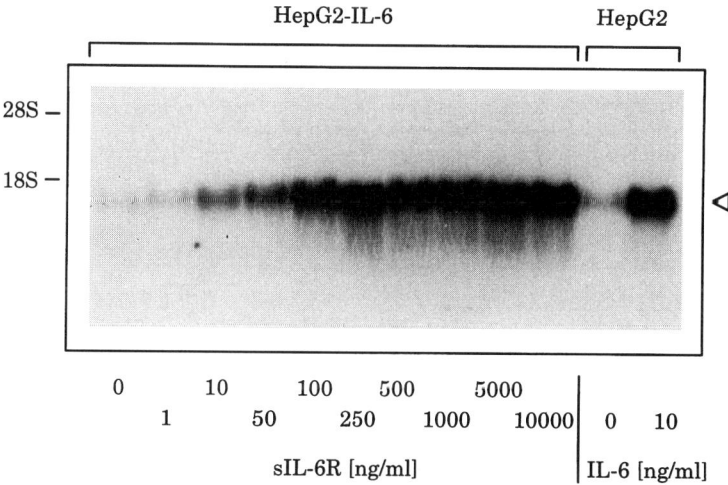

FIGURE 3. Biological activity of the soluble IL-6 receptor purified from baculovirus-infected insect cells. HepG2-IL-6 cells were incubated with soluble IL-6 receptor (sIL-6-R) at increasing concentrations. Haptoglobin mRNA induction (*open arrowhead*) was analyzed by Northern blotting and autoradiography. HepG2 cells stimulated with IL-6 served as a control.

to a continuous cellulose-membrane support covering the complete sequence of IL-6. FIG. 4 shows that distinct peptides bound the [^{125}I]-soluble gp80. Peptides 56 to 59 correspond to the C-terminus of IL-6 (amino acids 166 to 184) which we have previously shown to be required for the interaction with the IL-6 receptor.[25] Peptides 30 to 33 covering part of the predicted B-helix and the BC-loop (amino acids 88 to 108) of IL-6 also interacted with the soluble IL-6 receptor (FIG. 4). A similar observation was previously made by Ekida *et al.*[26]

ACUTE-PHASE RESPONSE FACTOR (APRF)

One of our major interests during the last years has been to elucidate the signal transduction pathway of IL-6 in liver cells. As schematically shown in FIGURE 5, IL-6 as well as the cytokines IL-11, LIF, OM and CNTF interact with their respective plasma membrane receptors from where the signal is transduced to the nucleus, and acute phase protein genes are induced.

α_2-Macroglobulin is the major acute phase protein of the rat. Several years ago we and others identified an IL-6 response element in the rat α_2-macroglobulin promoter.[27–29] This element contains two hexanucleotides, CTGGAA and CTGGGA, homologous to motifs in the promoters of the fibrinogen and other acute-phase protein genes.[30–32] To identify transcription factors involved in the regulation of the α_2-macroglobulin gene, we induced an acute phase response in rats by intraperitoneally injecting LPS and analyzed liver nuclear proteins isolated from these animals for binding to the α_2-macroglobulin IL-6 response element. By gel retardation assays using a [^{32}P]-labeled synthetic oligonucleotide containing the CTGGGA motif of the α_2-macroglobulin promoter, the transient activation of a nuclear factor which we call APRF (acute-phase response factor) after LPS injection was observed (FIG. 6). Injection of IL-6 caused an even more rapid activation of APRF. Furthermore, APRF activation was also observed in hepatoma (HepG2) cells in culture after incubation with IL-6.[33] Here, activation of APRF occurred within 5 min after the addition of IL-6, and was maximal after 15 min. Purification of APRF from rat livers yielded a single polypeptide of approximately 87 kD.[34] Further characterization of APRF demonstrated its activation by IL-6 in various cell types indicating a ubiquitous occurrence of this transcription factor. We could also demonstrate that all other cytokines acting through the signal transducer gp130 (*i.e.*, LIF, OM, CNTF, and IL-11) are able to activate APRF as well.[34]

In addition to binding to the α_2-macroglobulin promoter, APRF binds to IL-6 response elements of various other acute phase protein genes, for example, the genes for haptoglobin, α_1-acid glycoprotein, γ-fibrinogen, and α_1-antichymotrypsin.[33] By comparison of these binding sites, we deduced a palindromic APRF binding consensus sequence, TT^A/$_C$CNG^G/$_T$AA (FIG. 7). Using this consensus sequence we were able to identify APRF binding sites also in IL-6 response elements of several IL-6–induced immediate-early genes.[35] These data suggest that APRF plays a central role in the transcriptional regulation not only of the α_2-macroglobulin gene but also of many other IL-6 target genes.

APRF is different from other transcription factors known to be activated by interleukins–*e.g.*, NF-IL6 or NF-κB.[33] However, the binding consensus for APRF as defined above is reminiscent of binding sites for GAF (interferon-γ activation factor), a transcription factor activated by interferon-γ.[36,37] In fact, we recently demonstrated that APRF and GAF possess almost identical binding sequence specificities, and that

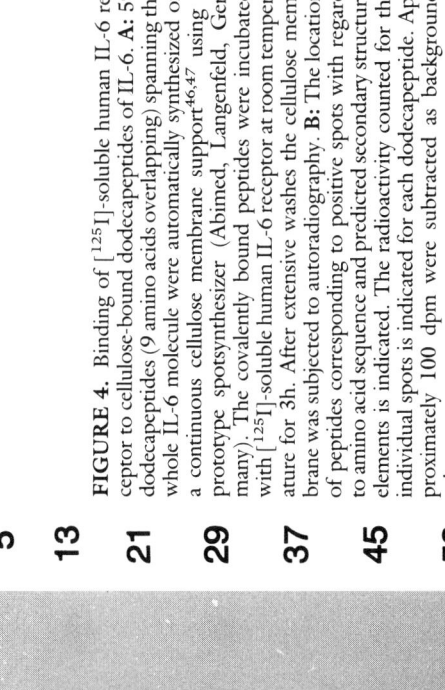
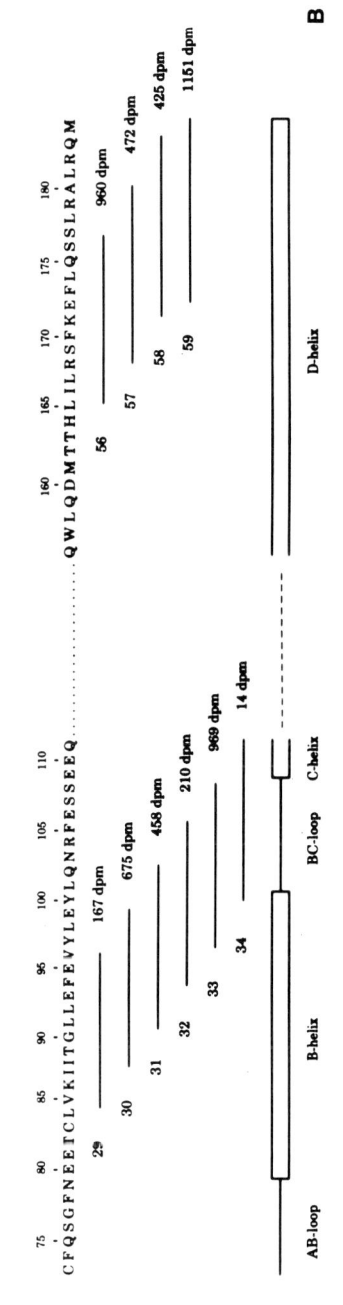
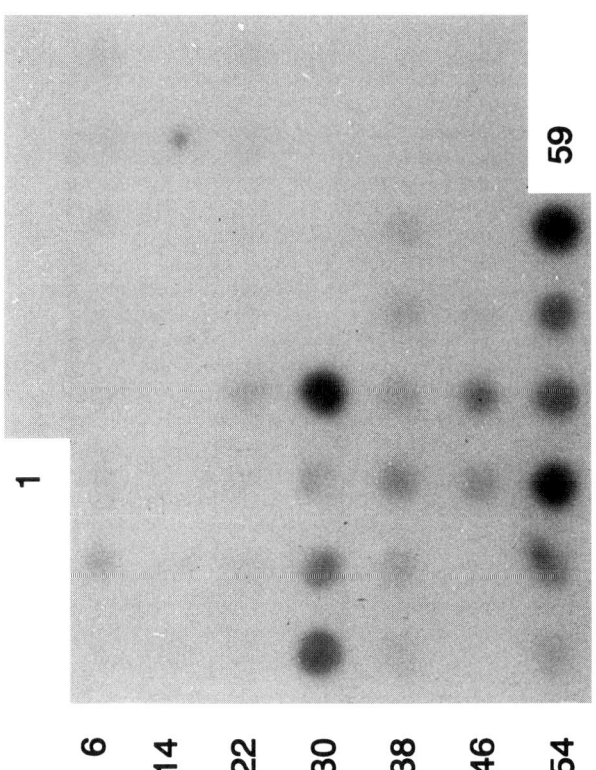

FIGURE 4. Binding of [^{125}I]-soluble human IL-6 receptor to cellulose-bound dodecapeptides of IL-6. **A:** 59 dodecapeptides (9 amino acids overlapping) spanning the whole IL-6 molecule were automatically synthesized on a continuous cellulose membrane support[46,47] using a prototype spotsynthesizer (Abimed, Langenfeld, Germany). The covalently bound peptides were incubated with [^{125}I]-soluble human IL-6 receptor at room temperature for 3h. After extensive washes the cellulose membrane was subjected to autoradiography. **B:** The location of peptides corresponding to positive spots with regard to amino acid sequence and predicted secondary structure elements is indicated. The radioactivity counted for the individual spots is indicated for each dodecapeptide. Approximately 100 dpm were subtracted as background values.

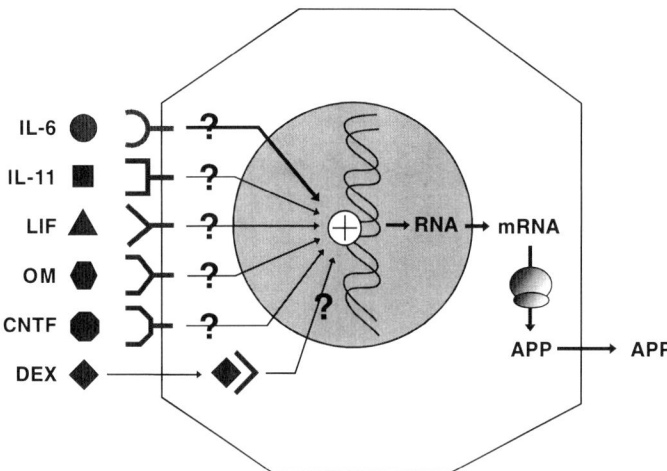

FIGURE 5. Induction of acute phase protein synthesis in hepatocytes by IL-6-type cytokines. All IL-6-type cytokines, *i.e.* IL-6, IL-11, LIF, OM, and CNTF, bind to plasma membrane receptors containing the signal transducer gp130 and induce the synthesis of acute phase proteins (APP) in hepatocytes. Glucocorticoids (dexamethasone, DEX) have permissive effects for the IL-6-induction of some but not all acute phase proteins.

binding sites for these factors represent regulatory elements responsive to both IL-6 and interferon-γ.[35] GAF is formed by a homodimer of the Stat91 protein, a member of the STAT (for: signal transducer and activator of transcription) family of transcription factors. Interferon-γ induces the rapid tyrosine phosphorylation of this protein which preexists in an inactive monomeric form in the cytoplasm.[38] The similar binding specificities of APRF and GAF suggested a relatedness of the two factors. We therefore

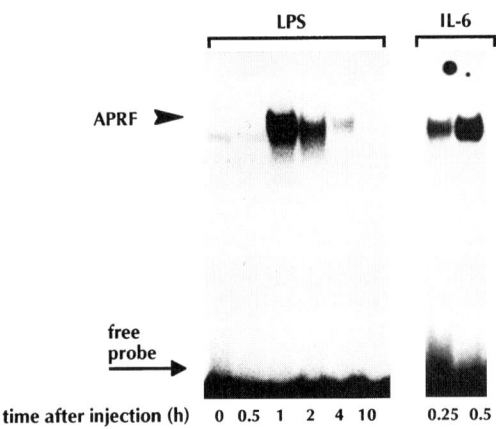

FIGURE 6. Activation of APRF by LPS and IL-6 in rat liver. Rats were intraperitoneally injected with LPS (10 mg/kg of body weight) or recombinant human IL-6 (60,000 B-cell stimulatory factor 2 units/kg). After the times indicated, livers were removed and nuclear extracts prepared. 1 μg nuclear protein was subjected to a gel retardation assay using a [^{32}P]-labeled oligonucleotide containing the CTGGGA-motif of the rat α_2-macroglobulin promoter as a probe. The position of the retarded APRF-DNA complex is indicated.

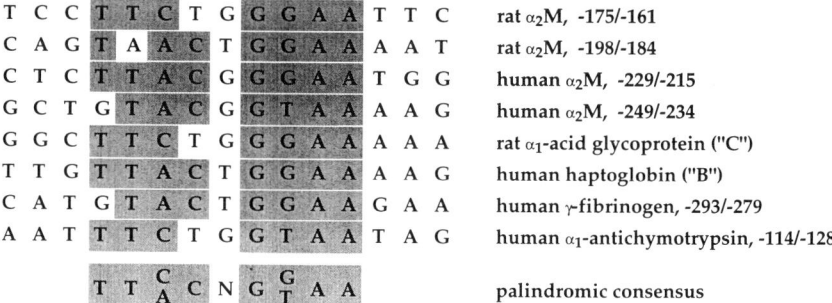

FIGURE 7. Definition of a palindromic consensus binding sequence for APRF. APRF binding sites localized in the promoters of the rat and human α_2-macroglobulin (α_2M) genes, the C-element of the rat α_1-acid glycoprotein,[32] the B-element of the human haptoglobin gene,[31] and the IL-6 response elements of the human γ-fibrinogen and α_1-antichymotrypsin genes[33] were aligned. Homologies to the palindromic consensus are indicated by grey boxes.

tested various antisera raised against known members of the Stat family for a potential cross-reactivity with APRF. As shown in FIGURE 8, an antiserum raised against the amino-terminus of Stat91 and its splice variant, Stat84, supershifted the APRF-DNA complex in a gel retardation assay. Other antisera to Stat91, Stat84, or Stat113 did not recognize APRF indicating that APRF is very likely related to but different from Stat91.[34]

In fact, recent cloning of cDNAs for APRF confirmed that the factor, now also called Stat3, is a novel member of the STAT family with about 50% homology to Stat91.[39,40]

MECHANISM OF APRF ACTIVATION

By preincubation of HepG2 cells with the protein synthesis inhibitor cycloheximide we could demonstrate that APRF activation by IL-6 does not require *de novo* protein synthesis and therefore occurs at the posttranslational level.[33] Activated APRF was first observed in the cytosolic fractions indicating that an inactive, cytoplasmic form of the factor is rapidly activated in response to IL-6 and is then translocated to the nucleus.[33] Protein tyrosine kinase inhibitors blocked the activation of APRF indicating the involvement of tyrosine phosphorylations in the IL-6 signaling pathway leading to APRF activation.[34] In fact, when APRF was incubated with monoclonal antibodies to phosphotyrosine, the DNA-binding activity of the factor was inhibited (FIG. 9). When the antibodies were saturated by adding phosphotyrosine, APRF activity was not affected in the gel retardation assay proving the specificity of this interaction. We conclude that activated APRF contains phosphorylated tyrosine residues. Phosphoamino acid analysis of APRF immunoprecipitated from IL-6–treated, [^{32}P]-phosphate-labeled HepG2 cells confirmed the presence of both phosphoserine and phosphotyrosine in activated APRF.[41]

By immunoprecipitation of APRF and Stat91 from HepG2 cells using antibodies to Stat91/84 we examined whether the observed APRF tyrosine phosphorylation is

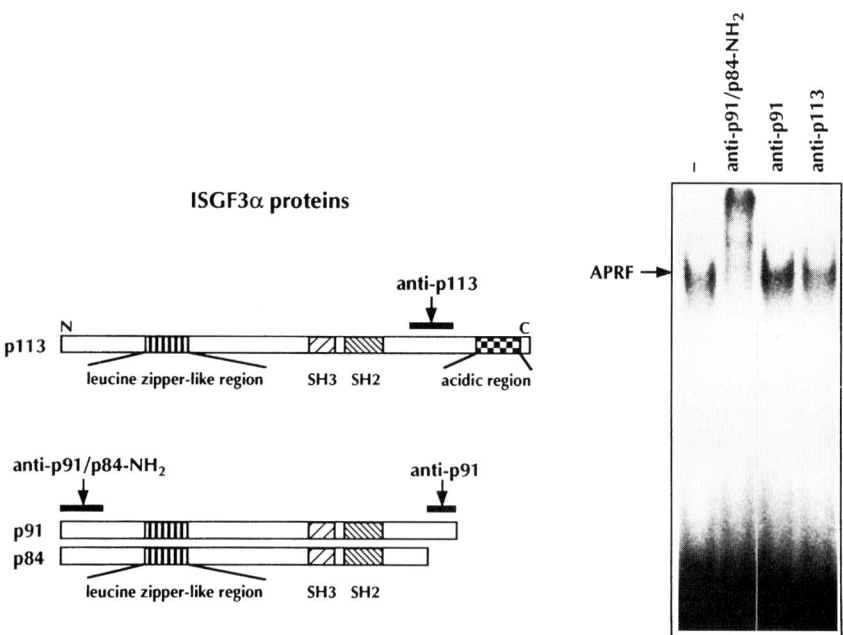

FIGURE 8. APRF is recognized by an antiserum to the amino-terminus of Stat91. Polyclonal antisera raised against the indicated portions of the Stat113 (p113), Stat91 (p91), and Stat84 (p84) proteins were incubated with 1 μg liver nuclear extract from LPS-treated rats. APRF DNA-binding was then measured in a gel retardation assay (*right*).

induced by IL-6. When immunoprecipitates from either untreated HepG2 cells or cells incubated with IL-6 or interferon-γ were subjected to SDS-polyacrylamide electrophoresis and subsequently analyzed by immunoblotting with antibodies to phosphotyrosine, an IL-6–induced tyrosine phosphorylation of APRF became apparent (FIG. 10). In addition, IL-6 triggered the tyrosine phosphorylation of Stat91 whereas interferon-γ induced only the Stat91 tyrosine phosphorylation but not that of APRF. When the same experiment was carried out with immunoprecipitates from HepG2 cells treated with IL-6 for various periods, three tyrosine-phosphorylated bands appeared with different time courses (FIG. 11). While the 91-kD band corresponds to Stat91, the 89- and 87-kD bands both represent APRF.[34] As we could show recently, APRF is serine phosphorylated between 10 and 15 min after IL-6 stimulation of HepG2 cells.[42] The mobility shift of APRF observed in FIGURE 11 is due to this additional posttranslational modification. Our data show that the tyrosine phosphorylation of APRF is required for nuclear translocation and DNA binding of the factor while the function of the IL-6–induced serine phosphorylation is not yet known. It is of interest, however, that the latter modification can be inhibited by the protein serine/threonine kinase inhibitor H7,[42] which is known to also block the induction of target genes by IL-6.[43] Therefore, APRF serine phosphorylation may be necessary for nuclear functions of the transcription factor.

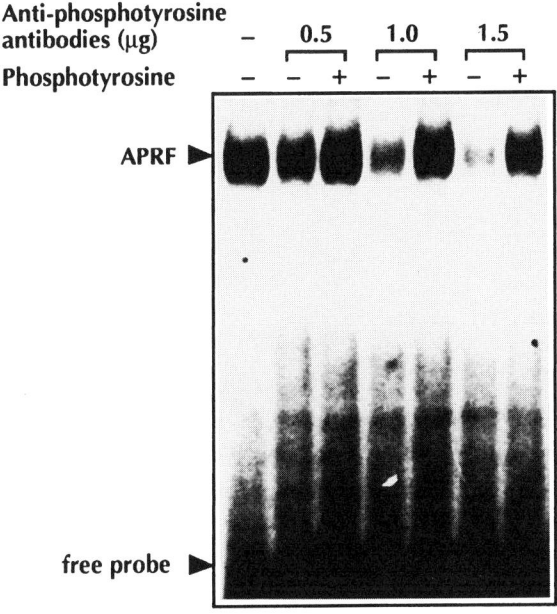

FIGURE 9. Inhibition of APRF DNA-binding activity by antibodies to phosphotyrosine. Nuclear extracts (5 μg) from HepG2 cells treated with 100 units/ml IL-6 for 15 min were incubated with monoclonal antibodies to phosphotyrosine at the concentrations indicated and without or with 1 mM phosphotyrosine. Then, DNA-binding of APRF was measured by a gel retardation assay as described for FIGURE 6.

IL-6 SIGNAL TRANSDUCTION

IL-6 induces the rapid tyrosine phosphorylation of gp130. Furthermore, a protein tyrosine kinase activity was reported to be coprecipitated with gp130 from IL-6-treated cells.[11] Since this tyrosine kinase may also be involved in APRF activation, it was of great interest for us to identify protein tyrosine kinases regulated by IL-6.

Tyk2, a protein tyrosine kinase of the JAK family, had been demonstrated to play an important role in the signal transduction pathway of interferon-α.[44] By immunoprecipitation of Tyk2 from IL-6–treated HepG2 cells we could demonstrate that IL-6 triggers the rapid tyrosine phosphorylation of Tyk2 in HepG2 cells indicating a function of the kinase in IL-6 signaling as well.[41] Furthermore, the two other known members of the JAK family, Jak1 and Jak2 were also shown to be activated in response to IL-6.[41,45] These tyrosine kinases are constitutively associated with gp130[41,45] and are likely to be activated by the ligand-induced homodimerization of gp130.

At present, it is not known whether Jak kinases directly phosphorylate APRF or Stat91. However, our recent observation that IL-6 induces the transient association of APRF with gp130[41] shows that by the action of IL-6 APRF is brought in close proximity to the activated Jak kinases and thus is in favor of that assumption.

FIGURE 12 summarizes the findings on IL-6 signaling. After binding of IL-6 to gp80 the IL-6/gp80-complex associates with two gp130 molecules. Jak kinases bound

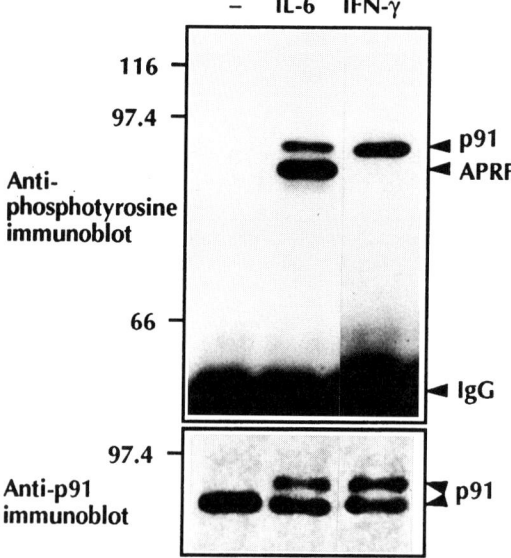

FIGURE 10. IL-6–induced tyrosine phosphorylation of APRF and Stat91. HepG2 cells were incubated for 15 min with either IL-6 (100 units/ml) or interferon-γ (IFN-γ, 25 ng/ml). Cell lysates were immunoprecipitated using an antiserum against the amino-terminus of Stat91/84, and the immune complexes subjected to SDS-polyacrylamide electrophoresis. Proteins were transferred to polyvinyldifluoride membrane and analyzed by immunoblotting with antibodies to phosphotyrosine (*top*) or Stat91, (p91, *bottom*).

to the cytoplasmic part of gp130 are activated and both the Jak kinases themselves and gp130 are tyrosine-phosphorylated. Subsequently, APRF and Stat91 associate with gp130, possibly through their SH2 domains. After phosphorylation at tyrosine the transcription factors dimerize and translocate to the nucleus where they bind to IL-6 response elements in the promoters of acute phase protein genes and other IL-6 target genes inducing their transcription.

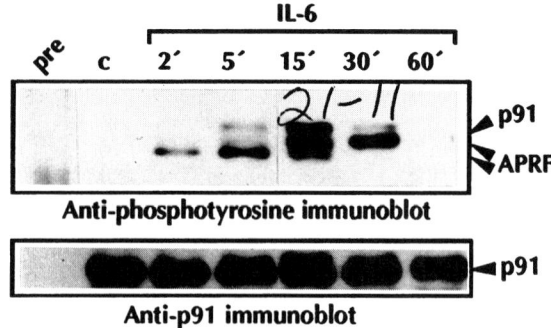

FIGURE 11. Time course of APRF tyrosine phosphorylation. HepG2 cells incubated for various periods with 100 units/ml IL-6 were lysed, immunoprecipitated with antiserum against the amino-terminus of Stat91/84, and immunoblotted with anti-phosphotyrosine or anti-Stat91. The positions of Stat91 (p91) and of APRF before and after serine phosphorylation (lower and upper APRF band, respectively) are indicated.

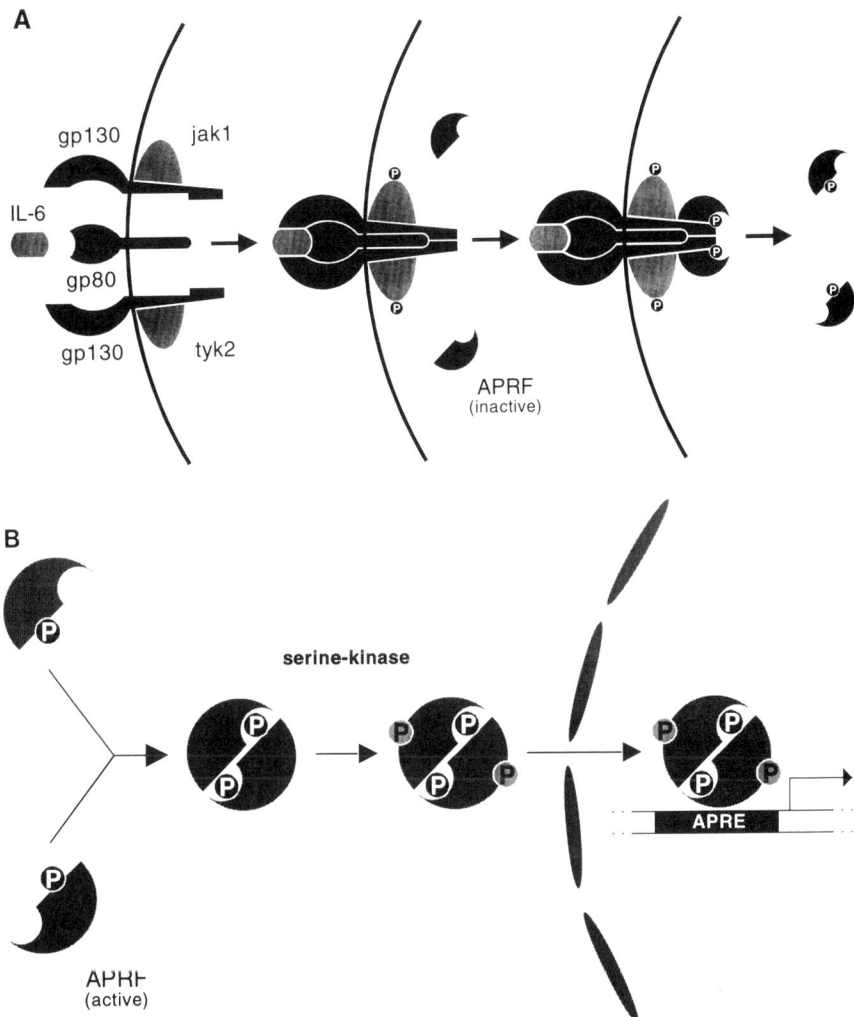

FIGURE 12. Current model of IL-6 signal transduction. Binding of IL-6 to gp80 triggers the homodimerization of gp130 and the activation of associated Jak protein tyrosine kinases. APRF transiently interacts with gp130, is tyrosine-phosphorylated, dimerizes, and translocates to the nucleus. An additional phosphorylation of APRF at serine occurs about 10 min later and may be important for nuclear functions of APRF. In the nucleus, APRF binds to its binding sites in the promoters of IL-6 target genes and induces their transcription.

ACKNOWLEDGMENTS

We thank C. Schindler (New York) for the gift of antisera to Stat proteins. We also acknowledge the help of M. Robbertz with artwork and D. Kocak and S. Cottin with the preparation of the manuscript.

REFERENCES

1. BAZAN, J. F. 1990. Haemopoietic receptors and helical cytokines. Immunol. Today **11**: 350–354.
2. DE VOS, A. M., M. ULTSCH & A. A. KOSSIAKOFF. 1992. Human growth hormone and extracellular domain of its receptor: crystal structure of the complex. Science **255**: 306–312.
3. WLODAVER, A., A. PAVLOVSKY & A. GUSTCHINA. 1992. Crystal structure of human recombinant interleukin-4 at 2.25 A resolution. FEBS Lett. **309**: 59–64.
4. HILL, C. P., T. D. OSSLUND & D. EISENBERG. 1993. The structure of granulocyte-colony-stimulating factor and its relationship to other growth factors. Proc. Natl. Acad. Sci. USA **90**: 5167–5171.
5. HIRANO, T. & T. KISHIMOTO. 1990. Interleukin-6. *In* Peptide growth factors and their receptors I. M. B. Sporn and A. B. Roberts, Eds.:633–665. Berlin: Springer.
6. VAN SNICK, J. 1990. Interleukin-6: An overview. Ann. Rev. Immunol. **8**: 253–279.
7. HEINRICH, P. C., J. CASTELL & T. ANDUS. 1990. Interleukin-6 and the acute phase response. Biochem. J. **265**: 621–636.
8. YAMASAKI, K., T. TAGA, Y. HIRATA, H. YAWATA, Y. KAWANISHI, B. SEED, T. TANIGUCHI, T. HIRANO & T. KISHIMOTO. 1988. Cloning and expression of the human interleukin-6 (BSF-2/IFN beta 2) receptor. Science **241**: 825–828.
9. HIBI, M., M. MURAKAMI, M. SAITO, T. HIRANO, T. TAGA & T. KISHIMOTO. 1990. Molecular cloning and expression of an IL-6 signal transducer, gp130. Cell **63**: 1149–1157.
10. BAZAN, J. 1990. Structural design and molecular evolution of a cytokine receptor superfamily. Proc. Natl. Acad. Sci. USA **87**: 6934–6938.
11. MURAKAMI, M., M. HIBI, N. NAKAGAWA, T. NAKAGAWA, K. YASUKAWA, K. YAMANISHI, T. TAGA & T. KISHIMOTO. 1993. IL-6-induced homodimerization of gp130 and associated activation of a tyrosine kinase. Science **260**: 1808–1810.
12. BRAKENHOFF, J. P. J., M. HART, E. R. DE GROOT, F. DI PADOVA & L. A. AARDEN. 1990. Structure-function analysis of human IL-6. Epitope mapping of neutralizing monoclonal antibodies with amino- and carboxy-terminal deletion mutants. J. Immunol. **145**: 561–568.
13. EHLERS M., J. GRÖTZINGER, F. D. DE HON, J. MÜLLBERG, J. P. J. BRAKENHOFF, J. LIU, A. WOLLMER & S. ROSE-JOHN. 1994. Two regions of interleukin-6 responsible for binding and signal transduction. J. Immunol. In press.
14. ZOHLNHÖFER, D., L. GRAEVE, S. ROSE-JOHN, H. SCHOOLTINK, E. DITTRICH & P. C. HEINRICH. 1992. The hepatic interleukin-6 receptor. Down-regulation of the interleukin-6 binding subunit (gp80) by its ligand. FEBS Lett. **306**: 219–222.
15. DITTRICH, E., S. ROSE-JOHN, C. GERHARTZ, J. MÜLLBERG, T. STOYAN, K. YASUKAWA, P. C. HEINRICH & L. GRAEVE. 1994. Identification of a region within the cytoplasmic domain of the interleukin-6 signal transducer gp130 important for ligand-induced endocytosis of the IL-6 receptor. J. Biol. Chem. **269**: 19014–19020.
16. HOPKINS, C. R. 1992. Selective membrane protein trafficking: Vectorial flow and filter. Trends Biochem. Sci. **17**: 27–31.
17. LETOURNEUR, F. & R. D. KLAUSNER. 1992. A novel di-leucine motif and a tyrosine-based motif independently mediate lysosomal targeting and endocytosis of CD3 chains. Cell **69**: 1143–1157.
18. FARRAR, M. A. & R. D. SCHREIBER. 1993. The molecular cell biology of interferon-gamma and its receptor. Annu. Rev. Immunol. **11**: 571–611.
19. TROWBRIDGE, I. S., J. F. COLLAWN & C. R. HOPKINS. 1993. Signal-dependent membrane protein trafficking in the endocytic pathway. Annu. Rev. Cell Biol. **9**: 129–161.

20. MURAKAMI, M., M. NARAZAKI, M. HIBI, H. YAWATA, K. YASUKAWA, M. HAMAGUCHI, T. TAGA & T. KISHIMOTO. 1991. Critical cytoplasmic region of the interleukin 6 signal transducer gp130 is conserved in the cytokine receptor family. Proc. Natl. Acad. Sci. USA **88:** 11349–11353.
21. NOVICK, D., H. ENGELMANN, D. WALLACH & M. RUBINSTEIN. 1989. Soluble cytokine receptors are present in normal human urine. Jem **170:** 1409–1414.
22. NARASAKI, M., K. YASUKAWA, T. SAITO, Y. OHSUGI, H. FUKUI, Y. KOISHIHARA, G. D. YANCOPOULOS, T. TAGA & T. KISHIMOTO. 1993. Soluble forms of the interleukin-6 signal-transducing receptor component gp130 in human serum possessing a potential to inhibit signals through membrane-anchored gp130. Blood **82** 1–7.
23. MÜLLBERG, J., H. SCHOOLTINK, T. STOYAN, M. GÜNTHER, L. GRAEVE, G. BUSE, A. MACKIEWICZ, P. C. HEINRICH & S. ROSE-JOHN. 1993. The soluble interleukin-6 receptor is generated by shedding. Eur. J. Immunol. **23:** 473–480.
24. MACKIEWICZ, A., H. SCHOOLTINK, P. C. HEINRICH & S. ROSE-JOHN. 1992. Complex of soluble human IL-6-receptor/IL-6 up-regulates expression of acute-phase proteins. J. Immunol. **149:** 2021–2017.
25. KRÜTTGEN, A., S. ROSE-JOHN, C. MÖLLER, B. WROBLOWSKI, A. WOLLMER, J. MÜLLBERG, T. HIRANO, T. KISHIMOTO & P. C. HEINRICH. 1990. Structure-function analysis of human interleukin-6. Evidence for the involvement of the carboxy-terminus in function. FEBS Lett. **262:** 323–326.
26. EKIDA, T., C. NISHIMURA, S. MASUDA, S. I. ITOH, I. SHIMADA & Y. ARATA. 1992. A receptor-binding peptide from human interleukin-6: Isolation and a proton nuclear magnetic resonance study. Biochem. Biophys. Res. Commun. **189:** 211–220.
27. KUNZ, D., R. ZIMMERMANN, M. HEISIG & P. C. HEINRICH. 1989. Identification of the promoter sequences involved in the interleukin-6 dependent expression of the rat α_2-macroglobulin gene. Nucleic Acids Res. **17:** 1121–1138.
28. HATTORI, M., L. J. ABRAHAM, W. NORTHEMANN & G. H. FEY. 1990. Acute-phase reaction induces a specific complex between hepatic nuclear proteins and the interleukin 6 response element of the rat alpha 2-macroglobulin gene. Proc. Natl. Acad. Sci. USA **87:** 2364–2368.
29. ITO, T., H. TANAHASHI, Y. MISUMI & Y. SAKAKI. 1989. Nuclear factors interacting with an interleukin-6 responsive element of rat alpha 2-macroglobulin gene. Nucleic Acids Res. **17:** 9425–9435.
30. FOWLKES, D. M., N. T. MULLIS, C. M. COMEAU & G. R. CRABTREE. 1984. Potential basis for regulation of the coordinately expressed fibrinogen genes: Homology in the 5'flanking regions. Proc. Natl. Acad. Sci. USA **81:** 2313–2316.
31. OLIVIERO, S. & R. CORTESE. 1989. The human haptoglobin gene promoter: Interleukin-6-responsive elements interact with a DNA-binding protein induced by interleukin-6. EMBO J. **8:** 1145–1151.
32. WON, K. A. & H. BAUMANN. 1990. The cytokine response element of the rat alpha 1-acid glycoprotein gene is a complex of several interacting regulatory sequences. Mol. Cell. Biol. **10:** 3965–3978.
33. WEGENKA, U. M., J. BUSCHMANN, C. LÜTTICKEN, P. C. HEINRICH & F. HORN. 1993. Acute-phase response factor, a nuclear factor binding to acute-phase response elements, is rapidly activated by interleukin-6 at the posttranslational level. Mol. Cell. Biol. **13:** 276–288.
34. WEGENKA, U. M., C. LÜTTICKEN, J. BUSCHMANN, J. YUAN, F. LOTTSPEICH, W. MÜLLER-ESTERL, C. SCHINDLER, E. ROEB, P. C. HEINRICH & F. HORN. 1994. The interleukin-6-activated acute-phase response factor is antigenically and functionally related to members of the signal transducer and activator of transcription (STAT) family. Mol. Cell. Biol. **14:** 3186–3196.
35. YUAN, J., U. M. WEGENKA, C. LÜTTICKEN, J. BUSCHMANN, T. DECKER, C. SCHINDLER, P. C. HEINRICH & F. HORN. 1994. The signaling pathways of interleukin-6 and interferon-γ converge by the activation of different transcription factors which bind to common responsive DNA elements. Mol. Cell. Biol. **14:** 1657–1668.
36. DECKER, T., D. J. LEW, J. MIRKOVITCH & J. E. DARNELL, JR. 1991. Cytoplasmic activation of GAF, an INF-γ-regulated DNA-binding factor. EMBO J. **10:** 927–932.

37. EILERS, A., M. BACCARINI, F. HORN, R. A. HIPSKIND, C. SCHINDLER & T. DECKER. 1994. A factor induced by differentiation signals in cells of the macrophage lineage binds to the gamma interferon activation site. Mol. Cell. Biol. **14:** 1364–1373.
38. SHUAI, K., C. SCHINDLER, V. R. PREZIOSO & J. E. DARNELL, JR. 1992. Activation of transcription by IFN-γ: Tyrosine phosphorylation of a 91-kD-DNA binding protein. Science **258:** 1808–1812.
39. ZHONG, Z., Z. WEN & J. E. DARNELL, JR. 1994. Stat3: A STAT family member activated by tyrosine phosphorylation in response to epidermal growth factor and interleukin-6. Science **264:** 95–98.
40. AKIRA, S., Y. NISHIO, M. INOUE, X.-J. WANG, S. WEI, T. MATSUSAKA, K. YOSHIDA, T. SUDO, M. NARUTO & T. KISHIMOTO. 1994. Molecular cloning of APRF, a novel IFN-stimulated gene factor 3 p91-related transcription factor involved in the gp130-mediated signaling pathway. Cell **77:** 63–71.
41. LÜTTICKEN, C., U. M. WEGENKA, J. YUAN, J. BUSCHMANN, C. SCHINDLER, A. ZIEMICKI, A. G. HARPUR, A. F. WILKS, K. YASUKAWA, T. TAGA, T. KISHIMOTO, G. BARBIERI, S. PELLEGRINI, M. SENDTNER, P. C. HEINRICH & F. HORN. 1994. Association of transcription factor APRF and protein kinase JAK1 with the IL-6 signal transducer gp130. Science **263:** 89–92.
42. LÜTTICKEN, C., P. COFFER, J. YUAN, C. SCHWARTZ, C. SCHINDLER, W. KRUIJER, P. C. HEINRICH & F. HORN. 1995. Interleukin-6-induced serine phosphorylation of transcription factor APRF: Evidence for a role in interleukin-6 target gene induction. FEBS Lett. **360:** 137–143.
43. NAKAJIMA, K. & R. WALL. 1991. Interleukin-6 signals activating junB and TIS11 gene transcription in a B-cell hybridoma. Mol. Cell. Biol. **11:** 1409–1418.
44. VELAZQUEZ, L., M. FELLOUS, G. STARK & S. PELLEGRINI. 1992. A protein tyrosine kinase in the interferon α/β signaling pathway. Cell **70:** 313–322.
45. STAHL, N., T. G. BOULTON, T. FARRUGGELLA, N. Y. IP, S. DAVIS, B. A. WITTHUHN, F. W. QUELLE, O. SILVENNOINEN, G. BARBIERI, S. PELLEGRINI, J. N. IHLE & G. D. YANCOPOULOS. 1994. Association and activation of Jak-Tyk kinases by CNTF-LIF-OSM-IL-6 β receptor components. Science **263:** 92–95.
46. FRANK, R. 1992. Spot synthesis: an easy technique for the positionally addressable, parallel chemical synthesis on a membrane support. Tetrahedron **48:** 9217–9232.
47. KRAMER, A., A. SCHUSTER, U. REINEKE, R. MALIN, R. VOLKMER-ENGERT, C. LANDGRAF & J. SCHNEIDER-MERGENER. 1994. Combinatorial cellulose-bound peptide libraries: Screening tool for the identification of peptides that bind ligands with predefined specificity. Methods (Comp. Meth. Enzymol.) **6:** 388–395.

DISCUSSION OF THE PAPER

T. HIRANO (*Osaka University Medical School, Osaka, Japan*): You have shown that anti-p91/p84 immunoprecipitates contain tyrosine-phosphorylated molecules with a molecular weight corresponding to gp130. You also said that gp130 and APRF form a complex. What is the final proof that this molecule is really gp130?

P. C. HEINRICH: We have dissociated the gp130/APRF complex after immunoprecipitation with anti-p91/p84 and performed a second immunoprecipitation with an antiserum against gp130. After SDS-PAGE and anti-phosphotyrosine immunoblotting, gp130 was identified. This was demonstrated on the left two lanes of the slide I showed.

A. RAY: (*Yale University School of Medicine, New Haven, CT*): Do you have any evidence that APRF or p91 is a direct substrate for either Jak1, Jak2, or Tyk2?

HEINRICH: Since the Jak kinases are activated very rapidly (within 2 minutes) after IL-6 is bound to its receptor, and APRF as well as p91 are also tyrosine-phosphorylated with similar kinetics, we think that it is very likely that both transcription factors are substrates for the Jak kinases.

RAY: Have you tried co-immunoprecipitation of Jak kinases and APRF or p91?
HEINRICH: We have tried this co-immunoprecipitation, but we could not demonstrate any association.

M. REVEL (*Weizmann Institute of Science, Rehovot, Israel*): I would like to make a comment. When you use an α_2-macroglobulin probe, you have shown us one complex. Other gel conditions, however, can resolve this one complex in different forms. I will talk about that tomorrow.

G. CILIBERTO (*Istituto di Ricerche Biologia Moleculare P. Angletti, Pomezia (Rome), Italy*): My question relates to the first part of your talk. You showed a mutant in the cytoplasmic domain of gp130 which is deleted by 136 amino acids from the C-terminal end. This mutant is not internalized well. According to what Heinz Baumann has described before, such a mutant should still be able to signal because it contains boxes 2 and 3. So, what can you deduce from that?

HEINRICH: A deletion mutant lacking 136 amino acids from the C-terminal end of the cytoplasmic domain of gp130 does not internalize IL-6 any more, but as a chimeric receptor with the G-CSF extracellular domain is still able to signal when measured with a β-fibrinogen CAT construct. Box 3 of Heinz Baumann does not contain the internalization sequence which we have defined as a leucine motif at positions Leu145-Leu146. Thus, one may conclude that internalization and signaling are different processes.

Transcription Factors as Targets of Cytokine Signals[a]

WARREN S.-L. LIAO,[b] SZU-YAO LU, JIANYI HUANG, LI LI, AND ZHANYONG BING

Department of Biochemistry and Molecular Biology
The University of Texas M. D. Anderson Cancer Center
1515 Holcombe Boulevard
Houston, Texas 77030

INTRODUCTION

Transcription initiation in eukaryotic cells depends on the interaction of many transcription factors with an array of *cis*-regulatory elements and with each other.[1,2] In response to cellular or environmental signals, these transactivators increase the rate of transcription initiation, presumably by interacting with and recruiting of general transcription factors to the initiation complex.[3-6] These interactions together confer on a promoter its characteristic strength and specific pattern of expression.[2,7]

While transcription activation plays a central role in the up-regulation of gene expression, factors that interfere with their function are also important for controlling these cellular responses. Similarly, active repression of transcription is required to suppress the expression of genes in tissues where they should be silent.[8,9] One of the mechanisms for such negative transcriptional control is selective repression by sequence-specific DNA-binding proteins. Such transcription repressors[1,10-18] were shown to negatively regulate transcription by a variety of mechanisms, including interfering with the binding of transactivators by competing for DNA-binding sites.[11,15,17] Additionally, the repressors may block the activity of the basal transcription complex directly.[10,18] Consequently, the expression pattern of a target gene is ultimately determined by the combined effects of transactivators and repressors.[11,17]

For studies of the interplay between transactivators and transrepressors on inducible gene control, the regulation of acute-phase genes by inflammatory mediators represents an excellent model.[19,20] While the acute-phase genes are normally expressed at low levels, they are dramatically and transiently induced in response to acute inflammation. The magnitude and transient nature of the induction suggest potential involvement of activation and repression mechanisms in turning these genes on and off.[19,21] The level of serum amyloid A (SAA), one of the major acute-phase proteins, is increased up to 1000-fold in response to inflammation and tissue damage.[22,23] This large increase in hepatic SAA synthesis is mainly as a consequence of a 200-fold increase in SAA gene transcription.[22]

To understand the molecular mechanisms of SAA gene regulation during inflammation, we have analyzed the 5′-flanking regions of the rat SAA1 gene and have identified five *cis*-regulatory elements, including two C/EBP-binding sites and one

---

[a] This work was supported by National Institutes of Health Research Grant AR3885 to W.S.-L.L.

[b] Address correspondence to Dr. Liao at Box 117 at the above address; Tel: (713) 792-2556; Fax: (713) 790-0329.

NFκB-binding site.[24] Transient transfection analysis of the promoter demonstrated that a 65-bp DNA fragment (positions -135 to -71) could confer cytokine responsiveness on a heterologous promoter in liver and nonliver cells.[24,25] This fragment thus functions as a non-cell-specific cytokine response unit (CRU). Within the CRU we have identified binding sites for C/EBP and NFκB transcription factors as well as the ubiquitous transcription factor YY1. While site-specific mutations of either C/EBP- or NFκB-binding sites completely abolished the promoter activity, mutations of the YY1-binding site resulted in derepression of the SAA1 promoter, suggesting that YY1 may function as a repressor to repress SAA1 expression. Consistent with this notion is that conversion of YY1-binding site into a stronger site completely repressed both basal and cytokine-induced SAA1 expression. Thus, in the rat SAA1 promoter, YY1 functions as a repressor, not only contributing to SAA1's low basal expression, but may also play a role in the transiency of its expression in response to cytokine induction.

MATERIALS AND METHODS

Cell Culture and Conditioned Medium

Hep3B cells were cultured in basal medium consisting of modified Eagle's medium and Waymouth MAB (3:1, v/v, pH 7.0) plus 2% fetal bovine serum and 8% equine serum. Conditioned medium (CM) was prepared from activated mixed lymphocyte cultures as described by Huang *et al.*[25] and was used as a mixture with an equal volume of basal medium.

Plasmid Constructs

pSAA1(-301) and pSAA1(-117) were constructed by inserting DNA fragments containing different lengths of the 5' flanking sequences of the rat SAA1 promoter into the *Sma*I site of pSVoCAT vector.[24,25] Three site-specific mutant constructs, pSAA1(-117mG$_2$), pSAA1(-110mG$_2$), and pSAA1(-117mG$_5$) each with mutations that affect YY1 binding, were constructed using oligonucleotides that contained the indicated mutations as primers in the polymerase chain reactions and the pSAA1 (-117) DNA as template. All constructs were examined by gel electrophoresis and verified by DNA sequencing.

Transient Transfection and Chloramphenicol Acetyltransferase Assay

Hep3B cells (10^6 cells/100-mm dish) were incubated for 16 to 24 h at 37°C before being transfected with 20 µg of plasmid DNA as described.[24] To elicit the acute-phase response, cells were treated with 50% CM approximately 16 to 20 h after transfection. As controls, transfected cells were treated in parallel with the basal medium. Approximately 18 to 24 h after treatment, the cells were harvested, cell extracts prepared, and the protein content in extracts were measured.[26] The CAT activity was subsequently determined[25,27] and quantified by measuring the radioactivity of [^{14}C]chloramphenicol spots corresponding to the acetylated and nonacetylated forms by liquid scintillation spectrometry or by ImageQuant (Molecular Dynamics).

Nuclear Extracts and Whole Cell Extracts

For nuclear extract preparations, cells were lysed in hypotonic buffer by homogenization with a Dounce homogenizer and the extracts were prepared as described.[24,28] For whole cell extracts, cells were lysed for 5 min on ice in 4.6 volumes of Triton buffer (1% Triton, 100 mM KCl, 50 mM Tris, pH 8.0, 0.1 mM EDTA, 1 mM DTT, 12.5 mM $MgCl_2$, 20% glycerol) with freshly added protease inhibitors (1 μg/ml leupeptin, 1μg/ml pepstatin, and 1 μg/ml aprotinin). The extracts were then clarified by centrifugation at 10,000 × g for 10 min and used immediately or stored in aliquotes at −80°C. For the latter part of these experiments we employed a modified method for nuclear extract preparations that preserved YY1 protein intact. In this improved procedure, cells were first lysed in hypotonic buffer by homogenization as described.[28] The isolated nuclei were subsequently lysed in the Triton buffer containing the protease inhibitors as for the whole cell extracts. Nuclear debris was removed by centrifugation and nuclear extracts were then stored at −80°C.

Electrophoretic Mobility Shift Assay and Methylation Interference Analysis

For mobility shift assays, 2×10^4 cpm (0.2 to 1 ng) of ^{32}P-labeled DNA fragments and 2.5 μg of nuclear protein were mixed in the reaction buffer.[29] Following a 15-min incubation at room temperature, samples were then loaded onto a 5.5% polyacrylamide gel (19:1 cross-linking ratio) in 1 X Tris-glycine buffer (0.38 M glycine, 50 mM Tris, 2 mM EDTA) and subjected to electrophoresis. The gel was then dried and autoradiographed. In oligonucleotide competition experiments, nuclear extracts were preincubated with an excess amount of competitor for 5 min before the probe was added. When antibodies were included in the supershift experiments, nuclear extracts were preincubated with the probe for 5 min before addition of preimmune or polyclonal antibodies. Reaction mixtures were incubated for an additional 10 min before being loaded onto the gel.

For the methylation interference experiments, the DNA probe was partially methylated with dimethyl sulfate. The protein-bound and free DNAs were separated on gels, extracted, purified, and subsequently cleaved by piperidine. The samples were heated at 90°C for 2 min in 95% formamide before electrophoresis on a 10% polyacrylamide gel.

Oligonucleotides and Antibodies

The following oligonucleotides and their complements were used as competitors in gel retardation assays: wild-type NFκB binding sequence, 5'-AGTTGAGGGGAC-TTTCCCAGGC-3' (Promega) and mutant NFκB biding sequence, 5'-GATCCGCT-CACTTTCCG-3'; wild-type C/EBP binding sequence, 5'-CGATGCCTAGATGGC-GCAATCTGGTTAT-3' and mutant C/EBP binding sequence 5'-CGATGCCTA GATGGGATATCCTGGTTAT-3'.[30] YY1 binding sequence from chicken α-actin promoter (5'-CGTCGCCATATTTGGGTG-3') and rabbit polyclonal antibodies against recombinant human YY1 were kindly provided by Drs. Robert Schwartz and Te-Chung Lee.[31,32] Antibodies against C/EBPβ and the p50 subunit of NFκB are from Dr. Steve McKnight and Promega, respectively.

RESULTS

A Ubiquitous Cytokine Response Unit–binding Factor Identified as YY1

Our previous studies have demonstrated that NFκB and C/EBP interact with the 65-bp CRU [HinfI(-135)/AvaII(-71) fragment] of the rat SAA1 promoter and are required for promoter function (FIG. 1A).[24,25] However, when CRU was used as a probe in gel mobility shift assays, additional DNA-protein complexes—a major complex (C_1) and a much weaker complex (C_2)—were detected. To determine the DNA sequences involved in the formation of complexes C_1 and C_2, we performed methylation interference studies. Analysis of the C_1 complex showed that, on the coding strand, methylation of any one of the six guanidine residues from bp -96 to -86 interfered with protein binding. On the noncoding strand, two guanidines (positions -84 and -94) were found to interfere with DNA-protein complex formation when methylated (FIG. 1B). Identical methylation interference patterns were observed for the C_2 complex (FIG. 1B), suggesting that it might be a degradation product of C_1 protein. It is noteworthy that this protein apparently bound to a region that overlaps with the NFκB-binding site. Indeed, the methylation interference patterns showed that this protein shared not only binding regions with NFκB, but also significant base contacts (FIG. 1B, bottom panel). Thus, this protein could interfere with NFκB binding through competition for overlapping binding sites.

Examination of the DNA sequences required to bind C_1 and C_2 revealed a close homology to that of the ubiquitous cellular factor YY1 (FIG. 2A).[33–36] To determine whether the protein in the C_1 and C_2 complexes is actually YY1 or a YY1-related factor, and whether YY1 can bind to CRU, several approaches were taken. First, the specificity of C_1 and C_2 binding was tested by oligonucleotide competition with a known YY1-binding sequence. As shown in FIGURE 2B, the YY1-binding site, as well as the wild-type oligo-G sequence, specifically inhibited formation of the C_1 and C_2 complexes, while mutant oligo-mG_3 did not have any effect on complex formation.

In addition to the C_1 and C_2 complexes, a slower-migrating complex, C_3, was detected. Formation of this complex was similarly inhibited by oligo-G and YY1-binding site oligonucleotides (FIG. 2B). Given that the protein in the C_1 complex was highly susceptible to degradation and that complex C_3 was not observed until the extract was prepared using the modified procedure, it is likely that the protein in the C_3 complex is related to the protein in C_1 complex and may represent the intact form of the protein. Indeed, in some extracts when the preparation time was shortened, the C_3 complex became the most prominent complex (see below).

Since YY1 is a zinc finger-containing protein and requires zinc for its DNA-binding activity,[32,35] we tested the zinc requirement for the formation of these complexes. When the zinc chelator 1,10-phenanthroline was added the formation of all three complexes was inhibited, whereas the formation of DNA-NFκB and DNA-C/EBP complexes was not affected (FIG. 2C). This inhibitory effect could be partially relieved by the addition of 1 mM zinc, but not by other divalent cations such as Ca^{2+} and Mg^{2+}. These results further suggest that all three complexes (C_1, C_2, and C_3) are formed by the same or very similar protein and their DNA-binding characteristics are similar to YY1.

To examine whether YY1 can bind the CRU, recombinant YY1 and YY1 synthesized *in vitro* were used in gel mobility shift experiments. Bacterially produced recombinant HisYY1 and *in vitro* synthesized YY1 both could bind to the CRU and formed complexes with the same mobility as the C_1, C_2, and C_3 complexes (FIG. 2D). Formation of these complexes was specifically inhibited by addition of an excess of YY1-

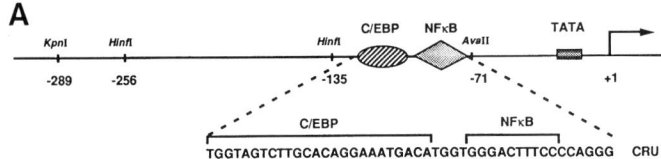

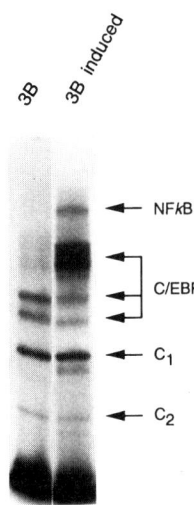

FIGURE 1. Binding of a ubiquitous nuclear factor to the cytokine response unit. **A:** *Top*, schematic of the 5'-flanking region of the rat SAA1 gene with the nucleotide sequence spanning part of the CRU shown. Positions of NFκB- and C/EBP-binding sites, as well as the TATA motif, are indicated. *Bottom*, gel mobility shift assays. End-labeled CRU [*Hin*fI(-135)/*Ava*II (-71)] was incubated with Hep3B nuclear extracts (2.5 μg) prepared from unstimulated (3B) and CM-stimulated (3B-induced) cells. Positions of specific DNA-protein complexes are indicated by arrows.

binding sequences and thus represent the intact (C_3) and the degraded (C_1 and C_2) forms of YY1.

Lastly, specific antibodies against YY1 were utilized in gel retardation assays to unequivocally confirm that the protein in complexes C_1, C_2, and C_3 is indeed YY1. As shown in FIGURE 2E, while preimmune sera had no effect on DNA-protein complex formation, anti-YY1 antibodies specifically diminished the formation of complexes C_1, C_2, and C_3. These results indicated that protein in complexes C_1, C_2, and C_3 and YY1 share common antigenicity. On the basis of these results, we concluded that the proteins in these three complexes represent YY1 and degraded forms of YY1 and that they bind to CRU in a highly sequence-specific manner.

YY1 Functions as a Repressor on SAA1 Promoter

Since YY1 could repress or activate transcription of many mammalian and viral genes,[32-37] we were intrigued with its effects on SAA1 transcription. To test the

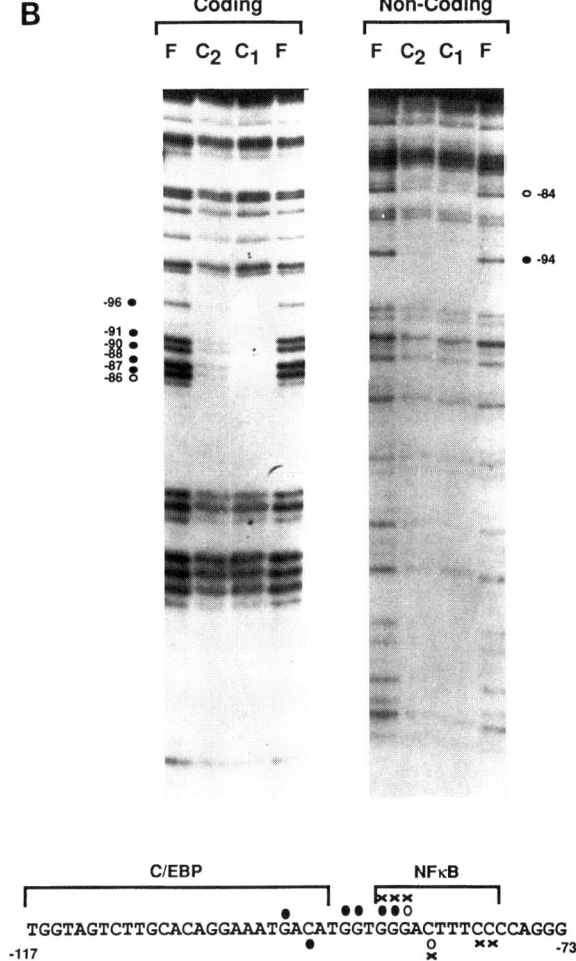

FIGURE 1. *(Continued).* **B:** Methylation interference analysis of complexes C_1 and C_2. The coding or the noncoding strand of CRU was radioactively labeled, partially methylated by dimethylsulfoxide, and then used in scaled-up gel retardation assays with Hep3B nuclear extracts. The DNA-protein complexes C_1 and C_2 and the free DNA (F) bands were excised and treated as described in MATERIALS AND METHODS. Positions of methylated guanidine residues that interfered with complex formation are indicated by filled circles. Open circles represent partial interference. Methylation interference patterns for complex C_1 and NFκB (X)[48] are summarized at the bottom. Binding sites for NFκB and C/EBP are indicated by brackets.

functional role of YY1, SAA1 promoter constructs containing site-specific mutations at the YY1-binding site were examined in transient transfection assays. Four reporter constructs were generated: a wild-type construct—pSAA1(-117), two mutant constructs—pSAA1(-117mG$_2$) and pSAA1(-110mG$_2$) containing a 3-bp mutation in

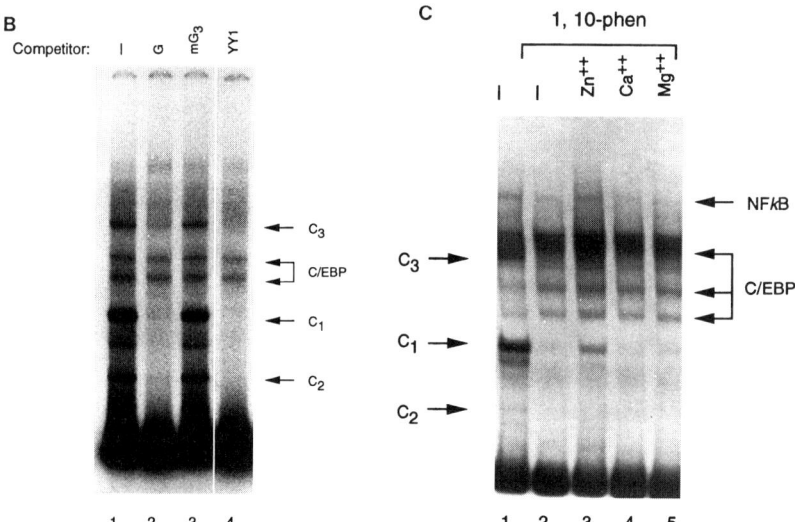

FIGURE 2. YY1 participates in complex C_1 formation. **A:** Binding sites for NF-E1/δ/YY1. Sequence comparison of DNA-binding site for complex C_1 in the rat SAA1 promoter with known YY1-binding sequences. The CCAT core sequence is highlighted. **B:** Oligonucleotide competition. Labeled CRU was incubated with Hep3B nuclear extracts in gel retardation assays. Specific DNA-protein interactions were competed with 100-fold molar excess of oligo-G (lane 2), oligo-mG$_3$ (lane 3), and YY1-binding sequence (YY1) from the α-actin promoter.[32] **C:** Zinc requirement of DNA-binding activity. Binding reactions were performed in the absence (lane 1) or presence (lanes 2 to 5) of 3 mM 1, 10-phenanthroline (1, 10-phen). Divalent cations were added (lanes 3 to 5) to a final concentration of 1 mM.

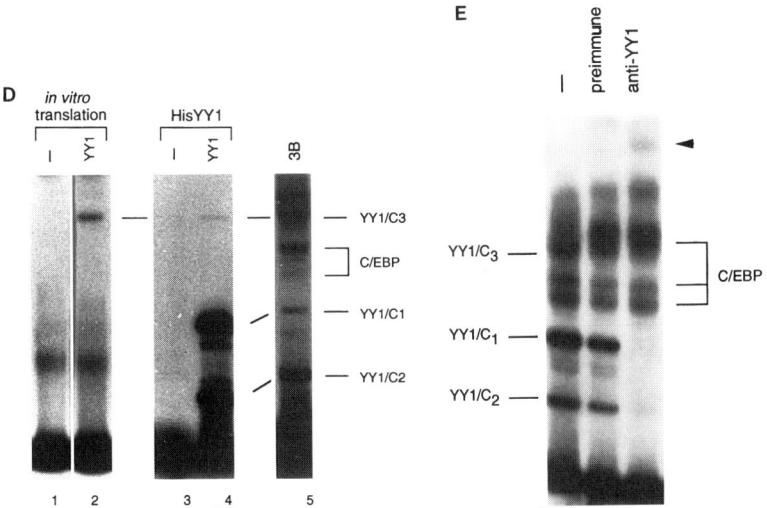

FIGURE 2. *(Continued).* **D:** Binding of recombinant YY1 to CRU. Labeled CRU probe was incubated with control reticulocyte lysate (lane 1), *in vitro* translated YY1 (lane 2), control bacterial lysate (lane 3), bacterially produced HisYY1 protein (lane 4), or Hep3B nuclear extract (lane 5). **E:** Supershift of complexes C_1, C_2, and C_3 by anti-YY1 antibodies. Hep3B nuclear extracts were preincubated with labeled CRU before adding the preimmune antibodies (preimmune) or polyclonal anti-YY1 antibodies (anti-YY1). Specific DNA-protein complexes are indicated. The supershift caused by anti-YY1 antibodies is indicated by the arrowhead.

the YY1-binding site that diminished YY1-binding activity and pSAA1(-117mG$_5$) containing a 4-bp change which converted the YY1-binding site into a strong binding site (FIG. 3A). Both types of mutation did not affect C/EBP-binding activity (data not shown). As shown in FIGURE 3B, when transfected into Hep3B cells, the wild-type construct pSAA1(-117) exhibited the expression pattern characteristic for the SAA1 promoter.[24,25] However, pSAA1(-117mG$_2$) and pSAA1(-110mG$_2$) constructs consistently showed 2- to 4-fold the basal expression level of the wild-type construct. Furthermore, their induced activities were also increased, though to a lesser extent. Thus, mutations that prevented YY1 binding actually resulted in higher promoter activity. These results are consistent with a derepression model for the regulation of the SAA1 promoter.

To further confirm that YY1 exerts a negative effect on SAA1 expression, a third mutant construct, pSAA1(-117mG$_5$), was generated in which the YY1-binding site has been mutated resulting in a 20-fold increase in YY1-binding affinity (data not shown). When transfected into Hep3B cells, pSAA1(-117mG$_5$) showed lower basal activity than that of the wild-type construct. Moreover, this construct is completely unresponsive to stimulation by the conditioned medium. A likely explanation for the lack of response is that more efficient binding of YY1 to the high-affinity YY1-binding site precludes activated NFκB from binding to the NFκB binding site and thus prevents transcription activation of the SAA1 promoter.

NFκB and YY1 Compete for Overlapping Binding Sites in the CRU

Our transient transfection studies and methylation interference experiments raised an interesting possibility that the regulatory mechanism for SAA1 transcription in-

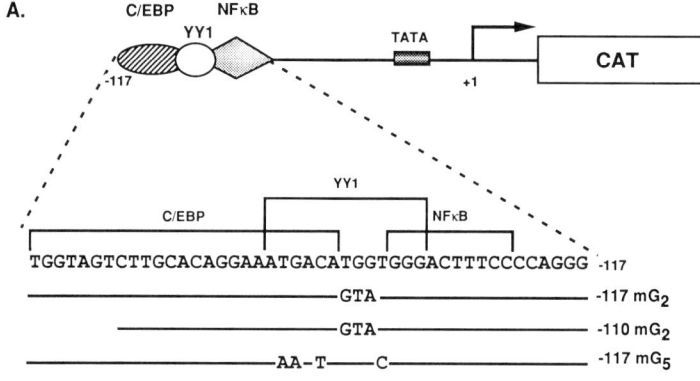

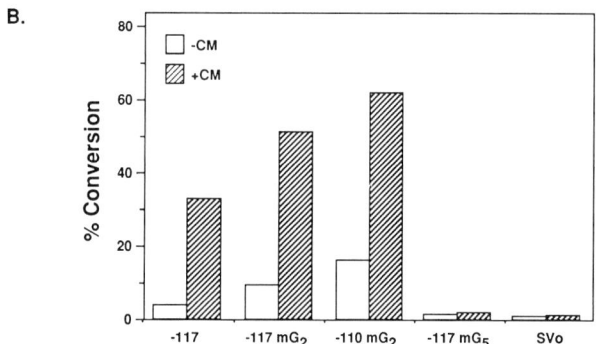

FIGURE 3. Effects of YY1-binding site mutation on SAA1 promoter activity. **A:** Schematic of CAT constructs containing the wild-type or mutated YY1-binding site. The nucleotide sequence spanning C/EBP-, YY1-, and NFκB-binding sites are shown. Mutated nucleotides in three mutant constructs, pSAA1(-117mG$_2$), pSAA1(-110mG$_2$), and pSAA1(-117mG$_5$) are indicated. **B:** Effect of YY1-binding site mutation on SAA1 promoter activity. Hep3B cells were transiently transfected with reporter constructs containing the wild-type or mutated YY1-binding site. pSVoCAT vector (SVo) was included as control. Approximately 24 h after transfection, cells were treated with basal medium (−CM) or 50% CM (+CM). Protein concentration and CAT activity were determined after 18 h of stimulation.

volves an on-off switch in which YY1 exerts its negative effects by interfering with NFκB binding to the CRU. Conversely, transcription activation by NFκB can be achieved by displacing YY1 from the CRU. Thus, the state of transcription repression or activation may depend on the relative binding efficiencies of YY1 and NFκB. To test this hypothesis, gel retardation assays were performed under probe-limiting conditions, to allow YY1 and NFκB to compete for limited amounts of target DNA. As shown in FIGURE 4, when the amount of NFκB p50 subunit was increased, its binding activity was correspondingly elevated to high levels, whereas YY1-binding activity was concomitantly reduced. These results indicate that NFκB and YY1 bind to CRU in a mutually exclusive manner.

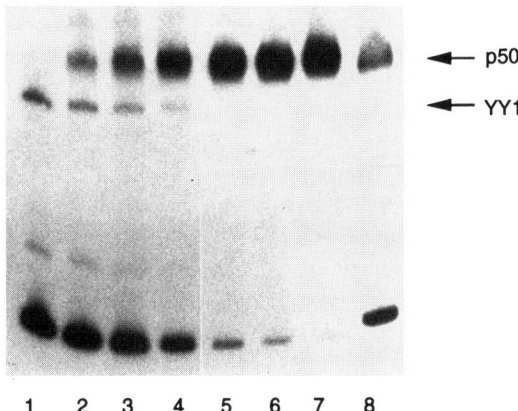

FIGURE 4. Mutually exclusive binding of NFκB and YY1 to CRU. Gel-retardation assays were performed with labeled CRU in probe-limiting conditions (3×10^3 cpm, 100 pg). Indicated amounts of recombinant NFκB p50 subunit (Promega) were added to the DNA probe and constant amounts (25 μg) of Hep3B whole cell extracts which served as source of YY1. The Hep3B whole cell extract was omitted in lane 8. Specific protein-DNA complexes are indicated by arrows.

DISCUSSION

Previous studies on rat SAA1 promoter have shown that the 65-bp CRU (positions -135 to -71) could confer cytokine responsiveness on a heterologous promoter. The induction of SAA1 by cytokines apparently depends on the synergistic interaction between NFκB- and C/EBP-binding sites within the CRU. In addition to C/EBP and NFκB, a third transcription factor was shown to interact with the CRU. We identified this factor as YY1 based on its binding site specificity, gel mobility, dependence on zinc for DNA-binding activity, functional role, and immunological cross-reactivity. Methylation interference and protein competition experiments indicated that YY1 and NFκB shared overlapping binding sites and that the binding of one factor interfered with the binding of the other. Consistent with the notion that YY1 plays a repressive role in SAA1 expression, site-specific mutations that abolished YY1 binding elevated the basal and cytokine-induced activities of SAA1 promoter. Moreover, introduction of a strong YY1-binding site specifically reduced SAA1 expression in transient cotransfection assays. Therefore, YY1 functions as a negative regulator, repressing the SAA1 promoter through competition with NFκB for overlapping binding sites.

Based on these findings, we propose a model depicting the transcriptional repression and activation of rat SAA1 gene in control cells and in response to cytokine induction (FIG. 5). Activation of the rat SAA1 promoter is achieved through combina-

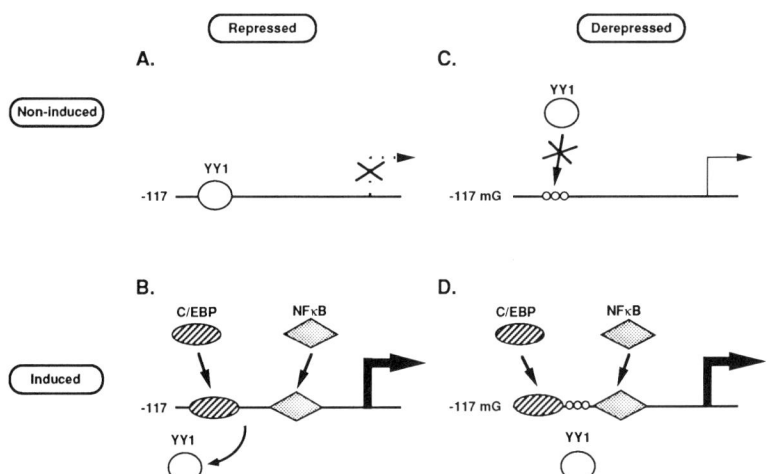

FIGURE 5. Model for transcriptional repression and activation through the interplay of YY1, NFκB, and C/EBP. A two-stage occupancy model (A and B) is proposed for the rat SAA1 promoter. **A:** In noninduced cells, YY1 functions as a transcription repressor contributing to the low level of SAA1 basal expression. **B:** Upon cytokine induction, elevated C/EBP- and NFκB-binding activities not only displace YY1 or prevent YY1 from binding, but also transactivate the SAA1 promoter, thus converting the promoter from a transcriptionally silent state to one that is highly active. **C:** Mutation of YY1-binding site results in the derepression of SAA1 promoter in control cells and **D:** even greater response in cytokine-stimulated cells. Potential protein-protein interactions of YY1, NFκB, and C/EBP with each other or with transcription factors in the initiation complex are not shown.

torial changes in the binding activities of the cytokine-induced NFκB and C/EBP transactivators and the ubiquitously expressed YY1 repressor. In noninduced cells, NFκB exists in a latent form and is retained in the cytoplasm.[38,39] On the other hand, YY1 is found in the nucleus, capable of binding to the CRU. Thus YY1 exerts its repressive effects on the SAA1 promoter, contributing to the very low basal activity (FIG. 5A). In response to cytokine stimulation, binding activities of nuclear NFκB and C/EBP are elevated, while that of YY1 remains constant.[40] Increased NFκB- and C/EBP-binding activities displace YY1 from the CRU, converting the SAA1 promoter from a transcriptionally silent state to one that is highly active (FIG. 5B). At the end of the acute-phase response, NFκB- and C/EBP-binding activities return to basal levels, allowing YY1 to reoccupy its binding site and shutoff SAA1 transcription. The ability of YY1 to reoccupy CRU may contribute to the transiency of SAA1 expression. Mutations that abolish YY1 binding result in derepression of the SAA1 promoter (FIG. 5C). Because NFκB and C/EBP transactivators are not activated in nonstimulated cells, this derepression only elevates the promoter activity two- to fourfold. Subsequent stimulation with cytokines further increases promoter activity to levels that are higher than the controls (FIG. 5D), presumably owing to the absence of YY1-binding site for YY1 to compete with NFκB for DNA-binding. Therefore, the expression of SAA1 is strictly regulated by the interplay between repressor and activators to ensure it is expressed under appropriate physiological conditions.

YY1 is a multifunctional transcription factor that plays a key role in the expression of many mammalian and viral genes.[34–37,41,42] Although the diverse effects of YY1 remain to be analyzed, our studies indicated that one of the mechanisms by which YY1 represses SAA1 transcription is through competition with the transcription activator NFκB for overlapping binding sites. Interestingly, YY1 has also been shown to exert negative effects on other gene regulatory elements (α-actin[31,32,37]; ϵ-globin[43]; β-casein[44]) by competing for overlapping binding sites with transactivators. Thus, competing with distinct transcription activators for overlapping cis-acting elements is one mechanism by which YY1 represses transcription. It is noteworthy that in contrast to SAA1 gene transcription, which is transiently induced in response to acute inflammation, the expression of α-actin, ϵ-globin, and β-casein genes is developmentally regulated and has more long-term effects. Interestingly, our binding studies showed that the YY1-binding site in the CRU is a much weaker site than that in the serum response element of the α-actin promoter (unpublished results). The weak YY1-binding site in CRU may allow inflammation-induced NFκB to displace YY1 more readily, resulting in more efficient activation of SAA1 promoter. Thus, a weak YY1-binding site in the SAA1 promoter may be a necessity for SAA1 induction, whereas a strong YY1-binding site is necessary for more long-term repression of α-actin gene in myoblasts.

Our studies showed that increasing amounts of NFκB can displace YY1 form CRU. However, given the transcriptional synergism between NFκB and C/EBP,[25,45] it remains possible that *in vivo* both NFκB and C/EBP are required to efficiently displace YY1. This cooperative displacement may involve protein-protein interactions between these activators and the repressor. Interestingly, two recent studies[46,47] demonstrated functional and physical association between the ATF bZIP proteins and NFκB. Thus, cross-family interaction between Rel family and bZIP family proteins, in which one transcription factor can modulate the activity of another by direct physical interaction, may constitute a novel mechanism for regulating the potent transcription factor NFκB. Since NFκB can respond to a variety of stimulating agents in many cell types and serve as a potent transcriptional activator for many inducible genes,[38,39] its interactions with C/EBP and YY1 may represent an additional strategy to ensure that the acute-phase mediators can cause the specific induction of SAA through NFκB-activating pathways.

ACKNOWLEDGMENTS

We are grateful to Drs. Robert Schwartz and Te-Chung Lee for providng YY1-binding sequence and rabbit polyclonal antibodies against recombinant human YY1, and to Drs. Tom Shenk and Eduardo Montalvo for providing HisYY1 plasmid and human YY1 cDNA. Alisha Tizenor's assistance with the graphics is greatly appreciated.

REFERENCES

1. JIANG, J., C. A. RUSHLOW, Q. ZHOU, S. SMALL & M. LEVINE. 1992. EMBO J. **11:** 3147–3154.
2. MANIATIS, T., S. GOODBOURN & J. A. FISCHER. 1987. Science **236:** 1237–1245.
3. ARNOSTI, D. N., A. MERINO, D. REINBERG & W. SCHAFFNER. 1993. EMBO J. **12:** 157–166.
4. GOODRICH, J. A., T. HOEY, C. J. THUT, A. ADMON & R. TJIAN. 1993. Cell **75:** 519–530.
5. PTASHNE, M. 1988. Nature (London) **335:** 683–689.
6. XU, X., C. PROROCK, H. ISHIKAWA, E. MALDONADO, Y. ITO & C. GELINAS. 1993. Mol. Cell. Biol. **13:** 6733–6741.

7. MITCHELL, P. J. & R. TJIAN. 1989. Science **245:** 371–378.
8. PONTA, H., A. C. B. CATO & P. HERRLICH. 1992. Biochim Biophys Acta **1129:** 255–261.
9. RENKAWITZ, R. 1990. Trends in Genet. **6:** 192–196.
10. FONDELL, J. D., A. L. ROY & R. G. ROEDER. 1993. Genes Dev. **7:** 1400–1410.
11. HOCH, M., N. GERWIN, H. TAUBERT & H. JACKLE. 1992. Science **256:** 94–97.
12. JAYNES, J. B. & P. H. O'FARRELL. 1991. EMBO J. **10:** 1427–1433.
13. LEVINE, M. & J. L. MANLEY. 1989. Cell **59:** 405–408.
14. LICHT, J. D., M. J. GROSSEL, J. FIGGE & U. M. HANSEN. 1990. Nature (London) **346:** 76–79.
15. LIU, Y., N. YANG & C. T. TENG. 1993. Mol. Cell. Biol. **13:** 1836–1846.
16. PAULWEBER, B., F. SANDHOFER & B. LEVY-WILSON. 1993. Mol. Cell. Biol. **13:** 1534–1546.
17. STANOJEVIC, D., S. SMALL & M. LEVINE. 1991. Science **254:** 1385–1387.
18. TENHARMSEL, A., R. J. AUSTIN, N. SAVENELLI & M. D. BIGGIN. 1993. Mol. Cell. Biol. **13:** 2742–2752.
19. FEY, G. H. & G. M. FULLER. 1987. Mol. Biol. Med. **4:** 323–338.
20. KUSHNER, I. 1982. Ann. N. Y. Acad. Sci. **389:** 39–48.
21. GAULDIE, J. & H. BAUMANN. 1991. *In* Cytokines and Inflammation. E. S. Kimball, Ed. : 275–305. Boca Raton, Ann Arbor, Boston, London: CRC Press.
22. LOWELL, C. A., R. S. STEARMAN & J. F. MORROW. 1986. J. Biol. Chem. **261:** 8453–8461.
23. RIENHOFF, H. Y., JR., J. H. HUANG, X. LI & W. S. L. LIAO. 1990. Mol. Biol. Med. **7:** 287–298.
24. LI, X. & W. S. L. LIAO. 1991. J. Biol. Chem. **266:** 15192–15201.
25. LI, X. & W. S. L. LIAO. 1992. Nucleic Acids Res. **20:** 4765–4772.
26. BRADFORD, M. M. 1976. Anal. Biochem. **72:** 248–254.
27. GORMAN, C. M., L. F. MOFFAT & B. H. HOWARD. 1982. Mol. Cell. Biol. **2:** 1044–1051.
28. SHAPIRO, D. J., P. A. SHARP, W. W. WAHLI & M. J. KELLER. 1988. DNA **7:** 47–55.
29. KADONAGA, J. T. & R. TJIAN. 1986. Proc. Natl. Acad. Sci. USA **83:** 5889–5893.
30. HUANG, J. H. & W. S.-L. LIAO. 1994. Mol. Cell. Biol. **14:** 4475–4484.
31. LEE, T.-C., K.-L. CHOW, P. FANG & R. J. SCHWARTZ. 1991. Mol. Cell. Biol. **11:** 5090–5100.
32. LEE, T.-C., Y. SHI & R. J. SCHWARTZ. 1992. Proc. Natl. Acad. Sci. USA **89:** 9814–9818.
33. FLANAGAN, J. R., K. G. BECKER, D. L. ENNIST, S. L. GLEASON, P. H. DRIGGERS, B.-Z. LEVI, E. APPELLA & K. OZATO. 1992. Mol. Cell. Biol. **12:** 38–44.
34. HARIHARAN, N., D. E. KELLEY & R. P. PERRY. 1991. Proc. Natl. Acad. Sci. USA **88:** 9799–9803.
35. PARK, K. & M. L. ATCHISON. 1991. Proc. Natl. Acad. Sci. USA **88:** 9804–9808.
36. SHI, Y., E. SETO, L.-S. CHANG & T. SHENK. 1991. Cell **67:** 377–388.
37. GUALBERTO, A., D. LEPAGE, G. PONS, S. L. MADER, K. PARK, M. L. ATCHISON & K. WALSH. 1992. Mol. Cell. Biol. **12:** 4209–4214.
38. BAEUERLE, P. A. & D. BALTIMORE. 1988. Science **242:** 540–546.
39. BEG, A. A. & A. S. BALDWIN, JR. 1993. Genes Dev. **7:** 2064–2070.
40. LU, S. Y., M. RODRIGUEZ & W. S.-L. LIAO. 1994. Mol. Cell. Biol. **14:** 6253–6263.
41. HAHN, S. 1992. Current Biol. **2:** 152–154.
42. RIGGS, K. J., S. SALEQUE, K.-K. WONG, K. T. MERRELL, J.-S. LEE, Y. SHI & K. CALAME. 1993. Mol. Cell. Biol. **13:** 7487–7495.
43. PETERS, B., N. MEREZHINSKAYA, J. F. X. DIFFLEY & C. T. NOGUCHI. 1993. J. Biol. Chem. **268:** 3430–3437.
44. RAUGHT, B., B. KHURSHEED, A. KAZANSKY & J. ROSEN. 1994. Mol. Cell. Biol. **14:** 1752–1763.
45. STEIN, B. & A. S. BALDWIN, JR. 1993. Mol. Cell. Biol. **13:** 7191–7198.
46. DU, W., D. THANOS & T. MANIATIS. 1993. Cell **74:** 887–898.
47. KASZUBSKA, W., R. HOOFT VAN HUIJSDUIJNEN, P. GHERSA, A.-M. DERAEMY-SCHENK, B. P. C. CHEN, T. HAI, J. F. DELAMARTER & J. WHELAN. 1993. Mol. Cell. Biol. **13:** 7180–7190.
48. BAEUERLE, P. A. 1991. Biochim. Biophys. Acta **1072:** 63–80.
49. HUANG, J. H., H. Y. REINHOFF, JR. & W. S. L. LIAO. 1990. Mol. Cell. Biol. **10:** 3619–3625.

DISCUSSION OF THE PAPER

I. KUSHNER (*Case Western Reserve University, Cleveland, OH*): Warren, that was a beautiful presentation. I want to follow up on your initial statement that IL-1 is a major inducer of SAA. You are working with a rat model, and I am thinking particularly of studies with human SAA; many people have found that IL-6 plays a substantial role and indeed in some cells it is the only cytokine that can do it. So I wanted you to comment whether you were willing to admit that IL-6 may play a role and whether there is any possibility that APRF might be involved in that.

W. LIAO: Yes, in our studies of the rat SAA-1 gene IL-1 does play a major role. What I did not talk about is our studies with SAA-3. In that case the regulatory mechanism is completely different. The SAA-1 is not responsive to IL-6 and the addition of IL-6 to IL-1 does not activate it further. However, for SAA-3 IL-1 again is a major activator. But in that case, addition of IL-6 synergizes with IL-1 and gives higher activity. In our studies we have looked at the cytokine response element and found again that C/EBP is one of the transcription factors required. In addition, we have found a novel factor which we call SEF-1, but this factor is a constitutive factor and does not change following cytokine treatment. Interestingly, right in the middle of SEF-1 binding site there is a consensus APRF binding site; now we are checking whether this site indeed can function as an APRF binding site and therefore confirm these synergistic effects with IL-6.

Isolation of Two Interleukin-6 Response Element Binding Proteins from Acute Phase Rat Livers[a]

JÜRGEN RIPPERGER,[b] STEFAN FRITZ,[b] KARIN RICHTER,[b]
BIRGIT DREIER,[b] KURT SCHNEIDER,[b] KLAUS LÖCHNER,[b]
ROLF MARSCHALEK,[b] GERTRUD HOCKE,[b]
FRIEDRICH LOTTSPEICH,[c] AND GEORG H. FEY[b]

[b]*University of Erlangen-Nürnberg*
D 91058 Erlangen, Germany

[c]*Max Planck Institute for Biochemistry*
D 82152 Martinsried, Germany

INTRODUCTION

Hepatic acute phase genes have been divided into two classes according to the cytokines, that are their main inducers.[1–3] Class 1 genes are regulated by both interleukin-1 (IL-1) and interleukin-6 (IL-6) and their transcription is enhanced by glucocorticoids. Class 2 genes are controlled by IL-6 and glucocorticoids. Class 1 includes the hemopexin, haptoglobin, α_1 acid glycoprotein, human C-reactive protein, serum amyloid A and complement C3 genes. Some of these genes, such as the α_1 acid glycoprotein gene, are regulated synergistically by combinations of IL-1 and IL-6.[1,3,4] Tumor necrosis factor α (TNFα) has similar effects on class 1 genes as IL-1. For both classes interleukin-11 (IL-11), leukemia inhibitory factor (LIF) and oncostatin M (OSM) can substitute for IL-6, at least in cultured hepatic cells.[1,3,5–8] Representatives of class 2 are the β-fibrinogen, α_1 proteinase inhibitor (α_1 antitrypsin), cysteine-proteinase inhibitor (thiostatin), α_1 antichymotrypsin and rat α_2 macroglobulin (α_2M) genes. These genes can be induced by the IL-6-type cytokines (IL-6, IL-11, LIF and OSM), but not by IL-1.[1,3] IL-1 counteracts the induction of some class 2 genes, including the β-fibrinogen gene, by IL-6.[3,9,10] Class 1 genes utilize the transcription factor C/EBPβ (also referred to as NF-IL6) as their main cytokine-activated control factor.[11–14] The transcription factors regulating class 2 genes have not yet been fully identified. The factors APRF/Stat3 (acute phase response factor/singal transducer and activator of transcription 3) and p91/Stat1 are clearly involved in the regulation of class 2 genes.[15–19] The present study provides an indication for the participation of at least one additional DNA binding protein in the cytokine-induced transcription of class 2 genes.

The activation of class 2 genes follows a different time course under different experimental conditions. In hepatoma cell lines stably transfected with reporter con-

---

[a] This work was supported by a research grant from Deutsche Forschungsgemeinschaft (to G.H.F.) and a graduate student fellowship from the state of Bavaria (to J.R.).

Address for correspondence: Dr. Georg H. Fey, Chair of Genetics, University of Erlangen-Nürnberg, Staudtstrasse 5, D 91058 Erlangen, Germany. Tel: 0049-9131-858493; Fax: 0049-9131-858526.

structs, that carried the control regions of class 2 genes, increased transcription was observed within one hour after addition of the cytokine. Maximum transcriptional activity was reached approximately 3 to 4 hours after the addition of the cytokine.[20-23,27] In living rats the response was slower, and the time course depended on the nature of the stimulus and the route of its administration. When the acute phase response was triggered by an intraperitoneal injection of complete Freund's adjuvant (CFA), hepatic transcription rates of the α_2M gene reached a maximum 12 to 16 hours after the injection, and α_2M mRNA accumulated to peak concentrations after 18 to 20 hours.[24-26] The response was faster, when the stimulus was an intravenous injection of IL-6 or lipopolysaccharides (LPS).[15,17] Other investigators have successfully purified transcription factors mediating the effects of IL-6 from mouse livers after intravenous injection of recombinant IL-6. The factor APRF/Stat3 was discovered by such experiments.[17] Here we report the purification of two nuclear proteins binding at the IL-6 response element (IL-6 RE) of the α_2M gene from rat livers, that had been excised 8 to 12 hours after an intraperitoneal injection of CFA.

PURIFICATION OF IL-6 RE-BINDING PROTEINS

The IL-6 RE of the rat α_2M gene is a binding site for nuclear proteins, that interact with this element in a sequence-specific manner. Binding was detected by DNAseI footprinting, methylation interference and gel mobility shift experiments.[20,27,28] A highly characteristic protein-DNA complex (complex II, FIG. 1) was observed, when nuclear extracts from acute phase rat livers were reacted with a radiolabeled, double-stranded synthetic oligonucleotide (TB2, FIG. 1), that contained a tandem dimer of the IL-6 RE of the rat α_2M gene.[20,28] No corresponding complex was obtained with nuclear extracts from untreated control animals. The complex was sequence specific for the IL-6 RE as determined by competition gel mobility shift experiments.[20,28] A complex of indistinguishable mobility was also obtained with nuclear extracts from IL-6-treated rat and human hepatoma cells (FIG. 1). Nuclear extracts from untreated control cultures produced either only a very weak complex II or none (FIG. 1). The protein composition of these complexes was unknown when this study was initiated and may have differed for rat and human cells. However, the identical mobility of the complexes from both species was taken to indicate, that the proteins assembling these complexes were probably conserved and may thus be functionally important. Other protein-DNA complexes migrating faster than complex II were also detected (FIG. 1). They were not specific for the IL-6 RE and were therefore neglected in this context.

An additional indication for the potential importance of complex II was obtained from time course studies. Complex II was clearly detected with nuclear extracts from livers excised 2 hours after an intraperitoneal injection of CFA. Its intensity gradually increased and reached a maximum with extracts from livers excised 10 to 12 hours after the injection. Although the parallel increase of the transcriptional activity of the α_2M gene[24,25] and the intensity of this complex may have been coincidental, we interpreted this finding as an additional indication of a functional relevance of complex II. Therefore, it was decided to purify the protein(s) that assemble complex II from adult rat livers 8 to 12 hours after provoking an acute phase response by intraperitoneal injection of CFA.

Nuclei were prepared from the livers of adult male Sprague-Dawley rats (300 to 400 g body weight) after injection of CFA (0.4 ml per 100 g body weight). Livers were

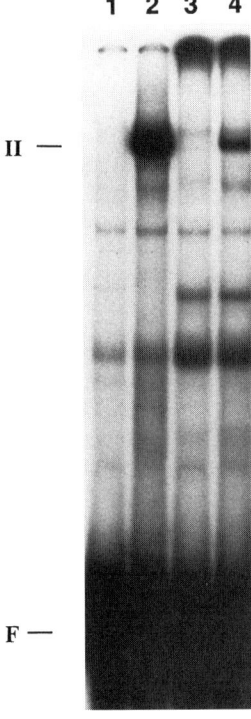

FIGURE 1. IL-6 RE binding proteins form a characteristic cytokine-induced protein-DNA complex revealed by gel mobility shift experiments. Nuclei were prepared from the livers of control animals (adult male Sprague Dawley rats) and from animals with an experimentally induced acute phase reaction (intraperitoneal injection of CFA). Livers were excised ten hours after the injection. Nuclear proteins were extracted following published procedures[29,30] and were incubated with the radiolabeled double-stranded oligonucleotide TB2, which contained two tandem copies of the IL-6 RE core element of the rat α_2M gene.[20,28] The sequence of TB2 was: 5' GAT CAT CCT T*CT GGG A*AT TCT GAT ATC CTT *CTG GGA* ATT CTG 3', where the nucleotides printed in italics represent the IL-6 RE core. TB2 was endlabeled with polynucleotide kinase and ^{32}P γ-ATP (adenosine triphosphate). The reaction mixtures were loaded on a nondenaturing polyacrylamide gel and separated by electrophoresis. The double-stranded free oligonucleotide migrated to position F. The characteristic cytokine-induced complex II is marked. This complex contained tyrosine-phosphorylated STAT factors binding at the IL-6 RE.[15,17,34] Other complexes migrating faster than complex II were shown to be non-specific.[20,28] Tracks 1,2: nuclear extracts from untreated rats and rats with an experimentally induced acute phase response. Tracks 3,4: Nuclear extracts from untreated and IL-6 treated Hep3B human hepatoma cells.[20–22] Similar results were also obtained with nuclear extracts from IL-6-treated FaO rat hepatoma cells.[21,27]

minced and homogenized in a custom-designed blender, and nuclei were collected by sedimentation through a sucrose cushion as described.[29,30] Nuclear proteins were extracted with 0.4 M lithium chloride and preciptiated with ammonium sulfate. The precipitate was resuspended, dialyzed and purified by three conventional column chromatography steps. The purification scheme was designed around a binding-site specific DNA affinity chromatography step as its central element.[31] However, pilot studies showed that the proteins building complex II copurified with a nuclease, that destroyed the affinity reagent. Therefore, conventional chromatographic media were tested in search of one, that removed the nucleolytic activity. No single medium achieved a complete separation, but a combination of three different columns produced satisfactory results. The optimized purification scheme is summarized in FIGURE 2. Purfication was monitored by performing gel-mobility shift experiments across the column profiles under similar conditions as in FIGURE 1. A significant removal of the proteins forming the non-specific complexes detected in FIGURE 1 was achieved. At the same time, the proteins capable of forming complex II copurified over all three columns, suggesting that either only a single polypeptide assembled the complex or several polypeptides with very similar chromatographic properties. After the final DNA affinity step, the purification was evaluated by electrophoresis in a sodium dodecyl sulfate (SDS)-polyacrylamide gel, followed by silver staining. Only three proteins of 92, 91 and 86 kD were visible at this point. The overall enrichment of

FIGURE 2. Purification scheme for IL-6 RE binding nuclear proteins from the livers of rats undergoing an acute phase response. Various parameters were optimized for the production of nuclear extracts, including the choice of a well-responding rat strain, the dose of the stimulus, the time-point for excision of the livers, conditions for the use of a custom-designed homogenizer (for the large scale homogenization of livers with 6 livers per batch), conditions for the sedimentation of nuclei through a sucrose cushion, conditions for optimal extraction of proteins from the nuclei (ionic strength, type of salt, choice of proteinase inhibitors and detergents, concentration of ammonium sulfate for precipitation of nuclear proteins, conditions for dialysis and resuspension). Optimized nuclear extracts were then applied to an SP-sepharose column and the relevant proteins were located in the flow-through. The flow-through was loaded onto a Q-sepharose column, which was step-eluted with increasing concentrations of potassium chloride. The proteins of interest were found in the 250 mM KCl fraction and were then applied directly to a phenyl-sepharose column. IL-6 RE binding proteins were released from this column by step elution with a buffer of very low ionic strength. DNA-affinity chromatography was performed next in two steps. First, the proteins were passed through an affinity column carrying a double-stranded oligonucleotide, mTB2, that contained a mutated IL-6 RE sequence. This sequence was no longer capable of specific binding, but still retained non-specific DNA binding proteins. The sequence of mTB2 was: 5' GAT CAT CCT T*GA TAT* CAT TCT GAT ATC CTT *GAT ATC* ATT CTG 3'.[20,28] The nucleotides printed in italics represent the mutated core of the IL-6 RE (see FIG. 1). Double-stranded mTB2 was multimerized by self-ligation and coupled to cyanogen-bromide (CNBr)–activated sepharose 4B following standard procedures.[31] The relevant proteins were then applied to a final affinity column with multimerized double-stranded TB2. The preparation of this column using self-ligated TB2 and CNBr-activated sepharose 4B and the elution conditions followed published procedures.[31]

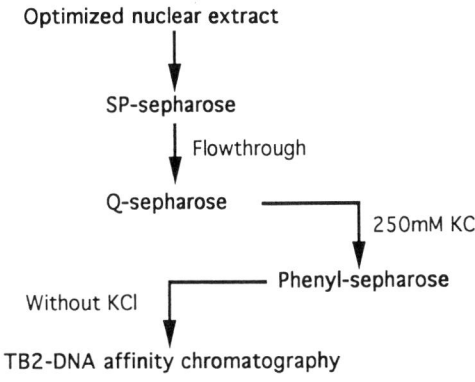

these proteins was greater than 6,000-fold. One large scale preparation (50 rats, 13 to 15 g per liver) typically yielded 10 μg of purified protein.

PARTIAL AMINOACID SEQUENCE ANALYSIS

In a first large-scale experiment the three polypeptides of 92, 91 and 86 kD were separated on a preparative polyacrylamide gel and electroblotted onto glossy bond (Biometra).[32] An attempt to determine the N-terminal sequences of all three proteins failed, because all had blocked N-termini. Therefore, it was necessary to produce and separate proteolytic fragments from each of the proteins for the purpose of sequence analysis. In a second large scale experiment, the three bands were excised and the proteins were partially digested inside the gel slices with lysyl endopeptidase.[33] The resulting peptide fragments were extracted from the gel and separated by reverse-phase high pressure liquid chromatography (HPLC). Well resolved peptides were then sequenced. As a result, one peptide sequence of 13 amino acid residues was obtained for the 86 kD protein and four sequences for the 91 kD species. All sequences showed strong similarity with the published mouse and human APRF/Stat3 se-

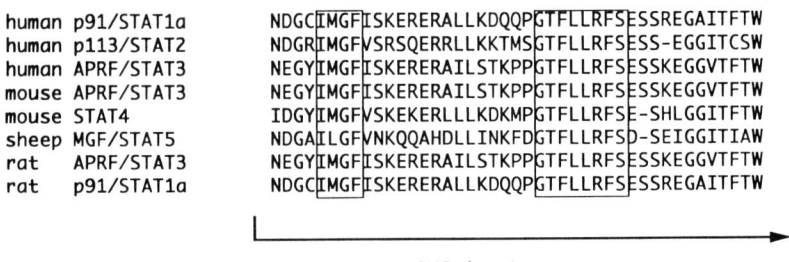

FIGURE 3. Conservation of the SH2 domain sequences in various Stat factors from humans, rodents and sheep. The boxed sequences are highly conserved. The human, mouse and sheep sequences are as published: human Stat1a and 2[35,36]; human and mouse APRF/Stat3[17]; mouse Stat4[37,38]; sheep MGF/Stat5.[39] The rat Stat1a and Stat3 sequences were determined from the cDNA clones described in the text and have not been previously published. The acute phase rat liver cDNA library was prepared in the vector λZapll (Stratagene Inc., La Jolla, California).

quences.[17] It was therefore concluded, that the peptides were fragments of rat APRF/Stat3. It is not clear, why rat Stat3 migrated at two positions corresponding to 86 and at 91 kD in an SDS polyacrylamide gel. The possibility, that different secondarily modified species were responsible for this result has to be considered.

The 92 kD protein produced two peptide sequences of 11 and 8 amino acid residues in length. A search of the available databases showed, that they were not related to Stats 1 and 3. Their sequences however did resemble a different Stat factor, and this interpretation was confirmed by additional experiments. A cDNA library was prepared with mRNA from acute phase rat livers. cDNA clones for Stats 1 and 3 and this 92 kD Stat factor were isolated and partially sequenced. The peptide sequences described above were contained in the cDNA-derived amino acid sequences. The sequences of each of these three cDNA species were then compared with the published sequences of mouse and human STAT factors. From this analysis it was concluded that the proteins purified were indeed rat Stat3 and another Stat factor distinct from rat Stats 1 and 3. A complete account of the identity and structure of this 92 kD Stat factor is in preparation. A comparison of the sequences of the SH2 domains (src-homology domains type 2) of mouse and human STAT factors, with those of rat Stats 1 and 3 derived from the cDNA clones described above is given in FIGURE 3.

DISCUSSION

Two IL-6 RE-binding proteins resulted from the purification described in this report: Stat3 and a 92 kD Stat factor distinct from Stats 1 and 3. This result was both reassuring and surprising. It was reassuring, because other authors had purified mouse Stat3 as one of the factors binding at an IL-6 RE.[17] It was surprising, because these other authors had not reported the purification of the murine equivalent of the 92 kD protein.[17] In addition, it was known, that rat Stat1 also binds at the IL-6 RE.[15,16,34,35] Therefore it was surprising, that Stat1 was not among the proteins purified by our procedure. Only tentative not definitive explanations of these results can be offered. One possibility is, that rat Stat1 may also have been among the proteins purified by our procedure, but conceivably its proteolytic peptide fragments were not among the few well-resolved species, that were selected for aminoacid sequence analysis. Alternatively, rat Stat1 may have been lost during the purification. It is known, that Stats 1 and 3 can bind either as homodimers or as heterodimers at the IL-6 RE.[15,17,34] If Stat1 had a weaker affinity for the site used in our procedure than Stat3 and the 92 kD factor, then it may have been separated from these two proteins during the purification and we may not have noticed it. In our purification those proteins were enriched, that formed the strongest complex II. If Stat1 either bound weakly at this site or was present in much smaller amounts than the other two factors and eluted at a different position in the column profiles, then we may have disregarded it while focusing on the material, that produced the strongest complex II. We cannot comment on why other authors have not reported the purification of the mouse homolog of the rat 92 kD Stat factor. In one report, peptides from factors other than APRF/STAT3 were also obtained, but not identified.[17] The murine homolog of the 92 kD rat Stat may have been one of those factors. Alternatively, the different results may have been the consequence of differences in the design of the two experiments. These other authors injected recombinant IL-6 intraveneously into mice and excised the livers 15 min after the injection. They also purified proteins by using a synthetic oligonucleotide representing the IL-6 RE of the rat α_2M gene, but the sequence of their oligonucleotide differed from ours. Their oligonucleotide was designed to represent the consensus IL-6 RE with a sequence modified for palindromic symmetry.[17,23] Our oligonucleotide consisted of two tandem copies of the core site in its original sequence. Thus, the different results may be due to species-specific differences in the abundance of the 92 kD STAT factor between rats and mice or to the different time points in the acute phase response, at which the livers were excised. Finally, they may also be due to different affinities of the 92 kD Stat factor for the two different oligonucleotide sequences used in these two studies. While all three STAT factors bind at the IL-6 RE of the α_2M gene, they conceivably do so with different affinities. The consensus binding sites and binding affinities of these three factors have not yet been measured directly. Thus, the two data sets do not contradict but rather complement each other.

The main new result of this study was the discovery of the 92 kD Stat factor in acute phase rat livers as one of the IL-6 RE binding proteins. We have not yet known, that it functions as a cytokine-induced transcription factor to mediate the IL-6 induced transcription of the α_2M gene. To show this would require additional functional studies—for example, the transfection of expression constructs for this factor into hepatoma cells and the demonstration that the factor enhances the IL-6-induced transcription of cotransfected reporter constructs carrying an IL-6 RE. Such experiments are planned, but have not yet been performed. However, the 92 kD factor is a member of the family of Stat factors, which are recognized transcription factors, and at least Stat3 has the capability, demonstrated by transfection studies, to mediate the effect of IL-6 on the transcriptional induction of the α_2M gene promoter (T. Kishimoto, personal communication). Therefore the 92 kD Stat factor probably is not only an IL-6 RE binding protein, but a transcription factor, that mediates the effect of IL-6 on the α_2M gene.

It has not yet been demonstrated, that the 92 kD factor is part of complex II. To demonstrate this would require specific antisera against the 92 kD factor, and such sera are not yet available. If the 92 kD factor were a functionally relevant factor and participated in the formation of complex II, as we suspect, then this would open interesting new possibilities. It would then become necessary to determine, whether it forms a complex II only as a homodimer, or also as a heterodimer and whether complexes with different heterodimerization partners mediate different functions. With the cloned cDNA for the 92 kD Stat factor now available it is possible to address these questions in the future.

SUMMARY

Proteins binding at the IL-6 response element of the rat α_2 macroglobulin gene were purified by a combination of conventional chromatographic procedures and binding-site specific DNA affinity chromatography. The proteins were purified from the nuclei of rat livers, excised at the peak of an experimentally induced acute phase response. By this procedure three polypeptides of 92, 91 and 86 kD were enriched more than 6,000-fold. Partial proteolysis with lysyl endopeptidase and aminoacid sequence analysis of proteolytic peptides identified the 86 and 91 kD species as the transcription factor Stat3 and the 92 kD species as a Stat factor distinct from Stats 1 and 3. cDNA clones for Stats 1, 3 and this 92 kD factor were isolated from a cDNA library prepared with mRNA from acute phase rat livers. Parts of their DNA sequences were determined and the sequences of the purified peptides were found in these cDNA sequences. Thus, the identity of the factors as Stat3 and a Stat factor different from Stats 1 and 3 was confirmed. These results suggest, thast APRF/Stat3 and p91/Stat1 are not the only factors mediating the effects of IL-6 on class 2 acute phase genes. The 92 kD Stat factor binding at the IL-6 RE probably also functions as a transcription factor in the cytokine-induced activation of the α_2M gene.

ACKNOWLEDGMENTS

We thank Drs. Daniel Lavery and Uli Schibler for advice on the purification of transcription factors and for providing blueprints for a homogenizer. We are indebted to Ward Coppersmith and colleagues from the instrument shop of the Scripps Research Institute for building the homogenizer. Prof. Hannappel made valuable suggestions for chromatographic procedures, and the generous gift of the proteinase inhibitor aprotinin (Trasylol™) by Drs. E. Möller and M. Mardin from Bayer AG, Germany, is gratefully acknowledged.

REFERENCES

1. BAUMANN, H. & J. GAULDIE. 1990. Regulation of hepatic acute phase plasma protein genes by hepatocyte stimulating factors and other mediators of inflammation. Mol. Biol. Med. **3:** 147–159.
2. BAUMANN, H., C. RICHARDS & J. GAULDIE. 1987. Interaction among hepatocyte-stimulating factors, interleukin-1 and glucocorticoids for regulation of acute phase plasma proteins in human hepatoma (HepG2) cells. J. Immunol. **139:** 4122–4128.
3. KOJ, A., J. GAULDIE & H. BAUMANN. 1993. Biological perspectives of cytokine and hormone networks. *In* Acute Phase Proteins. Molecular Biology, Biochemistry, and Clinical Applications. A. Mackiewicz, I. Kushner & H. Baumann, Eds.: 275–288. Boca Raton, FL: CRC Press.
4. BAUMANN, H., K. R. PROWSE, K.-A. WON & S. MARINKOVIC-PAJOVIC. 1993. Regulation of α_1-acid glycoprotein genes and relationship to other type 1 acute phase plasma proteins. *In* Acute Phase Proteins. Molecular Biology, Biochemistry, and Clinical Applications. A. Mackiewicz, I. Kushner & H. Baumann, Eds.: 409–423. Boca Raton, FL: CRC Press.
5. BAUMANN, H. & P. SCHENDEL. 1991. Interleukin-11 regulates the hepatic expression of the same plasma protein genes as interleukin-6. J. Biol. Chem. **266:** 20424–20427.
6. YANG, Y.-C. 1993. Interleukin-11: Molecular biology, biological activities, and possible signaling pathways. *In* Acute Phase Proteins. Molecular Biology, Biochemistry, and Clinical Applications. A. Mackiewicz, I. Kushner & H. Baumann, Eds.: 309–319. Boca Raton, FL: CRC Press.

7. RICHARDS, C. D., T. J. BROWN, M. SHOYAB, H. BAUMANN & J. GAULDIE. 1992. Recombinant oncostatin M stimulates the production of acute phase proteins in HepG2 cells and primary rat hepatocytes in vitro. J. Immunol. **148:** 1731–1736.
8. RICHARDS, C. D. & M. SHOYAB. 1993. The role of oncostatin M in the acute phase response. *In* Acute Phase Proteins. Molecular Biology, Biochemistry, and Clinical Applications. A. Mackiewicz, I. Kushner & H. Baumann, Eds.: 321–327. Boca Raton, FL: CRC Press.
9. GAULDIE, J., C. RICHARDS, D. HARNISH, P. LANSDORP & H. BAUMANN. 1987. Interferon-$\beta 2$ shares identity with monocyte-derived hepatocyte-stimulating factor and regulates the major acute phase response in liver cells. Proc. Natl. Acad. Sci. USA **84:** 7251–7255.
10. KOJ, A., A. KURDOWSKA, D. MAGIELSKA-ZERO, H. ROKITA, J. D. SIPE, J. M. DAYER, S. DEMCZUK & J. GAULDIE. 1987. Limited effects of recombinant human and murine interleukin-1 and tumor necrosis factor on production of acute phase proteins by cultured rat hepatocytes. Biochem. Internat. **14:** 553–560.
11. AKIRA, S., H. ISSHIKI, T. SUGITA, O. TANABE, S. KINOSHITA, Y. NISHIO, T. NAKAJIMA, T. HIRANO & T. KISHIMOTO. 1990. A nuclear factor for IL-6 expression (NF-IL6) is a member of the C/EBP family. EMBO J. **9:** 1897–1906.
12. POLI, V., F. P. MANCINI & R. CORTESE. 1990. IL6-DBP, a nuclear protein involved in interleukin-6 signal transduction, defines a new family of leucine zipper proteins related to C/EBP. Cell **63:** 643–653.
13. WILLIAMS, S. C., C. A. CANTWELL & P. F. JOHNSON. A family of C/EBP-related proteins capable of forming covalently linked leucine-zipper dimers in vitro. Genes & Develop. **4:** 1404–1415.
14. RAMJI, D. P., A. VITELLI, F. TRONCHE, R. CORTESE & G. CILIBERTO. 1993. The two C/EBP isoforms, IL-6 DBP/NF-IL6 and C/EBPδ/NF-IL6β, are induced by IL-6 to promote acute phase gene transcription via different mechanisms. Nucl. Acids. Res. **21:** 289–294.
15. WEGENKA, U. M., C. LÜTTICKEN, J. BUSCHMANN, J. YUAN, F. LOTTSPEICH, W. MÜLLER-ESTERL, C. SCHINDLER, E. ROEB, P. C. HEINRICH & F. HORN. 1994. The Interleukin-6-activated acute-phase response factor is antigenically and functionally related to members of the signal transducer and activator of transcription family. Mol. Cell. Biol. **14:** 3186–3196.
16. SADOWSKI, H. B., K. SHUAI, J. E. DARNELL JR. & M. Z. GILMAN. 1993. A common nuclear signal transduction pathway activated by growth factor and cytokine receptors. Science **261:** 1739–1744.
17. AKIRA, S., Y. NISHIO, M. INOUE, X.-J. WANG, S. WEI, T. MATSUSAKA, K. YOSHIDA, T. SUDO, M. NARUTO & T. KISHIMOTO. 1994. Molecular cloning of APRF, a novel IFN-stimulated gene factor 3 p91-related transcription factor involved in the gp130-mediated signaling pathway. Cell **77:** 63–71.
18. KISHIMOTO, T., T. TAGA & S. AKIRA. 1994. Cytokine signal transduction. Cell **76:** 253–262.
19. DARNELL, J. E. JR., I. M. KERR & G. R. STARR. 1994. Jak-STAT pathways and transcriptional activation in response to IFNs and other extracellular signaling proteins. Science **264:** 1415–1421.
20. HOCKE, G. M., D. BARRY & G. H. FEY. 1992. Synergistic action of interleukin-6 and glucocorticoids is mediated by the interleukin-6 response element of the rat $\alpha_2$macroglobulin gene. Mol. Cell. Biol. **12:** 2282–2294.
21. HOCKE, G. M., M.-Z. CUI, J. A. RIPPERGER & G. H. FEY. 1993. Regulation of the rat $\alpha_2$macroglobulin gene by interleukin-6 and leukemia inhibitory factor. *In* Acute Phase Proteins. Molecular Biology, Biochemistry, and Clinical Applications. A. Mackiewicz, I. Kushner & H. Baumann, Eds.: 467–494. Boca Raton, FL: CRC Press.
22. FEY, G. H., G. M. HOCKE, D. R. WILSON, J. A. RIPPERGER, T. S.-C. JUAN, M.-Z. CUI & G. J. DARLINGTON. 1994. *In* The Liver: Biology and Pathobiology, Third Edition. I. M. Arias, J. L. Boyer, N. Fausto, W. B. Jakoby, D. A. Schachter & D. A. Shafritz, Eds.: 113–143. New York: Raven Press, Ltd.
23. HORN, F., U. M. WEGENKA & P. C. HEINRICH. 1993. Regulation of the $\alpha_2$macroglobulin gene. *In* Acute Phase Proteins. Molecular Biology, Biochemistry, and Clinical Applica-

tions. A. Mackiewicz, I. Kushner & H. Baumann, Eds.: 443–465. Boca Raton, FL: CRC Press.
24. NORTHEMANN, W., M. HEISIG, D. KUNZ & P. C. HEINRICH. 1985. Molecular cloning of cDNA for $\alpha_2$macroglobulin and measurements of its transcription during experimental inflammation. Eur. J. Biochem. **137:** 257–262.
25. BIRCH, H. E. & G. SCHREIBER. 1986. Transcriptional regulation of plasma protein synthesis during inflammation. J. Biol. Chem. **261:** 8077–8082.
26. GEHRING, M. R., B. R. SHIELS, W. NORTHEMANN, M. H. L. DEBRUIJN, C.-C. KAN, A. C. CHAIN, D. NOONAN & G. H FEY. 1987. Sequence of rat liver $\alpha_2$macroglobulin and acute phase control of its messenger RNA. J. Biol. Chem. **262:** 446–454.
27. HATTORI, M., L. J. ABRAHAM, W. NORTHEMANN & G. H. FEY. 1990. Acute phase reaction induces a specific comlex between hepatic nuclear proteins and the interleukin-6 response element of the rat $\alpha_2$macroglobulin gene. Proc. Natl. Acad. Sci. USA **87:** 2364–2369.
28. BRECHNER, T., G. HOCKE, A. GOEL & G. H. FEY. 1991. The interleukin-6 response factor of the rat $\alpha_2$macroglobulin gene binds cooperatively at two adjacent sites in the promoter upstream region. Mol. Biol. Med. **8:** 267–285.
29. GORSKI, K., M. CARNEIRO & U. SCHIBLER. 1986. Tissue-specific in-vitro transcription from the mouse albumin promoter. Cell **47:** 767–776.
30. SIERRA, F. 1990. A laboratory guide to in vitro transcription. Basel, Switzerland: Birkhäuser Verlag.
31. KADONAGA, J. & R. TJIAN. 1986. Affinity purification of sequence-specific DNA binding proteins. Proc. Natl. Acad. Sci. USA **83:** 5889–5893.
32. ECKERSKORN, C., W. MEWES, H. GORETZKI & F. LOTTSPEICH. 1988. A new siliconized glass fiber as support for protein chemical analysis of electroblotted proteins. Eur. J. Biochem. **176:** 509–519.
33. ECKERSKORN, C. & F. LOTTSPEICH. 1989. Internal amino acid sequence analysis of proteins separated by gel electrophoresis after tryptic digestion in a polyacrylamide matix. Chromatographia **28:** 92–94.
34. LÜTTICKEN, C., U. M. WEGENKA, J. YUAN, J. BUSCHMANN, C. SCHINDLER, A. ZIEMIECKI, A. G. HARPUR, A. F. WILKS, K. YASUKAWA, T. TAGA, T. KISHIMOTO, G. BARBIERI, S. PELLEGRINI, M. SENDTNER, P. C. HEINRICH & F. HORN. 1994. Association of transcription factor APRF and protein kinase Jak1 with the interleukin-6 signal transducer gp130. Science **263:** 89–92.
35. SCHINDLER, C., X.-Y. FU, T. IMPROTA, R. AEBERSOLD & J. E. DARNELL, JR. 1992. Proteins of transcription factor ISGF-3: One gene encodes the 91- and 84-kDa ISGF-3 proteins that are activated by interferon α. Proc. Natl. Acad. Sci. USA **89:** 7836–7839.
36. FU, X.-Y., C. SCHINDLER, T. IMPROTA, R. AEBERSOLD & J. E. DARNELL, JR. 1992. The proteins of ISGF-3, the interferon α-induced transcriptional activator, define a gene family involved in signal transduction. Proc. Natl. Acad. Sci. USA **89:** 7840–7843.
37. YAMAMOTO, K., F. W. QUELLE, W. E. THIERFELDER, B. L. KREIDER, D. J. GILBERT, N. A. JENKINS, N. G. COPELAND, O. SILVENNOINEN & J. N. IHLE. 1994. Stat4, a novel gamma interferon activation site-binding protein expressed in early myeloid differentiation. Mol. Cell. Biol. **7:** 4342–4349.
38. ZHONG, Z., Z. WEN & J. E. DARNELL, JR. 1994. Stat3 and Stat4: Members of the family of signal transducers and activators of transcription. Proc. Natl. Acad. Sci. USA **91:** 4806–4810.
39. WAKAO, H., F. GOUILLEUX & B. GRONER. 1994. Mammary gland factor (MGF) is a novel member of the cytokine regulated transcription factor gene family and confers the prolactin response. EMBO J. **13:** 2182–2191.

DISCUSSION OF THE PAPER

G. CILIBERTO (*Istituto di Ricerche di Biologia Molecolare P. Angeletti, Pomezia (Rome), Italy*): I wonder if you have tried tyrosine phosphatase to determine whether the mechanism of binding is similar to that of APRF?

G. H. FEY: No, we have not yet worked with anti-tyrosine phosphate antibodies or with tyrosine phosphatase. Such experiments are obviously to come in the future. The purification was achieved only a few weeks ago and we have not yet had time to do these experiments.

CILIBERTO: Also connected to this question—given the fact that it is likely to belong to the same family as the other proteins and given some cross-reactivity with available antibodies, have you tried to use anti-p91?

FEY: Yes, we have tried to use an anti-human p91 antibody, which we obtained from Dr. Darnell's lab, and it did not induce a supershift with our complex. This is not surprising, because Friedemann Horn has data saying that most of the anti-p91 antibodies recognized epitopes at the carboxy-terminus and would not cross-react with other Stat factors. You would have to use special antibodies that recognize epitopes at the N-terminus in order to see antigenic cross-reactivity between p91 and other members of that family. We have tried, but it did not work for us.

V. POLI (*Istituto di Ricerche di Biologia Moleculare P. Angeletti, Pomezia (Rome), Italy*): There is something I did not understand—perhaps I missed it. As far as I understood you used as a binding site for your gel retardation assay basically the same responsive element which was used at the beginning by Friedemann Horn to characterize APRF. Because the IL-6 core element was used at the beginning at least—and this is what I do not understand—why have you failed to see the activation of the APRF in your system, for example in rats?

FEY: We do not fail to see that. We see an early complex in rat hepatoma cells, but you do not see it fully developed in the whole rat liver at the level of resolution that I showed. If you overexposed these autoradiographs you would also see a complex II at one hour. But the early phase probably is exactly what they see within the first hour after IL-6.

P. C. HEINRICH (*Klinikum der RWTH Aachen, Germany*): Why do you not see an early complex here at 45 minutes or one hour 30 minutes that would correspond to that which you see in rat hepatoma cell or human hepatoma cell or in the mouse that you inject intravenously with LPS or IL-6?

FEY: Now this was not an intravenous injection; this was an intraperitoneal injection, and the pharmacokinetics was much slower. If you inject complete Freund's adjuvant into the peritoneum, the macrophages first need to have time to produce IL-6 and then the IL-6 needs to get out of the peritoneum and reach the blood stream. It is just a slower process than what you have if you inject IL-6 or LPS intravenously.

HEINRICH: In our case it did not matter how we applied LPS in rats. And, actually, at 10 hours we did not get any get shift as you have it. In your case it is really optimal or very strong. That is definitely a discrepancy.

FEY: We did not inject LPS, we injected complete Freund's adjuvant, and I do not see a discrepancy. We did get a weak complex I at 45 minutes and one hour 30 minutes, but it reached a maximum intensity only at 10 and 12 hours.

L. A. AARDEN (*Netherlands Red Cross Transfusion Service, Amsterdam*): It is good that we have a picnic soon to resolve all of these questions.

Functional Analysis of IL-6 and IL-6DBP/C/EBPβ by Gene Targeting

ELENA FATTORI,[a] CAROLINA SELLITTO,[a]
MANUELA CAPPELLETTI,[a] DOMENICO LAZZARO,[a]
DIANA BELLAVIA,[b] ISABELLA SCREPANTI,[c]
ALBERTO GULINO,[b] FRANK COSTANTINI,[d]
AND VALERIA POLI[a]

[a]*Istituto di Ricerche di Biologia Molecolare P. Angeletti*
via Pontina km 30.600
00040 Pomezia (Rome), Italy

[b]*Dipartimento di Medicina Sperimentale*
Universitá dell'Aquila
Aquila, Italy

[c]*Dipartimento di Medicina Sperimentale*
Universitá La Sapienza
Rome, Italy

[d]*Department of Genetics and Development*
Columbia University
New York, New York 10032

INTRODUCTION

Interleukin-6 (IL-6) is a cytokine with a broad spectrum of activities in the immune, hematopoietic and neuronal systems (reviewed in ref. 1), and it is considered one of the major mediators of the liver acute phase response (reviewed in ref. 2). IL-6–disregulated production has been associated with various diseases such as multiple myeloma, glomerulonephritis, and several autoimmune diseases.[3] Moreover, IL-6 has been shown to play an important role in the induction of osteoclastogenesis in the bone marrow of estrogen-depleted female mice.[4] The pathway of signal transduction from the specific membrane receptor to the activation of IL-6 specific genes is rather complex and has still to be fully clarified. Early events consist of the activation of members of the Jak-Tyk family of non-receptor tyrosine kinases,[5] which results in tyrosine phosphorylation and nuclear translocation of Stat transcription factors.[6,7] The ras pathway is also activated[8] and, through the activation of the C/EBP family,[9] is thought to be responsible for later events following IL-6 stimulation. All members of this family show a strong homology at their carboxy-terminal, which carries a basic and a leucine-zipper domain,[10] and are able to homo- or heterodimerize; thus the actual number of functional polypeptides is higher than the number of genes. It is generally believed that the ratio between homo- and heterodimers is important for the selective activation/inactivation of target genes.

C/EBPβ was originally isolated from a rat cDNA library as an IL-6–inducible transcription factor (IL6DBP; IL-6–dependent DNA binding protein) involved in the induction of several positive acute phase genes and in the transcription of the albumin gene,[11] and the human homolog was isolated as a transcription factor involved in the induction of the IL-6 gene in response to IL-1 and IL-6.[12] Since then,

C/EBPβ binding sites have been identified on the promoter of several cytokine genes such as IL-1β[13] and IL-8.[14]

Here we describe the results of the studies performed to clarify *in vivo* the role of different elements of this complex network making use of IL-6– and C/EBPβ-deficient mice.

EXPERIMENTAL PROCEDURES

Construction of Vectors

The construction of the IL-6 homologous recombination vector has been described.[15]

For the C/EBPβ replacement vector the 5' homology, a fragment containing 45 bp of 5' untranslated region and the first 673 bp of the coding region (up to aa 225), was cloned upstream of an MC1-Neo poly(A) cassette from Stratagene. An MC1 herpes simplex thymidine kinase (TK) cassette was inserted upstream of the 5' homology as described previously.[15] The 3' homology was a 5.4 Kb fragment carrying the 3' untranslated region of the gene starting from the stop codon, and was inserted downstream from the Neo cassette. The construct resulted in the deletion of the last 72 aminoacids of the protein.

Generation of IL-6– and C/EBPβ-deficient Mice

ES cell clones carrying either the IL-6 or the C/EBPβ mutation were injected into blastocysts of C57BL6 mice and transplanted into the uteri of F1 (CBA × C57BL6) foster mothers. Male chimeras were mated to MF1 females, and agouti offspring (representing germline transmission of the ES genome) were screened for the presence of the targeted locus by Southern blot analysis. Female offspring heterozygous for the mutation were bred once with mice of the 129/SV/EV strain,[16] the strain from which the CCE ES cells were derived. The resulting heterozygous offspring were bred together to generate mice homozygous for the mutation.

Animals and Treatments

Mice bred in our barrier facility were used. They were maintained in standard conditions under a 12 hour light-dark cycle and provided irradiated food and chlorinated water *ad libitum*. Procedures involving animals and their care were conducted in conformity with national and international laws and policies (EEC Council Directive 86/609, OJ L 358, 1, Dec. 12, 1987; Italian Legislative Decree 116/92, Gazzetta Ufficiale della Repubblica Italiana n. 40, Feb. 18, 1992; NIH Guide for the Care and Use of Laboratory Animals, NIH publication No. 85-23, 1985). LPS (From *E. coli* serotype 026:B6) was purchased from Sigma Chemical Co. (St. Louis, MO), resuspended in sterile pyrogen-free saline solution and injected ip at a dose of 1 mg/kg body weight. Steam-distilled turpentine was injected subcutaneously (sc). A single injection of 100 μl was given for the analysis of mRNAs. Two injections, one over each hind limb, were given for the analysis of body weight and food intake. Control mice were injected ip or sc with sterile pyrogen-free saline solution. Blood was collected from the retroorbital cavity.

For the body weight and food intake mice were weighed every 24 hours starting from the day and time of treatment (day 0). Food intake was measured for each group

(6 mice) at the same time intervals and mean food intake per mouse per day was calculated.

Northern Blotting Analysis, ELISA Assay and Western Blotting

Total RNA was isolated by the guanidine isothiocyanate method,[17] fractionated by electrophoresis (20 μg per lane), and transferred to a GeneScreen membrane (NEN). Poly(A)$^+$ mRNA was prepared using oligo d(T) columns (5 Prime...3 Prime, Inc. Boulder CO). Hybridization was carried out with the cDNAs for IL-6, C/EBPB, $\alpha_2$macroglobulin (α_2M),[18] serum amyloid P (SAP),[19] serum amyloid A (SAA),[20] α_1-acidic glycoprotein (AGP),[21] Haptoglobin (Hp),[21] hemopexin (Hpx),[22] and albumin (alb).[23] GAPDH (glyceraldehyde-3-phosphate-dehydrogenase)[24] was used as internal control. The relative abundance of the different mRNAs was measured by densitometric scanning of the autoradiographs.

IL-6 ELISA assay was performed using the rat anti-mouse IL-6 monoclonal MP5-20F3 from Pharmingen for capturing and a rabbit anti-mIL-6 polyclonal antibody for detection of the bound protein.

Liver nuclear extracts were prepared according to Gorsky et al.,[25] fractionated on a 12.5% SDS PAGE gel and transferred to nitrocellulose. The anti-NH$_2$ antibody (gift from U. Schibler) and the antibody against the full length protein were both rabbit polyclonal raised against the rat protein expressed in bacteria, and they were revealed with a polyclonal anti-rabbit IgG antibody conjugated with alkaline phosphatase (Promega).

Bone Histomorphometry

Four-month-old females were subjected to ovariectomies under ketamine anesthesia. On day 22 and on day 28 after surgery all the animals were injected intraperitoneally with oxytetracycline (30 mg/kg) and with calcein (20 mg/kg), respectively. On day 32, mice were sacrificed; one femur and one tibia per animal were fixed in 10% buffered formalin and processed undecalcified as previously described.[15]

Histomorphometric analysis was carried out as described.[15] The number of animals studied was respectively: IL-6$^{+/+}$ N-OVX: n = 5; IL-6$^{+/+}$ OVX: n = 5; IL-6$^{-/-}$ N-OVX: n = 6; IL-6$^{-/-}$ OVX: n = 7.

Phenotypic Analysis of Lymphoid Organs

Cell suspensions obtained from the thymuses, spleens, and lymph nodes were single or double stained with different monoclonal antibodies (MAbs). The following MAbs were used in the flow cytometric analysis: FITC-conjugated anti-CD3 (clone 145-2C11) was obtained from Boehringer Mannheim (Mannheim, Germany). PE-conjugated anti-CD3 (clone 145-2C11), PE-conjugated anti-B220 (clone RA3-6B2), FITC-conjugated anti-IgG1 (clones G1-6.5), FITC-conjugated anti-dg (clone GL3), PE-conjugated anti-ab (clone H57-597), and PE- and FITC-conjugated rat and hamster IgG immunoglobulin standard antibody, used as control of immunofluorescence, were obtained from Pharmingen (San Diego, CA). For staining, 3×10^5 to 10^6 cells were incubated 20 min on ice with saturating amounts of antibody, then washed in ice cold PBS, suspended in 0.3 ml of ice cold PBS and analyzed on FACScan (Becton Dickinson, Mountain View, CA), with at least 1×10^4 events scored. Dead cells were excluded from the analysis by propidium iodide staining. Fluorescence data were analyzed by FACScan or Consort 30 programs.

RESULTS

Generation of IL-6–deficient Mice

To abolish IL-6 function we constructed a replacement vector (FIG. 1A) in which a 2.1 kb fragment containing the proximal promoter and the first three exons of the

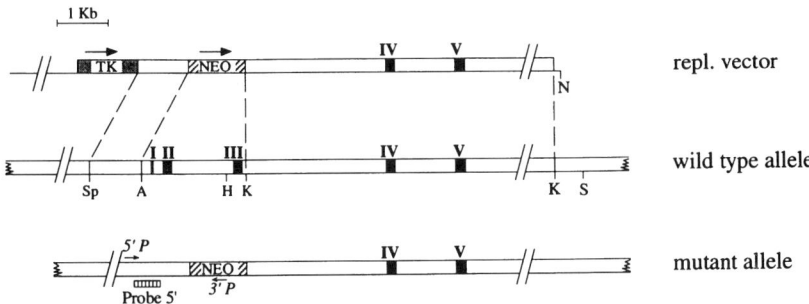

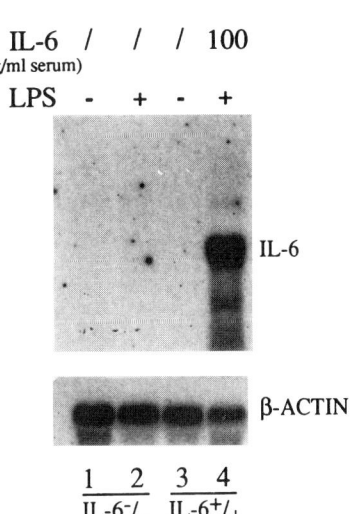

FIGURE 1. IL-6 gene disruption. **A:** strategy used to mutate the IL-6 gene: black boxes indicates the 5 exons of the IL-6 genes. The transcription orientations of the NEO and TK genes are shown by the arrows. 5'P and 3'P indicate the oligos used for the PCR analysis of the mutant clones while Probe 5' is the segment used for the Southern hybridization. **B:** Northern blot on total liver RNA (20 γ) from IL-6 $/_-$ and IL-6$^+/_+$ mice either untreated (−) or injected with LPS (+) hybridized with a murine IL-6 probe and a mouse β-actin probe as an internal control. The level of circulating IL-6 measured in the same mice by an ELISA assay are indicated above each lane.

gene were replaced by a MCI-Neomycin (Neo) poly(A) + cassette. This construct was used to mutate the endogenous mouse IL-6 as described.[15]

IL-6 mRNA was absent in the homozygous IL-6$^{-/-}$ mice, as shown by a Northern blot on total spleen mRNA before and after injection of bacterial lipopolysaccaryde (LPS), a potent inducer of IL-6 gene transcription (FIG. 1B). Serum IL-6 measured by an ELISA assay was present at a concentration of 100 ng/ml in the wild type mice after LPS treatment and was not detectable in the mutants.

Generation of IL-6DBP–deficient Mice

To mutate the C/EBPβ gene we used a replacement vector in which the carboxy-terminal part of the gene coding for the leucine zipper and part of the basic domain was substituted with an MCI-Neo poly(A) + cassette (FIG. 2A). C/EBPβ$^{-/-}$ mice were obtained and a Northern blot experiment on liver mRNA (FIG. 2B) showed

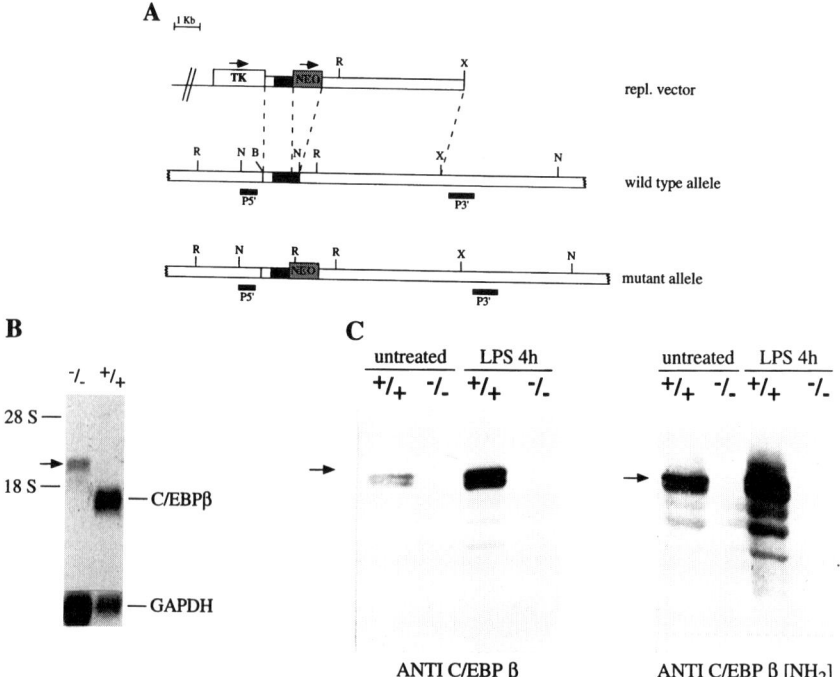

FIGURE 2. C/EBPβ gene disruption: **A:** strategy used to mutate the C/EBPβ gene: arrows indicate the transcription orientation of TK and Neo genes; P5' and P3' are the two probes used for the genotypic analysis through Southern blot. **B:** Northern blot analysis of poly(A) + mRNA from livers of C/EBPβ$^{+/+}$ and $^{-/-}$ mice treated for 2 hours with LPS. C/EBPβ cDNA was used as a probe and GAPDH as internal control. The arrow indicates the slower migrating band in the $^{-/-}$ mice. **C:** western blot analysis on liver nuclear extracts from C/EBPβ$^{-/-}$ and $^{+/+}$ mice untreated and treated for 4 hours with LPS. The antibodies used were raised against the whole protein (α-C/EBPβ) or against the N-terminal region (α-NH$_2$).

the absence of the C/EBPβ-specific mRNA. The slower migrating band can be detected also with a Neo probe and probably is a fusion RNA between the 5' region of the C/EBPβ gene and the Neo gene. To demonstrate the absence of the protein, we prepared liver nuclear extracts from untreated and LPS-treated wild type and C/EBPβ$^{-/-}$ mice and performed a Western blot analysis using two different polyclonal antibodies: one directed against the N-terminal portion of the molecule and one against the whole protein. The absence of any detectable signal excluded the possibility that a truncated or a fusion protein is produced from the fusion RNA.

IL-6$^{-/-}$ Mice

Effects of the IL-6$^{-/-}$ Mutation on Bone

Since several lines of evidence indicate that IL-6 could have a role in bone metabolism and in the pathogenesis of post-menopausal osteoporosis,[4,26,27] we compared bone structure and metabolism in IL-6–deficient female mice and wild-type littermates both under normal conditions and in an estrogen-depleted state caused by ovariectomy. FIGURE 3 shows the results of the static and dynamic analysis of the distal femoral metaphysis.

Independently from their estrogen status, IL-6$^{-/-}$ mice showed higher bone turnover than their wild type littermates. The osteoid surface, which represents the newly formed bone not yet mineralized (FIG. 3A), and the rate of bone formed per day

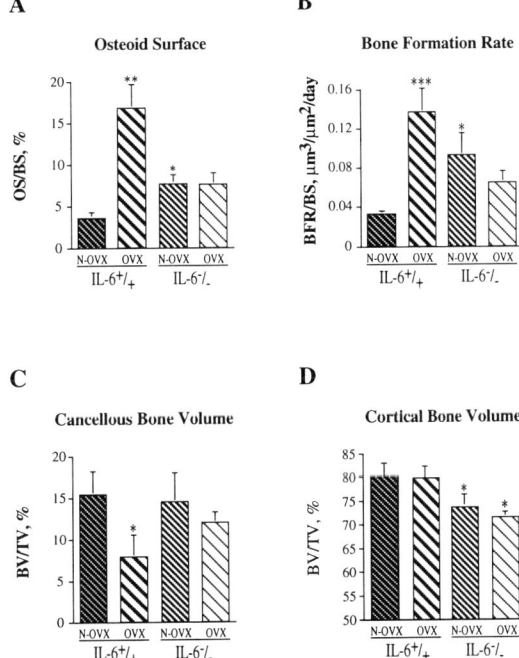

FIGURE 3. Bone parameters in femora from ovariectomized (OVX) and non-ovariectomized (N-OVX) IL-6$^{+/+}$ and IL-6$^{-/-}$ mice. Bars represent means ± SEM. **A:** Osteoid surface, expressed as a percentage of the total trabecular bone surface (OS/BS, %), *$p < 0.05$; **$p < 0.01$, significantly different from IL-6$^{+/+}$ N-OVX. **B:** Bone formation rate per unit of trabecular bone surface (BFR/BS, mm^3/mm^2/day). *$p < 0.05$; ***$p < 0.001$, significantly different from IL-6$^{+/+}$ N-OVX. **C:** Cancellous bone volume (BV/TV, %), expressed as the percentage of the metaphyseal area occupied by cancellous bone excluding the cortices. *$p < 0.05$, significantly different from IL-6$^{+/+}$ N-OVX. **D:** Cortical bone volume (BV/TV, %), expressed as the percentage of the cortical tissue area divided by the cross-sectional area × 100. *$p < 0.05$, significantly different from IL-6$^{+/+}$ N-OVX.

(FIG. 3B) were significantly higher in the IL-6$^{-/-}$ mice than in the wild-type littermates. This accelerated bone turnover did not, however, alter the total amount of trabecular bone (FIG. 3C); in contrast the amount of cortical bone was significantly reduced in IL-6$^{-/-}$ mice in comparison to their wild-type littermates (FIG. 3D). These results indicate that IL-6 is required for the maintenance of a physiological bone turnover and for the formation of a normal amount of cortical bone, while its absence does not influence the maintenance of a normal trabecular bone mass. Estrogen depletion following ovariectomy leads to high bone turnover (FIG. 3, A and B) and cancellous bone loss in normal mice (FIG. 3C). Interestingly, in IL-6–deficient female mice, ovariectomy did not cause significant changes in bone volume and turnover, indicating that IL-6 has a critical role in mediating the effects of estrogen depletion on bone loss.

Inflammatory Response in IL-6$^{-/-}$ Mice

Several reports indicated IL-6 as one of the major inducers of liver acute phase genes transcription during inflammation (reviewed in ref. 28). Bacterial infection (which can be mimicked by injection of LPS) or sterile tissue lesions such as cuts or burns (experimentally reproduced by subcutaneous injection of turpentine) are distinct inflammatory challenges that elicit different immunological responses but both lead to the activation of the same set of liver acute phase genes and to the same pathological manifestations such as hypoglycemia, loss of body weight and decreased food intake.

We decided to utilize the IL-6$^{-/-}$ mice to investigate the requirement for IL-6 in the host response to these different inflammatory stimuli. As shown in FIGURE 4A, the induction of AP mRNA was comparable in the livers of $^{+/+}$ and $^{-/-}$ mice

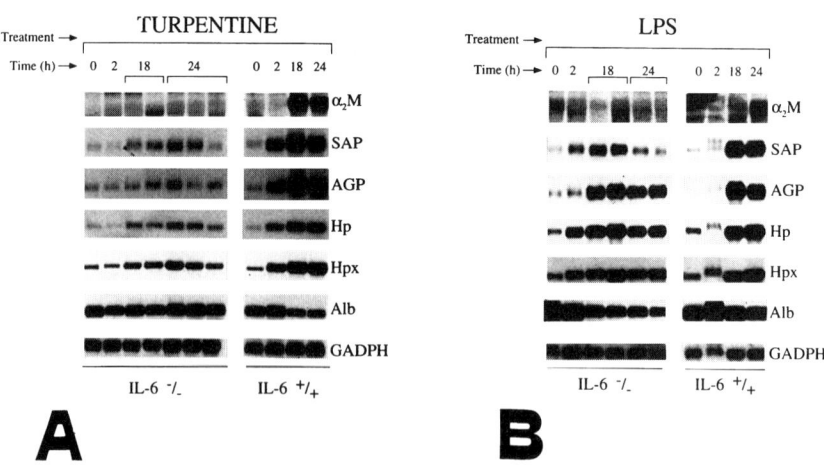

FIGURE 4. Liver acute phase genes induction in IL-6$^{+/+}$ and $^{-/-}$ mice. Northern blot analysis on total liver RNA (10 γ) from IL-6$^{-/-}$ and $^{+/+}$ mice treated with turpentine **(A)** or LPS **(B)** for 2, 18 and 24 hours. As probes we used the cDNAs for $\alpha_2$macroglobulin (α_2M), serum amyloid P (SAP), α_1-acidic glycoprotein (AGP), haptoglobin (Hp), Hemopexin (Hpx) and Albumin (alb). GAPDH (glyceraldehyde-3-phosphate-dehydrogenase) was used as internal control.

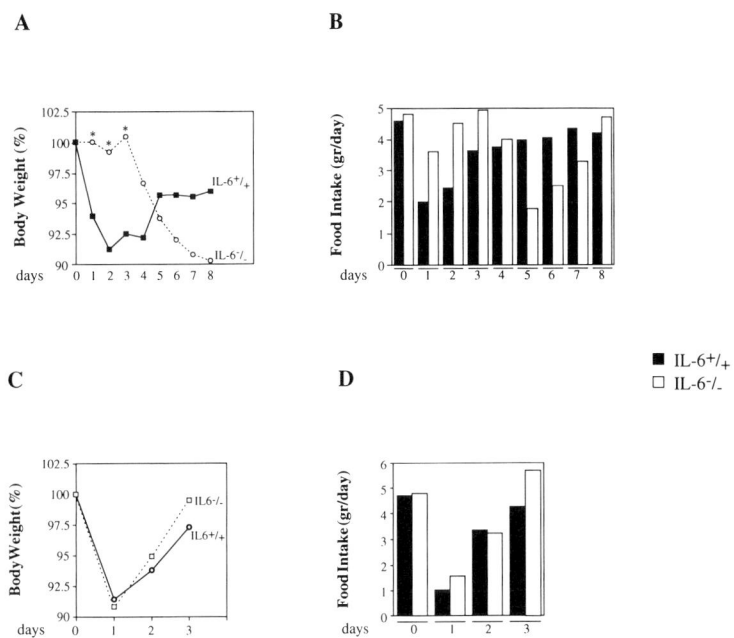

FIGURE 5. Changes in body weight and food intake after turpentine (**A** and **B**) and LPS (**C** and **D**) treatment. $*p < 0.01$, significantly different from IL-6$^{+/+}$ mice.

in response to LPS injection. Moreover, also symptoms of cachexia such as weight loss and food intake were comparable between $-/-$ and $+/+$ mice (FIG. 5, C and D). In contrast, upon turpentine injection not only were most of the acute phase genes poorly activated (FIG. 4B), but the mutant mice did not lose weight in the first 3 days after treatment and their food intake was not decreased (FIG. 5, A and B). Notably, the α_2m mRNA was not induced by either treatment, indicating that this gene is solely responsive to IL-6.

These findings suggest the existence of two different inflammatory pathways in response to systemic or localized tissue damage and indicate IL-6 as a key mediator in the latter.

$C/EBP\beta^{-/-}$ Mutant Mice

Acute Phase Response in C/EBPβ-deficient Mice

To analyze the pattern of activation of liver acute phase genes, we induced inflammation by a subcutaneous injection of turpentine and analyzed the mRNA levels for several positive acute phase genes at different time points. As shown in TABLE 1, the induction of haptoglobin (hp) and hemopexin (Hpx) genes was not altered in the mutant mice as compared to their wild type littermates. Serum amyloid P (SAP) and serum amyloid A (SAA) induction were altered in both amplitude and temporal extension. In particular, at 24 hours the mRNA levels for these acute phase genes were dramatically reduced in the mutant mice, while still at their maximum in the

TABLE 1. Induction of Liver Acute Phase Response Genes in C/EBP$^-$/$_-$ and $^+$/$_+$ Mice

	0	2 h	18 h	24 h	0	2 h	18 h	24 h
HP	2.5	19.2	68.7	100.0	2.1	13.0	73.3	88.0
HPX	7.5	30.9	72.0	100.0	10.6	20.3	77.3	70.1
SAP	—	—	94.6	100.0	—	—	78.0	15.5
SAA	—	—	52.9	100.0	—	—	21.6	26.0
	C/EBPβ$^+$/$_+$				C/EBP$^-$/$_-$			

Values are calculated as percentage of the maximal induction in the wild-type animals.

wild type mice. These results suggest that C/EBPβ function in the regulation of the induction of SAP and SAA genes transcription is required in the later phases of induction rather than at its onset.

Lymphoproliferative Alterations in C/EBPβ–deficient Mice

Homozygous C/EBPβ$^-$/$_-$ mice develop skin lesions, swelling of the mucosa, and lymphoadenopathy starting from around 16 weeks of age. Examination of the lymphoid organs after this age revealed a marked enlargement of the spleen (up to 10 times) and of peripheral lymph nodes (up to 1 cm in diameter). Histological analysis showed an expansion in the B-cell/plasma cell population in the lymph nodes and spleen and infiltration of plasma cells in the peribronchial region of the lung, in the portal areas of the liver and in the stroma of the kidney (not shown). Extramedullary hemopoiesis was found in spleen, liver and lymph nodes (not shown).

To better characterize these changes in the immune cell populations, the cell composition in lymphoid organs was analyzed at different ages. While the total cell recovery and immune cell distribution was unchanged in the thymus of $^-$/$_-$ mice as compared to the $^+$/$_+$ littermates (not shown), an evident alteration in the T/B cell distribution was revealed by fluorescence activated cell sorter (FACS) analysis in spleen and lymph nodes of mutant mice. This alteration started after the age of 16 weeks and its entity increased with age.

FIGURE 6 shows the analysis of the lymph nodes. The total cell yield is increased in $^-$/$_-$ mice after the age of 16 weeks and a rise in the B-cell population B220 positive (C) is accompanied by a relative decrease in the T-cell CD3 positive population (B). The same imbalance between B and T cells was observed also in the spleen (FIG. 7), where the increase in B-cell number was mostly due to memory B-cells characterized by the presence of surface IgG. It is important to notice that the decrease in T-cell number is only percentual and is due to the increase in the absolute cell number.

The expansion in the B-cell population in C/EBPβ$^-$/$_-$ mice is surprisingly reminiscent of that observed in transgenic mice overexpressing IL-6.[29,30,31] To investigate if the absence of C/EBPβ could result in an up-regulation of IL-6 production we measured IL-6 levels in C/EBPβ$^+$/$_+$ and $^-$/$_-$ mice by an ELISA assay. Interestingly, the basal levels of circulating IL-6 were significantly higher in $^-$/$_-$ than in $^+$/$_+$ mice, although individuals with low or even undetectable levels of IL-6 were present (data not shown). This finding suggests that disregulation of IL-6 production occurs in the C/EBPβ$^-$/$_-$ mice as a reactive phenomenon which needs to be triggered by antigenic stimuli that accumulate during the life span of the mice rather than as an intrinsic disregulation. Moreover, we propose that C/EBPβ might act, in certain conditions, as an inhibitor of IL-6 synthesis.

FATTORI et al.: GENE TARGETING

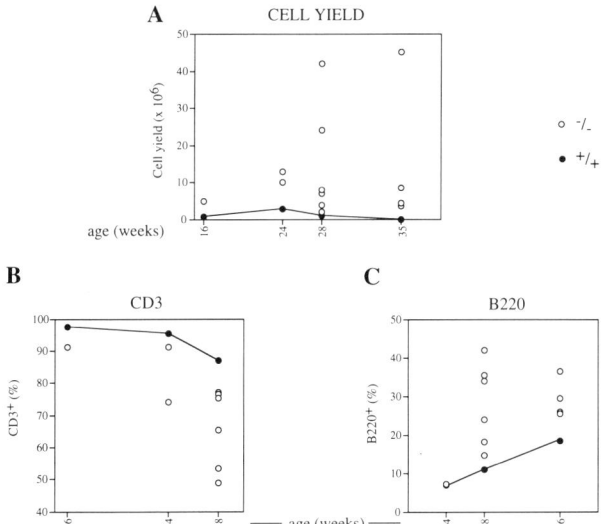

FIGURE 6. Phenotypic analysis of lymph node cells. C/EBPβ$^{-/-}$ mice: white circles; wild type mice: black circles. **A:** total lymph node cells recovered at different ages. **B:** and **C:** percentage of CD3+ and B220+ lymphocytes, respectively, recovered from lymph nodes of $^{+/+}$ and $^{-/-}$ mice at different ages.

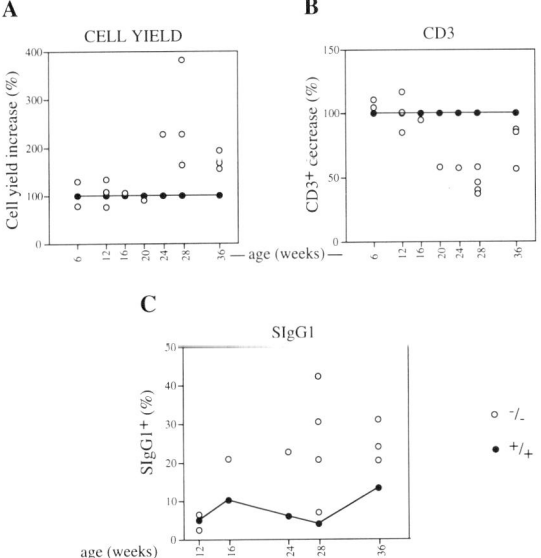

FIGURE 7. Phenotypic analysis of splenic lymphocytes. C/EBPβ$^{-/-}$ mice: white circles; wild type mice: black circles. **A:** Total splenic lymphocytes recovered at different ages. The results are expressed as percentage of increase of C/EBPβ$^{-/-}$ total splenic lymphocytes with respect to the total yield of control splenic lymphocytes for each specific age considered as 100%. **B:** percentage of decrease of CD3+ T lymphocytes in C/EBPβ$^{-/-}$ mice, with respect to the percentage of CD3+ cells from control mice, considered as 100% for each respective age. **C:** percentage of sIgG+ B lymphocytes recovered at each age.

CONCLUSIONS

We have tried to clarify *in vivo* some of the physiological and pathological roles of IL-6 and some aspects of its signal transduction pathway using IL-6– and C/EBPβ-deficient mice. In particular, we have demonstrated that IL-6 plays a key role in the regulation of bone metabolism and in the mechanism of inflammation. Moreover, we have shown that the absence of C/EBPβ results in hyperproliferation of B cells and hemopoietic cells and up-regulates IL-6 production. Conversely, the induction of acute phase response genes transcription is negatively affected in C/EBPβ-deficient mice. Taken together these results indicate that the function of the C/EBPβ transcription factor in the IL-6–induced phenomena can vary from one cell type to another, and is probably determined by the complex interaction with other members of the C/EBP family. More specifically, we propose that under certain conditions C/EBPβ might act as a repressor of IL-6 transcription, and not as an activator, as is generally believed.

ACKNOWLEDGMENTS

We wish to thank H. Baumann, U. Müller-Eberhard, S. Maeda, J. Sipe, and U. Shibler for the generous gift of probes and antibodies.

REFERENCES

1. VAN SNICK, J. 1990. Annu. Rev. Immunol. **8:** 253–278.
2. BAUMANN, H. & J. GAULDIE. 1994. Immunol. Today **15:** 74–80.
3. HIRANO, T., S. AKIRA, T. TAGA & T. KISHIMOTO. 1990. Immunol. Today **11:** 443–449.
4. JILKA, R. L., G. HAMGOC, G. GIRASOLE, G. PASSERI, D. C. WILLIAMS, J. S. ABRAMS, B. BOYCE, H. BROXMEYER & S. C. MANOLAGAS. 1992. Science **257:** 88–91.
5. STAHL, S., T. G. BOULTON, T. FARUGGELLA, N. Y. IP, S. DAVIS, B. A. WITTHUHN, F. W. SILVENNOINEN, G. BARBIERI, S. PELLEGRINI, J. N. IHLE & G. D. YANCOPOULOS. 1994. Science **293:** 92–97.
6. SADOWSKI, H. B., S. KE, J. E. DARNELL, JR. & M. Z. GILMAN. 1993. Science **261:** 1739–1744.
7. IHLE, J. N., B. A. WITTHUHN, F. W. QUELLE, K. YAMAMOTO, W. E. THIERFELDER, K. BRENT & O. SILVENNOINEN. 1994. TIBS **19:** 222–227.
8. SATOH, T., M. NAKAFUKU, N. TERADA, K. I. ARAI & A. MIYAIJMA. 1992. J. Biol. Chem. **267:** 24149–24152.
9. NAKAJIMA, T., S. KINOSHITA, T. SASAGAWA, K. SASATI, M. NARUTO, Y. KISHIMOTO & S. AKIRA. 1993. Proc. Natl. Acad. Sci. USA **88:** 11349–11353.
10. LANDSCHULZ, W. H., P. F. JOHNSON & S. L. MCKNIGHT. 1989. Science **243:** 1681–1688.
11. POLI, V., F. P. MANCINI & R. CORTESE. 1990. Cell **63:** 643–653.
12. AKIRA, S., H. ISSIHIKI, T. SUGITA, O. TANABLE, S. KINOSHITA, T. NAKAJIMA, T. HIRANO & T. KISHIMOTO. 1990. EMBO J **9:** 1897–1906.
13. ZHANG, Y. & W. ROM. 1993. Mol. Cell. Biol. **13:** 3831–3837.
14. MATSUSAKA, T., K. FUJIKAWA, Y. NISHIO, H. MUKAIDA, K. MATSUSHIMA, T. KISHIMOTO & S. AKIRA. 1993. Proc. Natl. Acad. Sci. USA **90:** 10193.
15. POLI, V., R. BALENA, E. FATTORI, A. MARKATOS, M. YAMAMOTO, H. TANAKA, G. CILIBERTO, G. A. RODAN & F. COSTANTINI. 1994. EMBO J. **13:** 1189–1196.
16. ROBERTSON, E. J. 1987. *In* Tetracarcinomas and Embryonic Stem Cells: A Practical Approach. E. J. Robertson, Ed. 71–192. Oxford: IRL Press.
17. CHOMCZYNSKI, P. & N. SACCHI. 1987. Annal. Biochem. **162:** 156–159.

18. NORTHEMANN, W., T. ANDUS, V. GROSS, M. NAGASHIMA, G. SHREIBER & P. C. HEINRICH. 1983. FEBS Lett. **161:** 319–322.
19. MURAKAMI, T., S. OHNISHI, S. NISHIGUCHI, S. MAEDA, S. ARAKI, K. SHIMADA. 1988. Biochem. Biophys. Res. Commun. **155:** 554–560.
20. SIPE, J. D., H. R. COLTEN, G. GOLDERGER, M. D. EDGE, B. F. TACK, A. S. COHEN & A. S. WHITEHEAD. 1985. Biochemistry **24:** 2931–2936.
21. BAUMANN, H., R. E. HILL, D. N. SAUDER & G. P. JAHREIS. 1986. J. Cell Biol. **102:** 370.
22. NIKKILA, H., J. D. GITLIN & U. MULLER-EBERHARD. 1991. Biochemistry **30:** 823–829.
23. KIOUSSIS, D., R. HAMILTON, R. W. HANSON, S. M. TILGHMAN & J. M. TAYLOR. 1979. Proc. Natl. Acad. Sci. USA **76:** 4370–4374.
24. PIECHACZYK, M., J. M. BLANCHARD, L. MARTY, CH. DANI, F. PANABIERES, S. EL SABOUTY, PH. FORD & PH. JEANTEUR. 1994. Nucleic Acids Res. **12:** 6951–6963.
25. GORSKI, K., M. CARNEIRO & U. SHIBLER. 1986. Cell **47:** 767–776.
26. MICHALEVZIC, R., D. LIFSHITZ & M. REVEL. 1989. Scanning Microsc. **3:** 1143–1150.
27. GIRASOLE, G., R. L. JILKA, G. PASSERI, S. BOSWELL, G. BODER, D. C. WILLIAMS & S. C. MANOLAGAS. 1992. J. Clin. Invest. **89:** 883–891.
28. POLI, V. & G. CILIBERTO. 1994. *In* Liver Gene Expression. F. Tronche & M. Yaniv, eds., pp 131–151 R. G. Landes Company.
29. SUEMATSU, S., T. MATSUDA, K. AOZASA, S. AKIRA, N. NAKANO, S. OHNO, J. MIYAZAKI, K. YAMAMYRA, T. HIRANO & T. KISHIMOTO. 1989. Proc. Natl. Acad. Sci. USA **86:** 7547–7551.
30. HAWLEY R. G., A. Z. FONG, B. F. BURNS & T. S. HAWLEY. 1992. J. Exp. Med. **176:** 1149–1163.
31. FATTORI, E., C. DELLA ROCCA, P. COSTA, M. GIORGIO, L. DENTE, L. POZZI & G. CILIBERTO. 1994. Blood **83:** 2570–2579.

DISCUSSION OF THE PAPER

M. KOPF (*Max-Planck-Institut für Immunobiologie, Freiburg, Germany*): You injected turpentine in two doses or you gave 2 times 75 µl. We gave 2 times 50 µl. I do not think that it really accounts for a difference. Did you titrate whether addition of more turpentine really induces more acute phase response?

V. POLI: No, we did not. The question was about our observation that after long-term treatment with turpentine (up to 6 days) the IL-6–deficient mice started to lose weight and one or two mice died; and then we just sacrificed them all. Manfred Kopf was telling me that he did the same experiment with his IL-6–deficient mice and he did not find any mortality and I think one reason might be that we gave more turpentine. I must say also that only 2 of 8 mice died. Maybe in the next experiment you might see zero. This is a possibility. We did not check whether the higher dose of turpentine would influence the induction of acute phase proteins. We checked the plasma levels of IL-1α and TNF and they were normal. At the moment we are in the process of checking SAA levels.

In Lethally Irradiated Mice Interleukin-12 Protects Bone Marrow but Sensitizes Intestinal Tract to Damage from Ionizing Radiation[a]

R. NETA, S. M. STIEFEL, AND N. ALI

Department of Experimental Hematology
Armed Forces Radiobiology Research Institute
Bethesda, Maryland 20889-5603

INTRODUCTION

Lethality after whole body exposure to ionizing radiation is due to a failure of several organ systems.[1-3] The hematopoietic system is the most sensitive, and death due to hematopoietic failure occurs more than a week after exposure to doses of radiation as low as 700 cGy for some strains of mice. The failure of the gastrointestinal system results at doses of radiation usually exceeding 1500 cGy and death due to such failure occurs within 4 to 7 days. Administration of the cytokines interleukin-1 (IL-1), stem cell factor (SCF), and tumor necrosis factor (TNF), prior to irradiation of mice in the range of doses causing hematopoietic failure, protects mice from death.[4-6] Antibodies to any one of these three cytokines abrogate LPS-induced radioprotection and render untreated mice more sensitive to radiation lethality.[7-9] The above findings indicate that endogenous production of these three cytokines in untreated mice and in mice radioprotected with LPS is the basis for radioprotection. Furthermore, radioprotection with IL-1 is abrogated by anti-SCF antibody and radioprotection with SCF is reduced by anti-IL-1R antibody, suggesting that radioprotection with either cytokine requires interaction with the other.[10,11] Consistent with the requirement for interaction of IL-1, SCF, and TNF in radioprotection, combined administration of IL-1 and TNF or IL-1 and SCF results in synergistic radioprotection.[5,10,11]

Interleukin-12 is a recently identified cytokine produced by monocytes/macrophages and lymphocytes challenged with bacteria or their products.[12] Originally identified as natural killer cell stimulatory factor (NKSF),[13,14] IL-12 has been recognized as playing a role in the generation of T_h1 cells from T_h0 cells.[14-16] More recently, IL-12 has been shown to have hematopoietic effects, as indicated by its ability to synergize with hematopoietic growth factors in increasing the number and the size of hematopoietic colonies.[17-19] The ability of IL-12 to promote the growth of hematopoietic progenitor cells, suggested the evaluation of IL-12 for its ability to protect from lethal irradiation.

---

[a] This work was supported by the Armed Forces Radiobiology Research Institute, Defense Nuclear Agency, under Research Work Unit 00129. The opinions contained herein are the private views of the author; no endorsement by the Defense Nuclear Agency has been given or should be inferred. The research was conducted according to the principles enunciated in the *Guide for the Care and Use of Laboratory Animals* prepared by the Institute of Laboratory Animal Resources, National Research Council.

MATERIALS AND METHODS

Mice

B6D2F1 mice, 8–10 wks old, were purchased from Jackson Laboratories (Bar Harbor, ME). Mice were handled as previously described.[5] All animal use protocols were approved by Institutional Animal Use and Care Committee.

Antibodies

Rat monoclonal IgG1, anti-murine IL-1 receptor antibody, (35F5) and anti-murine IL-6 (20F3) were generous gifts from Dr. Richard Chizzonetti (Hoffmann-LaRoche, Nutley, NJ), and Dr. John Abrams (DNAX, Palo Alto, CA), respectively. A rat IgG_1 mAb to β-galactosidase (GL113) was used as a control. Anti-murine TNF (TN3.19.12.) was a generous gift from Dr. Robert Schreiber (Washington University, St. Louis, MO). Rat IgG_1 anti-IFN-γ mAb (XMG-6) was purified from ascites by $(NH_4)_2SO_4$ precipitation and DE-52 ion exchange chromatography and was generously provided by Dr. Fred Finkelma (USUHS, Bethesda, MD). A polyclonal rabbit anti-murine SCF antibody was generously provided by Dr. Douglas Williams (Immunex, Seattle, WA) along with rabbit preimmune control serum. Chromatographically purified rat IgG (Sigma, St. Louis, MO) was used as an additional control. R-phycoerythrin (R-PE) conjugated rat anti mouse c-kit monoclonal antibody 3C1 (IgG2b), and PE-conjugated rat IgG2b (control) were purchased from Pharmingen (San Diego, CA).

Treatment

Recombinant murine IL-12 (batch MRB 021693-1.2, bioactivity of 5.6×10^6 units/mg) was received from Genetics Institute, human IL-1 (rHu IL-1α 117-271 Ro 24-5008 lot IL 1 2/88 activity 3×10^8 units/mg) was kindly provided by Dr. Peter Lomedico, (Hoffmann-LaRoche, Nutley, NJ). The antibodies and recombinant cytokines were diluted in pyrogen-free saline on the day of injection. Antibodies or control immunoglobulin were given i.p. 6-20 h prior to i.p. injection of cytokines.

Irradiation

Mice were randomized, placed in ventilated Plexiglass containers and bilaterally irradiated using the AFRRI ^{60}Co whole body irradiator as described.[11] The number of surviving mice was recorded daily for 30 days.

FACS Analysis

Bone marrow cells (BMC) were obtained by flushing femurs into RPMI media containing 5% FCS. After washing, cells were counted and resuspended in Dulbecco PBS with 2% FCS at the concentration of 2×10^6/ml. Cells were stained for 30 min with 10 μg/ml of either Phycoerythrin (PE) conjugated anti-murine c-kit antibody (3C1) or PE-conjugated, control IgG2b. The cells were washed twice and resuspended in 1 ml of 2% FCS-Dulbecco PBS. The % c-kit$^+$ cells was calculated by subtracting the % of cells stained with control antibody from % of cells stained with c-kit antibody.

Immunofluorescence analysis was performed with an EPICS ELITE flow cytometer (Coulter Cytometry, Miami, Fl) utilizing logarithmic amplification. RBCs, platelets and debris were excluded from the analysis based on light scatter criteria. Twenty five thousand cells were counted for each histogram.

Statistical Analysis

Statistical evaluation of the results was carried out using χ^2 analysis.

RESULTS

Radioprotection by IL-12 Administered Prior to Irradiation

The stimulatory effect of IL-12 on hematopoietic progenitors,[17-19] similar to those reported for SCF and IL-1,[20] instigated experiments to compare IL-12 with IL-1 as a potential radioprotector. A single dose of 1 μg/mouse of IL-12 given ip 18 to 24 hours prior to a ^{60}Co-γ whole body lethal irradiation (950 cGy) protected 77% of B6D2F1 mice from death. The radioprotective effect of IL-12 was comparable to that of IL-1 (75%). The mice treated with IL-12 had increased numbers of nucleated bone marrow cells (BMC) (8.4×10^5/femur in IL-12 treated vs 1.8×10^5/femur in control mice) at 6 days following 950 cGy radiation.

The Effect of Anti-IL-1R, Anti-SCF and Anti-IFNγ Antibody in IL-12–induced Radioprotection

Our previous work showed that SCF and IL-1 are interdependent radioprotectors.[10,11] Whereas there is no evidence that IL-12 induces SCF or IL-1, IL-12 is an inducer of IFN-γ and a number of its effects are attributed to IFN-γ. A hundred μg/mouse of antibody to IFN-γ did not affect IL-12 radioprotection whereas antibody to IL-1R and SCF brogated IL-12 radioprotection, indicating that the radioprotective effect of IL-12 is not mediated by IFN-γ, but does require IL-1 and SCF cooperation.

IL-12 Sensitizes Mice to Lethal Effects of Radiation

IL-1 and SCF given in combination are synergistic in protecting mice from lethal radiation.[10,11] In those studies the treatment with the combination of the two cytokines resulted in $LD_{50/30}$ of 1273 cGy. Because IL-12, like IL-1 and SCF, has a costimulatory effect on BM progenitor cell growth and, as shown above, is also radioprotective by itself, we tested the possibility that IL-12 may enhance radioprotection by SCF or IL-1. Unexpectedly, combined administration of SCF and IL-12, as well as administration of IL-12 alone, resulted in accelerated death of mice exposed to 1200 cGy. B6D2F1 mice that received 1 μg/mouse of IL-12 succumbed within 4 days to radiation-induced death, consistent with death due to GI injury. This apparent sensitizing effect was dependent on the dose of IL-12 and was apparent at doses as low as 40 ng/mouse. Following administration of 1 μg/mouse of IL-12, a hundred percent of B6D2F1 mice were dead within 4 days after 1200 cGy. In the absence of IL-12 treatment, the same mice required doses greater than 1600 cGy. Similar sensitization of B6D2F1 mice was induced when IL-12 was given 18 hours before or within 2 days, but not 3 days, after irradiation. The sensitizing effect of IL-12 was abrogated with 100 μg/mouse of anti-IFN-γ antibody, indicating that IFN-γ was an essential mediator contributing to accelerated death.

Three days after irradiation with 1200 cGy mice treated with IL-12 had twofold higher numbers of nucleated BMC/femur that expressed c-kit$^+$, a phenotypic marker characteristic of BM progenitor cells, than control mice. This indicates that even at doses of radiation at which it causes gastrointestinal damage and death, IL-12 still radioprotects hematopoietic cells.

Gross necropsy 3 days after 1200 cGy radiation of mice treated with IL-12 revealed that the lumen of the small intestine was moderately distended with fluid ingests, suggesting the disruption in the absorption process. In mice treated with IL-12 and anti-IFN-γ antibody the gut appeared normal. Microscopically, treatment with IL-12 of 1200 cGy irradiation mice greatly exacerbated the histologically observed damage to the gut induced by radiation alone, with a much greater decrease in the number of crypts. The extent of damage caused by IL-12 and 1200 cGy was greater than that caused by 1600 cGy irradiation, a dose resulting within 6 days in death of B6D2F1 mice. Treatment with anti-IFN-γ antibody of the 1200 cGy irradiated, IL-12–treated mice, markedly reversed the damage. In contrast, megakaryocytes were absent from the spleens of 1200 cGy irradiated mice, but still found in the spleens of irradiated mice that received IL-12 as well as IL-12 plus anti-IFN-γ antibody, further confirming that hematopoietic components were protected by IL-12.

DISCUSSION

We have demonstrated that treatment of mice with IL-12 has opposite effects on the response to ionizing radiation of hematopoietic and intestinal tissue. The increased survival of IL-12 pretreated mice given lethal irradiation (which causes death from hematopoietic failure), is associated with increased numbers of nucleated BMC in IL-12–treated vs. control, saline-treated mice. Moreover, greater numbers of BMC expressing c-kit$^+$ (a phenotypic marker for hematopoietic progenitor cells) were detected in IL-12-treated mice compared to control mice, 3 days after radiation with 1200 cGy, even though IL-12-treated, but not control mice, succumbed to GI death one day later.

The protection of BMC by IL-12 in irradiated mice may be due to its hematopoiesis-stimulating effects. Although IL-12 by itself does not support the growth of colonies of progenitor cells, it acts synergistically with SCF and IL-1 to promote the growth of primitive hematopoietic stem cells.[17–19] Indeed, as indicated by abrogation of the radioprotection with anti-IL-1R and anti-SCF antibody, radioprotection with IL-12 requires the presence of IL-1 and SCF. This mutual interdependence of IL-12, IL-1, and SCF extends our previous findings on co-dependence of IL-1 and SCF in radioprotection.[10,11] In our studies, unlike many other effects of IL-12, its induction of protection from lethal effects of ionizing radiation is IFN-γ independent, since it is not abrogated with anti-IFN-γ antibody. This is consistent with the finding that IL-12 acts directly to stimulate proliferation of primitive stem cells.[17]

Concerning the mechanisms for these survival enhancing effects by IL-1, SCF and IL-12 in lethally irradiated mice, we hypothesize that these may be based in part on the ability of these cytokines to induce and/or promote cycling of early hematopoietic progenitors to reach a more radioresistant phase of the cell cycle. Both IL-1 and SCF, *in vivo*, stimulate expansion of early hematopoietic progenitor cells (21–24). Within 18 hours following administration of IL-1 progenitor BMC were much more sensitive to HU, that is selectively toxic to cells in S-phase, and had an increased proportion of cells in the S + G_2 + M phase of the cell cycle.[21,22] Moreover, the lag period greater than 4 but less than 48 hours that is required for optimal radioprotection with IL-1 (4), SCF (11), and IL-12 (data not shown), further suggests that entry into a specific phase of the cell cycle, rather than mere expansion of hematopoietic progenitors, may be critical for radioprotection. Studies with synchronized cultures of numerous mammalian cell lines established that the late S phase of the cell cycle is most radioresistant.[25] Similarly, *in vivo* synchronization of rapidly dividing crypt cells in mouse jejunum by 5 intraperitoneal injections of hydroxyurea (HU) followed by exposure at time intervals thereafter to 1100 cGy of γ-rays indicated that crypt cells irradiated during late-S phase were a hundredfold more resistant than the cells in G_1/S phase.[26] These observations predict that driving stem and progenitor cells to late S phase may contribute to myeloprotection.

The finding that a single dose of IL-12, even as low as 40 ng/mouse, renders irradiated mice more sensitive to death due to gastrointestinal damage was unexpected. Histologically, the damage to crypt cells observed in jejunal sections obtained 3 days following combined treatment with IL-12 and 1200 cGy from B6D2F1 mice, was even more extensive than the damage caused by 1600 cGy. Since anti–IFN-γ antibody abrogates this sensitizing effect of IL-12, IFN-γ is an important mediator for such sensitization.

SUMMARY

Administration of IL-12 prior to lethal irradiation, protected a significant fraction of mice from ^{60}Co-γ radiation-induced lethal hematopoietic syndrome. Radioprotection was associated with an increase in the number of c-kit⁺ bone marrow cells (BMC) in IL-12 treated mice compared to saline-treated mice. Even after supralethal doses of radiation (1200 cGy), IL-12-treated mice had twofold greater numbers of c-kit⁺ BMC than controls. However the mice receiving IL-12 and 1200 cGy died of the gastrointestinal (GI) syndrome, evident by gross necroscopy and histological evaluation, within 4 to 6 days after irradiation. Induction of the GI syndrome in mice not treated with IL-12 required radiation doses of 1600 cGy. Thus, at doses of radiation at which IL-12 still protects c-kit⁺ hematopoietic cells, it sensitizes the intestinal tract to damage. Radioprotection with IL-12 was abrogated by anti-IL-1R or anti-SCF antibody, but not anti-IFNγ antibody. In contrast, anti-IFNγ antibody abrogated sensitization of the intestinal tract by IL-12.

ACKNOWLEDGMENTS

We thank Mrs Lillie Heman-Ackah for preparing intestinal sections and Mark Moorman for flow cytometry analysis of BMC.

REFERENCES

1. HALL, E. J. 1988. Radiobiology for the radiologist. Philadelphia: Lippincott Co.
2. BOND, V. P., T. M. FLIEDNER & J. O. ARCHAMBEAU. 1965. Mammalian Radiation Lethality. A Disturbance in Cellular Kinetics. New York: Academic Press.

3. LORENZ, E., D. UPHOFF, T. R. REID & E. SHELTON. 1951. Modification of irradiation injury in mice and guinea pigs by bone marrow injections. J. Natl. Cancer Inst. **12:** 197.
4. NETA, R., S. D. DOUCHES & J. J. OPPENHEIM. 1986. Interleukin-1 is a radioprotector. J. Immunol. **136:** 2483.
5. NETA, R., J. J. OPPENHEIM & S. D. DOUCHES. 1988. Interdependence of the radioprotective effects of human recombinant IL-1, TNF, G-CSF, and murine recombinant GM-CSF. J Immunol. **140:** 108.
6. ZSEBO, K. M., K. A. SMITH, C. A. HARTLEY, M. GREENBLATT, K. COOKE, W. RICH & I. K. MCNIECE. 1992. Radioprotection of mice by recombinant stem cell factor. Proc. Natl. Acad. Sci. USA **89:** 9464.
7. NETA, R., J. J. OPPENHEIM, R. D. SCHREIBER, R. CHIZZONITE, G. D. LEDNEY & T. J. MACVITTIE. 1991. Role of cytokines (interleukin 1, tumor necrosis factor, and transforming growth factor β in natural and lipopolysaccharide-enhanced radioresistance. J. Exp. Med. **173:** 1177.
8. NETA, R. R., R. PERLSTEIN, S. N. VOGEL, G. D. LEDNEY & J. ABRAMS. 1992. Role of IL 6 in protection from lethal irradiation and in endocrine responses to IL 1 and TNF. J. Exp. Med. **175:** 689.
9. NETA, R., D. WILLIAMS, F. SELZER & J. ABRAMS. 1993. Inhibition of c-kit ligand/steel factor by antibodies reduces survival of lethally-irradiated mice. Blood **81:** 324.
10. NETA, R., J. M. WANG, J. J. OPPENHEIM, N. DAVIS & C. M. DUBOIS. 1993. Cytokine interactions in protection from lethal irradiation: Synergy of IL-1 and Kit Ligand. In The Negative Regulation of Hematopoiesis; From Fundamental Aspects to Clinical Applications. M. Guigon, F. Lemoine, N. Dainiak, A. Schechter & A. Najman, Eds. Montrouge, France: John Libbey Eurotext. In press.
11. NETA, R., J. J. OPPENHEIM, J. M. WANG, C. M. SNAPPER, M. A. MORMAN & C. M. DUBOIS. 1994. Synergy of IL-1 and c-kit Ligand (KL) in radioprotection of mice correlates with IL-1 upregulation of mRNA and protein expression for c-kit on bone marrow cells. J Immunol. **153:** 1536.
12. TRINCHERI, G. 1993. Interleukin-12 and its role in the generation of Th1 cells. Immunol. Today **14:** 335.
13. KOBAYASHI, M., L. FRITZ, M. RYAN, R. M. HEWICK, S. C. CLARK, S. CHAN, R. LOUDON, F. SHERMAN, B. PERUSSIA & G. TRINCHERI. 1989. Identification and purification of natural killer cell stimulatory factor (NKSF), a cytokine with multiple biologic effects on human lymphocytes. J. Exp. Med. **170:** 827.
14. STERN, A. S., F. J. PODLASKI, J. D. HULMES, Y.-C. E. PAN, P. M. QUINN, A. G. WOLITZKY, P. C. FAMILLETTI, D. L. STERMLO, T. TRUITT, R. CHIZZONITE & M. K. GATELY. 1990. Purification to homogeneity and partial characterization of cytotoxic lymphocyte maturation factor from human B-lymphoblastoid cells. Proc. Soc. Natl. Acad. Sci. USA **87:** 6808.
15. HEINZEL, F. P., D. S. SCHOENHAUT, R. M. RERKO, L. E. ROSSER & M. K. GATELY. 1993. Recombinant IL-12 cures mice infected with Leishmania major. J. Exp. Med. **177:** 1505.
16. LOCKSLEY, R. M. 1993. Interleukin 12 in host defense against microbial pathogens. Proc. Natl. Acad. Sci. USA **90:** 5879.
17. JACOBSEN, S. E. W., O. P. VEIBY & E. B. SMELAND. 1993. Cytotoxic lymphocyte maturation factor (Interleukin 12) is a synergistic growth factor for hematopoietic stem cells. J. Exp. Med. **178:** 413.
18. PLOEMACHER, R. E., P. L. VAN SOEST, H. VOORVINDEN & A. BOUDEWIJN. 1993. Interleukin-12 synergizes with interleukin-3 and steel factor to enhance recovery of murine hematopoietic stem cells in liquid culture. Leukemia **7:** 1381.
19. HIRAYAMA, F., N. KATAYAMA, S. NEBEN, D. DONALDSON, E. B. NICKBARG, S. C. CLARK & M. OGAWA. 1994. Synergistic interaction between interleukin-12 and steel factor in support of proliferation of murine lymphohematopoietic progenitors in culture. Blood **83:** 92.
20. MUENCH, M. O., J. G. SCHNEIDER & M. A. S. MOORE. 1991. Interactions among colony-stimulating factors, IL-1β, IL-6, and kit-ligand in the regulation of primitive murine hematopoietic cells. Exp. Hematol. **20:** 339.

21. NETA, R., M. B. SZTEIN, J. J. OPPENHEIM, S. GILLIS & S. D. DOUCHES. 1987. In vivo effects of IL-1. I. Bone marrow cells are induced to cycle following administration of IL-1. J. Immunol. **139:** 1861.
22. SCHWARTZ, G. N., T. J. MACVITTIE, R. M. VIGNEULLE, M. L. PATCHEN, S. D. DOUCHES, J. J. OPPENHEIM & R. NETA. 1987. Enhanced hematopoietic recovery in irradiated mice pretreated with interleukin-1 (IL-1). Immunopharmacol. Immunotoxicol. **9:** 371.
23. JOHNSON, C. S., D. J. KECKLER, M. I. TOPPER, et al. 1989. In vivo hematopoietic effects of recombinant interleukin 1a in mice: Stimulation of granulocytic, monocytic, megakaryocytic and early erythroid progenitors; suppression of late stage erythropoiesis, and reversal of erythroid suppression with erythropoietin. Blood **73:** 678.
24. FLEMING, W. H., E. J. ALPERN, N. UCHIDA, K. IKUTA & I. L. WEISSMAN. 1993. Steel factor influences the distribution and activity of murine hematopoietic stem cells in vivo. Proc. Natl. Acad. Sci. USA **90:** 3760.
25. SINCLAIR, W. K. & R. A. MORTON. 1966. X-ray sensitivity during the cell generation cycle of cultured Chinese hamster cells. Radiat. Res. **29:** 450.
26. WITHERS, H. R., K. MASON, B. O. REID, N. DUBRAVSKY, H. T. BARKLEY, B. W. BROWN & J. B. SMATHERS. 1974. Response of mouse intestine to neutrons and gamma rays in relation to dose fractionation and cell cycle. Cancer **34:** 39.

DISCUSSION OF THE PAPER

A. KOJ (*Jagiellonian University, Krakow, Poland*): Do you have any clue how IL-12 may prime monocytes to produce TNF and IL-6? What would be the mechanism of action?

R. NETA: The priming probably occurs via induction of IFN-γ by IL-12. Such priming would be in accord with Monte Meltzer's original model of two signal activation of macrophage, involving IFN and LPS. Findings somewhat similar to ours were observed by Dr. Gianni Garotta of Hoffmann-LaRoche, who, using IL-12, sensitized mice to LPS-induced lethal Shwartzman reaction.

KOJ: Could IL-12 be replaced by something else?

NETA: Not in our system. We have tried several cytokines, including IFN-γ, which is clearly a mediator of this effect. According to Dr. Finkelman, IFN-γ is a much less stable cytokine when injected exogenously than is IL-12. Probably, the endogenously produced IFN-γ is much more potent than the injected.

A. RAY (*Yale University School of Medicine, New Haven, CT*): What is the reason for the difference in the lag period in radiation-induced lethality?

NETA: I did not have time to present this in the introduction of how radiation damage is generated. Radiation damages different tissues depending on the dose, and subsequently three distinct syndromes are recognized. Hematopoietic syndrome occurs at the lowest doses of radiation with death from 10 to 30 days in a mouse and 60 days in humans. Gastrointestinal syndrome in mouse occurs at doses exceeding 1600 cGy with death within 4 to 7 days after irradiation. It apparently takes this long for the gut damage to contribute to animal death. The third syndrome, known as cerebrovascular syndrome, is due to neurological and vascular failure and occurs within hours to 2 to 3 days after doses exceeding 10,000 cGy.

M. KUBIN (*Philadelphia, PA*): Did you ever try to reverse the effect of IL-12 by IL-10?

NETA: We are actually in the process of setting up these experiments. We will also try IL-4 in this system.

KUBIN: And how would you explain the effects of exogenously added IL-12 since it has been shown that it is constitutively produced and it exists in the serum of mice and humans?

NETA: I can only speculate that there are factors, IL-10 for example, that counteract IL-12 activity. Obviously, anti-IL-12 antibody could be used to establish the effect of endogenous IL-12. We do not know yet if the available antibody is sufficiently reliable *in vivo*.

KUBIN: What antibody do you use?

NETA: We have used a limited quantity of antibody obtained from Genetics Institute. I do not remember how it was made. I can also mention that we have tried injecting a NOS inhibitor to test whether it can block sensitization by IL-12. So far, we have not succeeded. On the other hand, using spin-label technique with gut tissue, we have some preliminary indications that nitric oxide may be involved in this process.

Adenovirus Vectors for Cytokine Gene Expression

CARL D. RICHARDS,[a] TODD BRACIAK,[a] ZHOU XING,[a] FRANK GRAHAM,[b] AND JACK GAULDIE[a]

[a]Department of Pathology
[b]Department of Biology
McMaster University
1200 Main Street W.
Hamilton, Ontario, Canada L8N 3Z5

INTRODUCTION

The cytokine interleukin-6 (IL-6) is a mediator of communication between various tissues and cells. Its functions include those in hematopoietic, immunologic and inflammatory processes (reviewed extensively elsewhere[1–3]). A major role of IL-6 *in vivo* is that of a mediator of hepatocyte acute phase protein production.[3,4] IL-6 has been identified as a monocyte and fibroblast-derived product that regulates liver acute phase gene transcription and protein expression *in vitro* and *in vivo*. Although other cytokines including IL-1, TNF (tumor necrosis factor) and IL-6-type cytokines such as LIF (leukemia inhibitory factor) IL-11 and oncostatin M regulate this response *in vitro*,[5,6] it appears that IL-6 is the major regulator in inflammatory responses due to particular stimuli *in vivo*.

In studying physiologic actions of IL-6, a major problem is presented by the short $T_{1/2}$ of injected recombinant or purified protein *in vivo*. As shown by Castell *et al.*,[7] injected recombinant IL-6 in rats shows a half-life of approximately 10 minutes. Searching for systems which allow significant and more prolonged presence of IL-6 and other cytokines in circulation has led to the development of transgenes and transfecting DNA vectors to express inserted IL-6 DNA in particular tissues. Although transgenic animals provide information about the effects of high levels of expression, they may not provide relevant data regarding the function of IL-6 overexpression in a local environment. Naked DNA or liposomal DNA transfer results in inefficient DNA incorporation or penetration to nuclei. Recombinant retrovirus vectors have been used successfully to transfer genes to certain tissues however retroviral product expression depends on replicating cells as targets for gene incorporation (reviewed elsewhere[8,9]). Thus, the progeny of replicating cells have virus-encoded genes which are expressed. Hawley *et al.*[10] have shown that a retrovirus-IL-6 gene transfer to bone marrow cells *in vitro*, which were transplanted into irradiated mice, led to a strong prolonged overexpression of IL-6. This resulted in lethal myeloproliferative disease as well as a pronounced increased in serum acute phase protein and serum immunoglobulin levels.

Adenoviruses (reviewed extensively elsewhere[11,12]) were first reported as distinct viruses that infected epithelial-like cells. Multiple serotypes have been identified in humans (grater than 40) and isolated from outbreaks of various diseases such as acute fibrile respiratory syndromes, epidemic keratoconjunctivitis and acute hemorrhagic cystitits. Adenovirus type 12 was shown to cause tumors in rodents; however, there are still no data associating tumors with adenoviral infection in humans. Intensified research on adenoviruses led to discoveries on RNA splicing and eukaryotic DNA replication *in vitro*, as well as techniques such as S1 nuclease mapping. Thus, many aspects of adenovirus replication and expression of viral proteins have been studied, providing a useful model to examine eukaryotic cell function.

Human adenoviruses show efficient infectivity, efficient passage to the nucleus where it exists as episomal DNA, high levels of transgene expression, and no or low incorporation of viral DNA into host genome. In addition to its natural tropism for the epithelium, adenovirus can infect a variety of non-replicating cell types. Adenovirus is characterized by a non-enveloped virion shaped in a regular icosahedron with a fiber structure projecting from each of its 12 vertices. The fiber structure is composed of a complex of penton base and fiber protein, both of which appear to play a role in attachment and/or internalization of the virus upon infection. This appears to also involve cell surface proteins such as α_v integrins[13] and a 50 kD unidentified receptor for fiber. The DNA sequence has been completed for Adenovirus 2 (Ad2) and Adenovirus 5 (Ad5) and has been divided into 4 early gene regions (E1 to E4, expressed before viral DNA replication) and late genes which are predominately virus structural proteins and are controlled by the major late promoter (MLP). Adenovirus type 5 (Ad5) has been used extensively by our laboratory and others as vectors for transfer of genes of interest and for use as vaccines.[12,14-19] We have infected rodents at various sites with Ad5 encoding IL-6 and analyzed IL-6 production and subsequent effects. This has provided a model of transient-gene transfer through which the biologic functions of IL-6 can be assessed in context of local tissue expression *in vivo*.

MATERIALS AND METHODS

The techniques used to construct adenovirus type 5 recombinant virus that express inserted cytokine have been described.[12,15] In the design of recombinant Ad5 vectors it is possible to fit inserts in the E3 or E1 region, either of which can drive expression of IL-6 cDNA. The E1 and E3 regions are non-essential for virus protein expression in cells in culture, and E3 is not essential for replication of viral DNA. Since the E1 region is necessary for viral replication in tissue culture, E1-deleted mutants or constructs can be rescued in the transformed 293 cell line[14] which supplies E1 in trans. IL-6 cassettes inserted into the E3 region contain the SV40 promoter as well as the SV40 polyadenylation site. IL-6 cassettes inserted into the E1 region contains human CMV promoter sequence as well as the SV40 polyadenylation signal. All viruses were purified on CsCl gradients and dialyzed thoroughly against 4 changes of autoclaved Tris-HCL pH 7.4 containing 10% glycerol, and stored frozen at $-75°C$.

Animals (Sprague-Dawley rats or Balb/c mice) were infected with the various Ad5 viruses (diluted to the indicated pfu in 300 μl of sterile endotoxin-free PBS, pH 7.4), anaesthetized and sacrificed at the times indicated. Serum samples were taken from the abdominal aorta, and bronchoalveolar lavage (BAL) was performed by infusing 3 ml PBS aliquots (total of 30 ml). The first aliquot was kept separate. IL-6 bioactivity in the serum samples and BAL fluid (first aliquot) was measured using the B9 proliferation assay. Cellular content of BAL were analyzed after collection by centrifugation and cytocentrifuge smear preparation. Serum levels of acute phase proteins were analyzed by rocket electrophoresis and comparison to a standard curve.[15]

The Ad5luc3 construct has been previously described.[21] Luciferase activity of tissues was measured 24 hours after infection when organ samples were placed in 100 mM potassium phosphate (containing 1 mM PMSF and 10 μg/ml aprotinin). After homogenation and sonication, cell debris was pelleted by centrifugation and the supernatant was assayed for luciferase activity.[15,21]

Northern blot analysis was completed by standard techniques using snap-frozen (liquid nitrogen) right lung tissue. The left lung was fixed by perfusion with 4% paraformaldehyde for histology. Constructs containing the lacZ gene have been described by others[22,23] and our construct is designated Ad5LacZA1.[24] Detection of LacZ gene product was performed as described.[22,24] After infection, lungs of rats were infused with fixative (2% formaldehyde, 0.2% glutaraldehyde in PBS at 4°C) for 1 hour. The fixative was poured out, the lungs were washed with PBS and then infused with the staining solution (5 mM $K_4Fe(CN)_6$, 5 mM $K_3Fe_3(CN)_6$, 2 mM $MgCl_2$ and 0.5 mg/ml of X-gal stain at 37°C overnight. Lung tissues could then be paraffin-embedded, sectioned, and counterstained.

RESULTS AND DISCUSSION

We have constructed recombinant human Ad5 viruses containing murine IL-6 cDNA (Ad5-mIL-6) inserted into the E3 region (Ad5E3-mIL6) or E1 region (Ad5E1-mIL6). These constructs can infect various cell types such as HeLa cells or 293 cells (shown in FIG. 1) and cause expression of high amounts ($\mu g/10^6$ cells/24 hrs) of virus-encoded IL-6 *in vitro*. Wild-type, or virus constructs containing glycoprotein B8 from Herpes HSV-1 (Ad5-gB8)[19] did not cause any detectable IL-6 production by 293 cells or HeLa cells. These Ad5 virus constructs have also been used to infect mice by various routes.

When Balb/c mice are infected intraperitoneally with E1 or E3 recombinant Ad5-mIL-6 viruses, systemic IL-6 is detected at significant and prolonged levels while Ad5-gB8 infected, or saline injected animals were within normal levels of plasma IL-6

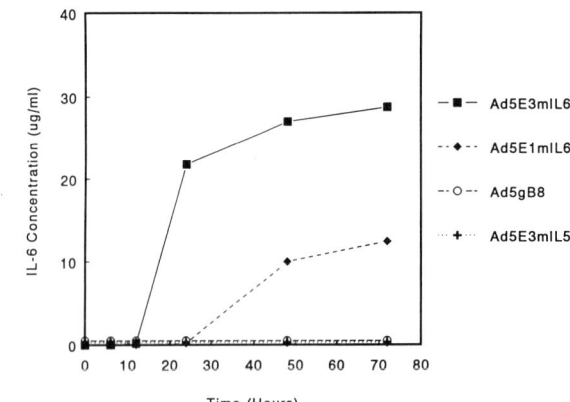

FIGURE 1. *In vitro* biological activity. To establish that the IL-6 cDNA-containing recombinant Ad5 viruses expressed biologically active protein, a B9 hybridoma growth assay for IL-6 was performed. Supernatants from the various recombinant infected and uninfected 293 cells were added to B9 cells plated in a 96-well tissue culture dish and growth was measured by the colorimetric MTT (tetrazolium) assay. Only supernatants from the IL-6 cDNA-containing recombinant viruses (Ad5E3-mIL-6 and Ad5E1-mIL-6) demonstrated enhanced IL-6 activity. No activity was detectable in supernatants from recombinant Ad5 viruses that express HSV gB8 (Ad5-gB8) or murine IL-5 (Ad5E3-mIL-5).

(FIG. 2a). Upon intraperitoneal infection, serum IL-6 is raised on days 1 to 3 (peaking on day 1) using either Ad5E3-mIL-6 or Ad5E1-mIL-6 viruses. This is also associated with enhanced acute-phase protein levels in serum, evident on days 1 through to day 7 of the Ad5-IL-6 virus infections but not Ad5-gB8 or saline-injected mice (FIG. 2b and c). Haptoglobin levels peaked on day 2–3 and were still markedly elevated on day 7, while α_1-AGP levels peaked on day 2–3, still elevated at day 5 and receded on day 7. The profile of these acute phase protein levels most likely reflect the amount of IL-6 expressed over time by Ad5-mIL-6.

A striking feature of Ad5-mIL-6 infected mice was the increase in size and weight (4-fold) of spleens that was most prominent at day 7 of infection. This did not occur with Ad5-gB8 or saline-injected animals. When examined histologically, the germinal centers and trabecular areas of the Ad5-mIL-6 spleens showed lymphoid expansion apparently of both B and T cell compartments. This is similar to the effects on spleen reported for exogenous recombinant IL-6 administration for 3 days.[20] Histological examination of the liver after ip infection showed small nodules at day 7 that appeared to be composed of mononuclear and lymphoid-like cells. These lymphoid nodules resolved by days 16–20 and were not seen at all in Ad5-gB8 infected animals (even at 10 times pfu).

With the use of an Ad5 construct encoding the cDNA for firefly luciferase (Ad5-Luc3), one can examine for specific tissue expression of virus encoded inserts.[21] Intraperitoneal injection of 10^9 pfu of Ad5-Luc3 into Sprague-Dawley rats (or 1×10^8 pfu into mice) and examination 24 hours later resulted in the greatest luciferase expression in liver, followed by spleen and then peritoneum (FIG. 3). Highest levels were found on the outer peritoneal edges of each organ. Quite small amounts were seen in thymus, kidney and lung. In contrast, after intratracheal instillation (i.t. infection), lung tissue was far the highest in luciferase expression whereas luciferase assayed in other organs such as the liver was much less (FIG. 3b). Injection of Ad5-Luc3 into right hind footpads of rats resulted in detectable luciferase levels in the right popliteal lymph node and right foot but not the left node or foot. Thus, infection with Ad5 at different sites in the rat can lead to specific organ and/or tissue expression of virus-encoded genes.

Adenovirus 5 vectors containing the *E. coli* lacZ gene (β-galactosidase) have been used previously[22,23] to examine tissues histologically for the cells that express virus-encoded genes. In our experiments, i.t. infection of Sprague-Dawley rats with 1×10^8 pfu of Ad5-lacZA1 (prepared as described elsewhere[24]) caused large amounts of significant expression of lacZ in the lung as detected by colorimetric conversion of the substrate stain X-gal. The stained lacZ product was found on the surface and throughout the right and left lungs. Tissue sectioning and examination showed that the major sites of lacZ expression were the epithelial cells of small and respiratory bronchioles as well as alveoli in close juxtaposition. This is consistent with adenovirus tropism for epithelial cells.

In examining the expression of IL-6 in this model of lung infection, northern analysis was performed at different times after Ad5-rIL-6 (rat IL-6 cDNA inserted into the E3 region) or Ad5-lacZA1 instillation. Total lung RNA showed strong expression of viral IL-6 mRNA (distinct in size from endogenous IL-6 mRNA) that was evident at 12 hours and maximal at days 1 and 3 while levels waned by day 7 (FIG. 4). The mRNA signals in Ad5-rIL-6 infection were many fold higher than those seen in LPS-treated rat lungs, which showed a characteristic pattern of 1.3 kb and 2.5 kb mRNA species. No significant IL-6 mRNA signals were seen in lungs from Ad5-lacZA1 infected animals. Furthermore, *in situ* hybridization showed that bronchial epithelial cells localized mRNA for IL-6 at day 3 of infection.[24] Ad5-lacZA1 infected animals were negative for IL-6 signal by *in situ* hybridization. These experi-

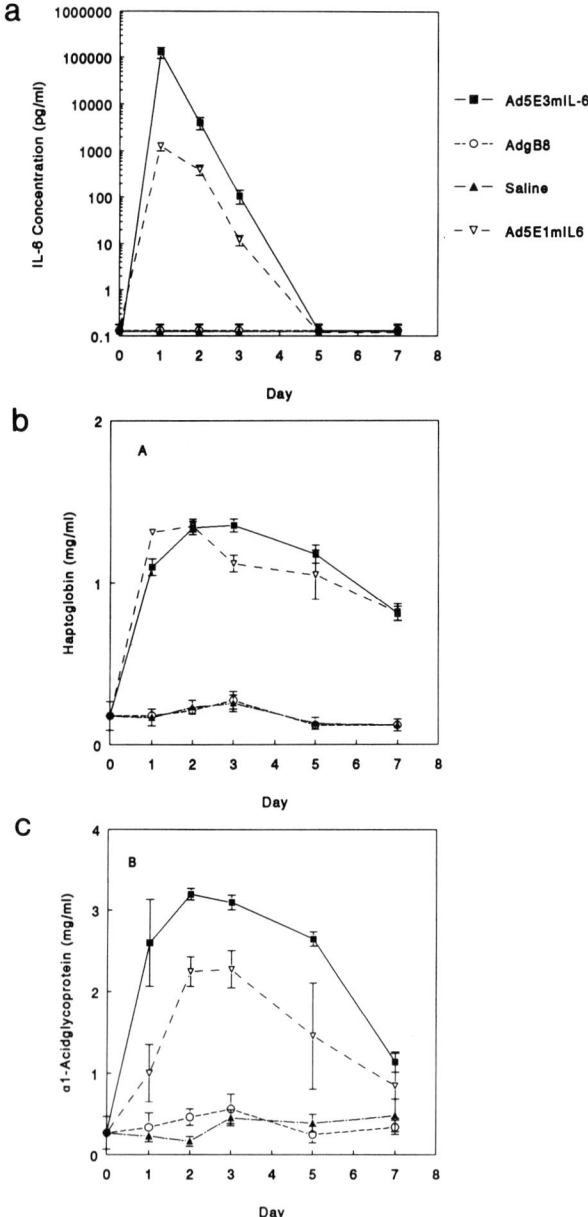

FIGURE 2. *In vivo* biological activity. To test the effects of Ad5-mIL-6 infection *in vivo*, 2×10^8 pfu of Ad5E3-mIL-6 and 5×10^8 pfu of Ad5E1-mIL-6 recombinant viruses were injected i.p. into Balb/c mice. At the indicated times after infection, animals were sacrificed (n = 5) and circulating IL-6 serum levels **(a)** were measured as well as levels for the serum acute phase proteins haptoglobin **(b)** and α_1-acid glycoprotein **(c)**.

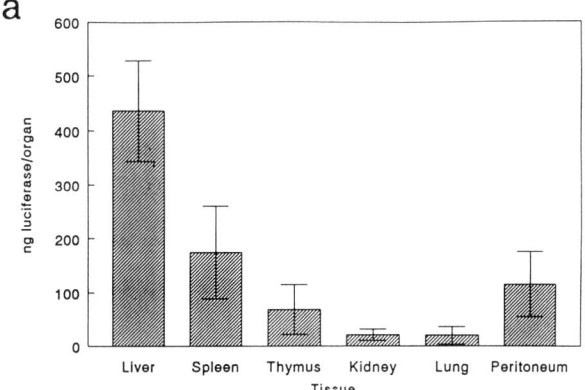

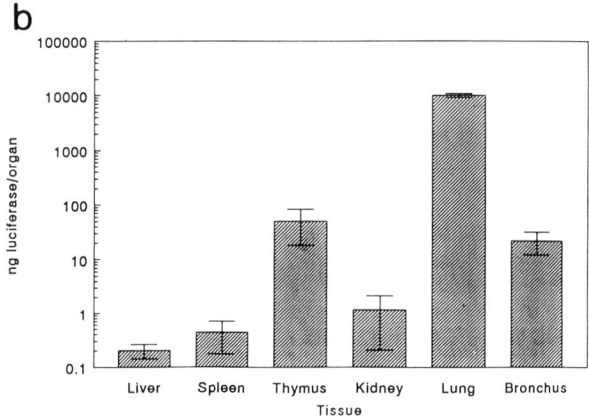

FIGURE 3. Expression of Ad5Luc3 in organs of Sprague-Dawley rats. Twenty four hours after infection, individual organs were removed and processed for luciferase activity as previously described.[21] **a:** i.p. infection on a linear ordinate. **b:** i.t. infection on a logarithmic ordinate. Data were expressed as the mean and SE from individual tissue samples (n = 3). (Reproduced from Braciak et al.[15] with permission.)

ments utilized 2×10^8 pfu in 300 µl of sterile-saline which in dose-response experiments was shown to result in minimal immediate inflammatory responses but significant levels of IL-6 expression.

Enhanced IL-6 protein levels were found in both the bronchoalveolar lavage (BAL) fluids and in serum of Sprague-Dawley rats infected i.t. with Ad5-rIL-6 (FIG. 5). This was dependent on dose (pfu) and showed substantial amounts of bioactive IL-6 in BAL and lower but significant amounts in serum at 24 hours after infection. Using 10^8 pfu, the levels of IL-6 were analyzed in Ad5-rIL-6 and Ad5-lacZA1 infected rats over time. Levels of IL-6 in BAL was markedly enhanced at days 1, 3 and 5 (peaking on day 3 at 100 ng/ml) after Ad5-rIL-6 but not Ad5-lacZA1 infections. This was also evident in serum where peak levels were also seen on day 3 (2 ng/ml).

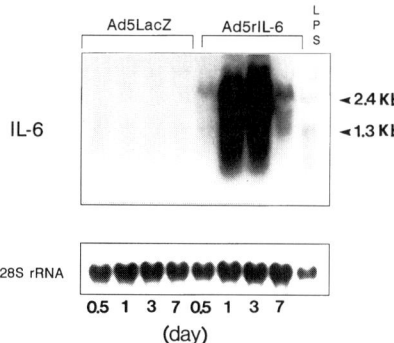

FIGURE 4. Kinetics of IL-6 transgene expression in total lung tissues. Sprague-Dawley rats infected i.t. with Ad5-laczA1 or Ad5-rIL-6 were sacrificed at the times indicated and RNA was extracted from lung tissue. Northern blot analysis was used to detect IL-6 mRNA species and endogenous IL-6 mRNA from rat lungs of LPS-challenged rats was used as a size marker. Note that the Ad5-rIL-6–infected lungs produced specific IL-6 RNA signal at a distinct size from the endogenous transcripts of 1.3 and 2.5 kb. Ethidium bromide stained 28S RNA is shown below as a control for RNA loading. (Reproduced from Xing et al.[24] with permission.)

We suggest the serum levels resulted from spill-over into the circulation from the lung. Measurement of α_1-CPI levels (a major acute phase protein in rat) in the serum at days 1, 2 and 3 showed raised levels (3, 6 and 8 fold respectively) in Ad5-rIL-6 infected animals but not in Ad5-lacZA1 animals. Thus, a typical acute phase response was seen associated with the over-expressed IL-6 in lung and raised serum levels of IL-6 in the Ad5-rIL-6 infected animals.

Since intraperitoneal infection of mice with Ad5-mIL-6 resulted in alterations in cellular composition of spleens and liver, the cellular component of the BAL and lung tissue of rats infected i.t. with Ad5-rIL-6 (and Ad5-lacZA1 as a comparison) was examined. Alveolar macrophages were the main component of BAL at 12 hours after infection, while at days 1, 2 and 3, small increases in numbers of neutrophils, monocytes and lymphocytes were seen in both Ad5-rIL-6 and Ad5-lacZA1 infections. These levels decreased in Ad5-LacZA1 treated animals thereafter, whereas Ad5-rIL-6 infection showed a marked increase in lymphocytes in BAL peaking at day 7, where greater than 10-fold of lymphocytes were observed in Ad5-rIL-6 infections over that in Ad5-lacZA1 infections (FIG. 6). Moderate increases in total numbers of macrophages and neutrophils were also seen at day 7 and levels of all cells declined at day 12 and were near basal levels at day 14.

To assess the subtypes of lymphocytes in this expansion, day 7 BAL cells were analyzed by FACS using specific monoclonal antibody to CD3 (T cell receptor component), CD4 (helper T cell), CD3a (cytotoxic T cell) and CD45R (pan B cell marker). The lymphocyte population was approximately 30% CD3$^+$ CD4$^+$, 47% CD3$^+$ CD8$^+$ and 2–4% CD45R$^+$ in either Ad5-rIL-6 or in Ad5-lacZA1 infections. However, Ad5-rIL-6 virus led to 8–10 times greater absolute numbers of each lymphocyte phenotype. The ratio of CD4$^+$ to CD8$^+$ cells remained similar in Ad5-rIL-6 infection, thus the marked expansion in lymphocytes did not appear to be subtype specific.

Histologically there was a mild to moderate inflammatory response in Ad5-lacZA1 or Ad5-rIL-6–infected lungs. This was marked by hyperemia, neutrophil and mononuclear cell infiltration in peribronchial, perivascular and interstitial spaces, as well as enlargement of bronchial associated lymphoid tissue (BALT) up to day 5. However, on day 7, Ad5-rIL-6–infected lungs showed severe lymphocytic hyperplasia in alveolar and interstitial spaces. The local BALT increased dramatically so that some sites expanded from the submucosa into the epithelium and formed intrabronchial protrusions. Diffuse lymphocytic infiltration was also seen throughout the lung and in some instances hyperplasia of bronchial and type II alveolar epithelial cells was observed.

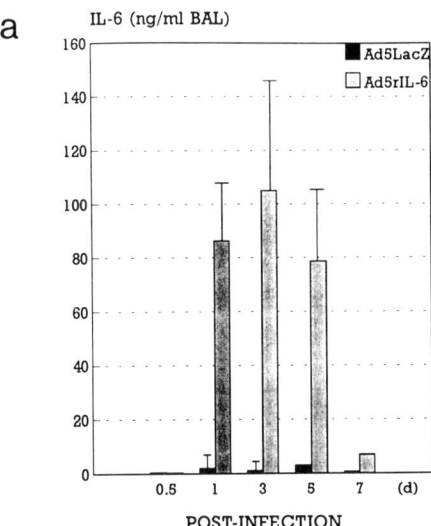

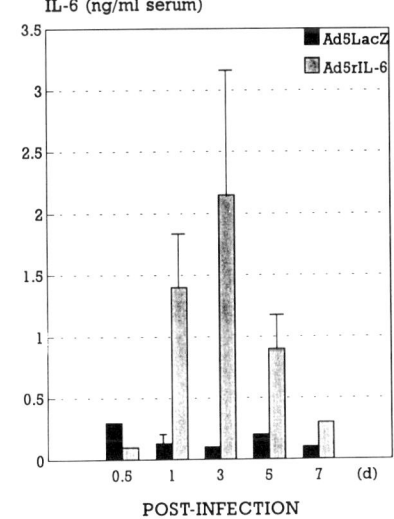

FIGURE 5. Kinetics of bioactive IL-6 protein content in BAL and serum. Sprague-Dawley rats were infected i.t. with Ad5-LacZA1 or Ad5-rIL-6 and sacrificed at the indicated time after infection. Samples of BAL fluid (a) and serum (b) were assayed for IL-6 content by the B9 hybridoma proliferation assay. (Reproduced from Xing et al.[24] with permission.)

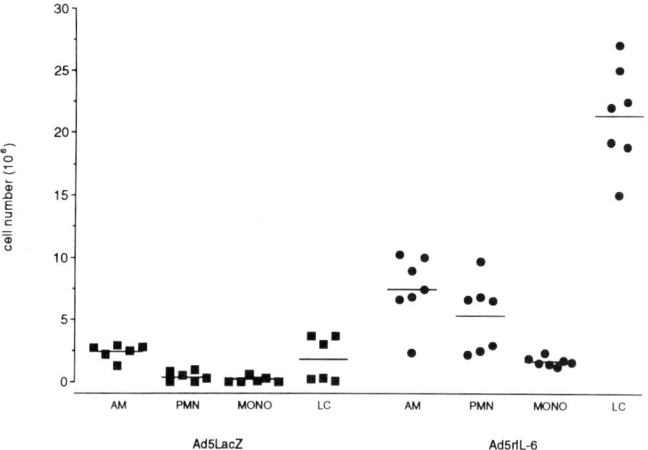

FIGURE 6. Cellular components of BAL fluid at day 7 after infection with Ad5-lacZA1 or Ad5-rIL-6. Data represent numbers of indicated cells from individual animals infected with Ad5-lacZA1 (squares) or Ad5-rIL-6 (dots). After 7 days of infection, animals were sacrificed and BAL samples were analyzed for alveolar macrophages (AM), neutrophils (PMN), monocytes (MONO) or lymphocytes (LC). The bars represent means of data.

These effects were much less evident on day 12 and the inflammatory changes in the lung were resolved to normal.

SUMMARY AND CONCLUSIONS

Recombinant Adenovirus type 5 constructs containing IL-6 cDNA can be used to infect cells *in vitro* and obtain a high level of IL-6 expression and secretion into culture media. Furthermore, Ad5-IL-6 viruses can also be used to infect Balb\c mice or Sprague-Dawley rats and obtain a high level of IL-6 expression that is sustained over a period of 3–5 days. Intratracheal infection was accompanied by dramatic increases in virus-encoded IL-6 mRNA levels in rat lung tissue, raised levels of IL-6 detected in bronchoalveolar lavage fluids and in serum, and IL-6–dependent sequelae such as liver acute phase responses. This occurs in a tissue-specific manner, depending on routes of infection by the virus. Rat lungs showed a prominent expansion (10 fold in numbers) of all classes of lymphocytes, including B cells, T helper cells (CD4+) and CTL (CD8+) at day 7 after infection which resolved significantly by day 12. Thus the associated biological effects of viral vector mediated IL-6 over-expression was also transient in nature. Other tissues can be infected with Ad5 and thus can also be induced to express selected genes in a transient fashion. We are currently examining the potential for Ad recombinant cytokine vectors in therapy for cancer and for bone marrow reconstitution after transplantation. Thus the use of recombinant Ad5 vectors may have a broad application in the study of cytokine function and possibly in future therapy as a transient gene transfer approach.

REFERENCES

1. REVEL, M. 1989. Host defense against infections and inflammations: Role of the multifunctional IL-6/IFN-beta2 cytokine. Experientia **45:** 549–557.

2. HIRANO, T., S. AKIRA, T. TAGA & T. KISHIMOTO. 1990. Biological and clinical aspects of interleukin 6. Immunol. Today **11:** 443–449.
3. HEINRICH, P. C., J. V. CASTELL & T. ANDUS. 1990. Interleukin-6 and the acute phase proteins. Biochem. J. **265:** 621–636.
4. BAUMANN, H. & J. GAULDIE. 1990. Regulation of hepatic acute phase plasma protein genes by hepatocyte stimulating factors and other mediators of inflammation. Mol. Biol. Med. **7:** 147–159.
5. RICHARDS, C. D., J. GAULDIE & H. BAUMANN. 1991. Cytokine control of acute phase protein expression. Eur. Cyt. Net. **2:** 89–98.
6. RICHARDS, C. D., T. J. BROWN, M. SHOYAB, H. BAUMANN & J. GAULDIE. 1992. Recombinant oncostatin-M stimulates the production of acute phase proteins in hepatocytes in vitro. J. Immunol. **148:** 1731–1736.
7. CASTELL, J. V., T. ANDUS, D. KUNZ & P. C. HEINRICH. 1989. Interleukin-6: The major regulator of acute-phase protein synthesis in man and rat. Ann. N. Y. Acad. Sci. **557:** 86–101.
8. ROEMER, K. & T. FRIEDMANN. 1992. Concepts and strategies for human gene therapy. Eur. J. Biochem. **208:** 211–225.
9. TEPPER, R. I. & J. J. MULÉ. 1994. Experimental and clinical studies of cytokine gene-modified tumor cells. Human Gene Therapy **5:** 153–164.
10. HAWLEY, R. G., A. Z. C. FONG, B. F. BURNS & T. S. HAWLEY. 1992. Transplantable myeloproliferative disease induced in mice by an interleukin 6 retrovirus. J. Exp. Med. **176:** 1149.
11. GINSBERG, H. S. 1984. The Adenoviruses. New York: Plenum.
12. GRAHAM, F. L. & L. PREVEC. 1991. Manipulation of adenovirus vectors. In Methods in Molecular Biology. E. J. Murray, Ed.:109–128. Clifton, NJ: The Humana Press Inc.
13. NEMEROW, G. R., D. A. CHERESH & T. J. WICKHAM. 1994. Adenovirus entry into host cells: A role for α_v integrins. Trends Cell Biol. **4:** 52–55.
14. GRAHAM, F. L., S. SMILEY, W. C. RUSSEL & R. NAIRN. 1977. Characterization of a human cell line transformed by DNA from human adenovirus type 5. J. Gen. Virol. **36:** 59–72.
15. BRACIAK, T. A., S. K. MITTAL, F. L. GRAHAM, C. D. RICHARDS & J. GAULDIE. 1993. Construction of recombinant human type 5 adenoviruses expressing rodent IL-6 genes. An approach to investigate in vivo cytokine function. J. Immunol. **151:** 5145–5153.
16. ROSENFELD, M. A., W. SIEGFRIED, K. YOSHIMURA, K. YONEYAMA, M. FUKAYAMA, L. E. STIER, P. K. PÄÄKKÖ, P. GILARDI, L. D. STRATFORD-PERRICAUDET, M. PERRICAUDET, S. JALLAT, A. PAVIRANI, J. P. LECOCQ & R. G. CRYSTAL. 1991. Adenovirus-mediated transfer of a recombinant α1-antitrypsin gene to the lung epithelium in vivo. Science **252:** 431–434.
17. ROSENFELD, M. A., K. YOSHIMURA, B. C. TRAPNELL, K. YONEYAMA, E. R. ROSENTHAL, W. DALEMANS, M. FUKAYAMA, J. BARGON, L. E. STIER, L. STRATFORD-PERRICAUDET, M. PERRICAUDET, W. B. GUGGINO, A. PAVIRANI, J. P. LECOCQ & R. G. CRYSTAL. 1992. In vivo transfer of the human cystic fibrosis transmembrane conductance regulator gene to the airway epithelium. Cell **68:** 143–155.
18. BETT, A. J., L. PREVEC & F. L. GRAHAM. 1993. Packaging capacity and stability of human adenovirus type 5 vectors. J. Virol. **67:** 5911–5921.
19. JOHNSON, D. C. 1991. Adenovirus vectors as potential vaccines against herpes simplex virus. Rev. Infect. Dis. **13:** S912–S916.
20. PURI, R. K. & P. LELAND. 1992. Systemic administration of recombinant interleukin-6 in mice induces proliferation of lymphoid cells *in vivo*. Lymphokine Cytokine Res. **11:** 133–139.
21. MITTAL, S. K., M. R. MCDERMOTT, D. C. JOHNSON, L. PREVEC & F. L. GRAHAM. 1993. Monitoring foreign gene expression by a human adenovirus-based vector using the firefly luciferase gene as a reporter. Virus Res. **28:** 67–90.
22. MASTRANGELI, A., C. DANEL, M. A. ROSENFELD, L. STRATFORD-PERRICAUDET, M. PERRICAUDET, A. PAVIRANI, J. P. LECOCQ & R. G. CRYSTAL. 1993. Diversity of airway epithelial cell targets for in vivo recombinant adenovirus-mediated gene transfer. J. Clin. Invest. **91:** 225–234.
23. ROESSLER, B. J., E. D. ALLEN, J. M WILSON, J. W. HARTMAN & B. L. DAVIDSON. 1993.

Adenoviral-mediated gene transfer to rabbit synovium in vivo. J. Clin. Invest. **92:** 1085–1092.
24. XING, Z., T. BRACIAK, M. JORDANA, K. CROITORU, F. L. GRAHAM & J. GAULDIE. 1994. Adenovirus-mediated cytokine gene transfer at tissue sites: Overexpression of IL-6 induces lymphocytic hyperplasia in the lung. J. Immunol. **153:** 4059–4069.

DISCUSSION OF THE PAPER

J. WEBER (*Cancer Center, University of California, Irvine, Orange, CA*): When you infected mice or rats with the adenoviral IL-6 construct did you see severe liver toxicity? You have indicated that there was a high concentration of virus-derived IL-6 production in the liver. What did the livers look like?

C. RICHARDS: The livers appeared pretty much normal with the exception of a little bit of lymphocytic expansion at different sites. So, again, it reflected what we were seeing in the lung. At this point we have not had the opportunity to assess the nature of which cell phenotype they are. Again, the liver showed relatively unremarkable pathology with the exception of an infiltration of lymphocytes.

P. SEHGAL (*New York Medical College, Valhalla*): I would like to make one comment just to complete the picture The adenovirus type 5 model has been used by Harry Ginsburg to show the rapid appearance of pneumonia in mice. Adnovirus type 5 does not replicate in rats or mice, and yet when he instills 10^{10} pfu per mouse intranasally there is a very rapid (within 2 days) cellular infiltration and exudation into the alveoli. It is a self-resolving disease state. It turns out that the very first cytokine which shows up in this situation is IL-6. Within 6 hours of Ad-5 installation you can see IL-6 in the lung.

WEBER: When cystic fibrosis patients have been treated with Ad-5 vector which contains CFTR they also get a very unusual syndrome that is very similar to what you are describing—severe pneumonitis.

SEHGAL: Fascinating. In the case of rat or mouse there is self-limiting pneumonitis. IL-1 and TNF show up a little later; Harry Ginsburg has found that if he now injects a cocktail of antibodies to IL-1, TNF, and IL-6 he can partially inhibit the pneumonitis. Steroids will inhibit the pneumonitis very well. I am concerned a little bit about this. Although I realize that the pfu per animal that you are using is at least an order of magnitude lower, if not 2 orders of magnitude lower, than in Dr. Ginsburg's experiments, I wonder if it is simply the adenovirus itself triggering some of the histological damage that you see.

RICHARDS: Yes, I think that this is a concern, although with our control adenoviruses that have been utilizing other genes inserted exactly the same way, we do not produce the same effect. This suggests that it is due to the IL-6 expressed by the inserted gene.

M. KOPF (*Max-Planck-Institut für Immunobiologie, Freiburg, Germany*): Did you assess the cellular content in the splenomegaly?

RICHARDS: No, we have not assessed that, but just by looking histologically it appears like lymphoid aggregation. So at this time that's all I can tell you.

KOPF: So far you have not immunized mice to check on the immune responses?

RICHARDS: Well, we have looked at the immune responses and we were hoping that we could actually modulate the immune response to the adenovirus by adding IL-6 in order to see what it does to the immune system. I think what Todd Barciak in our lab has shown at this point in time is that after primary infections of AD-IL-6 viruses versus other viruses there is no real difference in the antibody titer, for example to various different adenovirus proteins. In secondary infection there seems to be a little more of an effect; in other words, there is a twofold or so enhancement of antiviral titer in adenovirus type 5 constructs containing the IL-6 gene versus constructs that did not contain the IL-6 gene.

J. ELIAS (*Yale University School of Medicine, New Haven, CT*): Two questions. This is very nice work. As I am sure you know, there is a rising school of thought that latent viral infection can be a cause of many of the chronic inflammatory disorders that you see in the lung, everything from various interstitial diseases to even asthma are being considered now. Adenovirus is one of the viruses that have been implicated. Have you run your model chronically without the IL-6 genes in it? Have you gone beyond the 12-week time point to see what the vector itself does in terms of chronic effects?

RICHARDS: Yes, such work has been done over the last 5–10 years in Frank Graham's lab, and what I can say is that the mouse and the rat are not permissive for replication of Ad-5 viruses and we do not really see any long-term expression of viral proteins or viral DNA products in the animals.

ELIAS: That is exactly what you see in latent viral infection. You would not see replication of complete virus. You need to look for pathology that appears later.

RICHARDS: We have not seen obvious pathology in the mouse and rat. In humans, I'm not sure. We have also done repeated infections as well, looking at the IL-6 responses. What happens if we reinfect after 2 weeks, 1 month, 2 months, or 4 months after initial infection is that we actually lose all the IL-6–induced responses because we in fact immunized animals against adenoviruses and they are capable of clearing their viruses much faster.

ELIAS: That leads to the second question which I wanted to ask you to comment on: what is the mechanism of diminution between 7 days and 12 days?

RICHARDS: All I can say is that it is probably due to virus clearance because if you in fact look at plaque-forming units harvested from the lungs of these animals at this particular point of time, they are much decreased.

Interleukin-6-Type Cytokines in Myeloproliferative Disease[a]

ROBERT G. HAWLEY

Division of Cancer Biology
Reichmann Research Building, S-218
Sunnybrook Health Science Centre
2075 Bayview Avenue
Toronto, Ontario, Canada M4N 3M5

Interleukin (IL)-6, leukemia inhibitory factor (LIF), oncostatin M (OSM), ciliary neurotrophic factor (CNTF) and IL-11 make up a family of cytokines whose cognate receptors share a common signal-transducing component termed gp130.[1,2] With the exception of CNTF, the actions of which appear to be largely restricted to neuronal cells, cytokines signaling through gp130 display overlapping biologic activities on a variety of embryonic and adult tissues, including cells at various stages of differentiation within the hematopoietic system. Accumulated data, based largely on mapping studies of blast cell colony formation by Ogawa and colleagues,[3] have indicated that IL-6, LIF and IL-11 are among the factors that trigger dormant hematopoietic progenitors into cell cycle. In this paper, the evidence implicating IL-6-type cytokines in abnormal hematopoiesis is reviewed with the focus on the clonal hemopathies, the group of hematopoietic stem cell disorders which includes acute myelogenous leukemia (AML) and the myelodysplastic syndromes (MDS).[4]

ACTIONS OF THE IL-6 FAMILY OF CYTOKINES ON LEUKEMIC CELL LINES

Interleukin-6

A growth promoting effect of IL-6 on a myeloid leukemic cell line was initially reported by Caracciolo et al.[5] who showed that AML-193 monoblastic leukemic cells which die within five days in the absence of granulocyte-macrophage colony-stimulating factor (GM-CSF) can be supported by IL-6 for at least fifteen days in serum-free medium. Subsequently, IL-6 was found to inhibit the growth of U937 histiocytic leukemic cells[6] while inducing moderate (15% to 20%) differentiation.[7] The combination of IL-6 with GM-CSF or IL-1α results in enhanced growth inhibition of U937 cells and synergistic augmentation of differentiation.[7,8] IL-6 also interacts synergistically with GM-CSF to reduce colony number and suppress the growth of clonogenic cells formed by HL60 promyelocytic leukemic cells,[8] and it reduces granulocyte-CSF (G-CSF)–supported proliferation and colony formation by a subclone of the OCI/AML-1 cell line derived from a patient with M4 AML.[9] In the murine system, IL-6 stimulates proliferation of the IL-3-dependent NFS-60 myeloid leukemic cell line.[10]

---

[a] This work was supported by grants from the National Cancer Institute of Canada and the Medical Research Council of Canada. R.G.H. is a Career Scientist of the Ontario Cancer Treatment and Research Foundation.

Conversely, IL-6 induces differentiation of the M1 myeloid leukemic cell line, being the factor previously named macrophage-granulocyte inducer type 2A.[11] IL-6 also induces differentiation of WEHI-3B D$^+$ myelomonocytic leukemia cells but unlike its action on M1 cells, IL-6 does not reduce either the number or size of WEHI-3B D$^+$ colonies.[10]

Leukemia Inhibitory Factor

Originally discovered as a differentiation-inducing factor for murine M1 leukemic cells distinct from IL-6, LIF suppresses colony formation by the clonogenic cells and induces differentiation into a more mature macrophage-like phenotype.[12-14] LIF when acting alone has no observable effects on HL60 or U937 cells but in combination with GM-CSF, G-CSF or IL-6 reduces their clonogenicity.[8,15] LIF increases the doubling time and decreases the proportion of clonogenic populations in the G-CSF-dependent OCI/AML-1 cell line and in another AML cell line, factor-independent OCI/AML-3.[16] Despite functioning as a growth inhibitor for the aforementioned leukemic cell lines, LIF supports the proliferation of the murine IL-3–dependent DA-1a leukemic cell line[17] and is able to enhance the clonogenicity of certain murine *myc*-transformed erythroleukemic cell lines.[18]

Oncostatin M

OSM is very similar to LIF in its actions on leukemic cell lines. It enhances the differentiation of U937 cells in the presence of GM-CSF,[19] and it inhibits the proliferation and induces the differentiation of M1 cells.[20] An explanation for shared activities of OSM and LIF is provided by the finding that OSM binds to the high-affinity LIF receptor.[21]

Interleukin-11

Several myeloid leukemic cell lines, including M07E, MV4-11 and AML-193, display enhanced rates of proliferation to GM-CSF or IL-3 in the presence of IL-11.[22] IL-11 by itself stimulates the growth of the megakaryoblastic cell lines, CMK and Meg-J. In the case of CMK cells, IL-11-induced proliferation can be suppressed with an anti-IL-11 antibody.[23] Moreover, because IL-11 mRNA is expressed in CMK and Meg-J cells, and the growth of both lines can be inhibited by IL-11 antisense oligonucleotides, the data support the notion that IL-11 functions as an autocrine growth factor for these leukemic cell lines. IL-11 also stimulates proliferation of the GM-CSF-dependent TF-1 erythroleukemic cell line.[24] Unlike IL-6, LIF and OSM, IL-11 does not exhibit differentiation-inducing activity for murine M1 leukemic cells (T. Hawley, unpublished observations).

EFFECTS OF IL-6/LIF/IL-11 ON LEUKEMIC BLAST CELL GROWTH

Interleukin-6

Hoang *et al.*[25] were the first to examine the effects of IL-6 on the clonogenic progenitors from AML patients. They found that IL-6 alone had relatively little ability to support the *in vitro* growth of AML blasts, but enhanced colony formation by the blast cells from three of five AML patients in the presence of GM-CSF or IL-3. In a subsequent survey of forty AML patients, Akashi *et al.*[26] showed that IL-6 by itself could stimulate blast colony formation in one case. When AML blast populations were classified according to expression of the CD34 cell surface molecule, an antigen present on hematopoietic stem cells and early hematopoietic progenitors, IL-6 was found to enhance blast colony formation supported by IL-3 in ten of twelve $CD34^+$ AML cases and by IL-4 in seven of nine $CD34^+$ AML cases. On the other hand, among $CD34^-$ AML samples, synergism of IL-6 with IL-3 and IL-4 was seen in only one of twelve cases and three of seven cases, respectively. The ability of IL-6 to augment colony formation promoted by IL-3 was observed when purified $CD34^+$ blasts were used, indicating that the effects could be ascribed to the direct action of IL-6 on leukemic progenitors. Since IL-6 did not shorten the time course for the emergence of blast colonies nor affect the dose-response curves of blast colonies induced by IL-3, these data were interpreted to indicate the presence of clonogenic cell populations requiring simultaneous stimulation by IL-6 plus either IL-3 or IL-4 for their growth.[27]

In contrast to these results, Suzuki *et al.*[9] reported that of sixteen AML samples tested, IL-6 alone was capable of stimulating blast colony formation in eight cases while enhancing G-CSF-dependent proliferation of blasts in two cases; conversely, spontaneous blast colony formation was suppressed by IL-6 in two samples and G-CSF-dependent colony formation was reduced in one instance. In a follow-up study, IL-6 was found to reduce maximum blast colony formation in response to the combination of GM-CSF, G-CSF, IL-1β, and IL-3 in nine of ten AML patients.[28] A suppressive effect of IL-6 was observed by Givon *et al.*[29] where the growth of peripheral blood mononuclear cells from twenty-two AML patients in short-term liquid cultures was found to be lower in the presence of the cytokine. In addition, IL-6 produced a decrease in the proportion of blasts with an increase in more mature myeloid elements in thirteen of eighteen AML cases. Synergism of IL-6 with GM-CSF in supporting colony formation was demonstrated, however, in three of eight AML cases tested in the blast colony assay.

Recently, Takanashi *et al.*,[30] using a serum-free culture system, reported that IL-6 alone stimulated colony growth in five of eleven AML cases. When IL-6 was added together with GM-CSF or IL-3, increased colony numbers were obtained in five and four of eleven cases, respectively. Only in two of five M2 AML cases where there was spontaneous colony formation were the number of colonies reduced by addition of IL-6. Contrary to the findings of Givon *et al.*,[29] no alteration of cellular phenotype or morphology was observed, indicating that IL-6 did not suppress growth by inducing differentiation in these instances. While the reasons for the discrepancies among the various studies may be related in part to differences in isolation procedures, purity of the blast populations or the assay conditions employed, collectively, the findings demonstrate a marked heterogeneity in the IL-6 responsiveness of primary leukemic blast cells from AML patients.

Leukemia Inhibitory Factor

Takanashi *et al.*[30] also examined the effects of LIF on AML progenitors in the blast colony assay using their serum-free culture conditions. LIF by itself was found to weakly stimulate colony growth in two of eleven cases and to produce a significant increase in colony numbers in three, six and seven of eleven cases when added together with GM-CSF, IL-3 or IL-6, respectively. No differences were seen in the percentage of cells positive for various cell surface molecules examined or with regards myeloperoxidase expression, nor was there any alteration in cellular morphology before and after culture with LIF compared to culture without the cytokine. An earlier report had noted a variable response to LIF, ranging from inhibition to stimulation, when blasts from three of six AML patients were tested for colony formation or growth in liquid cultures.[16] The data of Takanashi et al.,[30] revealing a marked stimulatory activity of LIF on the growth of primary leukemic blasts contrasts sharply with its growth-inhibitory and differentiation-inducing effects on the majority of human and murine leukemic cell lines.[8,12-16] These disparate findings serve as a reminder that caution needs to be exercised when extrapolating results obtained with leukemic cell lines to primary leukemic populations. Another intriguing observation made in this study is an apparent synergy between LIF and IL-6; both cytokines might have been predicted to trigger the same signal transduction pathway.[31]

Interleukin 11

Hu et al.[22] showed that IL-11 alone had no effect when tested on AML blasts; however, addition of IL-11 to GM-CSF-containing or IL-3-containing cultures resulted in a 2- to 4-fold increase in colony count in thirteen of fourteen AML cases. In seven samples, assayed under serum-free conditions, the results were essentially the same as those obtained from serum-containing cultures. IL-11 was demonstrated to enhance IL-3–supported colony formation by CD34+ blasts purified from leukemic cells of one AML patient, ruling out indirect mechanisms of action. Thymidine suicide experiments using leukemic populations from two AML patients revealed that a significant fraction of the blast cells were in S-phase when exposed for sixteen hours to IL-3 and the proportion was increased in response to IL-11. These investigators further demonstrated that increased cycling of blast cells and enhanced colony formation were similarly induced by either IL-11 or IL-6 in combination with IL-3 whereas no additional improvement was obtained by combining all three cytokines. Considered together, the results argue that there are certain AML blasts for which IL-11 can enhance proliferation through a pathway shared by IL-6 and the effects are direct and not mediated by accessory cells or factors in the serum.

MECHANISMS OF IL-6/LIF/OSM/IL-11 EXPRESSION AND ACTION IN AML

Interleukin 6

The responsiveness of both primary blast cells and established cell lines from AML populations to IL-6, LIF (OSM) and IL-11 raises the question as to whether any of these cytokines might be involved in paracrine or autocrine leukemic growth control in patients.[32-36] Inspection of AML samples by Oster et al.[34] revealed that enriched blast cells of 14 of 54 cases cultured *in vitro* for 24 to 72 hours produced IL-6 that was detectable at the RNA level by Northern blot analysis and at the protein level by bioassay. Five of the 14 leukemias also expressed IL-1β and tumor necrosis factor-α (TNFα). Except for four cases of AML that expressed only IL-6, the remaining samples coexpressed two or more of GM-CSF, G-CSF and macrophage-CSF (M-CSF). None of the AML specimens that expressed IL-6 and failed to produce CSFs was able to spontaneously form colonies in methylcellulose whereas AML samples that showed production of IL-6 and CSFs grew autonomously. In four other AML samples displaying autonomous *in vitro* colony formation but failing to produce IL-6, addition of IL-6 to the cultures augmented colony growth. Van der Schoot et al.[37] similarly screened leukemic cells from thirty patients with AML for ability to produce

IL-6. After eighteen hours of culture, IL-6 production could be detected by bioassay in twelve of fifteen AML samples with monocytic differentiation (M4 and M5 subtypes) but not in cases of undifferentiated subtypes (none of 15 M1 and M2 patients). In every case, IL-6 production was paralleled by IL-1 production, with the IL-1– and IL-6–producing cells found mainly in the more mature monocytic cell fractions, defined as $CD34^-$ $CD14^+$ adherent cells. Notably, when expression of IL-6 was examined in leukemic blast populations prior to their introduction into culture, it could not be not detected. On the other hand, Fiedler et al.[38] isolated peripheral blood mononuclear cells containing at least 90% myeloblasts from AML patients by density gradient centrifugation and detected de novo expression of IL-6 mRNA by Northern blot analysis in eight of eleven cases. Using an enzyme-linked immunosorbent assay for IL-6, Beauchemin et al.[39] observed IL-6 production in culture supernatants of 11 of 21 AML samples after a 24-hour in vitro incubation period. IL-6 levels were comparable regardless of whether the leukemic populations were cultured in serum-supplemented or serum-free medium. The results differ slightly from those of van der Schoot et al.[37] in that no obvious correlation between IL-6 expression and AML subtype was observed. A correlation was found, however, between the levels of IL-6 produced and the levels of IL-1β produced. Moreover, in 10 of 16 samples, exposure to exogenous IL-1α caused an increase in IL-6 production while neutralization of the endogenous source of IL-1β with anti-IL-1 antibody resulted in a decrease in IL-6 production in six of six AML blast populations. In one AML sample which coproduced GM-CSF, antibody-mediated neutralization of the endogenous source of IL-1β reduced the level of GM-CSF mRNA below detection by Northern blot analysis whereas the level of IL-6 mRNA was diminished but IL-6 mRNA sequences were still readily detectable. Further testing revealed that neutralization of the endogenous source of IL-6 with an anti-IL-6 antibody caused a reduction in clonogenic cells in five of seven AML samples tested whereas addition of IL-6 to two AML samples resulted in enhancement of GM-CSF or IL-3–supported colony formation. No effect on cell proliferation was observed upon exposure of the cells to anti-IL-6, suggesting that such endogenously produced IL-6 was not sufficient per se to maintain clonogenic blasts in cycle. Recently, Ferrari et al.[40] obtained blast populations by density gradient centrifugation and negative selection with a mixture of antibodies against CD2 and CD19 (lymphocytes) and CD14 (monocytes) from six patients with AML of M1–M4 subtypes and examined expression of IL-6 mRNA and IL-6 receptor mRNA by reverse-transcriptase polymerase chain reaction. In all six cases studied, IL-6 receptor mRNA could be detected but IL-6 mRNA could only be detected in blasts from one case of M2 AML and in leukemic monocytes from a patient with M5 AML. All samples coexpressed mRNA encoding receptors for IL-1, IL-3 and steel factor (SF, c-kit ligand) as well as mRNA for SF. Together, the data argue that IL-6 can function as a survival factor for certain leukemic blasts;[41] indirect evidence in support of this hypothesis comes from studies of the murine M1 myeloid leukemic cell line, where inhibition of programmed cell death by IL-6, first described by Sabourin and Hawley[42] for B9 hybridoma/plasmacytoma cells, is observed for cells induced to lose viability by an apoptotic stimulus.[43,44] The combined results implicate paracrine mechanisms of IL-6 growth stimulation in AML, with a possible source of IL-6 being "differentiated" monocytic elements in M4 and M5 AML subtypes. Whether autogenous production of IL-6 by AML blasts is truly constitutive in some instances, in addition to being secondarily upregulated by IL-1 or as a consequence of in vitro manipulation of the leukemic cell populations,[45] remains a point of contention. Nonetheless, it is clear that a proportion of AML cells are capable of producing IL-6, and thus the participation of autocrine IL-6 stimulatory mechanisms in AML cannot be ruled out.

Leukemia Inhibitory Factor, Oncostatin M and Interleukin-11

Whether these IL-6-type cytokines are aberrantly produced in leukemic states is not known yet. In a recent study of 59 adherent layer cultures derived from patients with AML, MDS (described below) and other hematologic diseases, Wetzler et al.[46] demonstrated that biologically active LIF is produced by bone marrow stromal cells from all of the studied subjects. LIF levels in conditioned media from adherent layers were elevated in samples from patients with a spectrum of hematological neoplasms, including AML (median level, 3.0 ng/ml; range, 1.6–11.0 ng/ml) and MDS (median level, 4.5 ng/ml; range 1.4–15.5 ng/ml) as compared to samples from normal individuals (median level, 2.0 ng/ml; range, 0.7–4.6 ng/ml). OSM was originally identified as a factor produced by differentiated U937 histiocytic leukemic cells,[47] so it is not inconceivable that it might be expressed in certain cases of M4 and M5 AML. With regards IL-11 production, undifferentiated U937 cells, HL60 promyelocytic leukemic cells and K562 erythroleukemic cells all express IL-11 transcripts[23] although no information is available as to whether such expression occurs in primary AML cells.

INVOLVEMENT OF IL-6 IN MYELODYSPLASTIC SYNDROMES

MDS comprises a group of acquired disorders which are characterized by clonal, dysplastic growth of hematopoietic progenitors resulting in a varying degree of anemia, leukopenia and/or thrombocytopenia. Five classes of MDS have been described, namely refractory anemia (RA), RA with ring sideroblasts (RARS), RA with excess of blasts (RAEB), RA with excess of blasts in transformation (RAEBt), and chronic myelomonocytic leukemia (CMML).[4] CMML, characterized by monocytosis with greater than 20% bone marrow blast cells and lack of the Philadelphia chromosome of chronic myelogenous leukemia (CML), has a progression rate to AML of 30% to 40%. In contrast to the majority of AML blast cells which are routinely dependent on an exogenous source of factors for colony growth, spontaneous colony formation by the mononuclear cells from patients with CMML is frequently observed. In a survey of seven CMML patients, three AML patients and eight CML patients by Everson et al.,[48] 24-hour supernatants of T-cell–depleted mononuclear cells from all patients with CMML, but not AML or CML samples, or normal monocytes, contained substantial levels of IL-6. Conditioned medium from two of five CMML samples also contained GM-CSF. Spontaneous CMML colony formation could be partially inhibited by antibodies to GM-CSF or IL-6 in three cases studied whereas combination of these antibodies gave nearly complete (>93%) inhibition of spontaneous colony formation. Examination of fresh, uncultured CMML cells from one patient revealed constitutive GM-CSF expression but no detectable IL-6, implying that IL-6 production observed in the other samples might have been induced *in vitro*. Schipperus et al.[49] investigated the effects of IL-6 in combination with GM-CSF on colony formation of myeloid progenitors from eighteen patients with MDS (two RA, two RARS, seven RAEB, four RAEBt and three CMML) and five patients with leukemic transformation of MDS. IL-6 alone did not have colony-stimulating activity but an enhancing effect of IL-6 with GM-CSF was observed in 20 of 23 cases in all subtypes of MDS; in cases of reduced GM-CSF response, IL-6 was unable to increase colony numbers to normal values. In a survey of 45 patients with MDS, Herold et al.[50] found serum concentrations of IL-6 to range from undetectable to 150 pg/ml, with median and mean concentrations of 9 and 15 pg/ml, respectively. Elevated IL-6 concentrations were measured in 9 of 15 patients with RA, 11 of 17 patients with

RAEB, 7 of 7 patients with RAEBt and 5 of 6 patients with CMML. By comparison, no IL-6 could be detected in the serum of 20 healthy subjects tested. None of the MDS patients had shown any sign of infectious disease or other diseases associated with an acute-phase reaction, suggesting that elevated *in vivo* IL-6 levels are primarily MDS-associated. No correlation between IL-6 concentration and monocyte count was found in peripheral blood, arguing that elevated IL-6 levels in MDS patients are not simply caused by increased numbers of monocytes. The combined data implicate IL-6, possibly originating from aberrantly activated mononuclear cells, as a contributory factor in the *in vivo* proliferation of MDS progenitors.

ASSOCIATION OF IL-6 EXPRESSION WITH N-*RAS* GENE ACTIVATION

Mutated N-*ras* genes are the most commonly observed molecular alteration in AML, with the reported incidence ranging from 15% to 30%.[51] A high frequency (~40%) of N-*ras* gene involvement is also seen in MDS, with the highest incidence found in CMML cases that may evolve into AML.[52,53] An association between the expression of IL-6 by leukemic blast cells from AML patients and the presence of activating point mutations in the N-*ras* gene was first observed by Lübbert *et al.*[54] who analyzed leukemic cells from fifty AML patients using PCR and differential oligonucleotide hybridization. Clonal activation of N-*ras*, noted in the large majority of leukemic cells of six patients, was significantly correlated ($p = 0.0003$) with the ability of the cells to express IL-6 but not five other cytokines examined, including GM-CSF, G-CSF, M-CSF, IL-1β and TNFα, which were expressed with varying frequency in the AML cells. Oncogenic *ras* triggers an intracellular signal transduction pathway that results in the constitutive activation of transcription factors.[55,56] The promoter of the IL-6 gene contains several *cis*-acting elements that confer transcriptional inducibility by the factors AP-1, NF-IL6 and NF-κB.[57-59] Of these, *ras*-transformed cells have high activity of the AP-1 transcription factor complex, which can include hetero- and homodimers of proteins from the Fos and Jun families;[60,61] the transcriptional activity of NF-IL6 is also stimulated by activated *ras*.[2,62] Since the regulatory regions of the G-CSF, IL-1β and TNFα genes also contain NF-IL6-binding motifs,[63] it is unclear whether the selective expression of IL-6 in leukemic blasts harboring N-*ras* mutations would involve this factor. A recent report by Hsu *et al.*[64] showing that NF-IL6 can bind to AP-1 sites and that its binding affinity for NF-IL6 sites can be modulated through interaction with AP-1 family proteins suggests a mechanism by which promoter specificity might be conferred. Demetri *et al.*[65] directly tested the hypothesis that mutations in *ras* genes might contribute to constitutive expression of IL-6 and other cytokines. Human mesothelioma cells transfected with a mutated N-*ras* gene exhibited elevated IL-6 mRNA levels compared with controls. Upregulation of IL-6 in this experimental system was mediated predominantly by a post-transcriptional mechanism that resulted in increased stability of IL-6 mRNA transcripts.[66,67] Treatment of *ras*-transfectants with anti-IL-1 neutralizing antibody did not block IL-6 production, suggesting that the elevation in steady-state IL-6 mRNA levels was not a secondary event due to the enhanced expression of IL-1β that was also observed. These findings are sufficiently intriguing to encourage further investigations seeking to clarify the relationship between activated *ras* and IL-6 expression in AML and CMML.

IL-6-TYPE CYTOKINES AND MYELOPROLIFERATIVE DISEASE MODELS

Bone Marrow Chimera Models of IL-6 and IL-11 Excess

In the avian system, autocrine production of chicken myelomonocytic growth factor, a cytokine distantly related to IL-6, is a key step in induction of myeloid leukemia by the v-*myb* gene.[68] To investigate the effects of constitutive production of IL-6 by normal hematopoietic progenitors in a mammalian system, we engrafted lethally irradiated mice with bone marrow cells that had been infected *ex vivo* with a replication-defective recombinant retrovirus carrying an IL-6 gene.[69,70] Transplanted animals developed high circulating levels of IL-6 (7–130 ng/ml). Dysregulated synthesis of IL-6 provoked a myeloproliferative disease characterized by dramatically elevated peripheral neutrophil counts (up to 400×10^3 cells/mm^3) and enhanced splenic granulocyte-macrophage progenitor numbers (>60-fold increase). Eleven of 20 primary recipients died within 4 weeks of transplantation with massive splenomegaly (5- to 10-fold enlargement) and extensive neutrophil infiltration of the lungs and liver. All lethally irradiated secondary hosts receiving bone marrow from surviving primary animals presented with the myeloproliferative syndrome three to four weeks after transplant. By repeated serial transplantation, nine separate pedigrees comprising 43 animals were established. In the longest documented case, the progeny of a single retrovirally marked progenitor cell transferred the myeloproliferative disease to two secondary, four tertiary, and two quaternary recipients (for a total of 72 weeks). Spontaneous colony formation by granulocyte-macrophage progenitors in bone marrow and spleens of affected mice was observed. When pools of colonies were transferred to liquid culture, macrophage-like cells could be propagated for several weeks but permanent cell lines could not be established. No tumors formed when infected spleen cells were injected subcutaneously into sublethally irradiated syngeneic mice. Excessive IL-6 stimulation thus resulted in the development of a fatal yet nonneoplastic proliferative disorder, possibly involving committed myeloid progenitors with extensive self-renewal capacity.[71]

IL-6 transgenic mice of the same genetic background having lower serum IL-6 levels (0.1–5 ng/ml) survive for longer periods of time, allowing for the sporadic development of plasmacytomas with c-*myc* gene rearrangements.[72] Therefore, with the goal of assessing myeloid leukemia incidence in mice chronically exposed to low amounts of IL-6, we attempted to diminish the levels of circulating IL-6 achieved in bone marrow transplant recipients. A modified IL-6 gene was constructed containing the sequence Lys-Asp-Glu-Leu (KDEL) at its carboxy terminus for preferential intracellular accumulation of IL-6 within the endoplasmic reticulum or Golgi apparatus.[73] Although target cells infected with a recombinant retrovirus carrying the KDEL-modified IL-6 gene (IL-6-KDEL) were shown by bioassay to retain large amounts of IL-6 intracellularly, IL-6-KDEL expression by genetically modified bone marrow cells in engrafted mice evoked the fatal myeloproliferative syndrome with similar potency as wild-type IL-6.[1] In related studies, we introduced a *ras*-containing retroviral vector into hematopoietic progenitors in order to test the hypothesis that *ras* mutation can be an initiating event in myeloid leukemia. A marked leukocytosis was observed in the peripheral blood of lethally irradiated mice 4 to 8 weeks after engraftment with bone marrow cells constitutively expressing the v-H-*ras* gene. However, no myeloid malignancies were induced in any of 23 primary or secondary recipients. Instead, all of the mice developed precursor T- and B-cell acute lymphoblastic leukemia/lymphoma within 8 to 12 weeks of transplantation (Hawley *et al.*, manuscript submitted). Vector-directed expression of activated *ras* in myeloid progenitors promoted the formation of large macrophage colonies in day five methylcellulose cultures but continuous lines of more immature myeloid cells could only be established when large cell populations were infected. The data suggest that activated *ras* stimulates proliferation of myeloid progenitors without impeding terminal maturation and that secondary mutations blocking differentiation are necessary for neoplastic conversion to frank leukemia.[74,75] The cell lines derived should prove useful for investigation of the mechanisms controlling IL-6 production in myeloid cells harboring activated *ras* genes.

We have also used retroviral gene delivery to examine the consequences of enforced expression of IL-11 in the reconstituted hematopoietic systems of lethally irradiated mice.[76] High concentrations of IL-11 (>40 ng/ml) were detected in the plasma of all recipients receiving infected bone marrow cells. Despite the abnormally high plasma IL-11 levels, none of the mice (including 10 primary and 18 secondary recipients) died during the observation period (4 to 17 weeks). Chronic IL-11 exposure induced a 20- to 100-fold elevation in myeloid progenitor cell content and a two-fold enlargement of the spleen. Blood cell values in the majority of the mice remained within normal range except for a reproducible neutrophilic shift in the differential and a sustained rise in platelet counts (1.5-fold). The exceptions were two members of one transplant pedigree that presented with myeloid leukemia during the secondary transplant phase. A clonal origin of the disease was determined, with significant expansion of the marked clone, not overtly malignant at that time, having occurred in the spleen of the primary host. Bone marrow and spleen cells from the affected secondaries were leukemogenic within four weeks of transplant into sublethally irradiated tertiary recipients. Efforts to establish factor-dependent or autonomously growing cell lines in liquid culture from spleen cells of the tertiary animals were unsuccessful. Culturing of leukemic spleen cells from a quaternary recipient led to the establishment of an IL-11–producing yet IL-3–dependent myeloid progenitor cell line (PGMD1) that can be induced to differentiate into granulocytes and/or macrophages by GM-CSF and G-CSF. The PGMD1 cell line is leukemogenic when injected into sublethally irradiated syngeneic mice, with four of five mice developing myeloid leukemia, in one experiment, within six months of receiving an intravenous inoculum. The inability of autogenously produced IL-11 to support factor-independent growth of PGMD1 cells precludes a mechanism of transformation involving a classical autocrine loop;[23,77,78] indeed, it has not been demonstrated that the IL-11 synthesized by the leukemic cells is providing a growth stimulatory effect.[22–24] In any event, the results obtained in this experimental system would predict that abnormal IL-11 expression in human myeloid progenitors[23] could potentially contribute to leukemogenesis by expanding the target population at risk for transformation.

Cell Line Engraftment Model of LIF Excess

Metcalf and Gearing[79,80] examined the *in vivo* hematopoietic consequences of LIF by engrafting sublethally irradiated or unirradiated mice with the FDC-P1 myeloid cell line engineered to express this cytokine. The mice had high serum LIF levels (mean, 1270 units/ml) and developed a neutrophilic leukocytosis with extramedullary hematopoiesis in the spleen and liver. All became moribund with a myelosclerotic syndrome within twelve to seventy days of injection. When high doses of recombinant LIF (2 μg, three times daily for two weeks) were injected into mice, an elevation in myeloid progenitor numbers was observed in the spleen but the neutrophilia was not reproduced,[81] indicating that the latter phenomenon was probably not a direct effect of LIF.

CONCLUDING REMARKS

The message that emerges from studies of laboratory models and primary patient material is that IL-6-type cytokines can have opposing effects on myeloid leukemic cells. This is perhaps not surprising considering the spectrum of activities displayed by these factors on normal hematopoietic cells and the fact that AML is a heterogeneous group of malignancies with different etiology. However, there is considerable evidence implicating IL-6 as a synergistic factor supporting the *in vivo* growth of some AML blasts. With regards an "autocrine" mechanism of IL-6 action in leukemic growth control, it is important to bear in mind that only a minor proportion of AML blasts are self-renewing while the majority of the mononuclear cells are nonproliferating; whether the former population is a source of self-stimulatory IL-6 in certain instances has not been conclusively demonstrated. Regardless of the situation, it would be interesting to know what percentage of IL-6-producing leukemic cells carry N-*ras* mutations.

REFERENCES

1. HAWLEY, R. G. 1994. Hematopathology of interleukin 6-type cytokines. Stem Cells **12**(Suppl. 1): 155–171.
2. KISHIMOTO, T., T. TAGA & S. AKIRA. 1994. Cytokine signal transduction. Cell **76**: 253–262.
3. OGAWA, M. 1993. Differentiation and proliferation of hematopoietic stem cells. Blood **81**: 2844–2853.
4. WILLIAMS, W. J., E. BEUTLER, A. ERSLEV & M. A. LICHTMAN, Eds. 1990. Hematology, 4th edit. New York: McGraw-Hill.
5. CARACCIOLO, D., S. C. CLARK & G. ROVERA. 1989. Human interleukin-6 supports granulocytic differentiation of hematopoietic progenitor cells and acts synergistically with GM-CSF. Blood **73**: 666–670.
6. CHEN, L., Y. MORY, A. ZILBERSTEIN & M. REVEL. 1988. Growth inhibition of human breast carcinoma and leukemia/lymphoma cell lines by recombinant interferon-β_2. Proc. Natl. Acad. Sci. USA **85**: 8037–8041.
7. ONOZAKI, K., Y. AKIYAMA, A. OKANO, T. HIRANO, T. KISHIMOTO, T. HASHIMOTO, K. YOSHIZAWA & T. TANIYAMA. 1989. Synergistic regulatory effects of interleukin 6 and interleukin 1 on the growth and differentiation of human and mouse myeloid leukemic cell lines. Cancer Res. **49**: 3602–3607.
8. MAEKAWA, T., D. METCALF & D. P. GEARING. 1990. Enhanced suppression of human myeloid leukemic cell lines by combinations of IL-6, LIF, GM-CSF and G-CSF. Int. J. Cancer **45**: 353–358.
9. SUZUKI, T., T. MORIO, S. TOHDA, K. NAGATA, Y. YAMASHITA, Y. IMAI, N. AOKI, K. HIRASHIMA & N. NARA. 1990. Effects of interleukin-6 and granulocyte colony-stimulating factor on the proliferation of leukemic blast progenitors from acute myeloblastic leukemia patients. Jpn. J. Cancer Res. **81**: 979–986.
10. METCALF, D. 1989. Actions and interactions of G-CSF, LIF and IL-6 on normal and leukemic murine cells. Leukemia **3**: 349–355.
11. SHABO, Y., J. LOTEM, M. RUBINSTEIN, M. REVEL, S. C. CLARK, S. F. WOLF, R. KAMEN & L. SACHS. 1988. The myeloid blood cell differentiation-inducing protein MGI-2A is interleukin-6. Blood **72**: 2070–2073.
12. LIPTON, J. H. & L. SACHS. 1981. Characterization of macrophage- and granulocyte-inducing proteins for normal and leukemic myeloid cells produced by the Krebs ascites tumor. Biochim. Biophys. Acta **673**: 552–569.
13. TOMIDA, M., Y. YAMAMOTO-YAMAGUCHI & M. HOZUMI. 1984. Purification of a factor inducing differentiation of mouse myeloid leukemic M1 cells from conditioned medium of mouse fibroblast L929 cells. J. Biol. Chem. **259**: 10978–10982.

14. HILTON, D. J., N. A. NICOLA & D. METCALF. 1988. Purification of a murine leukemia inhibitory factor from Krebs ascites cells. Anal. Biochem. **173:** 359–367.
15. MAEKAWA, T. & D. METCALF. 1989. Clonal suppression of HL60 and U937 cells by recombinant human leukemia inhibitory factor in combination with GM-CSF or G-CSF. Leukemia **3:** 270–276.
16. WANG, C., M. LISHNER, M. D. MINDEN & E. A. MCCULLOCH. 1990. The effects of leukemia inhibitory factor (LIF) on the blast stem cells of acute myeloblastic leukemia. Leukemia **4:** 548–552.
17. MOREAU, J.-F., D. D. DONALDSON, F. BENNETT, J. WITEK-GIANNOTTI, S. C. CLARK & G. G. WONG. 1988. Leukaemia inhibitory factor is identical to the myeloid growth factor human interleukin for DA cells. Nature **336:** 690–692.
18. CORY, S., T. MAEKAWA, J. MCNEALL & D. METCALF. 1991. Murine erythroid cell lines derived with c-*myc* retroviruses respond to leukemia-inhibitory factor, erythropoietin, and interleukin 3. Cell Growth Diff. **2:** 165–172.
19. BRUCE, A. G., I. H. HOGGATT & T. M. ROSE. 1992. Oncostatin M is a differentiation factor for myeloid leukemia cells. J. Immunol. **149:** 1271–1275.
20. ROSE, T. M. & A. G. BRUCE. 1991. Oncostatin M is a member of a cytokine family that includes leukemia-inhibitory factor, granulocyte colony-stimulating factor, and interleukin 6. Proc. Natl. Acad. Sci. USA **88:** 8641–8645.
21. GEARING, D. P., M. R. COMEAU, D. J. FRIEND, S. D. GIMPEL, C. J. THUT, J. MCGOURTY, K. K. BRASHER, J. A. KING, S. GILLIS, B. MOSLEY, S. F. ZIEGLER & D. COSMAN. 1992. The IL-6 signal transducer, gp130: An oncostatin M receptor and affinity converter for the LIF receptor. Science **255:** 1434–1437.
22. HU, J. P., A. CESANO, D. SANTOLI, S. C. CLARK & T. HOANG. 1993. Effects of interleukin-11 on the proliferation and cell cycle status of myeloid leukemia cells. Blood **81:** 1586–1592.
23. KOBAYASHI, S., M. TERAMURA, I. SUGAWARA, K. OSHIMI & H. MIZOGUCHI. 1993. Interleukin-11 acts as an autocrine growth factor for human megakaryoblastic cell lines. Blood **81:** 889–893.
24. YIN, T., T. TAGA, M. L.-S. TSANG, K. YASUKAWA, T. KISHIMOTO & Y.-C. YANG. 1993. Involvement of IL-6 signal transducer gp130 in IL-11-mediated signal transduction. J. Immunol. **151:** 2555–2561.
25. HOANG, T., A. HAMAN, O. GONCALVES, G. G. WONG & S. C. CLARK. 1988. Interleukin-6 enhances growth factor-dependent proliferation of the blast cells of acute myeloblastic leukemia. Blood **72:** 823–826.
26. AKASHI, K., M. HARADA, T. SHIBUYA, T. ETO, Y. TAKAMATSU, T. TESHIMA & Y. NIHO. 1991. Effects of interleukin-4 and interleukin-6 on the proliferation of $CD34^+$ and $CD34^-$ blasts from acute myelogenous leukemia. Blood **78:** 197–204.
27. METCALF, D. 1993. Hematopoietic regulators: Redundancy or subtlety? Blood **82:** 3515–3523.
28. SUZUKI, T., M. BESSHO, K. HIRASHMA, S. TOHDA, K. NAGATA, Y. IMAI & N. NARA. 1992. Interleukin-6 reduces the optimal growth *in vitro* of leukemic blast progenitors from acute myeloblastic leukemia patients. Acta Haematol. **87:** 63–68.
29. GIVON, T., S. SLAVIN, N. HARAN-GHERA, R. MICHALEVICZ & M. REVEL. 1992. Antitumor effects of human recombinant interleukin-6 on acute myeloid leukemia in mice and in cell cultures. Blood **79:** 2392–2398.
30. TAKANASHI, M., T. MOTOJI, M. MASUDA, K. OSHIMI & H. MIZOGUCHI. 1993. The effects of leukemia inhibitory factor and interleukin 6 on the growth of acute myeloid leukemic cells. Leukemia Res. **17:** 217–222.
31. BOULTON, T. G., N. STAHL & G. D. YANCOPOULOS. 1994. Ciliary neurotrophic factor/leukemia inhibitory factor/interleukin 6/oncostatin M family of cytokines induces tyrosine phosphorylation of a common set of proteins overlapping those induced by other cytokines and growth factors. J. Biol. Chem. **269:** 11648–11655.
32. METCALF, D. 1989. The roles of stem cell self-renewal and autocrine growth factor production in the biology of myeloid leukemia. Cancer Res. **49:** 2305–2311.
33. DELWEL, R., C. VAN BUITENEN, M. SALEM, F. BOT, S. GILLIS, K. KAUSHANSKY, B. ALTROCK & B. LOWENBERG. 1989. Interleukin-1 stimulates proliferation of acute myelo-

blastic leukemia cells by induction of granulocyte-macrophage colony-stimulating factor release. Blood **74:** 586–593.
34. OSTER, W., N. A. CICCO, H. KLEIN, T. HIRANO, T. KISHIMOTO, A. LINDEMANN, R. H. MERTELSMANN & F. HERRMANN. 1989. Participation of the cytokines interleukin 6, tumor necrosis factor-α, and interleukin 1β secreted by acute myelogenous leukemia blasts in autocrine and paracrine leukemia growth control. J. Clin. Invest. **84:** 451–457.
35. HAEGEMAN, G., J. CONTENT, G. VOLCKAERT, R. DERYNCK, J. TAVERNIER & W. FIERS. 1986. Structural analysis of the sequence coding for an inducible 26-kDa protein in human fibroblasts. Eur. J. Biochem. **159:** 625–632.
36. JIRIK, F. R., T. J. PODOR, T. HIRANO, T. KISHIMOTO, D. J. LOSKUTOFF, D. A. CARSON & M. LOTZ. 1989. Bacterial lipopolysaccharide and inflammatory mediators augment IL-6 secretion by human endothelial cells. J. Immunol. **142:** 144–147.
37. VAN DER SCHOOT, C. E., P. JANSEN, M. POORTER, M. R. WESTER, A. E. G. K. VON DEM BORNE, L. A. AARDEN & R. H. J. VAN OERS. 1989. Interleukin-6 and interleukin-1 production in acute leukemia with monocytoid differentiation. Blood **74:** 2081–2087.
38. FIEDLER, W., E. SUCIU, C. WITTLIEF, W. OSTERTAG & D. K. HOSSFELD. 1990. Mechanisms of growth factor expression in acute myeloid leukemia (AML). Leukemia **4:** 459–461.
39. BEAUCHEMIN, V., L. VILLENEUVE, J. C. RODRIGUEZ-CIMADEVILLA, D. RAJOTTE, J. S. KENNEY, S. C. CLARK & T. HOANG. 1991. Interleukin-6 production by the blast cells of acute myeloblastic leukemia: Regulation by endogenous interleukin-1 and biological implications. J. Cell. Physiol. **148:** 353–361.
40. FERRARI, S., A. GRANDE, R. MANFREDINI, E. TAGLIAFICO, P. ZUCCHINI, G. TORELLI & U. TORELLI. 1993. Expression of interleukins 1, 3, 6, stem cell factor and their receptors in acute leukemia blast cells and in normal peripheral lymphocytes and monocytes. Eur. J. Haematol. **50:** 141–148.
41. SACHS, L. & J. LOTEM. 1993. Control of programmed cell death in normal and leukemic cells: New implications for therapy. Blood **82:** 15–21.
42. SABOURIN, L. A. & R. G. HAWLEY. 1990. Suppression of programmed death and G_1 arrest in B-cell hybridomas by interleukin-6 is not accompanied by altered expression of immediate early response genes. J. Cell. Physiol. **145:** 564–574.
43. YONISH-ROUACH, D., D. RESNITZKY, J. LOTEM, L. SACHS, A. KIMCHI & M. OREN. 1991. Wild-type p53 induces apoptosis of myeloid leukaemic cells that is inhibited by interleukin-6. Nature **352:** 345–347.
44. HOFFMAN, B. & D. A. LIEBERMANN. 1994. Molecular controls of apoptosis: Differentiation/growth arrest primary response genes, proto-oncogenes, and tumor suppressor genes as positive and negative modulators. Oncogene **9:** 1807–1812.
45. KAUFMAN, D. C., M. R. BAER, X. Z. GAO, Z. WANG & H. D. PREISLER. 1988. Enhanced expression of the granulocyte-macrophage colony stimulating factor gene in acute myelocytic leukemia cells following *in vitro* blast cell enrichment. Blood **72:** 1329–1332.
46. WETZLER, M., Z. ESTROV, M. TALPAZ, K. J. KIM & M. ALPHONSO, R. SRINIVASAN & R. KURZROCK. 1994. Leukemia inhibitory factor in long-term adherent layer cultures: Increased levels of bioactive protein in leukemia and modulation by IL-4, IL-1β, and TNF-α. Cancer Res. **54:** 1837–1842.
47. ZARLING, J. M., M. SHOYAB, H. MARQUARDT, M. B. HANSON, M. N. LIOUBIN & G. J. TODARO. 1986. Oncostatin M: A growth regulator produced by differentiated histiocytic lymphoma cells. Proc. Natl. Acad. Sci. USA **83:** 9739–9743.
48. EVERSON, M. P., C. B. BROWN & M. B. LILLY. 1989. Interleukin-6 and granulocyte-macrophage colony-stimulating factor are candidate growth factors for chronic myelomonocytic leukemia cells. Blood **74:** 1472–1476.
49. SCHIPPERUS, M. R., P. SONNEVELD, J. LINDEMANS, K. VAN LOM, M. VLASTUIN & J. ABELS. 1991. Interleukin-6 and interleukin-1 enhancement of GM-CSF-dependent proliferation of haematopoietic progenitor cells in myelodysplastic syndromes. Br. J. Haematol. **77:** 515–522.
50. HEROLD, M., F. SCHMALZL & H. ZWIERZINA. 1992. Increased serum interleukin 6 levels in patients with myelodysplastic syndromes. Leukemia Res. **16:** 585–588.
51. JANSSEN, J. W. G., A. C. M. STEENVOORDEN, J. LYONS, B. ANGER, J. U. BOHLKE, J. L.

Bos, H. Seliger & C. R. Bartram. 1987. *Ras* gene mutations in acute and chronic myelocytic leukemias, chronic myeloproliferative disorders, and myelodysplastic syndromes. Proc. Natl. Acad. Sci. USA **84**: 9228–9232.
52. Padua, R. A., G. Carter, D. Hughes, J. Gow, C. Farr, D. Oscier, F. McCormick & A. Jacobs. 1988. *Ras* mutations in myelodysplasia detected by amplification, oligonucleotide hybridization, and transformation. Leukemia **2**: 503–510.
53. Hirsch-Ginsberg, C., A. C. Lemaistre, H. Kantarjian, M. Talpaz, A. Cork, E. J. Freireich, J. M. Trujillo, M.-S. Lee & S. A. Stass. 1990. *Ras* mutations are rare events in Philadelphia chromosome-negative/bcr gene rearrangement-negative chronic myelogenous leukemia, but are prevalent in chronic myelomonocytic leukemia. Blood **76**: 1214–1219.
54. Lübbert, M., W. Oster, H. Knopf, F. McCormick, R. Mertelsmann & F. Herrmann. 1993. N-*ras* gene activation in acute myeloid leukemia: Association with expression of interleukin-6. Leukemia **7**: 1948–1954.
55. Egan, S. E. & R. A. Weinberg. 1993. The pathway to signal achievement. Nature **365**: 781–783.
56. Hill, C. S. & R. Treisman. 1995. Transcriptional regulation by extracellular signals: Mechanisms and specificity. Cell **80**: 199–211.
57. Tanabe, O., S. Akira, T. Kamiya, G. G. Wong, T. Hirano & T. Kishimoto. 1988. Genomic structure of the murine IL-6 gene. J. Immunol. **141**: 3875–3881.
58. Matsusaka, T., K. Fujikawa, Y. Nishio, N. Mukaida, K. Matsushima, T. Kishimoto & S. Akira. 1993. Transcription factors NF-IL6 and NF-κB synergistically activate transcription of the inflammatory cytokines, interleukin 6 and interleukin 8. Proc. Natl. Acad. Sci. USA **90**: 10193–10197.
59. Brach, M. A., H.-J. Gruss, T. Kaisho, Y. Asano, T. Hirano & F. Herrmann. 1993. Ionizing radiation induces expression of interleukin 6 by human fibroblasts involving activation of nuclear factor-κB. J. Biol. Chem. **268**: 8466–8472.
60. Smeal, T., B. Binetruy, D. A. Mercola, M. Birrer & M. Karin. 1991. Oncogenic and transcriptional cooperation with Ha-Ras requires phosphorylation of c-Jun on serines 63 and 73. Nature **354**: 494–496.
61. Derijard, B., M. Hibi, I.-H. Wu, T. Barrett, B. Su, T. Deng, M. Karin & R. J. Davis. 1994. JNK1: A protein kinase stimulated by UV light and Ha-Ras that binds and phosphorylates the c-Jun activation domain. Cell **76**: 1025–1037.
62. Nakajima, T., S. Kinoshita, T. Sasagawa, K. Sasaki, M. Naruto, T. Kishimoto & S. Akira. 1993. Phosphorylation at threonine-235 by a *ras*-dependent mitogen-activated protein kinase cascade is essential for transcription factor NF-IL6. Proc. Natl. Acad. Sci. USA **90**: 2207–2211.
63. Natsuka, S., S. Akira, Y. Nishio, S. Hashimoto, T. Sugita, H. Isshiki & T. Kishimoto. 1992. Macrophage differentiation-specific expression of NF-IL6, a transcription factor for interleukin-6. Blood **79**: 460–466.
64. Hsu, W., T. K. Kerppola, P.-L. Chen, T. Curran & S. Chen-Kiang. 1994. Fos and Jun repress transcription activation by NF-IL6 through association at the basic zipper region. Mol. Cell. Biol. **14**: 268–276.
65. Demetri, G. D., T. J. Ernst, E. S. Pratt II, B. W. Zenzie, J. G. Rheinwald & J. D. Griffin. 1990. Expression of *ras* oncogenes in cultured human cells alters the transcriptional and posttranscriptional regulation of cytokine genes. J. Clin. Invest. **86**: 1261–1269.
66. Ross, H. J., N. Sato, Y. Ueyama & H. P. Koeffler. 1991. Cytokine messenger RNA stability is enhanced in tumor cells. Blood **77**: 1787–1795.
67. Nair, A. P. K., S. Hahn, R. Banholzer, H. H. Hirsch & C. Moroni. 1994. Cyclosporin A inhibits growth of autocrine tumour cell lines by destabilizing interleukin-3 mRNA. Nature **369**: 239–242.
68. Metz, T., T. Graf & A. Leutz. 1991. Activation of cMGF expression is a critical step in avian myeloid leukemogenesis. EMBO J. **10**: 837–844.
69. Hawley, R. G., A. Z. C. Fong, B. F. Burns & T. S. Hawley. 1992. Transplantable myeloproliferative disease induced in mice by an interleukin 6 retrovirus. J. Exp. Med. **176**: 1149–1163.

70. HAWLEY, R. G., F. H. L. LIEU, A. Z. C. FONG & T. S. HAWLEY. 1994. Versatile retroviral vectors for potential use in gene therapy. Gene Therapy **1:** 136–138.
71. SCHROEDER, C., L. GIBSON, C. NORDSTROM & H. BEUG. 1993. The estrogen receptor cooperates with TGFα receptor (c-*erb*B) in the regulation of chicken erythroid progenitor self-renewal. EMBO J. **12:** 951–960.
72. SUEMATSU, S., T. MATSUSAKA, T. MATSUDA, S. OHNO, J. MIYAZAKI, K. YAMAMURA, T. HIRANO & T. KISHIMOTO. 1992. Generation of plasmacytomas with the chromosomal translocation t(12;15) in interleukin 6 transgenic mice. Proc. Natl. Acad. Sci. USA **89:** 232–235.
73. DUNBAR, C. E., T. M. BROWDER, J. S. ABRAMS & A. W. NIENHUIS. 1989. COOH-terminal-modified interleukin-3 is retained intracellularly and stimulates autocrine growth. Science **245:** 1493–1496.
74. PIERCE, J. H. & S. A. AARONSON. 1985. Myeloid cell transformation by *ras*-containing murine sarcoma viruses. Mol. Cell. Biol. **5:** 667–674.
75. SAWYERS, C. L., C. T. DENNY & O. N. WITTE. 1991. Leukemia and the disruption of normal hematopoiesis. Cell **64:** 337–350.
76. HAWLEY, R. G., A. Z. C. FONG, B. Y. NGAN, V. M. DE LANUX, S. C. CLARK & T. S. HAWLEY. 1993. Progenitor cell hyperplasia with rare development of myeloid leukemia in interleukin 11 bone marrow chimeras. J. Exp. Med. **178:** 1175–1188.
77. SPORN, M. B. & A. B. ROBERTS. 1985. Autocrine growth factors and cancer. Nature **313:** 745–747.
78. LANG, R. A. & A. W. BURGESS. 1990. Autocrine growth factors and tumourigenic transformation. Immunol. Today **11:** 244–249.
79. METCALF, D. & D. P. GEARING. 1989. Fatal syndrome in mice engrafted with cells producing high levels of the leukemia inhibitory factor. Proc. Natl. Acad. Sci. USA **86:** 5948–5952.
80. METCALF, D. & D. P. GEARING. 1989. A myelosclerotic syndrome in mice engrafted with cells producing high levels of leukemia inhibitory factor (LIF). Leukemia **3:** 847–852.
81. METCALF, D., N. A. NICOLA & D. P. GEARING. 1990. Effects of injected leukemia inhibitory factor on hematopoietic and other tissues in mice. Blood **76:** 50–56.

Pleiotropic Defects of IL-6–deficient Mice Including Early Hematopoiesis, T and B Cell Function, and Acute Phase Responses

MANFRED KOPF,[a] ALISTAIR RAMSAY,[b] FRANK BROMBACHER,[a]
HEINZ BAUMANN,[c] GIULIA FREER,[d] CHRIS GALANOS,[a]
JOSE-CARLOS GUTIERREZ-RAMOS,[e] AND GEORGES KÖHLER[a]

[a]Max-Planck-Institut für Immunobiologie
Postbach 1169
D-79111 Freiburg, Germany
[b]John Curtin School of Medical Research
Canberra, A.C.T. 2601, Australia
[c]Department of Molecular and Cellular Biology
Roswell Park Cancer Institute
Buffalo, New York 14263
[d]Experimentelle Immunologie
Universität Zürich
Zürich, Switzerland
[e]Center for Blood Research
Boston, Massachusetts 02115

Interleukin-6 (IL-6) is a cytokine produced by a variety of cells such as macrophages, T cells, B cells, fibroblasts, and endothelial cells in response to infection, trauma, and shock. It possesses a broad range of activities on the three major systems of the body, the immune system, the hematopoietic system and the nervous system.[1,2] Historically, IL-6 was given at least nine different names that were descriptive of individual biological activities of this cytokine. In the immune system it induces activated B cells to differentiate into antibody-secreting plasma cells[1,2] and to stimulate the proliferation and the differentiation of cytotoxic T cells.[3] In hematopoiesis, IL-6 acts synergistically with IL-3 to promote multilineage blast colony formation, probably by triggering the stem cells to enter the G_1 from the G_0 stage of the cell cycle.[4,5] Further, osteoclast formation from hemopoietic precursors is promoted by IL-6.[6] In addition, myeloid leukemic cell lines can be induced by IL-6 to differentiate into macrophages.[7] In the nervous system, IL-6 effects the hypothalamo-pituitary adrenal axis by stimulating the secretion of adrenocorticotropic hormone through corticotropine-releasing hormone.[8,9] In hepatocytes, IL-6 seems to be the major regulator of acute phase protein synthesis during an inflammatory response.[10] *In vitro*, other cytokines such as IL-11, Leukemia inhibitory factor (LIF), oncostatin M (OM), ciliary neurotrophic factor (CNTF), and IL-1 display partly overlapping activities with IL-6. Thus, IL-6 is a prototype cytokine with pleiotropic and redundant activities. More recently, the finding that specificity-determining α-components of receptors for IL-6, IL-11, CNTF, and LIF share a common signal-transducing component (gp130) suggests a molecular mechanism for redundant activities.[11] To elucidate the unique function of IL-6 *in vivo*, we have disrupted the IL-6 gene by homologous recombination and generated IL-6-deficient (IL-6 −/−) mice.[12]

THE GENERATION OF IL-6-DEFICIENT MICE

The IL-6 gene was disrupted in the second exon (first coding exon) by insertion of a neo^r cassette. F_1 mice (C57Bl/6 × 129 Sv) heterozygous for the mutation (IL-6$^{+/-}$) were interbred to obtain mice homozygous for the mutation. Loss of the wildtype alleles was confirmed by Southern analysis (not shown). IL-6 mRNA was assayed by reverse transcriptase PCR. Three sets of IL-6 primers from different exons were used to amplify cDNA from total RNA of LPS activated bone marrow macrophages from IL-6$^{+/-}$ and IL-6$^{-/-}$ mice. No amplification products were obtained from the latter, indicating the absence of spurious intact RNA or RNA splice products omitting exon 2. Consequently, neither a bioassay nor an ELISA performed with serum of LPS treated mice gave indication for an IL-6 protein.[12]

IL-6 IS NOT ESSENTIAL FOR EMBRYONIC DEVELOPMENT

IL-6 is expressed already in the preimplantation embryo.[14,15] Later in gestation, IL-6 is produced by extraembryonic tissue such as trophoblast or whole placental tissue and stimulates the release of chorionic gonadotropin (hCG).[16,17] Blood vessel supply of the uterine tissue stimulated by placental progesterone is regulated by hCG and, thus, indirectly may be by IL-6. More recently, LIF, an IL-6-type cytokine, was reported to be crucial for blastocyst implantation.[18] Interbreeding of IL-6 +/− heterozygous mice, however, resulted in inheritance of the defective IL-6 allele in a Mendelian pattern. Furthermore, interbreeding of IL-6$^{-/-}$ mice generated offspring in normal numbers and without obvious defects in development. Therefore, IL-6 appears not to be essential for embryonic development.

REDUCTION IN THE NUMBER OF UNCOMMITTED PROGENITOR CELLS (CFU-s)

In the steady state, the majority of the hematopoietic stem cells (HSC) are not in the cell cycle but reside dormant in the G_0 phase. Several factors, such as steel (SF), IL-3, IL-6, IL-11, M-CSF, and G-CSF have been shown to be required for the optimal maintenance an expansion of stem cell colonies, *in vitro*.[19] More recently, LIF-deficient mice were shown to have decreased numbers of stem cells in the bone marrow and spleen, which, however, remained multipotent.[13] IL-6, in synergy with IL-3, is known to accelerate the appearance of multilineage blast cells, probably by recruiting cells from G_0.[4,5] Using the well-documented effects of IL-6 on HSC and on early uncommitted progenitor cells *in vitro*, we have studied the consequence of IL-6-deficiency on the generation and maintenance of these cells.[20] Compared to controls, the numbers of primitive clonal progenitors in the bone marrow and spleen of IL-6-deficient mice was reduced by 55% and 70%, respectively, as determined by the ability to form spleen colonies (CFU-s d12) in lethally irradiated IL-6$^{+/+}$ recipient mice at day 12 post transfer (FIG. 1, a and b). Furthermore, the importance of IL-6 was examined by injecting bone marrow cells of IL-6$^{-/-}$ and IL-6$^{+/+}$ mice into lethally irradiated IL-6$^{-/-}$ mice (FIG. 1c). Again, the transfer of bone marrow cells from IL-6-deficient resulted in a 75% reduction of CFU-s d12. By contrast, the number of CFU-s d12 of bm cells from IL-6$^{+/+}$ mice that developed in a microenvironment devoid of IL-6 was only slightly reduced (FIG. 1c) compared to the colony number developing in IL-6$^{+/+}$ mice (FIG. 1a). The mean size of colonies of both groups and transfers was comparable. These data indicate the importance of IL-6 for the maintenance and/or

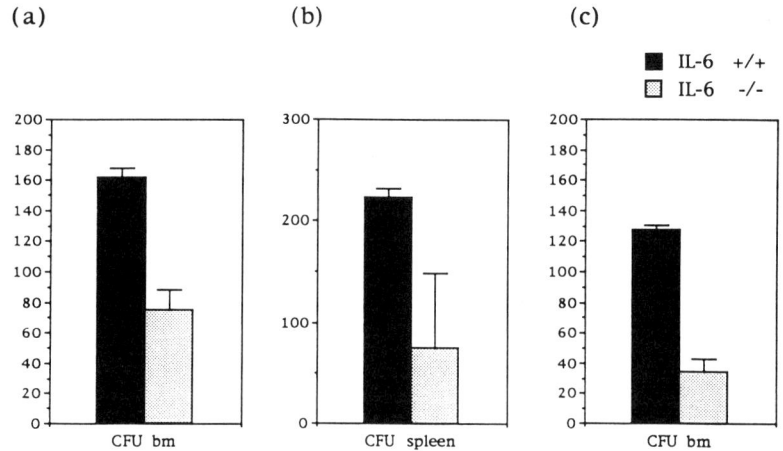

FIGURE 1. Hematopoiesis. Number of hematopoietic progenitors CFUs-day 12 per 10^5 cells in the bone marrow (**a,c**) and spleen (**b**) of 5 to 9 mice of each genotype (IL-6+/+ and IL-6−/− mice). Dissociated bone marrow and spleen cells of both groups were injected into lethally irradiated IL-6+/+ (**a**) and IL-6−/− recipient mice (**c**). Macroscopic spleen colonies were counted at day 12 after injection.

self renewal of uncommitted progenitor cells defined as CFU-s. The IL-6 activity seems to be mediated by the transferred cells with minor effects from the environment.

LOSS OF IL-6 RESULTS IN IMPAIRED GROWTH AND FUNCTION OF T CELLS

The development of the lymphoid compartment was investigated in 6- to 12-week old mice by cytofluorimetric analysis. The number of thymocytes (not shown) and peripheral T cells in IL-6$^{-/-}$ mice were consistently reduced by 30- to 50% as compared to controls (FIG. 2a). This is in agreement with results showing that IL-6 is a cofactor in the induction of T cell proliferation.[21,22] Thymocytes and peripheral T-cells, however, had normal expression patterns of T cell receptor α, β, γ, δ chains, CD4, CD8, CD44 (Pgp1), and CD24 (HSA). The B cell compartment in the bone marrow and spleen of IL-6$^{-/-}$ mice remained virtually unaffected, with normal expression of B220, IgM, IgD, and CD23. IL-6, in combination with IL-1, was suggested to activate resting purified T cells by moving cells from G_0 to G_1 through induction of the IL-2 receptor, and the initiation of IL-2 production. *In vitro*, CD4$^+$ T cells of splenic bulk cultures of IL-6$^{+/+}$ and IL-6$^{-/-}$ mice stimulated with ConA showed a comparable kinetic and magnitude of IL-2Rα expression (FIG. 2b), demonstrating that in cultures containing accessory cells IL-6 is not required for T cell activation. To assess T cell function *in vivo*, mice were infected with vaccinia virus. The generation and activity of cytotoxic T cells against vaccinia virus (VV)-WR showed a 3- to 10-fold reduction in mutant mice. They could not efficiently control virus replication as reflected in 10- to 1000-fold higher titers and became severely chachectic.[12] Meanwhile, there is compelling evidence that an important antiviral effector mechanism is mediated by cytokines such as interferons and tumor necrosis factor-α rather than by the cytolytic activity of CD8$^+$ T cells.[23,24] Thus, IL-6 may promote the production of antiviral cytokines. The reduction in CTL activity, which was only seen after infection with wildtype VV-WR, but not with an attenuated recombinant VV strain, may

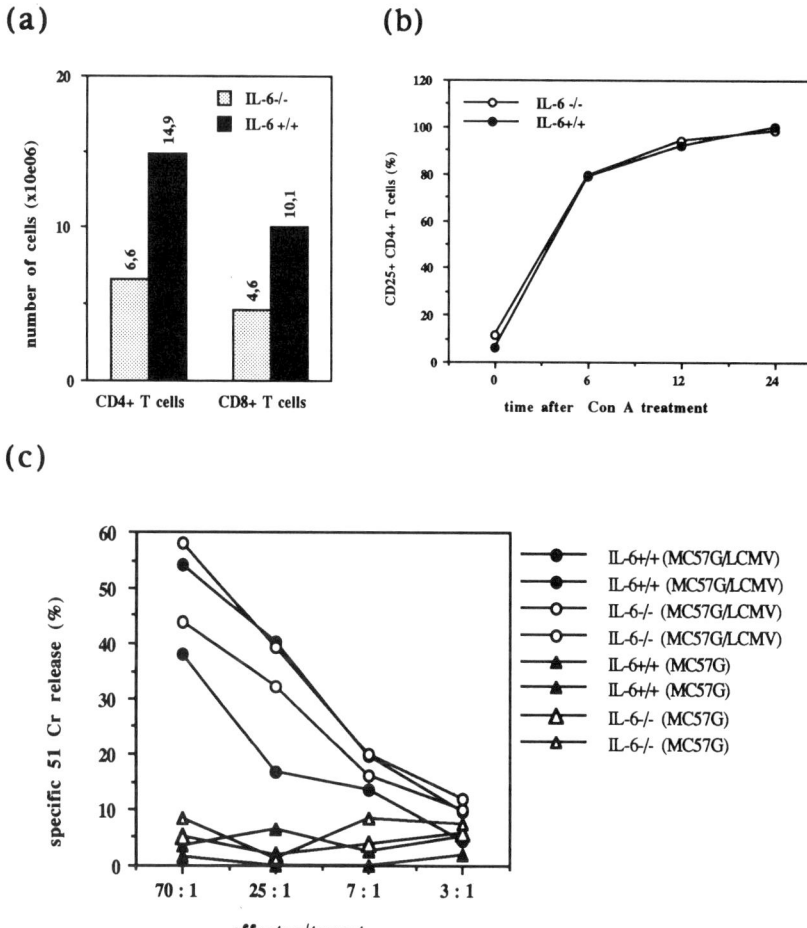

FIGURE 2. T cell development and function (a) Number of CD4+ and CD8+ T cells in the spleen of IL-6+/+ and IL-6−/− mice (8- to 10 week old; n = 5/group). (b) Percentage of CD4+ T cells expressing IL-2Rα (CD25) after stimulation with concanavalin A (Con A). Bulk spleen cells (2 × 10^6/ml) were stimulated with 5 μg concanavalin A for times indicated and analyzed by flow cytometry. (c) Cytotoxic T cell (CTL) response. Mice were infected i.v. with 2 × 10^3 plaque forming units (pfu) of lymphocytic choriomeningitis virus (LCMV-WE). Spleens were removed at day 8 and CTL activity determined by measuring ^{51}Cr release of target cells (MC57G) infected (circles) or uninfected (triangles) with LCMV.

be a secondary effect due to uncontrolled viral spread. This is further supported by the fact that CTL activity in IL-6–deficient mice against lymphocytic choriomeningitis virus (LCMV) was not affected (FIG. 2c).

THE ROLE OF IL-6 IN B CELL DIFFERENTIATION

IL-6 was originally identified as a lymphokine inducing final maturation of B cells into antibody secreting cells.[25,26] IL-6 overexpressing transgenic mice develop plasmacytosis and a massive increase in polyclonal IgG1.[27] Surprisingly, plasma cell numbers in the bone marrow and natural serum antibody levels in 8- to 12 week old mice were not different between IL-6 −/− and control mice. To assess B cell function during an immune response, bpo-specific antibody levels were determined at day 14 post primary (FIG. 3a). and day 7 post secondary immunization (FIG. 3b) with alum precipitated benzylpenicilloyl-keyholelimpethemocyanine (bpo-KLH). Serum levels of specific IgG1, IgG2a and IgG2b were reduced up to 10-fold as compared to controls. By contrast, IgM levels were comparable. This is in keeping with results of an infection with vesicular stomatitis virus (VSV). VSV is controlled both by virus-neutralizing IgM antibodies, which are T cell–help independent, and by IgG antibodies that are dependent on T cell help. Virus-neutralizing IgG was found to be 5- to 10-fold reduced in IL-6$^{-/-}$ mice during the course of VSV infection, whereas early (day 4) IgM titers are comparable to controls.[12] This suggests that B cell development and maturation to the stage of IgM secretion is not affected by the absence of IL-6. However, during a T cell help dependent antibody response, when B cells undergo the germinal center reaction, IL-6 seems to be required for the expansion of plasmablasts.

Mucosal surfaces represent the main route for the entry of pathogens. More than 95% of secretory IgA is locally produced by plasma cells in mucosal associated tissues (BALT, GALT).[28] It has been shown that surface IgA mucosal B cells express high levels of IL-6 receptor and respond to IL-6 with an increase in IgA secretion.[29] The availability of IL-6–deficient mice provides an ideal opportunity to study the importance of IL-6 on B cells in mucosal immune responses. IgA plasma cells in mesenteric lymph nodes, lung, and small intestine of naive IL-6$^{-/-}$ mice were reduced compared to controls. Intraperitoneal priming and subsequent local (intraduodenal) challenge with ovalbumin revealed a deficiency of IL-6$^{-/-}$ mice to mount antigen specific IgA responses in the intestines (FIG. 4a).[30] Moreover, after intranasal infection with a recombinant vaccinia virus (rVV) construct carrying the gene for hemagglutinin, specific antibody responses in the lungs were negligible in the absence of IL-6 (FIG. 4b), but could be restored with rVV expressing IL-6 (FIG. 4c).[30] By contrast, mucosal responses after oral immunization using ovalbumin in combination with cholera toxin, a potent adjuvant, did not reveal significant differences in specific antibody-producing cells (SABC) including IgA-SABC (N. Lycke, personal communica-

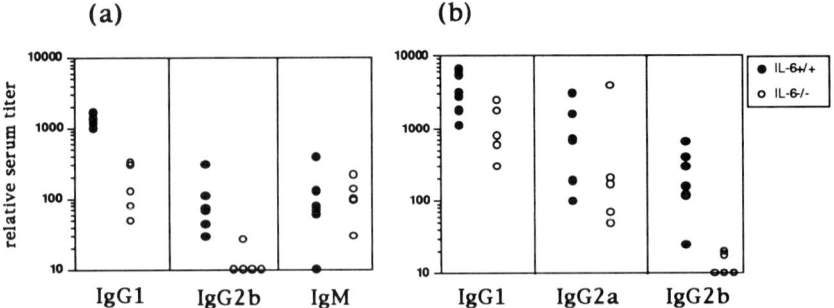

FIGURE 3. B cell responses after immunization. Relative serum titers of the different antibody isotypes binding bpo. Mice were immunized i.p. and subcutaneously with alum-precipitated bpo-KLH (40 μg) together with B. pertussis and boosted after 14 days. Serum was taken at day 14 after primary (**a**) and at day 7 after secondary immunization (**b**). Bpo-specific antibody levels were determined by ELISA. Results are expressed as the serum dilution where half-maximal absorbance values were obtained.

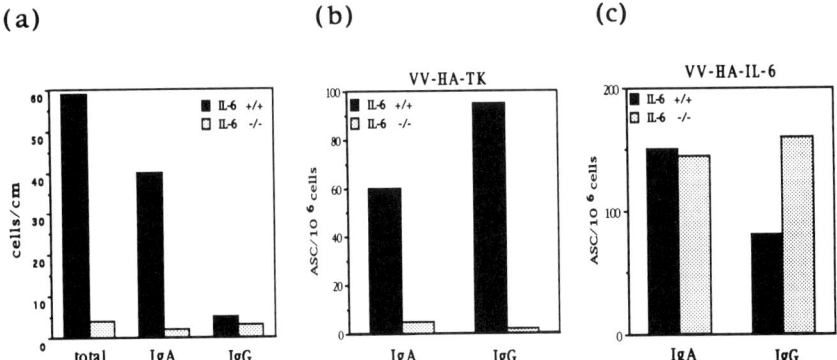

FIGURE 4. Mucosal responses. (a) Numbers and isotype distribution of cells in the intestines containing antibodies to ovalbumin after local immunization. (b,c) Numbers of hemagglutinin (HA) antibody secreting cells in the lungs of mice after intranasal infection with vaccinia virus expressing HA of influenza virus (a) and HA together with IL-6 (c). (Data are shown in ref. 30.)

tion.) These results suggest, that IL-6 becomes a crucial factor for mucosal responses dependent on the type of stimulation.

IL-6 REGULATES ACUTE PHASE PROTEIN SYNTHESIS AFTER TISSUE DAMAGE AND INFECTION

The acute phase response (APR) is a systemic reaction to inflammation and tissue damage.[31] The main features are fever, leukocytosis, increased vascular permeability, changes in steroid levels and the biosynthesis of acute phase proteins (APP) by hepatocytes. The macrophage or monocyte is usually the cell that elicits the APR cascade by secretion of a panel of inflammatory cytokines. *In vitro,* the known mediators of APP induction in hepatocytes are IL-1, TNF-α, IL-11, LIF, oncostatin M, CNTF, glucocorticoids, and IL-6, which was proposed to be one of the major stimulatory factors of APP synthesis. To elucidate the unique role of IL-6 in the liver acute phase protein response, IL-6 $-/-$ and control mice were challenged either with turpentine, LPS, or infection with the gram-positive bacteria *L. monocytogenes.* In IL-6$^{+/+}$ mice, both a local sterile tissue damage by subcutaneous injection of turpentine, and infection with gram-positive *L. monocytogenes* induced a particularly prominent increase in liver mRNA (FIG. 5a) and serum levels (FIG. 5b) for haptoglobin (HP), α_1 acid glycoprotein (AGP) and serum amyloid A (SAA), three representative APPs. In contrast, liver cells of IL-6–deficient mice reacted only weakly to these stimuli. This was particularly evident after tissue damage induced by turpentine, where the levels of SAA mRNA in IL-6–deficient mice were 100-fold reduced. Interestingly, after treatment with bacterial LPS, the induction of SAA, HP, and AGP mRNA was only slightly reduced in IL-6–deficient mice compared to controls (FIG. 5c). These results indicate that IL-6 is an important mediator of an acute phase protein response after tissue damage or infection with gram-positive intracellular bacteria but not gram-negative bacteria. Bacterial LPS has systemic rather than local effects and triggers inflammatory mediators from a variety of cell types such as fibroblasts, macrophages, and endothelial cells, which themselves induce hepatocytes in the absence of IL-6. There are more than 40 known APPs, which have a wide range of activities that contribute to host defense and tissue repair. Increase in complement cascade proteins, such as C2, C3, C4, C5, and C9 ultimately leads to the local accumulation of inflammatory cells, which participate in the elimination of pathogens. Coagulation components,

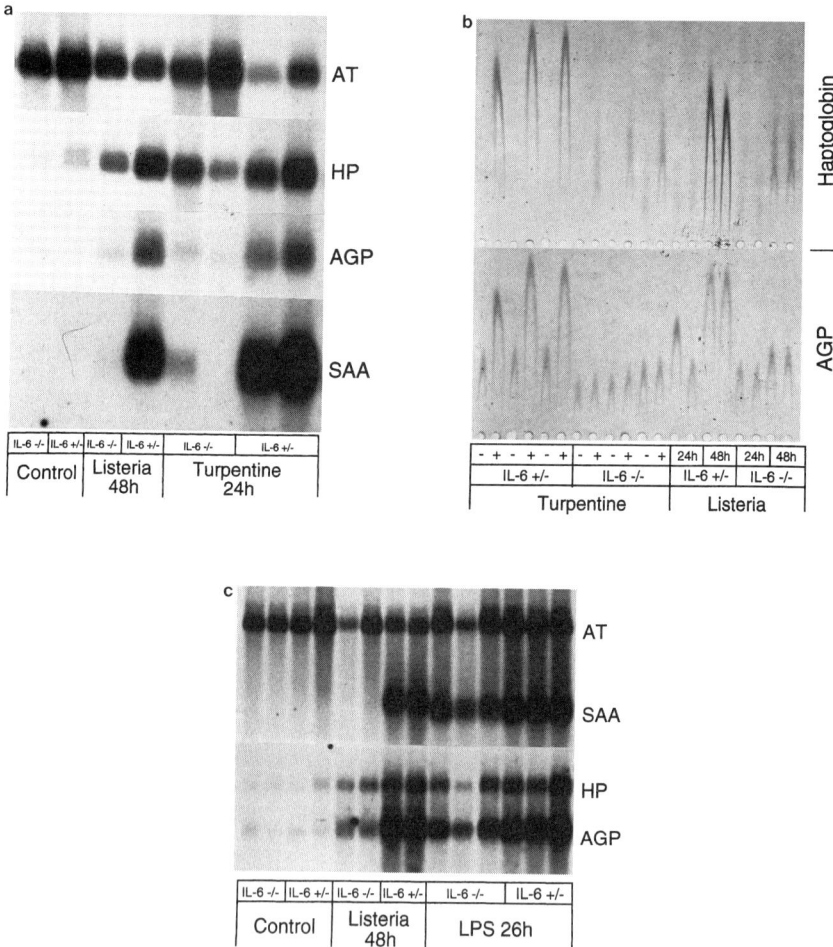

FIGURE 5. Liver acute phase response after inflammation. IL-6 $-/-$ and IL-6 $+/+$ mice were treated either by intravenous infection with L. monocytogenes (a,b c), or subcutaneous injection of 50 μl sterile turpentine (a,b) or intravenous injection of 1 μg LPS (c). Controls were untreated mice (**a,c**). Shown is the Northern blot analysis of liver RNA harvested at times indicated after treatment (**a,c**). Filters were hybridized with probes for haptoglobin (HP), α_1-acid glycoprotein (AGP), and serum amyloid A (SAA). α_1-anti-trypsin, an acute phase gene not affected by inflammation, was used for standardization, (**b**) AGP and HP protein serum levels as determined by rocket immuno-electrophoresis. The compiled results of this experiment were shown in ref. 12.

TABLE 1. Toxic Shock Response

Experiment	D-GalN (mg)	LPS (μg)	IL-6+/+ Lethality	IL-6-/- Lethality
1	20	0.05	4/4	4/4
	20	0.005	3/4	4/4
	20	0.0005	2/4	0/4
	20	—	0/4	0/4
2		600	nd	4/4
		400	4/4	0/4
		200	1/4	0/4
		100	0/4	0/4

Lethal toxicity after intravenous injection of LPS (*S. abortus equi*) alone or after sensitization with D-Galactosamine (D-GalN). D-GalN-sensitized mice died 6 to 8 hours after LPS challenge. Mortality of non-sensitized mice was recorded over 5 days.

such as fibrinogen and von Willebrand factor facilitate wound healing. Metal-binding proteins prevent loss of iron during infection and are scavengers of potentially dangerous free radicals. Determination of these APPs after infection with protozoan and metazoan parasites will help to elucidate the physiological role of the acute phase response and it's linkage to the immune response during infection.

IL-6 DOES NOT PLAY AN IMPORTANT ROLE IN LPS-INDUCED SEPTIC SHOCK

Toxic shock is a systemic response to infection with high mortality. Lipopolysaccharide (LPS, endotoxin)) from Gram-negative bacteria and enterotoxin from Gram-positive bacteria, such as *Staphylococcus aureus* A or B (SEB or SEA) enterotoxin, play an important role in the pathogenesis of septic shock.[32] Most of the toxic effects of LPS are mediated by inflammatory cytokines including TNF, IL-1, and IFN-γ,[33-35] whereas they are inhibited by IL-10.[36,37] Macrophages, which are the main source of the proinflammatory cytokines TNF, IL-1 and IL-6, were shown to be essential in mediating endotoxin reactions.[38] While the important role of TNF in the pathogenesis of toxic shock has been convincingly demonstrated,[33,39,40] the role of IL-6 has remained unclear. In man and mice, the IL-6 levels correlate well with toxic shock.[41,42] Blocking of IL-6 or IL-6R by monoclonal antibodies resulted in a dose-dependent protection to a lethal dose of mTNF.[43] However, protection was overcome, when the mTNF dose was slightly higher than the lethal dose. We studied a lethal challenge of high dose LPS and low dose LPS in combination with D-galactosamine (D-GalN), which enhances susceptibility to endotoxin by increasing the lethal activity of TNF. As shown in TABLE 1 injection of 400 μg LPS in IL-6+/+ mice resulted in lethality within 72 hours, whereas IL-6-deficient mice were cachectic but survived this dose. Injection of 600 μg LPS in IL-6-/- mice induced lethality. Sensitization with GalN and subsequent treatment with 0.5 ng LPS caused lethality in two out of four IL-6+/+ mice, while four of four IL-6-/- mice survived. Treatment with 5 ng LPS after GalN-sensitization, however, caused lethality in all IL-6-/- mice. Thus, IL-6-deficient mice are slightly, if at all, protected from LPS-induced lethality.

CONCLUSION

In vivo, absence of IL-6 affects the number of hematopoietic multilineage precursor cells (CFU-s), the number of T cells and their responses, B cell responses, macrophage activity, and acute phase responses of hepatocytes. In none of the cases is IL-6 crucially required. It seems that IL-6 is a systemic alarm signal that is indicative of tissue damage, infection, and/or inflammation and may coordinate early hematopoiesis, such as stem cell cycling and commitment, with specific immune responses. IL-6 optimizes these responses which have to act in concert.

REFERENCES

1. VAN-SNICK, J. 1989. Interleukin-6: An overview. Annu. Rev. Immunol. **8:** 253–278.
2. KISHIMOTO, T. 1987. The biology of interleukin-6. Blood **74:** 1–10.
3. HOUSSIAU, F. & J. VAN SNICK. 1992. IL6 and the T-cell response. Res. Immunol. **143:** 740–743.
4. IKEBUCHI, K., G. G. WONG, S. C. CLARK, J. N. IHLE, Y. HIRAI & M. OGAWA. 1987. Interleukin 6 enhancement of interleukin 3-dependent proliferation of multipotential hemopoietic progenitors. Proc. Natl. Acad. Sci. USA **84:** 9035–9039.
5. IKEBUCHI, K., J. N. IHLE, Y. HIRAI, G. G. WONG, S. C. CLARK & M. OGAWA. 1988. Synergistic factors for stem cell proliferation: Further studies of the target stem cells and the mechanism of stimulation by interleukin-1, interleukin-6, and granulocyte colony-stimulating factor. Blood **72:** 2007–2014.
6. LÖWIK, C. W. 1992. Differentiation Inducing Factors: Leukemia Inhibitory Factor and Interleukin-6. :300–324. Boca Raton, FL: CRC Press.
7. MIYAURA, C., K. ONOZAKI, Y. AKIYAMA, T. TANIYAMA, T. HIRANO, T. KISHIMOTO & T. SUDA. 1988. Recombinant human interleukin 6 (B-cell stimulatory factor 2) is a potent inducer of differentiation of mouse myeloid leukemia cells (M1). FEBS Lett. **234:** 17–21.
8. NAITOH, Y., J. FUKATA, T. TOMINAGA, Y. NAKAI, S. TAMAI, K. MORI & H. IMURA. 1988. Interleukin-6 stimulates the secretion of adrenocorticotropic hormone in conscious, freely-moving rats. Biochem. Biophys. Res. Commun. **155:** 1459–1463.
9. SPANGELO, B. L., A. M. JUDD, P. C. ISAKSON & R. M. MACLEOD. 1989. Interleukin-6 stimulates anterior pituitary hormone release in vitro. Endocrinology **125:** 575–577.
10. STADNYK, A. & J. GAULDIE. 1991. The acute phase protein response during parasitic infection. Immunol. Today **12:** A7–12.
11. KISHIMOTO, T., S. AKIRA & T. TAGA. 1992. Interleukin-6 and its receptor: A paradigm for cytokines. Science **258:** 593–597.
12. KOPF, M., H. BAUMANN, G. FREER, M. FREUDENBERG, M. LAMERS, T. KISHIMOTO, R. ZINKERNAGEL, H. BLUETHMAN & G. KOHLER. Impaired immune and acute-phase responses in interleukin-6-deficient mice. Nature **368:** 339–342.
13. ESCARY, J. L., J. PERREAU, D. DUMENIL, S. EZINE. P. BRULET. 1993. Leukemia inhibitory factor is necessary for the maintenance of haematopoietic sem cells and thymocyte stimulation. Nature **363:** 361–364.
14. MURRAY, R., F. LEE & C. P. CHIU. 1990. The genes for leukemia inhibitory factor and interleukin-6 are expressed in mouse blastocysts prior to the onset of hemopoiesis. Mol. Cell. Biol. **10:** 4953–4956.
15. ROTHSTEIN, J. L., D. JOHNSON, J. A. DELOIA, J. SKOWRONSKI, D. SOLTER & B. KNOWLES. 1992. Gene expression during preimplantation mouse development. Genes Dev. **6:** 1190–1201.
16. NISHINO, E., N. MATSUZAKI, K. MASUHIRO, T. KAMEDA, T. TANIGUCHI, T. TAKAGI, F. SAJI & O. TANIZAWA. 1989. Trophoblast derived IL-6 regulates human chorionic gonadotropin release through IL-6 receptor on human trophoblasts. J. Clin. Endocrinol. Metab. **71:** 536–541.
17. DUC-GOIRAN, P., C. CHANY & J. DOLY. 1989. Unusually large interferon-alpha-like mRNAs and high expression of interleukin-6 in human fetal annexes. J. Biol. Chem. **264:** 16507–16511.
18. STEWART, C. L., P. KASPAR, L. J. BRUNET, H. BHATT, I. GADI, F. KÖNTGEN & S. J. ABBONDANZO. 1992. Blastocyst implantation depends on maternal expression of leukaemia inhibitory factor. Nature **359:** 76–79.

19. ZIPORI, D. 1992. The renewal and differentiation of hemopoietic stem cells. FASEB J. **6:** 2691–2697.
20. BERNAD, A., M. KOPF, R. KULBACKI, N. WEICH, G. KÖHLER & J. C. GUTIERREZ-RAMOS. 1994. IL-6 is required in vivo for the regulation of stem cells and committed progenitors of the hematopoietic system. Immunity. **1:** 725–731.
21. UYTTENHOVE, C., P. G. COULIE & J. VAN SNICK. 1988. T cell growth and differentiation induced by interleukin-HP1/IL-6, the murine hybridoma/plasmacytoma growth factor. J. Exp. Med. **167:** 1417–1427.
22. LOTZ, M., F. JIRIK, P. KABOURIDIS, C. TSOUKAS, T. HIRANO, T. KISHIMOTO & D. A. CARSON. 1988. B cell stimulating factor 2/interleukin 6 is a costimulant for human thymocytes and T lymphocytes. J. Exp. Med. **167:** 1253–1258.
23. RAMSAY, A. J., J. RUBY & I. A. RAMSHAW. 1993. A case for cytokines as effector molecules in the resolution of virus infection. Immunol. Today **14:** 155–157.
24. SPRIGGS, M. K., B. H. KOLLER, T. SATO, P. J. MORRISELY, W. C. FANSLOW, O. SMITHIES, R. F. VOICE, M. B. WIDMER & C. R. MALISZEWSKI. 1992. β2-microglobulin-, CD8+ T cell deficient mice survive high doses of vaccinia virus and exhibit altered IgG responses. Proc. Natl. Acad. Sci. USA **89:** 6070–6074.
25. HIRANO, T., et al. 1986. Complementary DNA for a novel human interleukin (BSF-2) that induces B lymphocytes to produce immunoglobulin. Nature **324:** 73–76.
26. VAN SNICK, J., A. VINK, S. CAYPHAS & C. UYTTENHOVE. 1987. Interleukin-HP1, a T cell-derived hybridoma growth factor that supports the in vitro growth of murine plasmacytomas. J. Exp. Med. **165:** 641–649.
27. SUEMATSU, S., et al. 1989. IgG1 plasmacytosis in interleukin-6 transgenic mice. Proc. Natl. Acad. Sci. USA **86:** 7547–7551.
28. BRANDTZAEG, P. 1989. Overview of the mucosal immune system. Curr. Top. Microbiol. Immunol. **146:** 13–25.
29. BEAGLEY, K. W., J. H. ELDRIDGE, F. LEE, H. KIYONO, M. P. EVERSON, W. J. KOOPMAN, T. HIRANO, T. KISHIMOTO & J. R. MCGHEE. 1989. Interleukins and IgA synthesis. Human and murine interleukin 6 induce high rate IgA secretion in IgA-committed B cells. J. Exp. Med. **169:** 2133–2148.
30. RAMSAY, A. J., A. J. HUSBAND, I. A. RAMSHAW, S. BAO, K. I. MATTHAEI, G. KOEHLER & M. KOPF. 1994. The role of interleukin-6 in mucosal IgA antibody responses in vivo. Science **264:** 561–568.
31. KOJ, A. 1985. The acute phase response to injury and infection. A. H. Gordon & A. Koj, eds. :139–144. Amsterdam: Elsevier.
32. MORRISON, D. C. & J. L. RYAN. 1987. Endotoxins and disease mechanisms. Annu. Rev. Med. **38:** 417.
33. BEUTLER, B., I. W. MILSARK & A. C. CERAMI. 1985. Passive immunization against cachectin/tumor necrosis factor protects mice from lethal effect of endotoxin. Science **229:** 869–871.
34. CAR, B. D., V. M. ENG, B. SCHNYDER, L. OZMEN, S. HUANG, P. GALLAY, D. HEUMANN, M. AGUET & B. RYFFEL. 1994. Interferon gamma receptor deficient mice are resistant to endotoxic shock. J. Exp. Med. **179:** 1437–1444.
35. DINARELLO, C. A. 1992. Role of interleukin-1 in infectious diseases. Immunol. Rev. **127:** 119–146.
36. GERARD, C., C. BRUYNS, A. MARCHANT, D. ABRAMOWICZ, P. VANDENABEELE, A. DELVAUX, W. FIERS, M. GOLDMAN & T. VELU. 1993. Interleukin 10 reduces the release of tumor necrosis factor and prevents lethality in experimental endotoxemia. J. Exp. Med. **177:** 547–550.
37. HOWARD, M., T. MUCHAMUEL, S. ANDRADE & S. MENON. 1993. Interleukin 10 protects mice from lethal endotoxemia. J. Exp. Med. **177:** 1205–1208.
38. FREUDENBERG, M. A., D. KEPPLER & C. GALANOS. 1986. Requirement for lipopolysaccharide-responsive macrophages in galactosamine-induced sensitization to endotoxin. Infect. Immun. **51:** 891–895.
39. PFEFFER, K., et al. 1993. Mice deficient for the 55 kd tumor necrosis factor receptor are resistant to endotoxic shock, yet succumb to L. monocytogenes infection. Cell **73:** 457–467.

40. MIETHKE, T., C. WAHL, K. HEEG, B. ECHTENACHER, P. H. KRAMMER & H. T. WAGNER. 1992. Cell-mediated lethal shock triggered in mice by the superantigen staphylococcal enterotoxin B: Critical role of tumor necrosis factor. J. Exp. Med. **175:** 91–98.
41. WAAGE, A., A. HALSTENSEN, R. SHALABY, P. BRANDTZAEG, P. KIERULF & T. ESPEVIK. 1989. Local production of tumor necrosis factor alpha, interleukin 1, and interleukin 6 in meningococcal meningitis. Relation to the inflammatory response. J. Exp. Med. **170:** 1859–1867.
42. LIBERT, C., P. BROUCKAERT, A. SHAW & W. FIERS. 1990. Induction of interleukin 6 by human and murine recombinant interleukin 1 in mice. Eur. J. Immunol. **20:** 691–694.
43. LIBERT, C., A. VINK, P. COULIE, P. BROUCKAERT, B. EVERAERDT, J. VAN SNICK & W. FIERS. 1992. Limited involvement of interleukin-6 in the pathogenesis of lethal septic shock as revealed by the effect of monoclonal antibodies against interleukin-6 or its receptor in various murine models. Eur. J. Immunol. **22:** 2625–2630.

DISCUSSION OF THE PAPER

R. NETA (*Armed Forces Radiobiology Research Institute, Bethesda, MD*): Is it possible that differences between your lab and Valeria Poli's may be related to the strain differences of these animals? Are they the same strains of mice? Strains of mice may differ as much as the cell lines differ.

M. KOPF: Targeting of the IL-6 locus was done in the D3 ES cell line, which is derived from the 129Sv strain. The offspring of F2 C57Bl/6 × 129Sv interbreeding was backcrossed once with C57Bl/6. Mice for the analysis were taken from the offspring of IL-6 −/− and IL-6 +/+ homozygous breeding.

P. SEHGAL (*New York Medical College, Valhalla*): The organizers have realized that we had cut off the discussion yesterday on this critical issue. So we have requested Dr. Baumann from Buffalo to chair a roundtable discussion involving Drs. Poli, Kopf, Heinrich, and Fey at 4:30 this afternoon and they can discuss the differences in their experimental data.

NETA: So the next short question—a technical question. I was somewhat confused about the data you were presenting on hematopoiesis. Were you dealing with emergency hematopoiesis? Because when you showed us the model the mice were irradiated and you were recovering cells form irradiated mice.

KOPF: Donors of bone marrow and spleens were not irradiated. Recipient mice used to read out colony numbers in the spleen were lethally irradiated.

Interleukin-6-Type Cytokine–induced Changes in Acute Phase Protein Glycosylation[a]

WILLEM VAN DIJK

Department of Medical Chemistry
Faculty of Medicine, Vrije Universiteit
Van der Boechorststraat 7
1081 BT Amsterdam, The Netherlands

ANDRZEJ MACKIEWICZ

Department of Cancer Immunology
Academy of Medicine, Great Poland Cancer Center
Garbary 15
Poznań, Poland 61866

OCCURRENCE OF CHANGES IN GLYCOSYLATION

Human acute-phase proteins (APP), except for albumin and C-reactive protein, are glycoproteins which contain one or more asparagine-linked glycans of the complex type (see FIG. 1). The number of these glycans is dependent on the APP, thus α_1-acid glycoprotein (AGP) contains five and α_1-protease inhibitor (PI) three of these glycans. The type of branching, di-, tri- and/or tetraantennary (*cf.* FIG. 1), and the degree of fucosylation and sialylation is dependent on the APP and the (patho)physiological state (reviewed in refs. 1 and 3). Therefore, depending on the condition, various glycoforms can be found in serum for each glycosylated APP. Both the occurrence and the concentration of a glycoform can be easily detected by subjecting serum to crossed affinoimmunoelectrophoresis (CAIE) with a specific lectin as affinocomponent in the first dimension gel and a monospecific polyclonal antibody in the second dimension gel (FIG. 2). The degree of retardation of the APP by a lectin in the first electrophoresis direction is indicative for the number of diantennary glycans present on a glycoform (in case of the lectin concanavalin A (Con A)[3,4]), or its degree of fucosylation (in case of *Aleuria aurantia* lectin (AAL)[4,5]). The serum concentrations of the APP glycoforms can be calculated from the areas under the precipitin line. Thus, in the healthy state at least three different glycoforms are detectable for AGP by CAIE with Con A (FIG. 2a), C0, with only tri- and tetraantennary glycans, and C1 and C2 in which one, respectively, two of the glycans are replaced by a diantennary glycan.[3] Within apparently healthy individuals, no significant variation (less than 5%) was found for the relative occurrence of the three glycoforms when measured twice weekly during 1 month, but interindividual differences may occur (FIG. 3) (Van Ommen, E. C. R. and W. van Dijk, unpublished observations). With regard to the

---

[a] This research was supported by grants from the Dutch Organization for Scientific Research (900-523-063 and 900-512-164), from the II Maria Curie Sklodowska Fund (MZ-HHS-92-104), and from KBN (XIII.19).

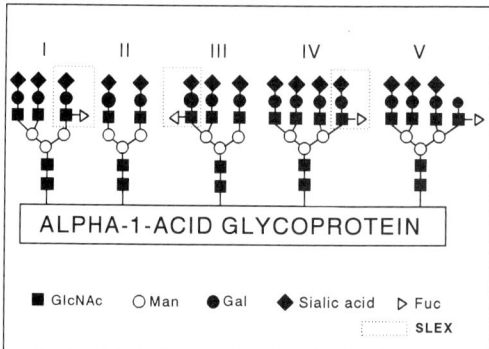

FIGURE 1. Schematic representation of possible glycan chains on AGP. The glycans can be of the diantennary (II), triantennary (I, III), or tetraantennary type (IV, V); the illustration represents only one of the various possible substitutions of AGP with these glycans. Fucosylation of sialylated antennae or branches of the glycans yields the sialyl Lewis^x (SLEX) blood group antigen (encadred structures in I, III, IV). In V the non-sialylated and fucosylated branch represent the Lewis^x (LEX) blood group antigen.

$\alpha 1 \rightarrow 3$-fucosylation of AGP CAIE revealed that one non-fucosylated (A0) and at least four fucosylated glycoforms (A1–A4) were detectable in serum in the healthy state (FIG. 2e). Since each of these glycoforms were present in the C0, C1 and C2 glycoforms (FIG. 4), at least 12 different glycoforms of AGP will be present in serum.[6]

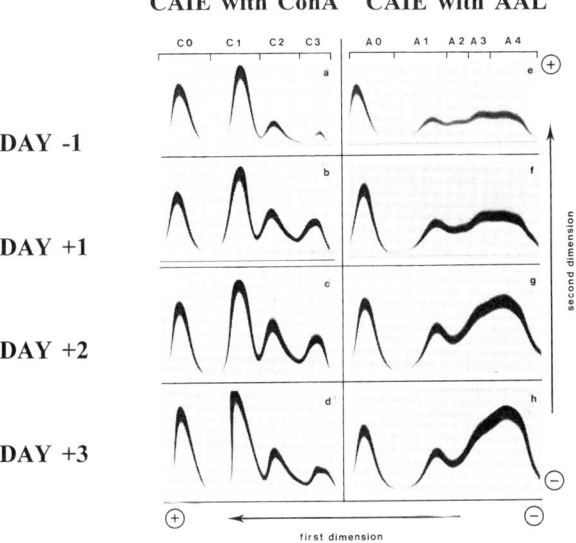

FIGURE 2. Reactivity of AGP with ConA and AAL before and at various days after surgery. Sera were obtained 1 day before **(a,e)**, and **(b,f)**, 2 **(c,g)** and 4 days **(d,h)** after laparotomy for the removal of a benign tumor of the uterus from a furthermore healthy woman. 1 µl serum was subjected to CAIE with Con A **(a–d)** or AAL **(e, f)** in the first-dimension gel, using anti-human AGP IgG for detection. Only the second dimension gels are shown; the application site in the first dimension gel coincides with the right hand side of each figure. C0 and A0, AGP non-reactive with Con A, respectively AAL; C1–C3 and A1–A4, AGP reactive with Con A, respectively, AAL in increasing order of reactivity.

FIGURE 3. Reactivity of AGP with Con A in the healthy state. Values are means ± SD for the sera of apparent healthy women who did (F+, n = 10) or did not use F−, n = 4) oral contraceptives or who were post-menopausal (FM, n = 4), and of apparent healthy men (M, n = 11). The relative distribution of the glycoforms was determined by planimetry of the corresponding surfaces under the precipitin lines.

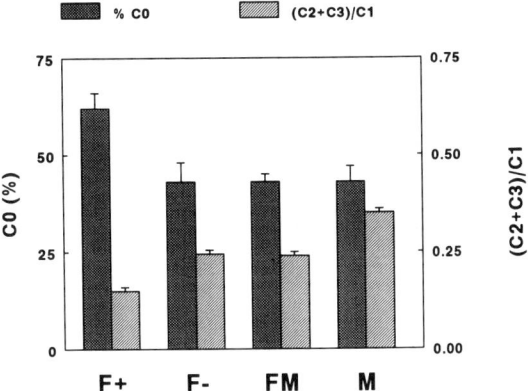

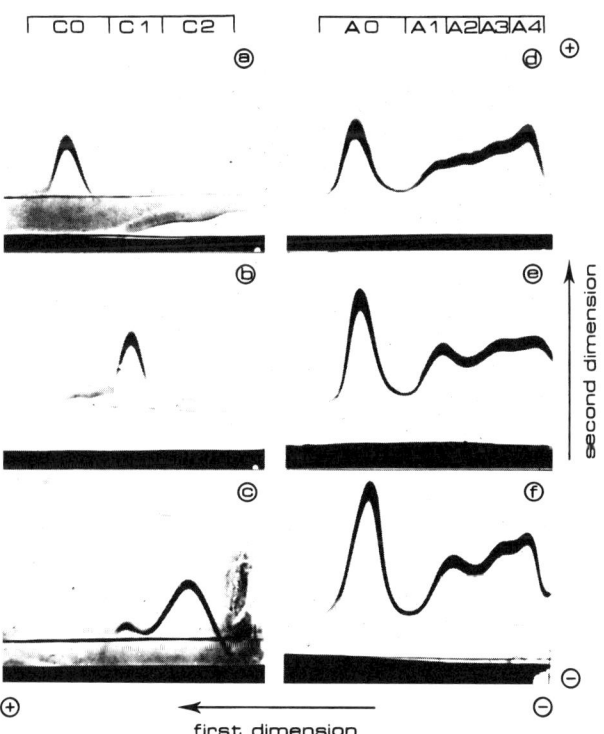

FIGURE 4. AAL reactivities of the C0, C1 and C2 glycoforms of AGP. C0 (**a**), C1 (**b**) and C2 (**c**) were isolated by preparative CAIE with Con A from normal serum human AGP (according to ref. 6), and were subjected to CAIE with AAL (**d–f**).

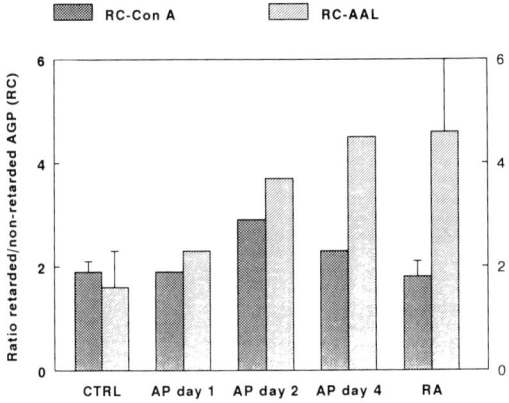

FIGURE 5. Reactivity of AGP with AAL and Con A in acute and chronic inflammation. CTRL, control sera; AP, acute-phase serum at several days after surgery (*cf.* FIG. 2); RA, sera of patients suffering from rheumatoid arthritis; RC, reactivity coefficient.

(Patho)physiological Changes in the Degree of Branching of APP

An acute-phase reaction induces a reversible increase in the diantennary containing glycoforms of APP.[1,2,5,7,8] This is illustrated by the time-dependent changes in the levels of the AGP glycoforms C0–C3 (FIG. 2, b–d) and the ratio $(C1+C2+C3)/C0$ (RC; FIG. 5) in the sera of a patient before and several days after surgery. Remarkably, a reversible decrease in diantennary containing glycoforms of AGP was found during pregnancy[9] and the usage of oral contraceptives (FIG. 2). This is most probably caused by increased plasma levels of estrogen, since treatment of males with this hormone resulted in the same type of changes[9] (Van Ommen, E. C. R. and W. van Dijk, unpublished observations). Decreases in diantennary containing glycoforms of AGP have also been found in rheumatoid arthritis (RA) Grades III and IV.[10] However, a transient increase of these glycoforms was manifest in RA during intercurrent infections (FIG. 6), showing that acute inflammatory conditions can reverse the RA-induced changes in glycosylation of AGP.[11] These results indicate that the factors involved in the induction of the changes in glycosylation are not identical in chronic

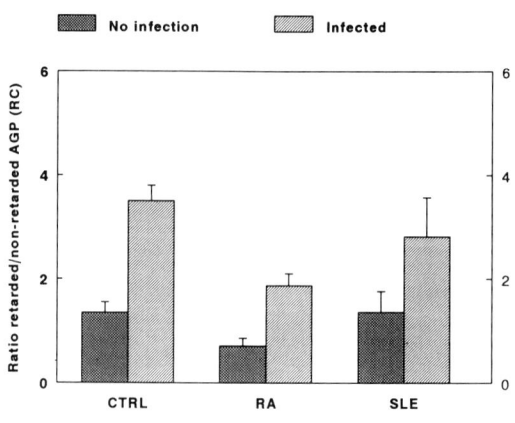

FIGURE 6. Con A reactivity of AGP in intercurrent infections in chronic inflammatory states; SLE, systemic lupus erythemathosis (see legend of FIG. 5 for other abbreviations).

and acute inflammation. Furthermore, additional factors to those regulating the mRNA-induction of AGP, or other routes of signal transduction, seems to be involved in the regulation of the changes, since they accompany, but are not dependent on changes in the concentration of total AGP.

(Patho)physiological Changes in Terminal Glycosylation of APP

The terminal glycosylation of APP investigated by us regards the $\alpha1\rightarrow3$-fucosylation of the Gal$\beta1\rightarrow3/4$GlcNAc (lactosamine) branches[3,5,6,12] and their sialylation[3,5,6,12,13] (cf. FIG. 1). On most APP sialic acid will be present in two types of linkages, $\alpha2\rightarrow3$ and $\alpha2\rightarrow6$ to the galactose residues of the lactosamine units. The presence of $\alpha2\rightarrow3$-linked sialic acid on a fucosylated lactosamine unit will result in the expression of the blood group determinant sialyl Le^x (SLEX; NeuAc$\alpha2\rightarrow3$-Gal$\beta1\rightarrow4$-(Fuc$\alpha1\rightarrow3$)GlcNAc-R). From a biological point of view, the SLEX structure is very important being the ligand for E- and P-selectin in the primary adhesion (rolling) of leukocytes to inflamed endothelium.[14-16] Therefore, it was no surprise that fucosylated structures of the type SLEX were expressed in very low amounts on AGP in control serum, despite the fact that approximately 60% of the AGP molecules were fucosylated to various extents.[3,5] However, increased expression of SLEX, in combination with an elevated fucosylation of AGP (i.e. strongly increased levels of AAL-reactive glycoforms) appeared to occur during acute inflammation.[5,6] This was already apparent at the first day after injury, but maximal values were reached at a later time, and prolonged much longer than the transient increase in diantennary containing glycoforms (FIG. 2, f–h). Although the increases in fucosylation and SLEX content were manifest in all Con A reactive glycoforms of AGP,[5] the extent of fucosylation appeared to be inversely related to the diantennary glycan content (cf. FIG. 4, d,e and f).[6] Increased fucosylation of APP was also detected under chronic inflammatory conditions.[12,17,18] In RA this coincided with increased levels of APP, and for AGP in a lower degree of sialylation.[12,13] A partial reversal of these anomalies was observed in patients responding to the treatment with low-dose methotrexate,[12] giving support to the idea that these changes in glycosylation were induced by chronic inflammatory factors.

Regulation of the Changes in Glycosylation in APP by Cytokines

In principle, changes in type of branching and increased sialylation and fucosylation of APP should have a biosynthetic origin.[19] However, it can not be excluded that differences in turnover of glycoforms, or glycosidases released during inflammation into the circulation[20] may have contributed to the changes found. The liver is the major source of APP, and the inflammation-induced changes in their serum levels result mainly from the effects of cytokines and other humoral factors on their biosynthesis by hepatocytes.[21-23] We have used primary cultures of isolated rat and human hepatocytes, and hepatoma cell lines to show that the changes in glycosylation of APP can have a hepatic origin and that they can be regulated by cytokines, glucocorticoids and growth factors. Indeed, human hepatocytes appeared to be able to secrete all AGP and PI glycoforms that were detectable by CAIE with Con A or AAL in control and patient sera.[24,25] Furthermore, the hepatoma cell lines Hep G2 and Hep 3B were able to secrete the various glycoforms of PI, α_1-antichymotrypsin (ACT), and haptoglobin detectable in human sera with CAIE with Con A.[26-29] Recombinant cytokines, dexamethasone and growth factors, alone and/or in combination, induced

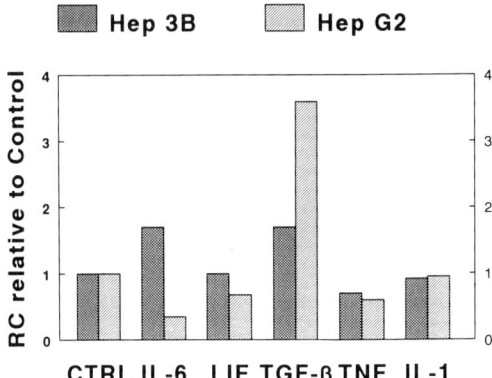

FIGURE 7. Regulation by cytokines of the Con A reactivity of PI in the human hepatoma cell lines Hep 3B and Hep G2. Cells were incubated for 2 days in the presence of IL-6 (50 U/ml), LIF (100 U/ml), TGFβ (10 ng/ml), TNFα (500 U/ml) and IL-1 (200 U/ml) in the presence of 1 μM dexamethasone. The RC's are given relative to control cells incubated in the presence of dexamethasone.

the synthesis and secretion of APP, and could provoke dose-dependent changes in the proportions of their different glycoforms as well.[30]

Detailed information about the inflammatory factors involved in the hepatic regulation of the changes in the proportions of diantennary containing glycoforms of AGP, PI and other APP was obtained in our studies with primary cultures of human hepatocytes and cultures of the human hepatoma cell lines Hep 3B and Hep G2. These studies supported clear evidence that the signal transduction pathways for the regulation of the changes in glycosylation of APP are at least partly independent of those governing protein synthesis. Despite the fact that the factors tested induced increased secretion of APP, or had no effect on it, two different types of change on the branching of the same APP were observed in the various model systems. Thus, the changes in branching induced by IL-6 in human hepatocytes and Hep-3B cells (FIG. 7) resembled those observed in sera of patients with acute inflammatory states, *i.e.* increased levels of the Con A–reactive glycoforms of AGP or PI.[24,26,28,29] The opposite effect was noted, however, for Hep G2 cells exposed to IL-6, leukemia inhibitory factor (LIF) or interferon-γ (FIG. 7), *i.e.* secreted PI displayed the changes observed in sera during pregnancy or in patients with RA grade III or IV.[26–30] On the other hand, exposure

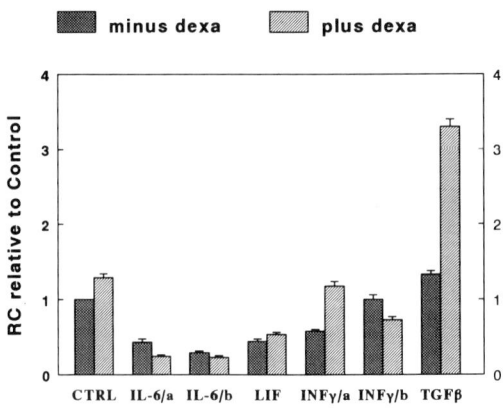

FIGURE 8. Effect of dexamethasone on the cytokine-induced changes in Con A reactivity of PI in Hep G2 cells. Cells were incubated for 2 days in the presence of IL-6 (10 (a) or 100 (b) U/ml), LIF (100 U/ml), TGFβ (2 ng/ml), INFγ (25 (a) or 100 (b) ng/ml) in the presence (plus dexa) or absense (minus dexa) of 1 μM dexamethasone. The RC's are given relative to control cells incubated in the absence of dexamethasone.

FIGURE 9. Effect of TGFβ and dexamethasone on cytokine-induced changes in Con A reactivity of PI in Hep G2 cells. Cells were incubated for 2 days in the presence of IL-6 (100 U/ml), LIF (100 U/ml) or INFγ (25 ng/ml) and, when indicated, TGFβ (2 ng/ml), in the presence (plus dexa) or absence (minus dexa) of 1 μM dexamethasone. The RC's are given relative to control cells incubated in the absence of dexamethasone.

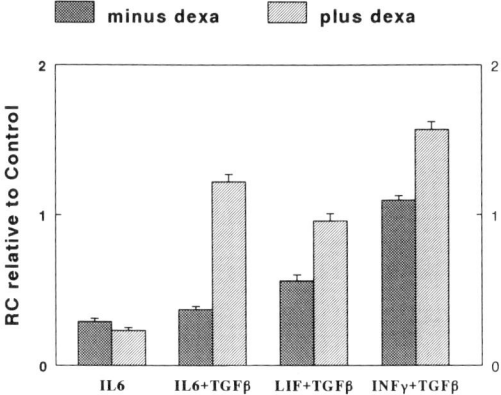

to transforming growth factor-β (TGFβ) and to dexamethasone caused increased secretion of the Con A–reactive glycoforms of PI in both the Hep 3B and the Hep G2 cells, but TNF-α led to a dose-dependent decrease in both cells.[27–30] IL-1 displayed no significant effects on the hepatoma cell lines, but stimulated the Con A reactivity of AGP secreted by human hepatocytes.[24,30]

The effects of cytokines on human hepatocytes were only found in the presence of dexamethasone. Although the effects of cytokines on Hep G2 cells were displayed without addition of the hormone, the concomitant exposure of these cells to dexamethasone did influence their inducing effects (FIG. 8). The specific induction of the Con A–reactive glycoforms of PI exerted by dexamethasone alone, strongly augmented the same effect of TGFβ in binary and also in more complex combinations with other cytokines[29] (FIGS. 8 and 9). Furthermore, dexamethasone appeared to antagonize the opposite actions of LIF and INFγ, but this effect could be overruled, in a dose-dependent way, by increasing their concentrations. Remarkably, dexamethasone further augmented the IL-6–induced decrease in Con A reactive glycoforms of PI. However, this action of dexamethasone was completely overruled by also exposing the Hep G2 cells to TGFβ (FIG. 9). This finding clearly illustrates that dexamethasone and TGFβ affect the glycosylation of PI along different routes, although, when present alone, they both exerted the same effect. The results further show, that the effects on the glycosylation of APP are strongly dependent on the composition of mixtures of cytokines, growth factors and hormones and their relative concentrations. This would explain the different glycosylation of APP observed under chronic and acute inflammatory conditions *in vivo*.

Effects of cytokines on changes in fucosylation and sialylation have not yet been thoroughly studied. Different fucosylated glycoforms of AGP are secreted by isolated human hepatocytes (FIG. 10), and increased fucosylation of PI and α_1-antichymotrypsin has been observed in Hep G2 cells [unpublished results].

MECHANISM OF ACTION

The biosynthesis of glycans is a post-translational multistep enzymatic process involving a series of highly specific glycosyltransferases and glycosidases.[19] Branching of N-linked glycans is regulated by at least four different GlcNAc transferases (GNTase), of which GNTase IV and V catalyze the formation of tri- and tetraantennary glycans.[31,32] Studies with liver cells have been hampered by difficulties in the assessment of these enzyme activities in hepatocytes, but changes have been noted in

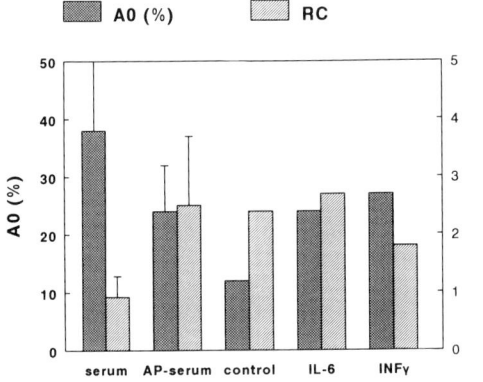

FIGURE 10. AAL reactivity of AGP secreted by monolayer cultures of human hepatocytes. Human hepatocytes were isolated and cultured as described,[8] in the presence of 10 μM dexamethasone for 72 hours and, when indicated, with IL-6 or INFγ (experiments performed in duplicate). The values for normal healthy serum (serum; = 8) and acute-phase serum (AP-serum; n = 7) are presented for purpose of reference (mean ± SD).

other components of the posttranslational biosynthetic pathways in the liver during inflammation.[2,33-36] Furthermore, Nakao et al.[37] have demonstrated that IL-6 can stimulate the activities of GNTase IV and V in human myeloma cells, resulting in an increased expression of tri- and tetraantennary glycans on the membrane-bound glycoproteins. Therefore, it is likely that inflammatory conditions will also affect the expression of glycosyltransferases in liver cells. Indeed, IL-6 and dexamethasone have been shown to regulate the expression and secretion of α2→6-sialyltransferase in rat and human hepatocytes.[20,35] This enzyme is involved in the sialylation of APP, but might also influence the fucosylation and the expression of SLEX-type structures on APP, because the action of α2→6-sialyltransferase is mutually exclusive to the actions of α2→3-sialyltransferase (sialic acidα2→3Gal-) and α1→3-fucosyltransferase (Fucα1→3GlcNAc-).[32,38] In addition, the branch specificities of these glycosyltransferases are non-identical, which results in differences in the terminal glycosylation of di-, and tri-, and tetraantennary glycans.[39] In conclusion, it is to be expected that the effects of cytokines, growth factors and glucocorticoids are exerted via changes in the expression of a small number of glycosyltransferases in the hepatocyte.

CONCLUDING REMARKS

Inflammation-induced changes in the glycosylation of APP occur throughout the animal kingdom and, therefore, appear to be an essential phenomenon in the general inflammatory reaction. These changes occur on several APP at approximately the same time. This will lead to a completely different carbohydrate-phenotype for the majority of the plasma proteins. Dependent on the state of inflammation—and thus on the temporary mixture of cytokines, glucocorticoids and growth factors—the plasma glycoproteins will express predominantly certain glycan chains, e.g., diantennary glycans in the early phase of acute inflammation, or highly fucosylated tri- or tetraantennary glycans towards the end of that condition, and in RA. These types of glycan structures play crucial roles in a number of biological processes, of which the selectin-mediated interaction between leukocytes and endothelial cells is manifest during acute as well as chronic inflammatory states.[14-16,40] Indeed, we and others have shown that AGP can modulate the immune system,[41-47] e.g., (i) inhibition of T-cell proliferation, and (ii) induction of an IL-1 inhibitor in macrophages. These effects are concentration dependent, reach optima in the physiological range of concentrations, and in many cases involve the carbohydrate portion of the molecule. The inflammation-induced expression of SLEX on AGP may result in a competition of AGP with the selectin-mediated influx of leukocytes into inflamed areas.[5,17,48] So, it is tempting to speculate that the cytokine-induced changes in glycosylation represent a humoral feed-back response of the hepatic acute-phase reaction to dampen down oligosaccharide-dependent cellular inflammatory reactions.

SUMMARY

The plasma levels and the glycosylation of acute-phase proteins (APP) are subject to marked changes during acute and chronic inflammation. The pathophysiological variations in different glycoforms of APP in serum most likely result from changes in the glycosylation process during their biosynthesis in the parenchymal cells of the liver. This is suggested from *in vitro* studies with isolated hepatocytes and hepatoma cell lines. Inflammatory cytokines appear to regulate the changes in glycosylation independent from the rate of synthesis of the APP. In addition, other humoral factors like corticosteroids and growth factors are involved. The interplay of these factors is determined by the stage of the disease (as in rheumatoid arthritis) or the physiological situation (as in pregnancy). The changes in glycosylation of specific APP might affect the operation of the immune system.

REFERENCES

1. TURNER, G. A. 1992. N-Glycosylation of serum proteins in disease and its investigation using lectins. Clin. Chim. Acta. **208:** 149–171.
2. VAN DIJK, W., G. A. TURNER & A. MACKIEWICZ. 1994. Changes in glycosylation of acute-phase proteins in health and disease: occurrence, regulation and function. Glycosyl. Disease **1:** 5–14.
3. BIERHUIZEN, M. F. A., M. DE WIT, C. A. R. L. GOVERS, W. FERWERDA, C. KOELEMAN, O. POS & W. VAN DIJK. 1988. Glycosylation of three molecular forms of human α_1-acid glycoprotein having different interactions with concanavalin A. Variations in the occurrence of di-, tri-, and tetraantenary glycans and the degree of sialylation. Eur. J Biochem. **175:** 387–394.
4. DEBRAY, H. & J. MONTREUIL. 1992. Specificity of lectins toward oligosaccharidic sequences belonging to N- and O-glycosylproteins. *In* Affinity Electrophoresis: Principles and Application. J. Breborowicz & A. Mackiewicz, Eds.: 23–57. Boca Raton, FL: CRC Press.
5. DE GRAAF, T. W., M. E. VAN DER STELT, M. G. ANBERGEN & W. VAN DIJK. 1993. Inflammation-induced expression of sialyl Lewis X-containing glycan structures on α_1-acid glycoprotein (orosomucoid) in human sera. J. Exp. Med. **177:** 657–666.
6. VAN DER LINDEN, E. C. M., T. W. DE GRAAF, M. G. ANBERGEN, R. M. DEKKER, E. C. R. VAN OMMEN, D. H. VAN DEN EIJNDEN & W. VAN DIJK. 1994. Preparative affinity electrophoresis of different glycoforms of serum glycoproteins. Application for the study of inflammation induced expression of sialyl-Lewis^x groups on alpha1-acid glycoprotein (orosomucoid). Glycosyl. Disease. **1:** 45–52.
7. NICOLLET, I., J.-P. LEBRETON, M. FONTAINE & M. HIRON. 1981. Evidence for α_1-acid glycoprotein populations of different pI values after Concanavalin A affinity chromatography. Study of their evolution during inflammation in man. Biochim. Biophys. Acta. **668:** 235–245.
8. POS, O., M. E., VAN DER STELT, G.-J. WOLBINK, N. W. M. NIJSTEN, G. L. VAN DER TEMPEL & W. VAN DIJK. 1990. Changes in the serum concentration and the glycosyla-

tion of human α_1-acid glycoprotein and α_1-protease inhibitor in severely burned patients: Relation to interleukin-6 levels. Clin. Exp. Immunol. **82:** 579–582.
9. WELLS, C., T. C. BØG-HANSEN, E. H. COOPER & M. R. CLASS. 1981. The use of Concanavalin A crossed immuno-affinoelectrophoresis to detect hormone-associated variations in α_1-acid glycoprotein. Clin. Chim. Acta. **109:** 59–67.
10. MACKIEWICZ, A., T. PAWLOWSKI, A. MACKIEWICZ-PAWLOWSKI, K. WIKTOROWICZ, & S. MACKIEWICZ. 1987. Microheterogeneity forms of α_1-acid glycoprotein as indicators of rheumatoid arthritis activity. Clin. Chim. Acta **163:** 185–190.
11. PAWLOWSKI, T., S. H. MACKIEWICZ & A. MACKIEWICZ. 1989. Microheterogeneity of α_1-acid glycoprotein in the detection of intercurrent infection in patients with rheumatoid arthritis. Arthr. Rheum. **32:** 347–351.
12. DE GRAAF, T. W., E. C. R. VAN OMMEN, M. E. VAN DER STELT, P. J. S. M. KERSTENS, A. M. TH. BOERBOOMS & W. VAN DIJK. 1994. Effects of low-dose methotrexate therapy on the concentration and the glycosylation of α_1-acid glycoprotein in the serum of rheumatoid arthritis patients: A longitudinal study. J. Rheumatol.:2209–2216.
13. PAWLOWSKI, T. & A. MACKIEWICZ. 1989. Minor microheterogeneity of alpha1-acid glycoprotein in rheumatoid arthritis. *In* Alpha1-acid glycoprotein: Genetics, biochemistry, physiological functions and pharmacology. P. Baumann, *et al.*, Eds.: 223–226. New York: A. R. Liss.
14. VARKI, A. 1993. Biological roles of oligosaccharides: All of the theories are correct. Glycobiology **3:** 97–130.
15. SHIMIZU, Y., W. NEWMAN, Y. TANAKA & S. SHAW. 1992. Lymphocyte interactions with endothelial cells. Immunol. Today **13:** 106–111.
16. LASKY, L. A. 1992. Selectins: Interpreters of cell-specific carbohydrate information during inflammation. Science **258:** 964–969.
17. VAN DER LINDEN, E. C. M., T. W. DE GRAAF, M. G. ANBERGEN, E. C. R. VAN OMMEN, M. E. VAN DER STELT & W. VAN DIJK. 1993. Expression of (sialyl)-Lewis X groups on human α_1-acid glycoprotein in acute and chronic inflammation. Glycoconjugate J. **10:** 316–317.
18. HAVENAAR, E. C., J. P. H. DRENTH, E. C. R. VAN OMMEN, J. W. M. VAN DER MEER & W. VAN DIJK. 1994. Glycosylation of α_1-acid glycoprotein in hyperimmunoglobulinemia D and periodic fever syndrome: Evidence for persistent inflammation. Clin. Immunol. Immunopathol. In press.
19. SCHACHTER, H. 1991. The yellow brick road to branched complex N-glycans. Glycobiology **1:** 453–461.
20. WOLOSKI, B. M. R. N. J., E. GOSPODAREK & J. C. JAMIESON. 1985. Studies on monokines as mediators of the acute-phase response. Effects on sialyltransferase, α_1-acid glycoprotein and β-N-acetylhexosaminidase. Biochem. Biophys. Res. Commun. **130:** 30–36.
21. SCHREIBER, G. & A. R. ALDRED. 1993. Extrahepatic synthesis of acute-phase proteins. *In* Acute-phase Proteins. Molecular Biology, Biochemistry and Clinical Applications A. Mackiewicz, I. Kushner & H. Baumann, Eds.: 39–76. Boca Raton, FL: CRC Press.
22. KUSHNER, I. & A. MACKIEWICZ. 1993. The acute phase response: An overview. *In* Acute-phase Proteins. Molecular Biology, Biochemistry and Clinical Applications A. Mackiewicz, I. Kushner & H. Baumann, Eds.: 3–19. Boca Raton, FL: CRC Press.
23. KOJ, A., J. GAULDIE & H. BAUMANN. 1993. Biological perspective of cytokine and hormone networks. *In* Acute-phase Proteins. Molecular Biology, Biochemistry and Clinical Applications. A. Mackiewicz, I. Kushner & H. Baumann, Eds.: 275–287. Boca Raton, FL: CRC Press.
24. POS, O., H. J. MOSHAGE, S.-H. YAP, J. P. M. SNIEDERS, L. A. AARDEN, J. VAN GOOL, W. BOERS, A. M. BRUGMAN & W. VAN DIJK. 1989. Effects of monocytic products, recombinant interleukin-1 and recombinant interleukin-6 on the glycosylation of α_1-acid glycoprotein: Studies with primary human hepatocyte cultures and rats. Inflammation **13:** 415–424.
25. VAN DIJK, W., O. POS, M. E. VAN DER STELT, H. J. MOSHAGE, S. H. YAP, L. DENTE, P. BAUMANN & C. B. EAP. 1991. Inflammation-induced changes in expression and glycosylation of genetic variants of α_1-acid glycoprotein (AGP): Studies with human sera, primary cultures of human hepatocytes and transgenic mice. Biochem. J. **276:** 343–347.

26. MACKIEWICZ, A., M. K. GANAPATHI & I. KUSHNER. 1987. Monokines regulate glycosylation of acute-phase proteins. J. Exp. Med. **166:** 253–258.
27. MACKIEWICZ, A. & I. KUSHNER. 1989. Interferon beta2/B-cell stimulating factor 2/interleukin 6 affects glycosylation of acute phase proteins in human hepatoma cell lines. Scand. J. Immunol. **29:** 265–271.
28. MACKIEWICZ, A. & I. KUSHNER. 1990. Transforming growth factor beta1 influences glycosylation of α_1-protease inhibitor in human hepatoma cell lines. Inflammation **14:** 485–487.
29. MACKIEWICZ, A., M. LACIK, G. GORNY & H. BAUMANN. 1993. Leukemia inhibitory factor, interferon gamma, and dexamethasone regulate N-glycosylation of α_1-protease inhibitor. Eur. J. Cell Biol. **60:** 331–336.
30. VAN DIJK, W. & A. MACKIEWICZ. 1993. Control of glycosylation alterations of acute-phase glycoproteins. *In* Acute-phase Proteins. Molecular Biology, Biochemistry and Clinical Applications. A. Mackiewicz, I. Kushner & H. Baumann, Eds.: 39–76. Boca Raton, FL: CRC Press.
31. PAULSON, J. C. & K. J. COLLEY. 1989. Glycosyltransferases: Structure, localization, and control of cell-type-specific glycosylation. J. Biol. Chem. **264:** 17615–17618.
32. VAN DEN EIJNDEN, D. H. & D. H. JOZIASSE. 1993. Enzymes associated with glycosylation. Curr. Opin. Struct. Biol. **3:** 711–721.
33. LOMBART, C., J. STURGESS & H. SCHACHTER. 1980. The effect of turpentine-induced inflammation on rat liver glycosyltransferases and Golgi complex ultrastructure. Biochim. Biophys. Acta **629:** 1–12.
34. KAPLAN, H. A., B. M. R. N. J. WOLOSKI, M. HELLMAN & J. C. JAMIESON. 1983. Studies on the effect of inflammation on rat liver and serum sialyltransferase. Evidence that inflammation causes release of Galβ1→4GlcNAc α2→6-sialyltransferase from rat liver. J. Biol. Chem. **258:** 11505–11509.
35. VAN DIJK, W., W. BOERS, W. SALA, A.-M. LASTHUIS & S. MOOKERJEA. 1986. Activity and secretion of sialyltransferase in primary monolayer cultures of rat hepatocytes cultured with and without dexamethasone. Biochem. Cell Biol. **64:** 79–84.
36. LAMMERS, G. & J. C. JAMIESON. 1988. The role of a cathepsin D-like activity in the release of Galβ1-4GlcNAc α2→6-sialyltransferase from rat liver Golgi membranes during the acute-phase response. Biochem. J. **256:** 623–631.
37. NAKAO, H., A. NISHIKAWA, T. KARASUNO, *et al.* 1990. Regulation of N-acetylglucosaminyltransferase III, IV and V activities and alteration of the surface oligosaccharide structure of a myeloma cell line by interleukin 6. Biochem. Biophys. Res. Commun. **172:** 1260–1266.
38. DE VRIES, T. & D. H. VAN DEN EIJNDEN. 1992. Occurrence and specificities of α3-fucosyltransferases. Histochem. J. **24:** 761–770.
39. NEMANSKY, M. & D. H. VAN DEN EIJNDEN. 1993. Enzymatic characterization of CMP-NeuAc:Galβ1→4GlcNAc-R α2→3-sialyltransferase from human placenta. Glyco. J. **10:** 99–108.
40. KOBATA, A. 1992. Structures and functions of the sugar chains of glycoproteins. Eur. J. Biochem. **209:** 483–501.
41. BENNETT, M. & K. SCHMID. 1980. Immunosuppression by human plasma α_1-acid glycoprotein: Importance of the carbohydrate moiety. Proc. Natl. Acad. Sci. USA **77:** 6109–6113.
42. CHIU, K. M., R. F. MORTENSEN, A. P. OSMAND & H. GERWURZ. 1979. Interactions of α_1-acid glycoprotein with the immune system. I. Purification and effects upon lymphocyte responsiveness. Immunology **32:** 997–1005.
43. COSTELLO, M., B. A. FIEDEL & H. GEWURZ. 1979. Inhibition of platelet aggregation by native and desialised α_1-acid glycoprotein. Nature **281:** 677–678.
44. DIRIENZO, W., G. F. STEFANINI, L. MIRIBEL, E. E. PAULLING, G. W. CANONICA & H. H. FUDENBERG. 1987. α_1-Acid glycoprotein on the membrane of human lymphocytes: Possible involvement in cellular activation. Immunol. Lett. **15:** 167–170.
45. POS, O., R. A. J. OOSTENDORP, M. E. VAN DER STELT, R. J. SCHEPER & W. VAN DIJK. 1990. Con A-nonreactive human α_1-acid glycoprotein (AGP) is more effective in modulation of lymphocyte proliferation than Con A-reactive AGP serum variants. Inflammation **14:** 133–141.

46. LYUTOV, A. G., V. A. ALESHKIN, L. I. NOVICOVA & A. L. PUKHALSKY. 1992. The influence of different forms of orosomucoid on immune reaction. Folia Histochem. Cytobiol. **30:** 211–212.
47. BORIES, P. N., J FEGER, N. BENBERNOU, J.-D. ROUZEAU, J. AGNERAY & G. DURAND. 1990. Prevalence of tri- and tetraantennary glycans of human α_1-acid glycoprotein in release of macrophage inhibitor of interleukin-1 activity. Inflammation **14:** 315–323.
48. WALZ, G., A. ARUFFO, W. KOLANUS, M. BEVILACQUA & B. SEED. 1990. Recognition by ELAM-1 of the sialyl-LeX determinant on myeloid and tumor cells. Science **250:** 1132–1134.

Co-ordinate Inhibition of the Production of TNF, IL-1, and IL-6 by Small Molecules

ANTHONY C. ALLISON

Dawa Corporation
2513 Hastings Drive
Belmont, California 94002

ELSIE M. EUGUI

Synthex Discovery Research
Palo Alto, California 94304

INTRODUCTION

TNF-α, IL-1β and IL-6 are major cytokines produced by cells of monocyte-macrophage lineage, although IL-6 is also produced by other cell types. It is generally accepted that TNF and IL-1 are proinflammatory. These cytokines induce the expression on endothelial cells of adhesion molecules that recruit leukocytes,[1] and they induce expression, in several cell types, of genes for phospholipases and cyclooxygenases required for production of lipid mediators of inflammation.[2] TNF-α and IL-1 augment expression in connective tissue type cells of neutral metalloproteinases that can degrade cartilage and bone matrix.[3]

The role of IL-6 in inflammation is less well defined. However, IL-6 is a co-factor in T-lymphocyte differentiation[4] as well as in the production of immunoglobulins by synovial tissue from patients with rheumatoid arthritis.[5] In this disease activated T-lymphocytes[6] and immune complexes[7] are thought to play a pathogenetic role. Furthermore, IL-6 augments degradation of bone induced by IL-1 and TNF,[8] and could contribute to bone erosion in rheumatoid arthritis and periodontal disease.[9]

The clinical benefits that might result from inhibiting the production and/or action of TNF-α and Il-1β are obvious. Attempts have been made to do this by the use of monoclonal antibodies against the cytokines, recombinant soluble receptors or recombinant IL-1 receptor antagonist (IL-1ra). Such experiments have provided valuable information about the roles of TNF-α and IL-1β in several experimental animal models of inflammation and septic shock. In some clinical trials (rheumatoid arthritis, Crohn's disease) promising results have been obtained, although in other trials (septic shock) the results have been disappointing. In any case, treatment requires large amounts of antibodies or recombinant proteins, which are expensive. The proteins must be administered by injection, and there is always the possibility that monoclonal antibodies will elicit anti-immunoglobulin responses.

For these reasons several laboratories have initiated research programs directed towards the identification of small molecules that inhibit the production and/or effects of TNF-α and IL-1β. By "small molecule" we mean a synthetic organic compound of relative molecular mass 400 or less, which is not a natural product such as a peptide, lipid or sugar. A drug suppressing the production of these cytokines might be useful as an anti-inflammatory agent lacking the gastrointestinal side effects of cyclooxygenase inhibitors and the many side effects of glucocorticoids. Several isolated reports of

TABLE 1. Inhibition by antioxidants of the Production of TNF-α and IL-1 in Monocytes and Macrophages

Cells Used	Compound	Cytokine Tested	References
Murine macrophages	Butylated hydroxyanisole	TNF	13
Murine macrophages	Probucol	IL-1	14
THP-1	Probucol α-tocopherol	IL-1β	15
Monocytes	N-acetylcysteine	TNF	16
Human whole blood	Dimethylsulfoxide, mannitol	IL-8	17

compounds inhibiting the production of these TNF-α or IL-1β have been published. During the past few years more systematic studies have identified drugs that inhibit the production of both TNF-α and IL-1β at the levels of transcription[10] or translation.[11] Our strategy has been to identify antioxidants which inhibit the activation of transcription factors which are required for the induced expression of the TNF-α, IL-1β and IL-6 genes in cells of the monocyte-macrophage lineage.[10] The same compounds do not inhibit the formation of IL-6 in fibroblasts, and they augment the expression of the gene for IL-1ra in monocytes.[12] Thus the effects of the drugs are both gene selective and cell-type selective, which is desirable therapeutically.

INHIBITION BY ANTIOXIDANTS OF THE TRANSCRIPTION OF GENES FOR PRO-INFLAMMATORY CYTOKINES

Several reports were published on the inhibitory effects of antioxidants on the production of individual cytokines by LPS-activated mouse peritoneal macrophages, human monocytes, THP-1 cells and human whole blood[13-17] (TABLE 1). We investigated the phenomenon systematically, comparing effects of different types of antioxidants on the production of TNF-α, IL-1β and IL-6 in cultured human peripheral blood mononuclear cells (PBM) activated by LPS and in other ways.[10] Some antioxidants, but not others, were found to be potent inhibitors of the production of all three cytokines. The molecular basis of antioxidant-mediated inhibition was analyzed, showing that antioxidants can inhibit the activation of transcription factors NF-κB and AP-1 and the transcription of cytokine genes. The *in vitro* observations were then confirmed by *in vivo* experiments in mice.

Initially a series of compounds was tested for capacity to inhibit the production of IL-1β in LPS-stimulated human peripheral blood mononuclear cell (PBM) cultures. Tetrahydropapaveroline (THP), a tetrahydroisoquinoline derivative, was found to be a potent inhibitor of IL-1β production (IC$_{50}$ about 1.5 μM, FIG. 1). Because they are structurally related to THP, 10,11-dihydroxyaporphine (apomorphine) and norapomorphine were tested, and found to inhibit IL-1 production efficiently (TABLE 2). The R(+) and R(−) stereoisomers of dihydroxyaporphine were equipotent in this assay, showing separation from dopamine against activity.

Antioxidants with widely different structures were then tested for capacity to inhibit the production of IL-1β in LPS-activated human PBM. IL-1β released into culture supernatants, as well as cell-associated protein (cell lysates) were evaluated using a two-site ELISA assay. Several moderately lipophilic antioxidants, including butylated hydroxyanisole (BHA) and nordihydroguaiaretic acid (NDGA), were found to be potent inhibitors of IL-1β production (IC$_{50}$ 4 μM or lower, TABLE 2).

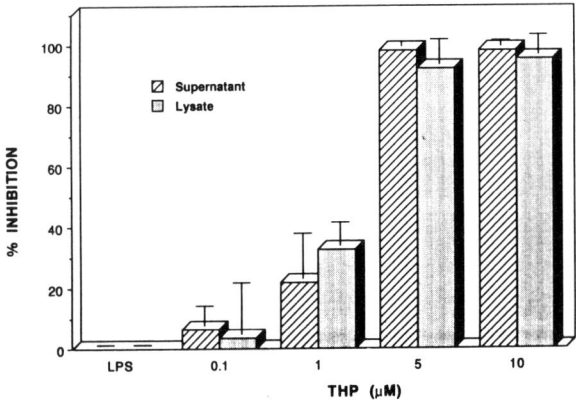

FIGURE 1. Dose-dependent inhibition by tetrahydropapaveroline (THP) of the production of IL-1β in human peripheral blood mononuclear cells activated by LPS. Means and standard errors of intracellular (lysate) and extracellular cytokines are shown.[10]

NDGA is an inhibitor of 5-lipoxygenase, as well as of lipid peroxidation. However, another redox 5-lipoxygenase inhibitor, Zileuton, did not affect IL-1β formation, suggesting that 5-lipoxygenase products are not involved in the signal transduction system leading to cytokine production in LPS-activated monocytes.

The more hydrophilic antioxidants tested, ascorbic acid and trolox, had no effect on IL-1β production in concentrations up to 200 μM. Mannitol, a hydroxyl radical scavenger, was inactive at 100 mM concentration. The same was true of the physiological lipophilic antioxidant α-tocopherol, as well as some classical antioxidants—butylated hydroxytoluene (BHT), quercetin and N,N'-diphenyl-p-phenylene diamine. N-

TABLE 2. Antioxidants Vary Widely in Potency as Inhibitors of Cytokine Formation[10]

High Activity	(IC$_{50}$ μM)
butylated hydroxyanisole (BHA)	2.9
tetrahydropapaveroline (THP)	1.0
apomorphine	2.6
norapomorphine	1.6
nordihydroguaiauretic acid (NDGA)	1.3
mepacrine	3.0
Low Activity (insignificant inhibition in the range 50–200 μM)	
atascorbic acid	
α-tocopherol	
mannitol	
trolox	
butylated hydroxytoluene (BHT)	
quercetin	
N,N'-diphenyl-p-phenylene diamine	
zileuton (5-lipoxygenase inhibitor)	

acetylcysteine had some inhibitory effect (IC_{50} 42 mM) but this was much lower than that of several lipophilic antioxidants (TABLE 2).

The question arose whether the inhibitory effect of THP is selective for the signaling pathway initiated by LPS or applies also to other effective inducers, such as silica and *Staphylococcus aureus* Cowan I (Pansorbin). THP proved to be equally potent in the inhibition of IL-1β production with all inducers tested. The drug also inhibited IL-1β production using a weaker inducer, Zymosan. These observations show that THP can inhibit the production of IL-1β by human PBM stimulated with several inducers. Similar observations were made with other antioxidants.

THP was also used to analyze the reversibility of the inhibitory effect. Adherent PHM were cultured with LPS and THP for two hours and repeatedly washed. Fresh medium containing the same amount of LPS was added and the cultures were incubated overnight. Duplicate cultures were maintained with LPS and THP for the same period without washing. Removal of the drug did not reverse its inhibitory effect, so the inhibition of IL-1β production by THP appears to be irreversible, at least until protein synthesis replaces inactivated molecules.

Tested in parallel with inhibition of cytokine synthesis, THP, 10,11-dihydroxyaporphine and BHA did not inhibit protein synthesis, as shown by incorporation of labeled leucine. Emetine, which is structurally related to THP, strongly inhibited protein synthesis in parallel experiments using monocytes.

BHA, THP, 10,11-dihydroxyaporphine and NDGA were further tested for effects

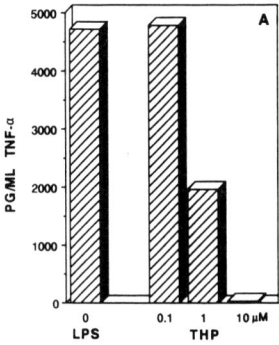

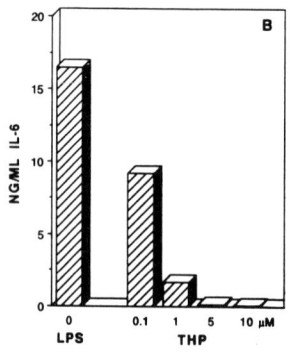

FIGURE 2. Dose-dependent inhibition by tetrahydropapaveroline (THP) of the production of TNF-α and of IL-6 by human peripheral blood mononuclear cells activated by LPS. Cytokines in the supernatant were assayed.[10]

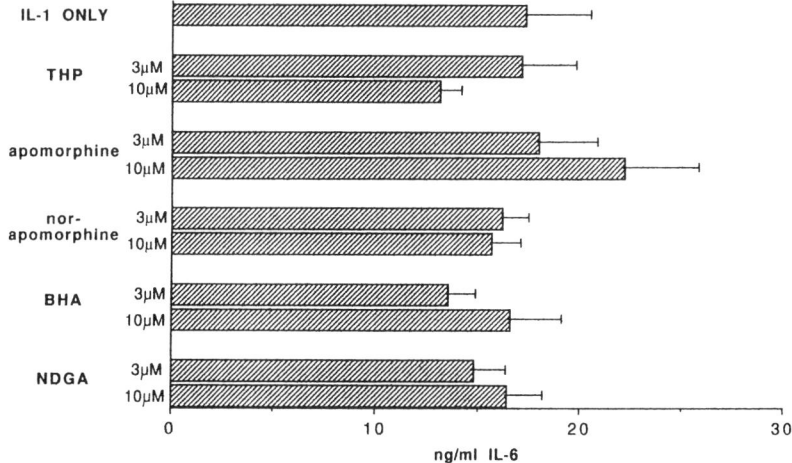

FIGURE 3. Lack of effect of antioxidants on the production of IL-6 in human dermal fibroblasts induced by IL-1β.[10]

on production of TNF-α and IL-6 by LPS-stimulated human PBM. All three compounds were found to be approximately equipotent as inhibitors of the production of the three cytokines (FIG. 2).

To ascertain whether this effect is exerted in all cell types, human dermal fibroblasts and fibroblast-type cells from synovial tissue of patients with rheumatoid arthritis were studied. In these cells IL-1 induces the production of IL-6. THP, BHA, 10,11-dihydroxyaporphine and norapomorphine, in concentrations higher than required to inhibit totally the production of IL-6 in PBM, had no demonstrable effect on IL-6 production in fibroblasts (FIG. 3). Thus antioxidant-mediated inhibition of cytokine production does not occur in all cell types.

Some of the compounds in TABLE 2 were selected for analysis of *in vivo* effects on cytokine production. Two different assays were used. In the first assay IL-1β production was measured using elicited peritoneal cells from mice, four hours after LPS challenge. The cytokine was measured in lysates of cells directly recovered from the peritoneal cavity (cell-associated IL-1β), as well as in the supernatants of cells after overnight culture (released IL-1β). Mice were pretreated with two doses of either THP or 10,11-dihydroxyaporphine (apomorphine, 50 mg/kg/dose) before LPS challenge (15 μg/mouse). The drugs were found to suppress the production of IL-1β by 53 to 86%.[10]

In the second assay, TNF-α and IL-1β were measured in serum following a lethal challenge with LPS (200 μg/mouse). Levels of TNF-α in circulating blood peak about 1½ hours and those of IL-1β 4 hours after LPS injection. Subcutaneous administration of a single dose of 10,11-dihydroxyaporphine, (100 mg/kg), given 30 minutes before challenge, inhibited TNF-α production by 95% (FIG. 4). Before IL-1β peak level, mice were given a second dose of dihydroxyaporphine (50 mg/kg), 2 hours after LPS and 2 hours before blood sampling. This treatment reduced the circulating levels of IL-1β by 88% (FIG. 4).[10] Thus *in vivo* cytokine production is strongly inhibited by THP and by dihydroxyaporphine.

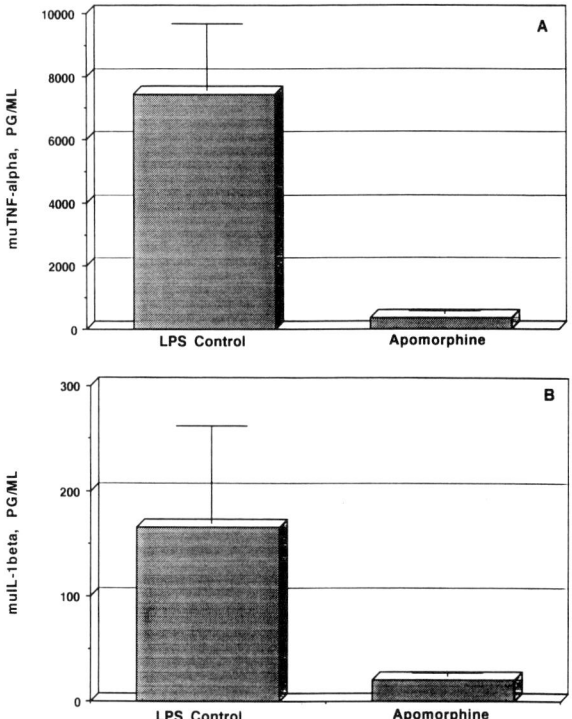

FIGURE 4. Apomorphine (10,11-dihydroxyaporphine) treatment of mice markedly decreases levels of TNF-α and of IL-1β in the circulation after challenge with LPS.[10]

MOLECULAR BIOLOGICAL EFFECTS OF ANTIOXIDANTS

To analyze the mechanism by which antioxidants suppress cytokine formation, levels of cytokine mRNAs were determined in LPS-stimulated PBM.[10] Previous studies had demonstrated that LPS markedly increases IL-1β mRNA. LPS also increases levels of TNF-α, IL-6 and IL-8 mRNAs in PBM. The antioxidants tested decreased TNF-α, IL-1β, and IL-6 mRNA levels to baseline expression, but had less effect on IL-8 mRNA.

To ascertain whether these effects are due to changes in transcription or changes in mRNA stability, nuclear transcription assays were performed. LPS markedly stimulated transcription of the IL-1β gene, and THP antagonized the stimulatory effect of LPS on transcription. In view of observations that antioxidants decrease AP-1 activity, one of the reference messages studied was *c-fos*. However, no effect of THP on transcription of the *c-fos* gene could be detected.

The experiments just described suggested that antioxidants inhibit LPS-stimulated transcription of some cytokine genes. To ascertain whether this is correlated with inhibited activation of transcription factors, electrophoretic mobility shift assays were performed. NF-κB and AP-1 were analyzed first because of reports that they are subject to redox regulation.[18–21] As shown in FIGURE 5, nuclear extracts of unstimulated PBM show NF-κB activity, which increases following LPS stimulation. Specificity of binding was shown by competition with unlabeled oligonucleotides. When PBM were treated with THP, in the presence or absence of LPS, nuclear NF-κB activity was markedly decreased or eliminated altogether. A higher concentration of THP did not affect the binding of NF-κB proteins to the DNA conserved sequence. Similar observations were made with AP-1.[10] Thus THP inhibited activation of NF-κB and AP-1 in intact cells but had no effect on the binding of these transcription complexes to cognate DNA recognition sequences. In cells treated with THP, no effect on several other transcription factors (SP-1, CRE, CTF/NF-1, OCT) could be demonstrated. Inhibition by antioxidants of the activation of transcription factors, including NF-κB and AP-1, could explain their suppression of cytokine gene transcription.

It is generally accepted that a *c-fos* serum responsive element and NF-κB play major roles in promoting expression of the IL-6 gene.[22] At least one member of the NF-IL-6 transcription factor complex also associates with the p50 subunit of NF-κB.[23] Evidence implicating κB sequences in LPS-induced expression of the TNF-α gene in

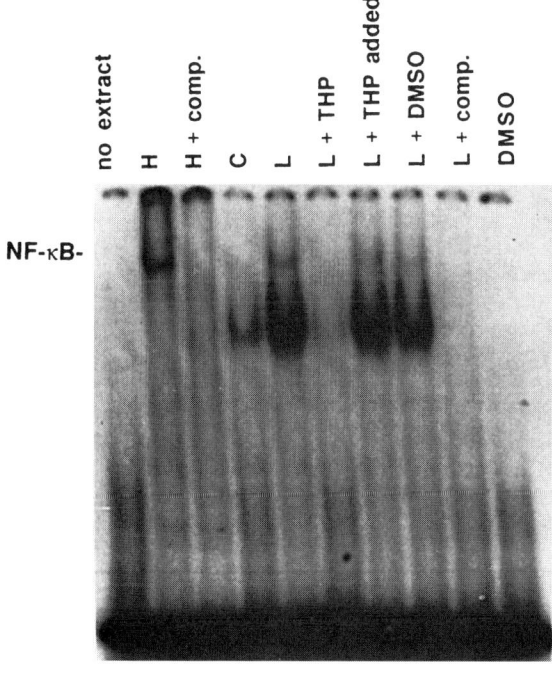

FIGURE 5. Gel mobility shift assays of monocyte nuclear extracts. Inhibition of NF-κB and binding to DNA sequences following LPS treatment in the presence of THP. LPS enhanced DNA-binding activity, which was significantly decreased by THP treatment. Legends: I, labeled oligo alone; H, positive control with HeLa nuclear extract; C, no treatment; COMP, oligo competitor; competition showed sequence specificity of the DNA binding L, LPS; Nuclear extracts were prepared 1 hour after treatment. THP decreased the activation of the transcription factor but had no direct effect on DNA binding.[10]

macrophages has also been presented.[24,25] NF-κB[26,27] and NF-IL-6[28,29] have also been shown to be required for induced expression of the human and murine IL-1β genes in cells of monocyte-macrophage lineage.

DISCUSSION

When cells of monocyte-macrophage lineage are activated by bacteria or bacterial products such as LPS or muramyl dipeptide, by lymphokines or by immune complexes, their production of superoxide is augmented.[30] At the same time, the concentrations of some transcription factors in their nuclei are increased. As reviewed in this paper, some lipophilic antioxidants can prevent such activation of transcription factors of the NF-κB, NF-IL-6 and AP-1 families, which are required for induced expression of the TNF-α, IL-1β and IL-6 genes in cells of the monocyte-macrophage lineage. The same antioxidants do not suppress IL-1 induced IL-6 expression in fibroblasts, in which non-oxidant activation of NF-κB, *e.g.* by protein kinase C,[22] may substitute for the oxidant activation of this transcription complex which occurs in monocytes and macrophages.

In the concentrations used, the antioxidants have no effect on protein synthesis and can augment the production of the IL-1ra and of lysosomal enzymes in monocyte-macrophage cultures.[12] Thus the effects are gene selective. Suppressing the production of pro-inflammatory cytokines while augmenting the production of IL-1ra is a novel strategy for anti-inflammatory therapy. The cell-type selectivity of suppressing IL-6 formation is therapeutically desirable. Inhibiting TNF-α, IL-1β and IL-6 formation locally, *e.g.* by drug in a mouthwash in periodontal disease, could decrease alveolar bone erosion. Inhibiting TNF-α, IL-1β and IL-6 formation in rheumatoid arthritis could decrease inflammation and joint erosion. Since IL-6 produced by bone marrow stromal cells is a co-factor in hematopoiesis, it would be therapeutically undesirable if the drug suppressing cytokine formation in cells of monocyte-macrophage lineage would have the same effect in fibroblast-type cells. Thus the cell-type selectivity of IL-6 suppression by the compounds now reviewed could add to their safety. During the past year antibodies against TNF-α have been found to improve the condition of patients with rheumatoid arthritis[31] and Crohn's disease.[32] It seems reasonable to postulate that drugs inhibiting, in a co-ordinate fashion, the production of TNF-α, IL-β and IL-6 will show at least comparable efficacy in these and other diseases in which inflammation plays a major pathogenetic role.

ACKNOWLEDGMENTS

We are indebted to collaborators in the research now reviewed—B. DeLustro, M. Ilnicka, S. Lee, S. Rouhafza and R. Wilhelm—and to Linda Miencier for preparation of the manuscript.

REFERENCES

1. POBER, J. S., M. P. BEVILACQUA, D. L. NEUDRIDO, L. A. LAPIERE, W. FIERS & M. A. GIMBRONE. 1993. Two distinct monokines, interleukin-1 and tumor necrosis factor, each independently induce biosynthesis and transient expression of the same antigen on the surface of cultured human vascular endothelial cells. J. Immunol. **136:** 1680–1687.

2. CROFFORD, L. J., R. L. WILDER, A. P. RISTIMÄKI, E. F. REMMERS, H. R. EPPS & T. HLA. 1993. Cyclooxygenase-1 and -2 expression in rheumatoid synovial tissues: Effects of interleukin-1β, phorbol ester and corticosteroids. J. Clin. Invest. **93**: 1095–1101.
3. MATRISIAN, L. M. 1990. Metalloproteinases and their inhibitors in matrix remodeling. Trends in Genetics **6**: 121–125.
4. TAKAI, Y., G. G. WONG, S. C. CLARK, S. J. BURKOFF & S. H. HERRMANN. 1988. B cell stimulatory factor-2 is involved in the differentiation of cytotoxic T lymphocytes. J. Immunol. **140**: 508.
5. NAWATA, Y., E. M. EUGUI, S. W. LEE & A. C. ALLISON 1989. IL-6 is the principal factor produced by synovia of patients with rheumatoid arthritis that induces B-lymphocytes to secrete immunoglobulin. Ann. N.Y. Acad. Sci. **557**: 230.
6. GASTON, J. S. H., S. STROBER, J. J. SOLVERA, et al. 1988. Dissection of the mechanisms of immune injury in rheumatoid arthritis using total lymphoid irradiation. Arthritis and Rheumatism **31**: 21–30.
7. MANNIK, M. & F. A. NARDELLA. 1983. Self-associating IgG rheumatoid factors. In New Horizons in Rhematoid Arthritis. Y. Shiokawa, T. Abe and Y. Yamauchi, Eds. 124–130. Amsterdam: Excerpta Medica.
8. ISHIMI, Y., C. MIUAURA, C. H. JIN, et al. 1990. IL-6 is produced by osteoblasts and induces bone resorption. J. Immunol. **145**: 3297–3303.
9. REINHARDT, R., M. MASADA, W. KALDAHL, et al. 1993. Gingival fluid IL-1 and IL-6 levels in refractory periodontitis. J. Clin. Periodontol. **20**: 225–231.
10. EUGUI, E. M., B. DELUSTRO, S. ROUHAFZA, M. ILNICKA, S. W. LEE, R. WILHELM & A. C. ALLISON. 1994. Some antioxidants inhibit, in a co-ordinate fashion, the production of TNF-α, IL-1β and IL-6 by human peripheral blood mononuclear cells. Internat. Immunol. **8**: 409–422.
11. LEE, J. C., A. M. BADGER, D. E. GRISWOLD, et al. 1993. Bicyclic imidazoles as a novel class of cytokine biosynthesis inhibitors. Ann. N.Y. Acad. Sci. **696**: 149–170.
12. WATERS, R. V., D. WEBSTER & A. C. ALLISON. 1993. Mycophenolic acid and some antioxidants induce differentiation of monocytic lineage cells and augment production of the IL-1 receptor antagonist. Ann. N.Y. Acad. Sci. **696**: 185–196.
13. CHAUDHRI, G. & I. A. CLARK. 1989. Reactive oxygen species facilitate the in vitro and in vivo lipopolysaccharide-induced release of tumor necrosis factor. J. Immunol. **143**: 1290–1294.
14. KU, G., N. S. DOHERTY, J. A. WOLOS & R. L. JACKSON. 1988. Inhibition by probucol of interleukin 1 secretion and its implication in atherosclerosis. Am. J. Cardiol. **62**: 77B–81B.
15. AKESON, A. L., C. W. WOODS, L. B. MOSHER, C. E. THOMAS & R. L. JACKSON. 1991. Inhibition of IL-1β expression in THP-1 cells by probucol and tocopherol. Atherosclerosis **86**: 261–270.
16. PERISTERIS, P., B. D. CLARK, S. GATTI, R. FAGGIANI, A. MANTOVANI, M. MENGOZZI, S. ORENCOLE, M. SIRONI & P. GHEZZI. 1992. N-acetylcysteine and glutathione as inhibitors of tumor necrosis factor production. Cell Immunol. **140**: 390–399.
17. DE FORGE, L. E., J. C. FANTONE, J. S. KENNEY & D. G. REMICK. 1992. Oxygen radical scavengers selectively inhibit interleukin 8 production in human whole blood. J. Clin. Invest. **90**: 2123–2129.
18. SCHRECK, R., P. RIEBER & P. A. BAUERLE. 1991. Reactive oxygen intermediates as apparently widely used messengers in the activation of NFκB transcription factor and HIV-1. EMBO J. **10**: 2247–2258.
19. ISRAEL, N., M.-A. GOUGERAT-POCIDALO, F. AILLET & J.-L. VIRELIZIER. 1992. Redox status influences constitutive or induced NF-κB translocation and HIV long terminal repeat activity in human T and monocytic cell lines. J. Immunol. **149**: 3386–3393.
20. DEVARY, Y., R. A. GOTTLIEB, L. F. LAU & M. KARIN. 1991. Rapid and preferential activation of the c-jun gene during the mammalian UV response. Mol. Cell. Biol. **11**: 2804–2811.
21. DATTA, R., D. E. HALLAHAN, S. M. KHARBANDA, E. RUBIN, M. L. SHERMAN, E. HUBERMAN, R. R. WEICHSELBAUM & D. W. KUFE. 1992. Involvement of reactive oxygen intermediates in the induction of c-jun gene transcription by ionizing radiation. Biochemistry **31**: 8300–8306.

22. HIRANTO, T., S. AKIRA, T. TAGA & T. KISHIMOTO. 1990. Biological and clinical aspects of interleukin 6. Immunol. Today **11**: 443–449.22.
23. LE CLAIR, K. P., M. A. BLANAR & P. A. SHARP. 1992. The p50 subunit of NF-κB associates with the NF-IL-6 transcription factor. Proc. Natl. Acad. Sci. USA **89**: 8145–8149.
24. SHAKHOV, A. N., M. A. COLLART, P. VASSALI, S. A. NEDOSPASOV & C. V. JONGENEEL. 1990. Kappa B-type enhancers are involved in lipopolysaccharide-mediated transcriptional activation of the tumor necrosis factor alpha gene in primary macrophages. J. Exp. Med. **171**: 35–47.
25. SUNG, S. J., J. A. WALTERS, J. HUDSON & J. M. GIMBLE. 1991. Tumor necrosis factor-α mRNA accumulation in human myelomonocytic cell lines. J. Immunol. **147**: 2047–2054.
26. HISCOTT, J., J. MEROIS, J. GAROUFALIS, et al. 1993. Characterization of a functional NF-κB site in the human interleukin-1β promoter: Evidence for a positive autoregulatory loop. Mol. Cell. Biol. **13**: 6231–6240.
27. COGSWELL, J. P., M. M. GODLEVSKI, G. B. WISELY, et al. 1994. NF-κB regulates IL-1β transcription through a consensus NF-κB binding site and a nonconsensus CRE-like site. J. Immunol. **153**: 712–722.
28. GODAMBE, S. A., D. CHAPLIN, T. TAKOVA & C. J. BELLONE. 1994. Upstream NFIL-6-like site located within a DNase 1 hypersensitivity region mediates LPS-induced transcription of the murine interleukin-1β gene. J. Immunol. **153**: 143–152.
29. SHIRAKAWA, F., K. SAITO, C. A. BONAGURA, D. L. GALSON, M. J. FENTON, A. C. WEBB & P. E. AURON. 1993. The human pro-interleukin β gene requires DNA sequences both proximal and distal to the transcription start site for tissue-specific induction. Mol. Cell Biol. **13**: 1332–1344.
30. JOHNSTON, R. B., JR. 1981. Enhancement of phagocytosis-associated oxidative metabolism as a manifestation of macrophage activation. *In* Lymphokines, Vol. 3: 33–52. E. Pick, Ed. New York: Academic Press.
31. ELLIOTT, M. J., R. N. MAINI, M. FELDMANN, R. O. WILLIAMS, F. M. BRENNAN & C. Q. CHU. 1993. Treatment of rheumatoid arthritis with chimeric monoclonal antibodies to TNF-α: Safety, clinical efficacy and control of the acute-phase response. J. Cell Biochem. **17B** (Suppl.):145.
32. VAN DEVENTER, S. Personal communication.

DISCUSSION OF THE PAPER

J. BIENVENU (*Lyon, France*): Can you comment on the specificity of such drugs? It was quite specific for TNF, but is it not in fact the case that to a lesser extent it is also active on IL-1, IL-6 production?

A. C. ALLISON: But that is the whole point. It is what we call co-ordinate inhibition of expression. There is some effect on IL-8, but less. But there is a strong effect on IL-1 and TNF production *in vivo* and *in vitro* by cells of monocyte-macrophage lineage.

BIENVENU: Is your drug active at micromolar concentrations?

ALLISON: Low micromolar.

BIENVENU: What is the pharmacological relevance of it *in vivo*?

ALLISON: For the first drug we have used in humans, we know from the pharmacokinetics that we can achieve relevant concentrations in the tissues concerned.

A. KOJ (*Jagiellonian University, Krakow, Poland*): I have two short questions. One concerns activation of monocytes and macrophages by LPS when you can block this with your drug—the anti-oxidative drug. What would be, in your opinion, the inhibition of respiratory burst of macrophages?

ALLISON: This is a very interesting question. There are two likely sources of oxidants. One of them is the B-cytochrome group, which is involved in superoxide production in endocytic vacuoles. Another is ubiquinone in mitochondia. At this stage we don't know which it is. But we have clearly been able to dissociate inhibition of the respiratory burst from inhibition of cytokine production.

KOJ: But did you not correlate the presence of respiratory burst and cytokine production?

ALLISON: No, but under conditions when you have activation you do have measurable production of superoxide.

KOJ: The second question concerns cells which produce cytokines and eventually respond to your drug. I understand that fibroblasts cannot be inhibited in cytokine production if they are stimulated by IL-1. And what about other factors?

ALLISON: I have to say that we have not really tested it systematically. We should do that and, after Dr. Elias's discussion the other day, we would be very intrigued to know whether IL-11 production in pulmonary cells is inhibited; he kindly consented to test some of our compounds. At this stage we do not know.

M. REVEL (*Weizmann Institute of Science, Rehovot, Israel*): I was under the impression that the failure of some of the drugs against septic shock is because the synthesis of TNF and IL-1 is so rapid that you always arrive afterwards. So how do you visualize that inhibitors of synthesis of TNF and IL-1 could be used in septic shock?

ALLISON: When you actually look at the times when people die it is quite a long time after they come in. These drugs turn off production of cytokine messenger RNA within 15 or 30 minutes. So we think that there is time. On the other hand, we think that you could use these drugs prophylactically in appropriate settings—in individuals who are likely to develop septic shock, *e.g.* if they are in intensive care.

P. B. SEHGAL (*Medical College of New York, Valhalla*): I have a question with respect to your cell-type specificity. I am having difficulty understanding how THP is supposed to work by interfering with NF-κB activation. The NF-κB activation pathway functions in fibroblasts and synoviocytes. How can you pin cell-type specificity on a mechanism such as that?

ALLISON: First of all, I am not sure that you need NF-κB in fibroblasts, because you and others have pointed out that there are so many other transcription factors acting on IL-6 expression in these cells.

SEHGAL: Well, we back-track on that one.

ALLISON: The second point is that you can activate NF-κB in other ways, through protein kinase, for example. And we may not be interfering with that. So, it is only where you have oxidant activation as the limiting factor, as we believe is the case in monocytes, that antioxidants suppress IL-6 production.

Interleukin-6: Effects on Tumor Models in Mice and on the Cellular Regulation of Transcription Factor IRF-1[a]

MICHEL REVEL,[b] ANNE KATZ,[b] LEA EISENBACH,[c]
MICHAEL FELDMAN,[c] NECHAMA HARAN-GHERA,[d]
SHEILA HARROCH,[b] AND JUDITH CHEBATH[b]

[b]*Department of Molecular Genetics and Virology*
[c]*Department of Cell Biology*
[d]*Department of Chemical Immunology*
Weizmann Institute of Science
Rehovot, Israel 76100

A number of studies have indicated that IL-6 exerts antitumoral activity *in vivo*, in some leukemias and against metastasing tumors (see refs. 1 and 2 for reviews). These studies in murine models would support applications of IL-6 therapy in specific clinical settings, such as prevention of metastases following resections of primary tumors or prevention of relapses in certain types of leukemias. However, such clinical studies have not yet materialized, due to the limited understanding of how IL-6 works on various cells, why it stimulates growth of some cells (*e.g.* myeloma and other hematopoietic cells) while inhibiting others, and due to the limited understanding of the mechanisms underlying the antitumor effects observed. This article reviews what we have learned from studies on murine models of leukemias and metastases and from *in vitro* studies on a gene regulatory effect of IL-6 that may be relevant to growth control in many cell types.

EFFECTS OF IL-6 IN MURINE TUMOR MODELS

Myeloid Leukemia Models

The recombinant human IL-6 glycoprotein produced in CHO-cells has been tested in radiation-induced acute myeloid leukemia (Rad-AML), either after intraperitoneal injection of tumor cells or during the primary induction period following irradiation.[3] The latter model allowed to study IL-6 action on bone marrow (BM) cells preceding the onset of overt leukemia. IL-6 was injected (1 μg/day/mouse, s.c.) for 10 days at 4–8 months after irradiation of SJL/J mice (300–350 rads, plus dexamethasone). The incidence of leukemia and death at 1 year after irradiation was reduced from 50% in the controls to 20% in the IL-6–treated mice.[3] Similar injections of GM-CSF increased, on the contrary, the leukemia incidence to 80%. A rapid disappearance of preleukemic cells present at 4 months in the BM of irradiated mice was observed 5 days after the end of the 10 days IL-6 treatment. These cells characterized by deletions

---

[a] Work supported by grants from InterPharm and Ares-Serono.

TABLE 1. Effect of IL-6 on Preleukemic Cells in Radiation-induced AML

Number of mice	Percentage of BM Cells with chr 2 Deletions				Mean/mouse
	1–10%	11–20%	21–30%	above 30%	
Control	1/15 (6%)	5/15 (33%)	3/15 (20%)	6/15 (40%)	27.8 ± 12.3
IL-6-Treated	10/15 (66%)	3/15 (20%)	2/15 (13%)	0/15 (0%)	9.3 ± 7.3 p < 0.001

SJL/J mice were irradiated (350 rad) and injected with dexamethasone (0.5 mg) and then treated 4 months later with rIL-6 (1 µg/d) for 10 days. Five days later, bone marrow cells were karyotyped (50–70 cells/mouse) and preleukemic cells characterized by chromosome 2 deletions were counted. Mice were classified in 4 groups according to frequency of abnormal cells. The last column is the mean percent of cells per mouse calculated for the 15 control and 15 IL-6 treated mice.

of chromosome 2 were reduced by a mean of 3-fold and only 13% of IL-6 treated mice had more than 20% of preleukemic cells in their BM population compared to 60% in the control irradiated mice (TABLE 1). This decrease was confirmed by injecting the BM cells to naive mice: leukemia developed in 73% of recipients of control mice BM but only in 33% of the IL-6–treated mice BM recipients. This decrease in preleukemic cells may result from immune mediated cell killing. IL-6 showed no effect on growth or differentiation of the Rad-AML cells *in vitro*. This contrasts with the growth-arrest and differentiation of myeloleukemic M1 cells[4] and human promonocytic U937 cells,[5] which also show apoptosis[6] in response to IL-6. Regarding clinical use of IL-6, a worry has been that IL-6 can synergize with GM-CSF or IL-3 to stimulate AML blast colonies in 30–50% of patients,[7,8] although IL-6 alone did not cause blast growth but rather enhanced AML cell differentiation.[3] The decrease in leukemia incidence observed in the murine Rad-AML model would suggest that the overall balance of IL-6 effects could still tilt to the therapeutic side in well chosen clinical settings of AML.

Metastasing Tumor Models

The F10.9 clone of B16 melanoma has a very high metastatic activity which appears related to its low immunogenicity *in vivo* and very low surface MHC-I levels. Our studies on the effect of rIL-6 were conducted in two models.[9] In experimental metastases produced by i.v. inoculation of F10.9 cells, mice die in 1–1.5 months with heavy lung metastatic loads. With a 3-week treatment by rIL-6 (1–10 µg/d, i.p) started at day 3, the mice survived and showed 90–95% reductions in metastases weight and number. The IL-6 treatment could be started as late as day 10, when metastases were present histologically, leading to survival and 80% metastases reductions.[9] Short 5-day treatments were not effective for F10.9 melanoma, although other reports on sarcoma metastastases used successfully such shorter treatments.[10]

In a second model of spontaneous metastases, F10.9 cells were injected into the footpad and the ensuing primary tumor was resected a month later. rIL-6 treatments (3 weeks, 10 µg/d) started 14 or 20 days after inoculation lead to 80% survival at 100 days, with 99% reduction of metastatic loads compared to control mice which all died between days 55 and 65.[9] IL-2 was not efficient in this model. IL-6 had only limited effects on the primary tumor but a strong action against metastases. In a recent experiment, we investigated the effect of rIL-6 therapy started after resection of the primary tumor. TABLE 2 shows that IL-6 still abrogated metastases, the mean load being reduced by over 90% as compared to controls who died of heavy metastases before day 57. This result would support a clinical approach based on the use of IL-6 for the prevention of metastatic growth following resection of primary tumors.

Similar studies on another highly metastatic murine tumor indicated that combinations of rIL-6 with tumor vaccines may be beneficial. The 3LL-D122 lung carcinoma cells are also very poorly immunogenic, a condition that can be corrected by transfection with H-2K genes following which a tumor antigen could be recovered from the MHC-I complex and identified as a mutated peptide of the gap junction connexin.[11] IL-6 therapy (carried out as in the melanoma studies above) did not suppress experimental D122 metastases, and had only a partial effect on spontaneous metastases.[12] However, when the 3-week course of rIL-6 was combined with 3 weekly injections of killed D122 cells, the lung metastases were completely inhibited. In fact rIL-6 appears to allow an immune response against the non-immunogenic parental D122 cells. A cytotoxic T-lymphocyte (CTL) activity could be clearly demonstrated in the immunized mice receiving the vaccine together with IL-6 but not in the controls with vaccine alone.[12] The CTL activity rose after the first week of IL-6 therapy, was D122 cell specific and responded to resensitization *in vitro* on D122 cells. The same effects could be achieved by injections of D122 cells transfected by IL-6 cDNA, the gene therapy vaccine inducing specific CTL activity (as well as increasing macrophages), and when started 11 days after tumor inoculation reduced the spontaneous metastases observed at 26 days.[13]

Induction of CTL activity against tumor cells seems to be an activity of IL-6 often observed in mice during antitumor therapy.[14] In the models that we have studied, IL-6 elicited CTL activity against tumor cells which by themselves were non-immunogenic suggesting that IL-6 might circumvent the absence of high MHC-I expression on the tumor cells. The type of immune cells involved seemed also to differ between tumors. In the F10.9 melanoma spontaneous metastases model,[9] a cytolytic activity of fresh splenocytes against the tumor cells was found to appear during IL-6 therapy. This lytic activity did not require resensitization, and preceded a peak of CTL activity dependent on resensitization *in vitro*. Differences between the F10.9 melanoma and D122 lung carcinoma models in term of IL-6–induced CTL response were further observed when mice were first depleted of CD4 or CD8 T-cells prior to challenge by tumor inoculation in the footpad. Depletion by injections of anti-CD4 (GK531)

TABLE 2. Late Treatment by IL-6 of F10.9 Melanoma Pulmonary Metastases

	Control Mice		IL-6–Treated Mice	
	Metastatic Load, mg	Number of Metastases	Metastatic Load, mg	Number of Metastases
Individual animals	905	>200	200	7
	645	>200	45	4
	455	>200	0	0
	395	>200	0	0
	360	>200	0	0
Mean (SEM)	550 (100)	200 (0)	49 (39)	2.2 (1.4)
			$p < 0.001$	$p < 0.0001$

Mice injected on day 0 by B16/F10.9 melanoma cells (2×10^5) in the footpad. Primary tumor removed by amputation at 26 days (mean size 8 mm). IL-6 given on days 28–31, 35–38, 42–45, at 10 μg/day i.p. divided in 3 daily injections. Lung weight and metastases counted at day 57 (when controls died).

and anti-CD8 (YTS) monoclonal antibodies was started on day 0 (i.v.), repeated 3 times at weekly intervals, and the depletion confirmed by FACS analysis of spleen cells at days 17 and 24. The IL-6 treatment of 3 weeks was started on day 14. With the F10.9 melanoma, depletion of either CD4 or of CD8 impaired the survival due to IL-6 (FIG. 1, upper panel). With the D122 lung carcinoma, a dependence on CD8 cells for the success of the IL-6 therapy combined with D122-vaccine was observed, but survival was less impaired by CD4 depletion. Even with CD8 depletion, the rIL-6 treatment still caused a marked delay in onset of death (FIG. 1, lower panel). The

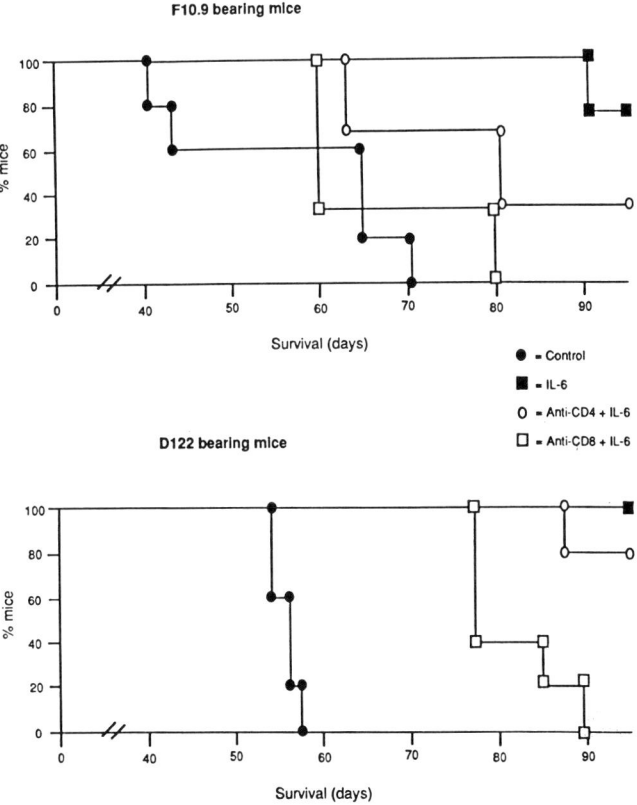

FIGURE 1. IL-6 therapy of spontaneous metastases in normal C57B1/6 mice and after depletion of CD4 or CD8 T-cell subsets. **Top:** Murine melanoma B16/F10.9 cells (2×10^5) were injected into the footpad of 6 mice/group on day 0. Anti-CD4 McAB GK531 was injected i.v. on day 0, and i.p. on days 20, 40, 60. Anti-CD8 McAB YTS was injected i.v. at day 0 and i.p at days 7, 14, 21 for optimal depletion as verified by FACS analysis. Undepleted mice *(closed squares)*, CD4 depleted *(open circles)* and CD8 depleted *(open squares)* received IL-6 on days 14–17, 21–24, 28–31 at 10 μg/day i.p.; control animals *(closed circles)* received PBS injections. The primary tumor was resected by amputation at day 52 and survival was followed until day 115. **Bottom:** Lung carcinoma 3LL/D122 cells were injected as above. Treatments were as above except that the IL-6–treated mice also received at days 14, 21 and 28, an injection i.p. of 2×10^6 killed D122 cells (irradiated at 5000 rads and mitomycin-C treated[12]) as vaccine.

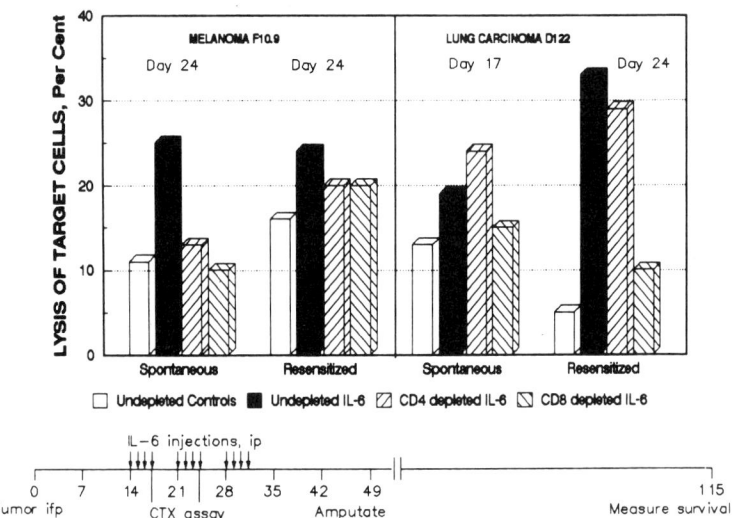

FIGURE 2. Induction of cytotoxic lymphocytes by IL-6 therapy in normal and CD4 or CD8 depleted tumor-bearing mice. Experimental conditions for melanoma B16/F10.9 *(left)* and lung carcinoma 3LL/D122 *(right)* as in FIGURE 1. At the end of the 1st and 2nd weeks of IL-6 therapy (days 17 and 24), two mice of each group were killed and the splenocytes incubated with ^{35}S-methionine labeled F10.9 or D122 cells respectively for 16 hours (Effector:Target, 100:1) and the percentage of specific lysis was determined[12] (spontaneous cytotoxic cells). Splenocytes were also cultured 5 days on monolayers of each tumor cell (killed by irradiation and mitomycin-C) to assay resensitized cytotoxic cells. Results at the day giving the highest CTL activity are shown. Other target cells used confirmed that the lysis is due to MHC-restricted CTL and not to NK cells.

CTL activities measured in these experiments are depicted in FIGURE 2. With F10.9 tumors, the IL-6 induced lytic activity without resensitization (spontaneous) was reduced in both CD4 and CD8 depleted mice (FIG. 2, left panel). With D122 tumors, the IL-6–induced activity was reduced by CD8 depletion but not by CD4 depletion. Therefore, CD8 CTL effector cells which are reactivated by *in vitro* sensitization, seem to be mainly involved in the antimetastatic effects on the D122 lung carcinoma. The response of melanoma F10.9 seems to be more complex and to involve CD4 and CD8 cells to generate mature lytic cells which do not need reactivation *in vitro*. In the melanoma-bearing mice, IL-6 also caused an increase in CD8 cells (9-fold) and in CD4 cells (2.5-fold) after the 2nd week of IL-6 injections, a phenomenon we did not observe in the lung carcinoma-bearing mice.

MECHANISMS OF IL-6 ACTION ON TUMORS AND CELLS

Does IL-6 Act on the Immune System or Also on Tumor Cells?

The requirement of CD4 and CD8 T-cells for the antitumor effects of IL-6 previously demonstrated by Mule *et al.*[15] for sarcoma tumors, and summarized above for the non-immunogenic melanoma and lung carcinoma, are not unique to this cytokine.

In fact, an intact immune system seems to be required for antitumoral effects of most cytokines, including interferons.[16] Undoubtedly, the immune system participates in the antimetastatic activity of IL-6, but this does not exclude that IL-6 may also have to affect directly the tumor cells. The apparent ability of IL-6 therapy to make non-immunogenic tumor cells trigger an immune response, may well be related to effects on the tumor cells, or on their interactions with helper or effector immune cells. Although we could not find an effect of IL-6 on growth or MHC-I contents when added *in vitro* to D122 or F10.9 cell cultures,[9,12] reduced growth and increased MHC-I were observed in IL-6 DNA transfected D122 cells which constantly secrete the cytokine.[13] Increases of MHC antigens and of other surface antigens such as CEA, have been documented in human colon carcinoma cell lines cultured for several days with IL-6 *in vitro*.[17] Increased adhesion to the extracellular matrix were observed in IL-6 DNA-transfected tumor cells along with increased integrin receptors for fibronectin, vitronectin, laminin, and collagen.[18]

IL-6 has complex and sometimes opposite effects on growth of various tumor cells (reviewed in ref. 1). Thus, decreased colony growth was observed in cells from human breast carcinomas along with loss of cell contacts.[5,19,20] IL-6 inhibits growth of cells from early stage melanomas,[21] but not of late stage cells where even stimulation may be seen.[21] Myeloma and B or T lymphoma cells are growth-stimulated by IL-6,[22,23] but chronic B-lymphocytic leukemia cells show a growth-inhibitory response.[24] A human early acute leukemia cell B1 with a pre-B/myeloid biphenotype is growth-inhibited by IL-6 and undergoes myeloid differentiation.[25] IL-6 induces complete growth arrest and differentiation of the murine M1 myeloleukemic cells,[4] an effect which may be partially seen or not at all in other myeloid leukemic cells.[1] These variable responses stress the need to better understand how IL-6 works on tumor cells and how its action may be regulated.

IRF-1 and IRF-2 as Molecular Probe of IL-6 Effects on Various Tumor Cells

The variability of tumor cell responses to IL-6 may of course be explained by abundance or scarcity of IL-6 receptors; for example the F10.9 and D122 tumors discussed above have very few receptors which may explain the absence of IL-6 response *in vitro*.[9,12] However, it is much more difficult to explain the opposite effects of IL-6 on growth of different cells which have abundant IL-6 receptor contents or situations in which addition of exogenous soluble IL-6 receptor enhance the opposite growth effects of IL-6.[26] As an approach to this question we compared two cell lines: growth-stimulated B9 murine hybridoma cells[27] and growth-inhibited T47D human breast carcinoma cells, which are both rich in IL-6 receptors.[9,20] We focused on the transcription factor IRF-1 and IRF-2 genes which appear to be involved in cell growth control[28,29] and to be modulated by IL-6 in M1 cells[30,31] and examined if the activities of these genes and their protein products differ with the type of growth response. IRF-1 (interferon regulatory factor-1) acts as a stimulatory transcription factor on enhancer sequences of the genes encoding type I interferons such as IFN-β, and of IFN-activated genes activated in response to IFN such as the MHC-I genes.[32-34] Both IRF-1 and IRF-2 bind to these enhancers, but IRF-2 acts as a repressor of IRF-1 function and binding.[28]

In both T47D and B9 cells, IL-6 caused a marked induction of IRF-1 mRNA and protein in 1 hour,[35] as had been previously seen in M1 cells,[36] indicating that this is a general activity of IL-6 in cells and is not specific of the differentiating myeloid cells. However, when the activity of the IRF-1 transcription factor was analyzed by DNA mobility shift assay, specific enhancer binding of IRF-1 was observed only in the IL-6–treated T47D breast cancer cells. In the B9 hybridoma cells, there was no IRF-1 binding but instead a strong constitutive binding of the IRF-2 repressor protein was observed.[35] This differential binding of IRF-1 and IRF-2 (confirmed by specific antibody blocking), was also seen when IL-6 sensitive and resistant clones of M1 cells were compared.[36] In sensitive M1 cells which stop growing and differentiate in response to IL-6, the IRF-1 enhancer binding activity was induced by IL-6. In an M1res clone, which grows normally in the presence of IL-6, no IRF-1 binding was seen and only constitutive IRF-2 binding was present.[36]

Transfections by IRF-1 and IRF-2 cDNA demonstrated that high IRF-2 expression correlates with growth stimulations and promotes malignant transformation, whereas IRF-1 expression produces opposite, growth-inhibitory effects.[29,37] Cell lines derived from IRF-1 knock out mice show that IRF-1 could be critical to prevent oncogenic transformation and to elicit programmed cell death.[38] The correlation that we observed between IL-6 growth inhibitory effects and induction of IRF-1 DNA-binding activity suggests that the surge of IRF-1 in response to IL-6 plays a role in growth regulation by IL-6, as illustrated in FIGURE 3. In cells in which the IRF-1 activity is repressed by high IRF-2 expression, the growth inhibitory effect of IL-6 would be blocked. Since IRF-2 binding appeared essentially constitutive and not IL-6 dependent, it is likely that other effects of IL-6 (e.g. junB induction) must be involved in the growth-stimulation of cells such as the B9 hybridoma.

Induction of IRF-1 is an activity common to IFN-α,β, IFN-γ and IL-6 and the effects of these cytokines on IRF-1 mRNA, protein and activity were very similar in T47D and B9 cells.[35] Since IRF-1 enhances the response to IFNs of IFN-stimulated genes such as MHC-I or $2'$–$5'$ A synthetase[33] or mimics IFN action,[32,34] IL-6 may exert similar effects on some tumor cells, decrease growth and increase immunogenicity. IL-6 may also synergize with low levels of IFN made by the cells since in M1 cells, some of the IFN-like effects of IL-6 were inhibited by blocking endogenous IFN with antibodies[31,39,40] and synergism between IL-6 and IFN was observed.[40] IFN-β mRNA is produced by the cells,[39] possibly due to IRF-1 induction (FIG. 3) but the amounts of IFN appear too small to account for the observed induction of MHC-I or $2'$–$5'$ A synthetase. The growth inhibition and the induction of many differentiation markers by IL-6 occurred in these cells even when IFN action was blocked.[31,40] Since IL-6 induces IRF-1 independently of IFN, the antioncogenic activities of IRF-1[29,38] could directly mediate most of IL-6 effects on the sensitive M1 cells as illustrated by FIGURE 3.

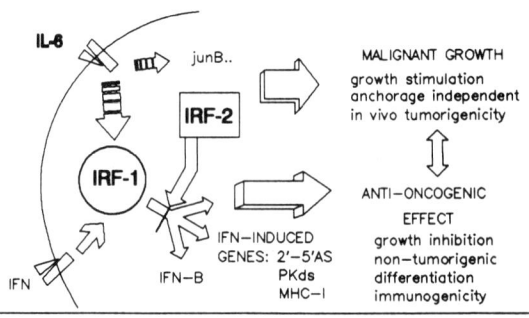

FIGURE 3. Schematic illustration of the potential roles of the IRF-1 transcription factor and IRF-2 repressor in the effects of IL-6. For details and references, see text.

TABLE 3. Sequences of Palindromic Interferon Response Elements pIRE and other GAS-like Sequences

Enhancer											
GAS consensus	N	T	T	N	C	N	N	N	A	A	N
pIRE/IRF-1	T	T	T	C	C	C	C	G	A	A	A
FcγR, pIRE/α₂M	T	T	T	C	C	C	A	G	A	A	A
ICSBP	T	T	T	C	C	G	A	G	A	A	A
Ly6E	A	T	T	C	C	T	G	T	A	A	G
GBP	A	T	T	A	C	T	C	T	A	A	A
α₂M human	A	T	T	C	C	C	G	T	A	A	G
α₂M rat	A	T	T	C	C	C	A	G	A	A	G
SIE/fos	G	T	T	C	C	C	G	T	C	A	A

FcγR: Fcγ Receptor gene; α₂M: α₂-Macroglobulin gene; ICSBP: Interferon control sequence binding protein, an IRF gene family member; Ly6E: a leukocyte protein gene; GBP: Guanosine nucleotide binding protein; SIE: serum-inducible element of the fos oncogene. The core sequence of the enhancers found in the above genes[35,46] is shown.

Activation of the IRF-1 Gene pIRE Enhancer by IL-6 and IFNs

Since rapid induction of IRF-1 mRNA appears to be a general effect of IL-6 in cells of lymphoid, myeloid or epithelial origin, we investigated if IL-6 controls the expression of this gene through activation of the enhancer element which is also involved in the response to IFNs. This enhancer sequence called palindromic IFN response element (pIRE, TABLE 3) is a member of the larger GAS (gamma-IFN activated sequence) family.[41,42] IFN-γ causes activation of transcription factor Stat91 (Stat1) which binds to GAS/pIRE elements as a dimer, and induces transcription of

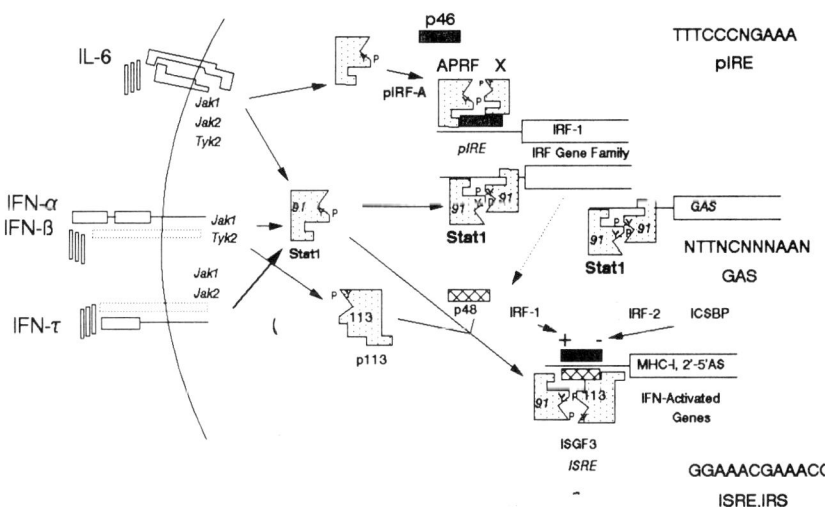

FIGURE 4. Schematic representation of the Stat transcription complexes activated in response to IL-6, IFN-β and IFN-γ as described in the text and in TABLE 4. The three receptor systems and associated Jak/Tyk tyrosine kinases are shown.

GAS/pIRE-reporter genes.[42,43] Stat1 is the p91 subunit of the ISGF3 transcription complex activated in response to IFN-α,β and which binds to ISRE sequences of IFN-activated genes such as MHC-I and 2'-5'A synthetase.[43] The relation between these Stat factors, the IFN-γ and IFN-α,β receptor systems and their associated Jak/Tyk tyrosine kinases[43] is illustrated in FIGURE 4.

IL-6 induced pIRE-luciferase gene expression in breast carcinoma T47D cells as strongly as did IFN-γ.[35] IL-6 activated binding of two types of transcription complexes on the pIRE/IRF-1 enhancer, both forming within 5 minutes of IL-6 treatment and requiring tyrosine phosphorylation but not protein synthesis (FIG. 5A). The faster migrating complex, which is also induced by IFN-γ, was identified as formed by Stat1(p91) by blocking with specific antibodies. In contrast, the slower complex pIRF-A induced by IL-6 did not contain Stat1.[35] The pIRF-A complex was found in the nucleus of IL-6–stimulated cells, at times when Stat1 activated by IL-6, or IFN-β or IFN-γ was still in the cytosol (FIG. 5A). pIRF-A was IL-6 dependent also in hybridoma B9 cells.[35] Enhancer competition experiments revealed that the IL-6–induced pIRF-A differs from Stat1 by being more specific for pIRE sequences such as found in the IRF-1, α_2-macroglobulin and FcγR genes than for GAS as found in the GBP and Ly6 genes[35,44] (see TABLES 3 and 4). These enhancers of the GAS family are not functionally identical since (FIG. 5B) the FcγR (pIRE/α_2m) sequence exhibited a different protein binding pattern than pIRE/IRF-1 from which it differs by one base pair only (TABLE 3). Thus, four distinct complexes were induced by IL-6 and by IFN-β, whereas IFN-γ still led to binding of Stat1 only. (FIG. 5B). The 3 upper complexes (pIRF-A, I and II) further differed from Stat1 by their sensitivity to N-ethyl maleimide (FIG. 5B) indicating that other proteins must be involved in these slower complexes. These studies[44] led to the identification of one of these proteins as Stat3/APRF which is the factor involved in activation of acute phase protein genes in liver cells following IL-6 treatment.[45,46] As summarized in TABLE 4, APRF was found by antibody blocking to be present in the 3 complexes pIRF-A, I and II induced by IL-6 in breast T47D cells. These results show that IL-6 activates APRF also in non-hepatic cells, in addition to Stat1 activation. They show also that IFN-β activates APRF.

TABLE 4. Four IL-6-dependent Complexes Formed with pIRE Probes

	pIRF-A	Complex I	Complex II	Complex III
Stat1C	No	No	Yes	Yes
Stat1N	No	No	No	Yes
Stat3/APRF	Yes	Yes	Yes	No
NEM	Sensitive	Sensitive	Sensitive	Resistant
Subunits	98,91 + 46	98,91		91
Affinity				
pIRE/IRF-1	+++	(+)	(+)	+++
FcγR	+++	+++	+++	+++
ICSBP	−	+++	+++	+++
Ly6E	−	(+)	(+)	+++
Inducer				
IL-6	+++	++	++	++
IFN-β	+	+	+	+
IFN-γ	(+)	−/+	−/+	+++
	Stat3 + X + small subunit	Stat3 dimer or Stat3 + X	Stat1/Stat3 heterodimer	Stat1 dimer

Stat1C or N indicates reaction with antibodies to carboxy- or amino-terminal domains of Stat1.

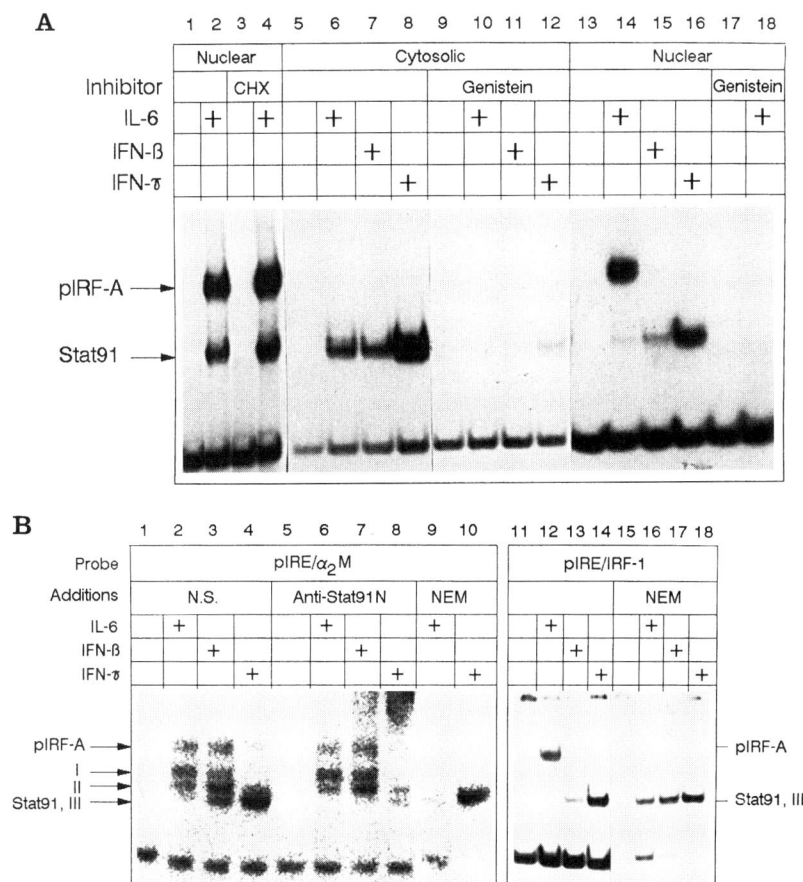

FIGURE 5. DNA-binding activities induced by IL-6 and IFNs on pIRE/IRF-1 and related enhancer sequences. **(A)** Nuclear and cytosolic extracts from breast carcinoma T47D cells after 15 minute treatments with IL-6 (20 ng, 100 U/ml), IFN-β or IFN-γ (500 U/ml) where indicated. In lanes 3,4 the cells were pretreated 30 minutes with cycloheximide (50 μg/ml) and in lanes 9–12, 17, 18 with genistein (100 μg/ml). Extracts were prepared and reacted as described[35,44] with the pIRE/IRE-1 sequence (TABLE 3). Positions of the complexes pIRF-A and Stat1 (Stat91, complex III) are shown by arrows. **(B)** Nuclear extracts from T47D cells after 45 minutes treatments with IL-6, IFN-β or IFN-γ where indicated, were reacted in mobility shift assays with pIRE/α$_2$M (FcγR) or pIRE/IRF-1 sequences (TABLE 3). In lanes 5–8, antibodies to Stat91N (amino acids 1–194) were preincubated with the extracts, and in lanes 9, 10, 15–18 the extracts were pretreated with N-ethyl maleimide (10 mM, 10 min) as described.[11] The positions of the 4 complexes pIRF-A, I, II and III (Stat1) are shown (see TABLE 4).

From DNA cross-linking experiments,[44] the IL-6–induced pIRF-A appears to be a large multimeric complex comprising 3 DNA-binding subunits of 98, 91 and 46 Kda (TABLE 4). Neither Stat2 (p113) nor ISGF3γ (p48) which form the ISGF3 complex mediating the IFN-α,β response, were found in pIRF-A but this complex seems to have a multimeric structure resembling that of ISGF3 (FIG. 4). Complex II contains both Stat1 and Stat3/APRF (TABLE 4). In analogy to the EGF-induced complexes A, B, C forming on GAS-like enhancers,[43] complex I, II and III may be Stat3 dimers, Stat3/Sta1 heterodimers and Stat1 dimers, respectively. None of these contained the p46 component, which appears unique to pIRF-A.

Conclusions

These studies show that the transcriptional activation of the IRF-1 gene produced by IL-6 in cells of various origins, involves a number of tyrosine phosphorylated transcription factors which also participate in the actions of IFNs and in the induction of acute phase protein genes by IL-6 in liver cells. Interestingly, IL-6 shares effects both with IFN-γ and with IFN-α,β, in line with the finding that all three kinases Jak1, Tyk2 and Jak2 can associate and respond to the IL-6/LIF/OSM/CNTF gp130 receptor component[47] (see FIG. 4). That through distinct receptor systems, different cytokines and growth factors (e.g. EGF, CSFs) can activate shared signal transduction JAK and STAT elements[43] may allow multiple synergistic as well as antagonistic actions which determine the ultimate biological outcome of the stimulus. The four different transcription complexes involved in IL-6 signaling show discrete enhancer sequence specificities, which can account for the diversity of gene responses to IL-6 as compared to other cytokines. It is of interest that besides IRF-1 and FcγR genes, the ICAM-1 gene[46] is controlled by a pIRE-like sequence that has high affinity for the IL-6 induced pIRF-A factor. ICAM-1 may well be involved in the effect of IL-6 on immunogenicity of tumor cells. The IRF-1 gene induction provides an interesting system to further understand IL-6 action on various cells, a system which may be relevant to the cell growth and immuno-regulatory effects of IL-6, and ultimately for its *in vivo* antitumoral effects.

ACKNOWLEDGMENTS

In vivo studies on Radiation induced leukemia were done by N. Haran-Ghera, A. Peled, P. Resnitzky. Studies on metastases by L. Eisenbach, M. Feldman and A. Katz. rIL-6 was provided by InterPharm and Ares-Serono. Gifts of anti Stat1 antibodies from Dr A. Larner and of anti-APRF from Dr S. Akira and T. Kishimoto are gratefully acknowledged.

REFERENCES

1. REVEL, M. 1992. Growth regulatory functions of IL-6 and antitumor effects. Forum in Immunology: IL-6. Research Immunol. **143**: 769–773.
2. MULE, J. J., S. G. MARCUS, J. C. YANG, J. S. WEBER & S. A. ROSENBERG. 1992. Clinical application of IL6 in cancer therapy. Forum in Immunology. Research Immunol. **143**: 777–779.
3. GIVON, T., S. SLAVIN, N. HARAN-GHERA, R. MICHALEVICZ & M. REVEL. 1992. Antitumor effects of human recombinant interleukin-6 on acute myeloid leukemia in mice and in cell cultures. Blood **79**: 2392–2398.
4. CHEN, L., D. NOVICK, M. RUBINSTEIN & M. REVEL. 1988. Recombinant interferon-$\beta 2$ (interleukin-6) induces myeloid differentiation. FEBS Letters. **239**: 299–304.
5. CHEN, L., Y. MORY, A. ZILBERSTEIN & M. REVEL. 1988. Growth inhibition of human

breast carcinoma and leukemia/lymphoma cell lines by recombinant interferon-$\beta 2$ (IL-6). Proc. Natl. Acad. Sci. USA. **85:** 8037–8041.
6. AFFORD, S. C., J. PONGRACZ, R. A. STOCKLEY, J. CROCKER & D. BURNETT. 1992. The induction by interleukin-6 of apoptosis in the promonocytic cell line U937 and human neutrophils. J. Biol. Chem. **267:** 21612–21616.
7. HOANG, T., A. HUMAN, O. GONCALVES, G. G. WONG & S. C. CLARK. 1988. Interleukin-6 enhances growth-factor dependent proliferation of the blast cells of acute myeloblastic leukemia. Blood **72:** 823–826.
8. AKASHI, K., M. HARADA, T. SHIBUYA, T. ETO, Y. TAKAMATSU, T. TESHIMA & Y. NIHO. 1991. Effects of interleukin-4 and interleukin-6 on the proliferation of CD34+ and CD34− blasts from acute myelogenous leukemia. Blood. **78:** 197–204.
9. KATZ, A., L. M. SHULMAN, A. PORGADOR, M. REVEL, M. FELDMAN & L. EISENBACH. 1993. Abrogation of B16 melanoma metastases by long-term low-dose interleukin-6 therapy. J. Immunother. **13:** 98–109.
10. MULE, J. J., J. K. MCINTOSH, D. M. JABLONS & S. A. ROSENBERG. 1990. Antitumor activity of recombinant IL-6 in mice. J. Exp. Med. **171:** 629–636.
11. MANDELBAUM, O., G. BERKE, M. FRIDKIN, M. FELDMAN, M. EISENSTEIN & L. EISENBACH. 1994. CTL induction by a tumor associated antigen octapeptide derived from a murine lung carcinoma. Nature **369:** 67–71.
12. KATZ, A., L. M. SHULMAN, M. REVEL, M. FELDMAN & L. EISENBACH. 1993. Combined therapy with IL-6 and inactivated tumor cells suppresses metastasis in mice bearing 3LL lung carcinomas. Intl. J. Cancer **53:** 812–818.
13. PORGADOR, A., E. TZEHOVAL, A. KATZ, E. VADAI, M. REVEL, M. FELDMAN & L. EISENBACH. 1992. Interleukin-6 gene transfection into Lewis lung carcinoma tumor cells suppresses the malignant phenotype and confers immunotherapeutic competence against parental metastatic cells. Cancer Res. **52:** 3679–3686.
14. KITAHARA, M., S. KISHIMOTO, T. HIRANO, T. KISHIMOTO & M. OKADA. 1990. The in vivo antitumor effect of human recombinant interleukin-6. Jap. J. Cancer. **81:** 1032–1038.
15. MULE, J. J., M. C. CUSTER, W. D. TRAVIS & S. A. ROSENBERG. 1992. Cellular mechanisms of the antitumor activity of recombinant interleukin-6 in mice. J. Immunol. **148:** 2622–2629.
16. GRESSER, I., C. MAURY, C. CARNAUD, E. DEMAEYER, M. T. MAUNOURY & F. BELLARDELLI. 1990. Antitumor effects of interferon in mice injected with IFN sensitive and IFN resistant Friend erythroleukemia cells—VIII. Role of the immune system in the inhibition of visceral metastases. Intl. J. Cancer **46:** 468–474.
17. DANSKY-ULLMANN, C., J. SCHLOM & J. W. GREINER. 1992. Interleukin-6 increases carcinoembryonic antigen and histocompatibility leukocyte antigen expression on the surface of human colorectal carcinoma cells. J. Immunother. **12:** 231–241.
18. SUN, W. H., R. A. KREISLE, A. W. PHILLIPS & W. B. ERSHLER. 1992. In vivo and in vitro characteristics of interleukin-6 transfected B16 melanoma cells. Cancer Res. **42:** 5412–5415.
19. TAMM, I., I. CARDINALE, J. KRUEGER, J. S. MURPHY, L. T. MAY & P. B. SEHGAL. 1989. Interleukin-6 decreases cell-cell association and increases motility of ductal breast carcinoma cells. J. Exp. Med. **170:** 1649–1669.
20. CHEN, L., L. M. SHULMAN & M. REVEL. 1991. IL-6 receptors and sensitivity to growth inhibition by IL-6 in clones of human breast carcinoma cells. J. Biol. Regul. Homeost. Agents **5:** 125–136.
21. LU, C., M. F. VICKERS & R. S. KERBEL. 1992. Interleukin-6: A fibroblast-derived growth inhibitor of human melanoma cells from early but not advanced stages of tumor progression. Proc. Natl. Acad. Sci. USA **89:** 9215–9219.
22. KLEIN, B., X. G. ZHANG, M. JOURDAN, J. CONTENT, F. HOUSSIAU, L. A. AARDEN, M. PIECHAZYCK & R. BATAILLE. 1989. Paracrine rather than autocrine regulation of myeloma-cell growth and differentiation by interleukin-6. Blood **73:** 517–525.
23. YEE, C., A. BIONDI, X. H. WANG, N. N. ISCOVE, J. DESOUSA, L. A. AARDEN, G. G. WONG & S. C. CLARK. 1989. A possible autocrine role for interleukin-6 in two lymphoma cell lines. Blood **74:** 798–804.
24. ADERKA, D., Y. MAOR, D. NOVICK, H. ENGELMAN, Y. KAHN, Y. LEVO, D. WALLACH

& M. REVEL. 1993. Interleukin-6 inhibits the proliferation of B-chronic lymphocytic leukemia cells that is induced by Tumor Necrosis Factor-α or -β. Blood **81:** 2076–2084.

25. COHEN, A., D. PETSCHE, T. GRUNBERGER & M. H. FREEDMAN. 1992. Interleukin-6 induces myeloid differentiation of a human biphenotypic leukemic cell line. Leukemia Res. **16:** 751–760.

26. NOVICK, D., L. M. SHULMAN, L. CHEN & M. REVEL. 1992. Enhancement of interleukin-6 cytostatic effect on human breast carcinoma cells by soluble IL-6 receptor from urine and reversion by monoclonal antibodies. Cytokine **4:** 6–11.

27. HELLE, M., L. BOIJE & L. A. AARDEN. 1988. Functional discrimination between interleukin-6 and interleukin-1. Eur. J. Immunol. **18:** 1535–1540.

28. TANAKA, N. & T. TANIGUCHI. 1992. Cytokine gene regulation: Regulatory cis-elements and DNA binding factors involved in the interferon system. Adv. Immunol. **52:** 263–281.

29. HARADA H., M. KITAGAWA, N. TANAKA, H. YAMAMOTO, K. HARADA, M. ISHIHARA & T. TANIGUCHI. 1993. Anti-oncogenic and oncogenic potentials of interferon regulatory factors-1 and -2. Science **259:** 971–974.

30. ABDOLLAHI, A., K. A. LORD, B. HOFMAN-LIEBERMAN & D. A. LIEBERMAN. 1991. Interferon regulatory factor-1 is a myeloid differentiation primary response gene induced by interleukin-6 and leukemia inhibitory factor: Role in growth inhibition. Cell Growth & Diff. **2:** 401–407.

31. GOTHELF, Y., J. RABER, L. CHEN, A. SCHATTNER, J. CHEBATH & M. REVEL. 1991. Terminal differentiation of myeloleukemic M1 cells induced by IL-6: Role of endogenous interferon. Lymphokine Cytokine Res. **10:** 369–375.

32. CHANG, C. H., J. HAMMER, J. E. LOH, W. L. FODOR & R. A. FLAVELL. 1992. The activation of major histocompatibility complex class I genes by interferon regulatory factor-1 (IRF-1). Immunogenetics **35:** 378–384.

33. REIS, L. F. L., H. HARADA, J. D. WOLCHOK, T. TANIGUCHI & J. VILCEK. 1992. Critical role of a common transcription factor, IRF-1, in the regulation of IFN-β and IFN-inducible genes. EMBO J. **11:** 185–193.

34. PINE, R. 1992. Constitutive expression of an ISGF2/IRF-1 transgene leads to interferon-independent activation of interferon-inducible genes and resistance to virus infection. J. Virol. **66:** 4470–4478.

35. HARROCH, S., M. REVEL & J. CHEBATH. 1994. Induction by interleukin-6 of interferon regulatory factor-1 (IRF-1) gene expression through the palindromic interferon response element pIRE and cell type-dependent control of IRF-1 binding to DNA. EMBO J. **13:** 1942–1949.

36. HARROCH, S., Y. GOTHELF, N. WATANABE, M. REVEL & J. CHEBATH. 1993. Interleukin-6 activates and regulates transcription factors of the interferon regulatory factor family in M1 cells. J. Biol. Chem. **268:** 9092–9097.

37. KIRCHHOFF, S., F. SCHAPER & H. HAUSER. 1993. Interferon regulatory factor 1 (IRF-1) mediates cell growth inhibition by transactivation of downstream target genes. Nucleic Acids Res. **21:** 2881–2889.

38. TANAKA, N., M. ISHIHARA, M. KITAGAWA, H. HARADA, T. KIMURA, T. MATSUYAMA, M. S. LAMPHIER, S. AIZAWA, T. W. MAK & T. TANIGUCHI. 1994. Cellular commitment to oncogene-induced transformation or apoptosis is dependent on the transcription factor IRF-1. Cell **77:** 829–839.

39. BICKEL, M., G. DVEKSLER, C. W. DIEFFENBACHER, S. RUHL, S. B. MIDURA & D. H. PLUZNICK. 1990. Induction of interferon-β and 2'5' oligoadenylate synthetase mRNAs by interleukin-6 during differentiation of murine myeloid cells. Cytokine **2:** 238–246.

40. COHEN, B., Y. GOTHELF, D. VAIMAN, L. CHEN, M. REVEL & J. CHEBATH. 1991. Interleukin-6 induces the 2',5' oligoadenylate synthetase gene in M1 cells through an effect on the interferon-responsive enhancer. Cytokine. **3:** 83–91.

41. SIMS, S. H., Y. CHA, M. F. ROMINE, P. Q. GAO, K. GOTTLIEB & A. B. DEISSEROTH. 1993. A novel interferon-inducible domain: Structural and functional analysis of the human regulatory factor 1 gene promoter. Mol. Cell. Biol. **13:** 690–702.

42. KANNO, Y., C. A. KOZACK, C. SCHINDLER, P. H. FRIGGERS, D. L. ENNIST, S. L. GLEASON, J. E. DARNELL & K. OZATO. 1993. The genomic structure of the murine ICSBP gene

reveals the presence of the gamma interferon-responsive element, to which an ISGF3-α subunit molecule binds. Mol. Cell. Biol. **13:** 3951–3963.
43. DARNELL, J. E., I. M. KERR, G. R. STARK. 1994. Jak-Stat pathways and transcriptional activation in response to interferons and other extracellular signaling proteins. Science **264:** 1415–1421.
44. HARROCH, S., M. REVEL & J. CHEBATH. 1994. Interleukin-6 signaling via four transcription factors binding palindromic enhancers of different genes. J. Biol. Chem. **269:** 26191–26195.
45. AKIRA, S., Y. NISHIO, M. NOUE, X. J. WANG, S. WEI, T. MATSUSAKA, K. YOSHIDA, T. SUDO, M. NARUTO & T. KISHIMOTO. 1994. Molecular cloning of APRF, a novel IFN-stimulated gene factor 3 p91-related transcription factor involved in the gp130-mediated signaling pathway. Cell **77:** 63–71.
46. YUAN, J. U. M. WEGENKA, C. LUTTICKEN, J. BUSCHMANN, T. DECKER, C. SCHINDLER, P. C. HEINRICH & F. HORN. 1994. The signaling pathways of interleukin-6 and gamma-interferon converge by the activation of different transcription factors which bind to common responsive DNA elements. Mol. Cell. Biol. **14:** 1657–1668.
47. STAHL, N., T. G. BOULTON, T. FARRUGELLA, N. Y. IP, S. DAVIS, B. A. WITTHUHN, F. W. QUELLE, O. SIVENNOINEN, G. BARBIERI, S. PELLEGRINI, J. IHLE & G. D. YANCOPOULOS. 1994. Association and activation of Jak-Tyk kinases by CNTF-LIF-OSM-IL-6 β receptor components. Science **263:** 92–95.

DISCUSSION OF THE PAPER

A. RAY (*Yale University of Medicine, New Haven, CT*): Are you looking at the antitumor effects of IL-6 in Taniguichi's IRF-1 knockout mice?

M. REVEL: No, not for the moment, but we should. It is a good suggestion. We are using the IL-6 knockout mice to do that.

G. CILIBERTO (*Istituto di Ricerche di Biologia Molecolare P. Angeletti, Pomezia (Rome), Italy*): First, my question is about the cell specificity of the pIRF-A complex. The second one is that the early activation of Stat factors occurs in the cytoplasm, so by preparing cytoplasmic extracts you can detect them. Can you detect pIRF-A in the cytoplasm?

REVEL: We have observed the cell specificity in epithelial breast carcinoma cells and B-9 hybridoma cells. pIRF-A is very strong in B-9 cells. It is in M-1 cells as well, and we do not think that it is cell specific. We are looking at non-liver cells only. Now, about the presence in cytoplasm, pIRF-A is found in the nuclear fraction. However, if you use genistein, an inhibitor of tyrosine kinase, you do not find it, and it is completely eliminated by phosphotyrosine antibody, showing that it contains phosphotyrosine. We believe that this phosphorylation occurs in the cytoplasm by receptor-associated kinases.

R. G. HAWLEY (*Sunnybrook Health Science Centre, Toronto, Ont., Canada*): The B-9 data are very nice. I would like to raise a point with regard to potential use of IL-6 as an inhibitor of myeloid leukemia. That is an interesting system in terms of its ability to inhibit during the induction phase, but most of myeloid leukemic cells are already blocked in differentiation, so you can induce some differentiation in them, but at the same time it is clear that you do provide some stimulation to a very primitive cell, the blast cell.

REVEL: You are absolutely right. It is easier to speak about what you see *in vitro*, so it may be that one involuntarily puts too much weight on *in vitro* effects on differentiation. When we look at the *in vivo* system in radiation-induced leukemia and we see disappearance of the preleukemic cells, it is most likely that they are eliminated by an immune response and not by differentiation. Actually, these cells *in vitro* will not differentiate. So they are probably eliminated by the fact that IL-6 allows the animal to detect preleukemic cells in its bone marrow that without IL-6 it could not detect. I do not know how it does it, or whether it can be applied in medicine.

HAWLEY: It is certain that there is a role of IL-6 as a positive growth factor in some instances of myeloid dysplastic syndromes, in particular chronic myelomonocytic leukemia.

REVEL: But, again, you do not want to put too much weight on growth effects for *in vivo* antitumor activity. I think that the growth stimulation you see *in vitro* may not always be the major effect you see *in vivo*. And if you can mount an immune response even at the price of risking growth stimulation, I think that the outcome of IL-6 use can still be quite positive for the host's response to the tumor. I just believe that clinical trials will have to be done to know whether there is any chance to use IL-6 in tumor therapy protocols or with tumor vaccines.

HAWLEY: I am not a clinician, but I can certainly see the potential utility in solid tumors, carcinoma of the breast or melanoma, for example, where you can definitely combine that with an inhibitory effect.

Clinical Trials with IL-6

JEFFREY S. WEBER

University of California, Irvine
Clinical Cancer Center
Orange, California 92668

A number of Phase I/II clinical trials have been conducted with IL-6 alone as an anticancer agent, or IL-6 following chemotherapy as a thrombopoetic agent. Initial studies of IL-6 given alone subcutaneously or after chemotherapy in patients with advanced cancer suggest that platelet counts are significantly increased, peaking 10 to 14 days after initiation of therapy. A number of other biologic effects were seen, including elevated C-reactive protein and fibrinogen levels, increased cortisol and ACTH, and a reversible normocytic, normochromic anemia of rapid onset that completely abated within 5 days of stopping therapy. No anti-tumor effects were seen in a phase II trial of IL-6 alone in patients with metastatic melanoma. Systemic symptoms including fevers, chills, nausea and fatigue were prominent at dose levels from 0.5 to 30 µg/kg daily. Unexpected toxicities included hyperglycemia requiring insulin therapy, atrial fibrillation, and reversible neurologic symptoms. No true MTD was seen with IL-6 alone, nor when IL-6 was administered to patients with metastatic sarcoma receiving MAID chemotherapy; doses of 25 to 30 µg/kg/day were tolerated without irreversible grade III–IV toxicity. When IL-6 was administered with MAID, or with ICE chemotherapy plus G-CSF, an accelerated recovery of platelet counts was seen in cycles with IL-6, compared with control cycles without cytokine.

DISCUSSION OF THE PAPER

A. MACKIEWICZ (*Academy of Medicine, Great Poland Cancer Center, Poznań, Poland*): Did you see any local changes at the site of subcutaneous injection of IL-6?

J. S. WEBER: Almost all the patients had transient erythema—that is, redness and warmth, but no abcess formation. Local cutaneous side effects faded quickly within several hours. At the doses we were using (up to 10 µg/kg/day), as long as you use indocin or acetaminophen these were very well tolerated. Minimal effects. It is only when you go to the higher doses that you begin to see the big systemic effects over a period of time.

R. HAWLEY (*Cancer Research Division, Sunnybrook Health Science Centre, Toronto, Ont., Canada*): I agree that one needs to be cautious in extrapolating results from mouse models to the human system, but there were a couple of toxicities that were reported earlier, first by Art Nienhuis at NIH using the model for Castleman's disease where he saw anemia with loss of iron storage in the marrow; also in our model we have significant anemia in addition to significant liver toxicity in mice that were over expressing IL-6. These are a couple of additional toxicities.

WEBER: I think that you could have predicted that qualitatively. I think that we were all surprised by how severe it was quantitatively. I mean, three or four patients out of fifty had severe liver toxicity as a real problem at high doses. And the other thing that I should add is that the cardiac side effects were completely unexpected. Finally, at the time there was no transgenic mouse model which showed that in some of those mice you can have severe neurologic effects; but in two of our patients who had i.v. IL-6 we had prominent neurologic side effects. For example, a patient who got his second dose of IL-6 called the nurse 4 hours later to say that he could not move the right side of his body. I went to see him at that point and he was literally completely paralyzed on the right side of his body. I lifted his arm and it was completely flaccid. Very impressive. An NMR scan of the head was normal and a lumbar puncture was completely unremarkable. The neurologic effects reversed over the next 24 to 48 hours, but he got no more IL-6. A second patient at his fifth dose, again at the highest dose, had severe ataxia—a terrible lack of coordination. He could not walk and he had such severe right-sided hand tremor that he could not hold a pen or use his right hand to eat. He used his left hand. Again, these effects were unexpected at that time.

P. SEHGAL (*New York Medical College, Valhalla*): Abe Mittelman has just completed a phase I study of IL-6 at New York Medical College in the same format using ICE followed by 10 days of IL-6 in *alternating* cycles. And, to summarize the data briefly, there have been instances where he had to stop IL-6 administration because of toxicity at doses in the range 5–10 to 25 µg/kg. Secondly, from the data I have seen from his study I am not terribly impressed yet that IL-6 had a significant effect on increase of platelet counts when compared to untreated controls. So that is the issue which will have to be evaluated more vigorously, more carefully.

WEBER: The big disappointment, Pravin, is that if you look at the mouse model that everybody has used, the doses administered of the nonglycosylated IL-6 are 5000 µg/kg, but we are limited in patients to 25 µg/kg, and that is one of our problems.

Phase IA/IB Evaluation of Mammalian Cell–derived Glycosylated Recombinant Human Interleukin (SIGOSIX) before and after Cytotoxic Chemotherapy

P. S. RITCH,[a] C. KEEVER,[a] J. SCHILLER,[b] S. RIVKIN,[a]
P. L. WITT,[a] S. E. GROSSBERG,[a] R. L. TRUITT,[a] H. BURRIS,[c]
D. D. Von HOFF,[d] L. VAICKUS,[e] D. DRECHSLER,[e] E. C. BORDEN,[a]
A. GALAZKA,[f] J. B. BREITMEYER,[e] AND A. ABDUL-AHAD[f,g]

[a]*Medical College of Wisconsin*
Milwaukee, Wisconsin

[b]*University of Wisconsin*
Madison, Wisconsin

[c]*University of Washington*
Seattle, Washington

[d]*University of Texas*
San Antonio, Texas

[e]*Serono Laboratories Inc.*
Boston, Massachusetts

[f]*Ares-Serono SA*
15 bis, Chemin des Mines
CH1202 Geneva, Switzerland

Interleukin-6 is a multifunctional pleiotropic cytokine that has demonstrated significant antineoplastic activity, immunoperturbation and biological response modifier effects, stimulation of the acute phase response and profound effects on hematopoiesis, particularly megakaryocyte maturation and thrombocytopoiesis. We have conducted a phase I evaluation of r-hIL-6 in patients with advanced neoplastic disease. Patient cohorts received escalating doses of r-hIL-6 subcutaneously at doses of 0.3, 1, 3 and 10 μg/kg/day, according to the following schema: cycle 0—r-hIL-6 daily × 7 days followed by washout recovery period: cycle 1—carboplatin 800 mg/m^2 IV; cycle 2—carboplatine 800 mg/m^2 IV, followed by daily r-hIL-6 for up to 21 days. Tolerance and toxicity were assessed to establish the maximum tolerated dose and define treatment-related toxicities. Serial monitoring included routine hematology and chemistry panels, acute phase proteins, immunophenotype and functional assays, hematopoietic colony assays, cytokine gene expression and induced proteins, pharmacokinetics and immunogenicity. Constitutional "cytokine" symptoms consisting variably of fever, chills and rigors, diaphoresis, headache, body aches, dizziness, anorexia,

---

[g] Author to whom correspondence should be addressed.

nausea and vomiting were seen frequently and were generally mild. Anemia was also commonly observed. At the highest dose level (10 μg/kg/day), confusion and hyperbilirubinemia were also seen occasionally. There was a profound stimulation of peripheral blood platelet counts and acute phase proteins in a dose-dependent fashion. Some patients demonstrated accelerated hematopoietic recovery of peripheral blood platelet counts following chemotherapy even at low doses of r-hIL-6 (0.3 μg/kg/day). There were no significant effects on major lymphocyte subsets or B-cell and T-cell subsets; however, r-hIL-6 significantly increased CD71 expression on monocytes (*i.e.* activation). At 10 μg/kg/day, r-hIL-6 stimulated increases in peripheral blood progenitor cells as determined by several hematopoietic colony assays. Preliminary analysis indicates no significant effect on serum neopterin or β-microglobulin levels. Patient accrual and further ancillary biological studies are continuing.

DISCUSSION OF THE PAPER

J. A. ELIAS (*Yale University School of Medicine, New Haven, CT*): Let me just ask a question that jumped out at me: some of the side effects which were reported with the non-glycosylated molecule were not seen by your group. Are we to believe that hepatic and neurologic abnormalities may be a function of the glycosylation of the molecule?

A. ABDUL-AHAD: In defense of *E. coli*–derived IL-6—we have not reached the levels that Dr. Weber has described. At the levels we used, we observed some hyperbilirubinemia at 10 μg/kg body weight, but it was not profound.

J. WEBER (*University of California, Irvine Clinical Cancer Center, Orange, CA*): We were giving 32–100 μg/kg/day, which is up to 10 times more than the Serono trial. So you may still see things.

J. BIENVENU (*Lyon, France*): Is the decrease of albumin you observed due to changing the endothelial permeability, as described for TNF?

ABDUL-AHAD: Unfortunately, I do not have the data.

G. FEY (*University of Erlangen-Nürnberg, Erlangen, Germany*): I am surprised that what you see among acute-phase proteins are increases in fibrinogen, CRP, and α_2-globulins. Nobody talked about changes in complement C3. Has that been seen to go up?

WEBER: We have looked at C3, but there were no significant changes up to 100 μg/kg/day of IL-6. A little surprising.

Interleukin-6-Type Cytokines and Their Receptors for Gene Therapy of Melanoma[a]

ANDRZEJ MACKIEWICZ,[b] MACIEJ WIZNEROWICZ,[b] ELKE ROEB,[c] JERZY NOWAK,[d] TOMASZ PAWLOWSKI,[e] HEINZ BAUMANN,[f] PETER C. HEINRICH,[c] AND STEFAN ROSE-JOHN[c]

[b]*Department of Cancer Immunology*
Chair of Oncology, Academy of Medicine
GreatPoland Cancer Center
61688 Poznań, Poland

[c]*Institute of Biochemistry*
RWTH Aachen
52100 Aachen, Germany

[d]*Institute of Human Genetics*
Polish Academy of Sciences
60476 Poznań, Poland

[e]*National Jewish Center for Immunology and Respiratory Medicine*
Denver, Colorado 802206

[f]*Department of Molecular and Cellular Biology*
Roswell Park Cancer Institute
Buffalo, New York 14263

INTRODUCTION

Cellular tumor vaccines have been used to treat patients with melanoma for the past few decades. They consisted of either tumor cell lysates, irradiated autologous or allogeneic tumor cells or irradiated virus-infected cells.[1] Immunization of patients with irradiated autologous cells resulted in clinical responses in 25% of patients[2] and stimulation of specific cytotoxic T-lymphocytes (CTL).[3] Polyvalent melanoma vaccine composed of three allogeneic cell lines induced IgM and IgG antibodies to melanoma associated antigens and in patients with stage IIIA and IV melanoma increased survival fourfold.[4]

Recently, there has been significant research carried out in generating so called genetic melanoma vaccines engineered to secret cytokines.[5] The strategy of action of these vaccines is to locally enhance tumor antigen presentation or to supply costimulation of the immune system for the activation of tumor-specific lymphocytes. The major concept is to deliver cytokines in high concentrations local to the tumor while systemic concentration should remain low. A number of cytokine genes such as IL-

---

[a] This work was supported by grants from the Deutsche Forschungsdgemeinschaft, the Fonds der Chemichen Industrie, the Stiftung Volkswagenwerk, and The State Committee for Scientific Research (Warsaw) KBN 4S402096.

1, IL-2, IL-4, IL-6, IL-7, IL-10, IL-11, TNFα, IFN-γ, granulocyte/macrophage CSF have been transfected into tumor cells with varying effects on tumorigenicity and immunogenicity.[6-16] Until now 8 clinical protocols based on preclinical studies using autologous (5) or allogeneic (3) melanoma cells utilizing TNF, IL-2, IFN-γ, IL-4 were approved (according to the list updated every month and published in *Human Gene Therapy*).

Significant antitumor potential has been demonstrated for IL-6. Original studies by Mule *et al.*[17] have shown that IL-6 injected into mice prevented melanoma growth and metastasis formation. Subsequent studies have demonstrated that transfection of the IL-6 gene into tumor cells of various origin had a more pronounced effect in tumor rejection and metastasis prevention than systemic IL-6 administration.[10] However, there are conflicting results showing that IL-6 cDNA transfected into murine lung carcinoma cells had no effect on tumor growth but increased mortality in mice.[18] Tumor inhibitory actions of IL-6 appear to be T-cell dependent; CD4+ and CD8+ cells were required for the regression of established pulmonary metastases of weakly immunogenic fibrosarcoma in mice following the systemic administration of IL-6.[10] Moreover, lung metastatic potential of a weakly immunogenic clone of Lewis lung carcinoma was significantly decreased following vaccination with tumor cells transfected with IL-6 cDNA.[10]

IL-6 acts through a receptor complex consisting of two different subunits, an 80 kD (gp80) IL-6 binding glycoprotein and a 130 kD (gp130) signal transducing protein.[19-21] Recently, it has been demonstrated that IL-6 initially binds to gp80 and then the complex associates with a dimmer of gp130 which is linked by disulfide bridges.[22,23] It has also been suggested that the complex may consist of two molecules of each IL-6, gp80 and gp130.[24] However, other groups were not able to demonstrate IL-6-IL-6 interactions (Dr. L. Aarden—this conference). Soluble forms of both receptor proteins have been described.[25-26] and shown to be generated by shedding.[27-29] Interestingly, a complex of a soluble form of gp80 (sIL-6R) in the presence of IL-6 can *in vitro* elicit a specific signal on cells which express gp130.[22,30-33] Moreover, it has been demonstrated that sIL-6R enhances IL-6 activity *in vitro*.[32,36] In our own studies[30] sIL-6R enhanced IL-6 activity in increasing gene expression of a number of acute phase proteins in human hepatoma cell line Hep G2. In addition, in the *in vitro* model of Hep G2 cells transfected with IL-6 cDNA in which gp80 is downregulated (what leads to homologous desensitization to IL-6) sIL-6R restored responsiveness of these cells to IL-6.[32] Both soluble forms of gp80 and gp130 were found in circulation but their biological role *in vivo* still remains obscure.[26,35] Recently, it was shown that IL-6 is present in the circulation in high molecular weight protein complexes, a component of which is the sIL-6R.[36,37] More recently it has been demonstrated that IL-6 in sera of patients with juvenile rheumatoid arthritis circulates as complex with sIL-6R.[38]

The gp130 was found to be a component of the receptors for number of cytokines such as leukemia inhibitory factor (LIF), oncostatin M, ciliary neurotrophic factor, IL-11 which accordingly were assigned as IL-6-type cytokines.[39,40] Although these cytokines share some biological functions, they play distinct roles in controlling homeostatic mechanisms[41] (also *Ann. N.Y. Acad. Sci.*, this volume). LIF for example has been suggested to act mainly locally,[42] whereas IL-6 is belied to have systemic effects.[39] Soluble forms of the LIF receptor (sLIF-R) were found in mice, but so far not in humans.[42] *In vitro* sLIFR inhibits LIF activity, but its biological role *in vivo* is still not known.

Accordingly, we undertook the studies described in this paper to evaluate antimelanoma activity of IL-6, LIF, sIL-6R and sLIFR. We used B-78 melanoma cells a subline of the widely used B16 cell line. B-78 cells are known not to express the class I MHC molecules ($H-2K^b$) which renders them to be low immunogenic and in consequence more tumorigenic than B16 cells.[43]

MATERIAL AND METHODS

Cell Culture and Transfection

B-78-H1 murine melanoma cells (kindly provided by Dr. L. H. Graf, Chicago, IL, USA) were maintained in MEM Eagle's medium (Biomed, Lublin, Poland) containing 10% fetal calf serum and tobramycin 50 µg/ml in 37°C in 5%CO_2/95% air. cDNAs coding for human IL-6 (kindly provided by Drs. T. Hirano and T. Kishimoto, Osaka, Japan), human LIF (kindly provided by Dr. Y. Janick, France) and murine sIL-6R (kindly provided by Dr. G. Ciliberto, Pomezia, Italy) were inserted into the XhoI site of the cloning vector pCDM8 (kindly provided by Dr. B. Seed, Boston, USA). SLIF-R inserted in pDC302 (pMLIFR3[44]) was generously provided by Dr. D. Gearing, Immunex Corp. For the establishment of stable cell lines cotransfections with the plasmid pSV2Neo were performed. Cells were transfected with CsCl purified plasmid DNAs using the calcium-phosphate precipitation method as described.[45] Resistant cell clones were selected in the presence of 500 µg/ml G418 and highly expressing cell clones were probed by Northern blotting. Control cells were transfected with pSV2Neo only.

Gen Expression Analysis

Northern blotting was carried out as described.[46] Nylon membranes were hybridized with a 1.1 kb EcoRI fragment of the human IL-6 cDNA,[47] a 0.7 kb XhoI fragment of human LIF cDNA,[48] a 1.0 kb Hind III/XbaI fragment of murine gp80 cDNA,[49] a 1.9 kb BamHI fragment of the murine gp130 cDNA,[50] and 2.8 kb fragment of murine LIF receptor, labeled by random priming.[51]

The IL-6 bioassay was performed using the IL-6-dependent murine plasmacytoma cell line B9 kindly provided by Dr. L. Aarden (Amsterdam, the Netherlands).[52] Moreover, human IL-6 secreted by transfected cells was determined by an ELISA (Genzyme, Cambridge, MA). LIF activity was measured using a bioassay based on human hepatoma cells Hep G2.[53] SIL-6R was estimated by radioimmunoassay.[54] To identify secretion of sLIF-R 2nd conditioned medium of transfected cells was collected, concentrated 50-fold and 20 µl separated on 7.5% SDS PAGE. The proteins were transferred to nitrocellulose and probed with polyclonal rabbit anti mouse LIF-R serum (provided by Immunex Corp.). The binding of antibodies on the Western blot was visualized by using ^{125}I-labeled goat anti rabbit Ig.

Surface expression of the IL-6R was measured using a [^{125}I]-IL-6 binding assay. [^{125}I]-IL-6, 4×10^5 dpm (specific activity of 10^5 dpm/ng IL-6) was added to 10^5 B-78 cells in the absence or presence of a 500-fold excess of unlabeled IL-6 for 2 h at 4°C. Cells were washed 5 times with icecold PBS containing 0.2% BSA, 0.1 mM $CaCl_2$ and 1 mM $MgCl_2$ and cell associated radioactivity was determined after a 2 h digestion in 1 M NaOH at 37°C and by gamma-counting.

Expression of $H-2K^b$ on transfected and untransfected cells was determined by FACS analysis using monoclonal biotinylated EH144 (anti H-2Kb) antibodies.[55]

Cell Proliferation Assay

Cell proliferation was measured by ^{3}H-thymidine incorporation as well as with a 3-[4,5-dimethylthiazol-2-yl]-2,5-di-phenyltetrazolium bromide (MTT) cell viability assay. Cells were cultured in 96-well microplates (5×10^5 cells per well) for 48 h and radioactivity or MTT was added for the last 4 h of culture.

Tumor Models

Eight to ten week old C57BL/6 × C3H (H-2 bxk) mice were obtained from the Institute of Immunology and Experimental Therapy (Wroclaw, Poland), severe combined immunodeficient (SCID) 6–8 week old CB17 (H-2b) mice were kindly provided by Dr. A. Mitchison (Berlin, FRG). Mice deficient of class I MHC molecules have been established by disruption of the β2-microglobulin (β_2m) genes and show a severe deficiency in the maturation of class I MHC-restricted CD8$^+$T cells.[56] They were used as homozygous ($-/-$) × C57BL/6 F3 as described.[57] Animals were injected subcutaneously (s.c.) with 5×10^5 viable (as determined by trypan blue dye exclusion) control (mock transfected) or cytokine and cytokine receptor transfected B-78 cells. Moreover, C57BL/6 × C3H severe combined immunodeficient (SCID) mice were injected intravenously (i.v.) into the tail vein with 5×10^5 control or transfected cells and after 4–5 weeks lung metastases were evaluated.

In another set of experiments C57BL/6 × C3H mice were primarily injected s.c. with transfected B-78 or control cells (left flank) and after 2 weeks challenged with parental B-78 cells (right flank). Mice were maintained for 4 months and tumor formation and survival were monitored. Moreover, the same strain of mice was primarily injected i.v. with B-78 parental cells and after 10 days subsequently challenged s.c. with B-78 or B-78-transfected cells. Animals were sacrificed 4–5 weeks following the first injection.

Presence of the lung metastases was analyzed using light microscopy. In order to quantify the extend of lung metastasis the following scale was introduced: 0 = no metastases found; 1 = melanoma cells found in blood vessels; 2 = one small metastatic focus; 3 = multiple metastatic foci; 4 = heavy metastatic tumor load.

RESULTS

Characterization of B-78 Cells and Transfectants

In order to characterize murine B-78 cells prior to transfection, we have analyzed the endogenous expression of IL-6, gp80, gp130, LIF and LIF-R. Northern blot analysis has demonstrated no detectable mRNA of IL-6, LIF and LIF-R and extremely low levels of gp80 and gp130 mRNAs (data not shown). IL-6 activity was determined in the culture medium and was estimated as corresponding to 70 pg/ml/24 h/10^7 cells. LIF activity was not detected by Hep G2 bioassay. When binding of [^{125}I]-IL-6 to B-78 cells was measured, 300–500 receptors per cell were detected (data not shown). Exposure of B-78 cells to various doses of exogenous IL-6 and dexamethasone did not influence mRNA expression of gp80 and gp130 (data not shown).

Untransfected B-78 cells were treated with increasing amounts of rhIL-6 (0–100 ng/ml) and LIF (0–100 ng) for 48 h and proliferation of the cells was studied. rhIL-6 caused slight increase of B-78 cells proliferation up to 35% above the control value at 100 ng/ml rhIL-6. LIF added to the culture did not affect cell proliferation (data not shown).

Cells were stably transfected with expression vectors containing cDNAs for human IL-6, human LIF, murine sIL-6R (gp80) and murine LIF-R. The transfected cells constitutively secreted 10–100 ng/ml/24 h/10^7 cells of IL-6, LIF and sIL-6R respectively (data not shown). Endogenous levels of gp80 and gp130 mRNA were unaffected by the transfection and selection procedures.

Proliferation of mock and IL-6, sIL-6R, LIF and sLIF-R transfected B-78 cells did not differ significantly between one another.

Analysis of Tumor Growth of B-78 and B-78 Transfected Cells

S.c. injections of melanoma cells into C57BL/6 × C3H mice resulted after 8 weeks in tumor formation in all but one animal studied. However, as shown in FIGURE 1, there were very significant differences in tumor size. B-78 cells transfected with sLIF-R formed tumors with diameters which exceeded those of the tumors formed by mock transfected cells. IL-6, sIL-6R, LIF and a combination of IL-6 and sIL-6R (1:1 mixture) caused a significant reduction of tumor diameters. The combination of IL-6 and sIL-6R was the most effective. Animals injected with B-78-LIF cells demonstrated significant weight loss (data not shown).

Kinetics of tumor growth and survival of C57BL/6 × C3H mice in the same experiment are demonstrated in FIGURE 2. As shown in FIGURE 2A all animals injected s.c. with control cells developed tumors at 4 weeks following injections. At this time point only half of the mice injected with B-78 transfected with IL-6, sIL-6R and LIF had tumors. Most of the animals injected with sLIF-R had tumors already 3 weeks after they were injected. Until the 7th week none of the animals injected with a mixture of B-78-IL-6 and B-78-sIL-6R cells (1:1) showed a palpable tumor (FIG. 2A). However, after 10 weeks both groups of mice injected with B-78-IL-6 cells and with a mixture of B-78-IL-6 and B-78-sIL-6R cells had tumors of comparable size. Survival analysis demonstrated increased survival time of mice injected with B-78-IL-

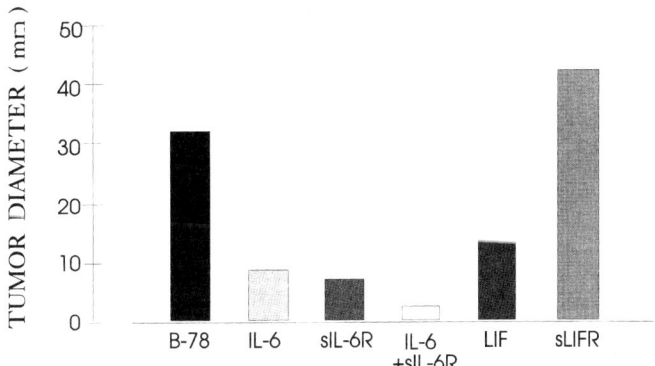

FIGURE 1. Tumor formation in mice injected subcutaneously with control and transfected B-78 cells. In each group 10 C57BL/6 × C3H mice were injected into the flank region with 5×10^5 cells and tumor size evaluated after 8 weeks.

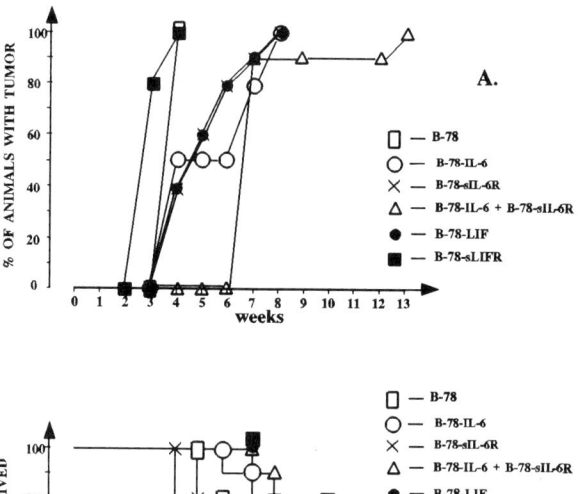

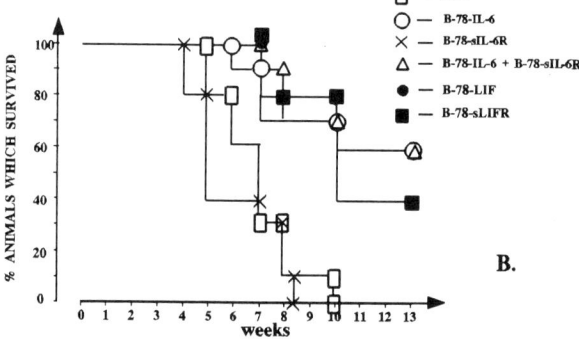

FIGURE 2. Kinetics of tumor incidence and survival of animals injected with B-78 mock and cytokine and their receptors transfected cells. In each group 10 animals were injected s.c. with 5×10^5 control and transfected B-78 cells. Weekly the animals were examined and tumor incidence (**A**) and survival (**B**) were scored.

6 and a mixture of B-78-IL-6 and B-78-sIL-6R cells when compared with mice injected with B-78 or B-78-sIL-6R cells alone (FIG. 2B). We have not established the cause of death of the injected animals.

In TABLE 1 the results of i.v. injections of melanoma cells into C57BL/6 × C3H mice 4–5 weeks after administration are shown. In mice injected with B-78 cells transfected with IL-6, sIL-6R and LIF expression vectors significantly fewer lung metastasis were found when compared with those injected with control cells. Animals injected with a mixture of cells transfected with IL-6 and sIL-6R cells showed almost no metastasis formation. Moreover, more animals injected with transfected cells than those injected with control cells survived 5 weeks.

Mice primarily injected s.c. with control and sIL-6R transfected cells challenged after 2 weeks with parental B-78 cells developed tumors after 8 weeks (FIG. 3A). However 80% of animals primarily injected with B-78-IL-6 cells and only 20% of injected with a mixture of IL-6 and sIL-6R transfected B-78 cells had tumors. This status has not changed throughout 16 weeks of observation. Survival analysis (FIG. 3B) has demonstrated significant differences between the groups studied: 90% of mice immunized with a mixture of IL-6 and sIL-6R B-78 compared to only 10% of control animals cells survived 16 weeks.

TABLE 1. Lung Metastasis Formation in C57BL/6 × C3H Mice

Cells	Number of Animals	Dead Animals[a]	Number of Animals with Lung Metastases[b]		
			0	1 + 2	3 + 4
B-78	17	5	2	2	8
B-78-IL-6	11	2	4	3	2
B-78-sIL-6R	11	3	7		1
B-78-IL-6 + B-78-sIL-6R	15	1	13	1	
B-78-LIF	10	3	4	2	1
B-78-sLIF-R	7	0	3	3	1

[a] Animals which did not survive 5 weeks.
[b] Metastases were evaluated using light microscopy according to the scale described in MATERIAL AND METHODS.

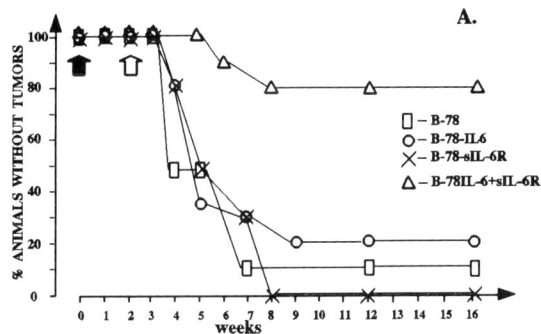

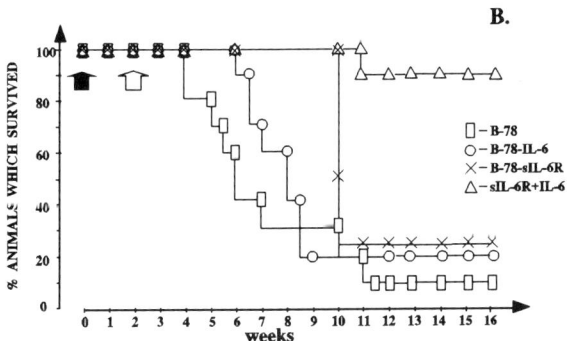

FIGURE 3. Stimulation of anti-melanoma immunity by cytokine transfected B-78 cells. 10 C57BL/6 × C3H mice were injected s.c. *(black arrow)* with 5×10^5 mock transfected and cytokine transfected B-78 cells. After 2 weeks mice were rechallenged s.c. *(white arrow)* with 5×10^5 parental B-78 cells and the tumor formation (**A**) and survival (**B**) analyzed.

TABLE 2. Lung Metastasis Formation in C57BL/6 × C3H Mice Challenged with B-78 Cells and Reinjected with B-78 or B-78 Transfected Cells

Cells	Number of Animals	Dead Animals[a]	Number of Animals with Lung Metastases[b]		
			0	1 + 2	3 + 4
B-78	12	7	1		4
B-78-IL-6	13	3	2	6	2
B-78-sIL-6R	11	3	2	5	3
B-78-LIF	13	1		4	8

[a] Legend as in TABLE 1.

Subsequent s.c. challenge of transfected melanoma cells into animals primarily injected i.v. with B-78 control cells resulted in a reduction of lung metastasis when compared to subsequent s.c. challenge with non-transfected cells (TABLE 2).

In order to elucidate the immunological mechanisms which might be induced by the transfected cells we have taken advantage of SCID mice, which are characterized by greatly reduced numbers of T and B cells.[58] TABLE 3 summarizes the results of i.v. injections of melanoma cells into SCID mice. All animals injected with control cells developed heavy lung metastasis and more than 50% of animals died within 5 weeks. Similarly B-78-IL-6 cells formed metastasis in the animals. Transfection of sIL-6R into B-78 cells resulted in reduced metastasis formation by these cells and increased survival of the animals. The combination of B-78-IL-6 with B-78-sIL-6R did not exceed the effect of B-78-sIL-6R alone.

All β2-m knockout mice injected s.c. with control cells developed tumors and died after two weeks following injection (TABLE 4). However, only 50% of animals injected with B-78-IL-6 cells had tumors which were significantly smaller. These mice died 4

TABLE 3. Lung Metastasis Formation in SCID Mice after Intravenous Injection with B-78 or B-78 Transfected Cells

Cells	Number of Animals	Dead Animals	Number of Animals with Lung Metastases[a]		
			0	1 + 2	3 + 4
B-78	7	4			3
B-78-IL-6	13	2		2	9
B-78-sIL-6R	15	2	8		5
B-78-IL-6 + B-78-sIL-6R	7	0	3	1	3

[a] Legend as in TABLE 1.

TABLE 4. Tumor Formation in β2-Microglobulin Knockout Mice Injected s.c.

Cells	Number of Animals	Dead Animals	No. of Animals with Tumor after Reinjection
B-78	8	8 (after 2 weeks)	
B-78-IL-6	8	4 (after 4 weeks)	0

weeks after cell injection. The remaining 50% of animals which did not develop tumors were injected s.c. with control cells. None developed a tumor.

DISCUSSION

The results obtained indicate that studied IL-6-type cytokines and their respective soluble receptors affect murine melanoma growth and metastasis formation. The major finding of our studies is that sIL-6R gene introduced into melanoma cells inhibits their growth, ability to metastasize, and stimulates potent, specific, and long lasting anti-melanoma immunity. The activity of the sIL-6R is linked to the presence of IL-6 either secreted by B-78 cells or produced by the host in response to injected tumor cells,[59] which is supported by the fact that in the system used the most pronounced biological effect of the sIL-6R was observed when sIL-6R–producing cells were combined with those producing IL-6.

In the studies presented LIF also showed potential antitumor effects. However, toxic effect of the doses used *(cachexia)* might dominate over the benefits of its action. Interestingly sLIF-R displayed diverse effects. It inhibited to some extend the metastatic potential of B-78 cells but promoted local tumor growth suggesting that sLIF-R may act both locally and systemically. Certainly this phenomenon needs further careful study.

As recently reported by others[16] transfection of the IL-6 gene into melanoma cells significantly inhibited their growth when injected into animals. Moreover, it increased survival time of injected mice. Surprisingly, transfection of a sIL-6R gene inhibited tumor incidence even to a higher degree than transfection with IL-6. However, it did not affect survival time when compared to mock transfected cells. The combination of IL-6 and sIL-6R transfectants demonstrated significantly different growth kinetics compared to those displayed by B-78-IL-6 or B-78-sIL-6R cells. In the initial phase of tumor growth a lag period in tumor formation of 3 weeks was observed when the combined injection was compared to single injections of B-78-IL-6 or B-78-sIL-6R cells. However, survival time experiments have demonstrated no difference between animals injected with B-78-IL-6 cells and the combination of IL-6 and sIL-6R secreting cells. However, preimmunization experiments have clearly shown a significantly higher potential of combination of IL-6 and its soluble receptor over IL-6 alone in stimulating specific and long lasting anti-melanoma immunity.

Similar inhibitory effects were observed when metastasis formation by transfected and mock transfected melanoma cells was studied in C57BL/6 × C3H mice 4–5 weeks after injection. In this *in vivo* bioassay transfection of sIL-6R into B-78 cells resulted in an even higher inhibitory effect of metastasis formation than transfection of IL-6 into B-78 cells. A spectacular effect was seen when cells transfected with IL-6 and with sIL-6R cDNA were injected together. These results are comparable to those were tumor growth after 5 weeks following s.c. injections of transfected B 78 cells was studied (FIG. 2).

It might be speculated that the biological action of IL-6-type cytokines and their soluble receptors, could be mediated by a direct growth inhibition of B-78 cells by the respective cytokine. However, this is certainly not the case since B-78 cells in the presence of high concentrations of IL-6 showed a rather increased proliferation rate when compared with control cells. Moreover, proliferation analysis of mock, cytokine and soluble receptor transfected cells showed no significant differences. In addition, the possibility of upregulation of $H-2K^b$ expression on the cell surface[60] by transfected factors was ruled out since the $H-2K^b$ molecule was not detectable in parental and transfected B-78 cells.

To evaluate the applicability of the studied factors for the construction of genetic cellular vaccines animals were primarily challenged i.v. with B-78 melanoma cells. Ten days later they were reinjected s.c. with the transfected cells. Such a procedure resulted in an increase in the number of animals surviving 5 weeks and in reduction in the number of lung metastasis. These results clearly indicate that cells transfected with IL-6, sIL-6R or LIF could be used in preparing cellular vaccines against cancer. In the present studies we did not irradiate the transfected cells in order to eliminate factors which could be affected by this procedure such as increased tumor immunogenecity.[6]

The obtained results suggest that IL-6 and IL-6 complexed with its soluble receptor may display diverse activities *in vivo*. Since combined secretion of IL-6 and sIL-6R inhibited melanoma growth in early phase it is possible that IL-6/sIL-6R complexes costimulate directly or indirectly NK cells. Such an activity has already been ascribed to IL-6[61]; however, in experiments with SCID mice lacking T and B lymphocytes but possessing NK cells, sIL-6R or IL-6/sIL-6R complexes were protective against the formation of lung metastasis while IL-6 alone was ineffective. Recent reports demonstrated that protection against tumors induced by the injection of plasmacytoma cells by a number of cytokines, T cells are not required during the first to 6–7 weeks.[6] This observation supports the hypothesis of significant stimulation of NK cells by IL-6/sIL-6R complexes. Costimulatory effects of a number of cytokines including IL-6 in antitumor activities were mainly linked to cytotoxic T lymphocytes.[5,9,10] This is supported by a recent demonstration that IL-6 can directly activate CD28 on T cells omitting B7 molecule.[62] Current experiments show that IL-6/sIL-6R complexes have even greater potential to stimulate specific antitumor immunity than IL-6. Results obtained with β2-microglobulin knockout mice lacking CD8$^+$ lymphocytes indicate however, significant involvement also of other cells than CD8$^+$ cells. The observed dissemination of the biological activity of IL-6 and the IL-6-sIL-6R complexes may be explained by the involvement of cells which do only express gp130 and are therefore non-responsive to IL-6 but respond to the complex of IL-6/sIL-6R.[30,33] The nature of these cells remains to be elucidated. Accordingly, biological functions ascribed to IL-6 might have to be verified since IL-6 complexes with its sIL-6R has been found in biological fluids.[36–38]

SUMMARY

B-78-H1 melanoma cells were stably transfected with cDNAs encoding human IL-6, human LIF, murine sIL-6R and murine sLIFR. The mock transfected and transfected cells demonstrated no detectable H-2K^b molecules. B-78 transfected cells were subcutaneously (s.c.) and intravenously (i.v.) injected to B57BL/6 × C3H mice. Control B-78 cells formed tumors and lung metastases in injected animals. Cells transfected with IL-6, LIF and sIL-6R showed greatly reduced tumor and metastases formation. Transfection of IL-6, sIL-6R or LIF had similar protective effects while the combination of IL-6 and sIL-6R was most effective. In contrast, cells transfected with sLIFR showed reduced metastasis formation but increased tumor growth compared to mock transfected cells. Kinetic analysis demonstrated a 3 weeks lag period between the formation of tumors by B-78 cells and the combination of B-78 cells transfected with IL-6 and sIL-6R. No such lag phase was seen when B-78-IL-6 or B-78-sIL-6R cells were injected alone. Mice primarily injected s.c. with a mixture of IL-6 and sIL-6R transfected cells and rechallenged after 2 weeks with parental B-78 cells demonstrated long-lasting antitumor immunity. IL-6 and sIL-6 transfected cells used alone for immunization had only limited effect. Injection of transfected cells into

SCID mice which are characterized by greatly reduced number of T and B cells, showed a protective effect of sIL-6R on metastasis formation by B-78 cells. β_2m knockout mice lacking CD8$^+$ T cells, injected with B-78 cells developed tumors and died after 2 weeks. However, B-78 cells transfected with IL-6 developed tumors in only 50% of animals. Mice without tumors rechallenged with B-78 cells demonstrated required immunity against parental melanoma cells. The results obtained indicate that studied IL-6-type cytokines and their respective soluble receptors affect murine melanoma growth and metastasis formation. The major finding of these studies is that IL-6 complexed with sIL-6R demonstrated qualitatively different biological activity than IL-6 alone especially in stimulating long lasting anti-melanoma immunity. The proposed mechanism of action of such complexes beside activation of cytotoxic T lymphocytes is activation of NK cells.

REFERENCES

1. BYSTRYN, J.-C., S. FERRONE & P. O. LIVINGSTON, Eds. 1993. Specific Immunotherapy of Cancer with Vaccines. Ann. N.Y. Acad. Sci. **690**.
2. BERD, D., H. C. MAGUIRE, JR. & M. J. MASTRANGELO. 1986. Cancer Res. **46:** 2572–2577.
3. MITCHELL, M. S., W. HAREL, R. A. KEMPF, E. HU, J. KAN-MITCHEL, G. DEAN & J. MORE. 1990. Clin. Oncol. 1–13.
4. MORTON, D. L., D. S. B. HOON, J. A. NIZZE, L. J. FOSHAG, E. FAMATIGA, L. A. WANEK, C. CHANG, R. F. IRIE, R. K. GUPTA & R. ELASHOFF. 1993. Ann. N.Y. Acad. Sci. **690:** 120–134.
5. TEPPER, R. I. & J. J. MULLE. 1994. Hu. Gene Ther. **5:** 153–164.
6. DRANOFF, G., E. JAFFEE, A. LAZENBY, P. GLUMBEK, P. LEVITSKY, K. BROSE, V. JACKSON, H. HAMADA, D. PARDOLL & R. C. MULLIGAN. 1993. Proc. Natl. Acad. Sci. USA **90:** 3539–3543.
7. OHE, Y., E. R. PODACK, K. J. OLSEN, Y. MIYAHARA, T. OHIRA, K. MIURA, K. NISHIO & N. SAIJO. 1993. Int. J. Cancer **53:** 432.
8. HOCK, H., M DORSCH, U. KUNZENDORF, Z. QIN, T. DIAMANTEIN & T. BLANKENSTEIN. 1993. Proc. Natl. Acad. Sci. USA **90:** 2774–2778.
9. MULLEN, C. A., M. M. COALE, A. T. LEVY, W. G. STETLER-STEVENSON, L. A. LIOTTA, S. BRANDT & R. M. BLAESE. 1992. Cancer Res. **52:** 6021–6024.
10. PORGADOR, A., E. TZEHOVAL, A. KATZ, E. VADAI, M. REVEL, M. FELDMAN & L. EISENBACH. 1992. Cancer Res. **52:** 3679–3686.
11. UCHIYAMA, A., D. S. B. HOON, T. MORSISAKI, Y. KANEDA, D. H. YUZUKI & D. L. MORTON. 1993. Cancer Res. **53:** 949–952.
12. GANSBACHER, B., R. BANNIERJI, B. DANIELS, K. ZIER, K. CRONIN & E. GILBOA. 1990. CANCER RES. **50:** 7820–7825.
13. ASHER, A. L., J. J. MULE, A. KASID, N. P. RESTIFO, J. C. SALO, C. M., REICHERT, G. JAFFE, B. FENDLY, M. KRIEGLER & S. A. ROSENBERG. 1991. J. IMMUNOL. **146:** 3227–3234.
14. GIAVAZZI, R., A. GAROFALO, M. R. BANI, M. ABBATE, P. GHEZZI, D. BORASCHI, A. MANTOVANI & E. DEJNA. 1990. Cancer Res. **50:** 4771–4775.
15. COLOMBO, M. P. & G. FORNI. 1994. Immunol Today **15:** 48–51.
16. SUN, W. H., A. KREISLE, A. W. PHILIPS & W. B. ERSHLER. 1992. Cancer Res. **52:** 5412–5415.
17. MULE, J. J., J. K. MCINTOSH, D. M. JABLONS & S. A. ROSENBERG. 1990. J. Exp. Med. **171:** 629–636.
18. OHE, Y., E. R. PODACK, K. J. OLSEN, Y. MIYAHARA, K. MIURA, H. SAITO, Y. KOISHIHARA, Y. OBSUGI, T. OHIRA, K. NISHIO & N. SAIJO. 1993. Br. J. Cancer **67:** 939–944.
19. YAMASAKI, K., T. TAGA, Y. HIRATA, H. YAWATA, Y. KAWANISHI, B. SEED, T. TANIGUCHI, T. HIRANO & T. KISHIMOTO. 1988. Science **241:** 825–828.
20. TAGA, T., M. HIBI, Y. HIRATA, K. YAMASAKI, K. MATSUDA, T. HIRANO & T. KISHIMOTO. 1989. Cell **58:** 573–581.

21. HIBI, M., M. MURAKAMI, M. SAITO, T. HIRANO, T. TAGA & T. KISHIMOTO. 1990. Cell **63**: 1149–1157.
22. MURAKAMI, M., M. HIBI, N. NAKAGAWA, T. NAKAGAWA, K. YASUKAWA, K. YAMANISHI, T. TAGA & T. KISHIMOTO. 1993. Science **260**: 1808–1810.
23. DAVIS, S., T. ALDRICH, N. STAHL, L. PAN, T. TAGA, T. KISHIMOTO, N. Y. IP & G. D. YANCOPOULOS. 1993. Science **260**: 1805–1808.
24. STOYAN, T., U. MICHALIS, H. SCHOOLTINK, M. VAN DAM, R. RUDOLPH, P. C. HEINRICH & S. ROSE-JOHN. 1993. Eur. J. Biochem. **216**: 239–245.
25. NOVICK, D., H. ENGELMANN, D. WALLACH & M. RUBINSTEIN. 1989. J. Exp. Med. **170**: 1409–1414.
26. NARAZAKI, M., K. YASUKAWA, T. SAITO, Y. OHSUGI, H. FUKUI, Y. KOISHIHARA, G. D. YANCOPOULOS, T. TAGA & T. KISHIMOTO. 1993. Blood **82**: 1120–1126.
27. MULLBERG, J., H. SCHOOLTINK, T. STOYAN, M. GUNTHER, L. GRAEVE, G. BUSE, A. MACKIEWICZ, P. C. HEINRICH & S. ROSE-JOHN. 1992. Eur. J. Immunol. **23**: 473–480.
28. MULLBERG, J., H. SCHOOLTINK, T. STOYAN, P. C. HEINRICH & S. ROSE-JOHN. 1992. Biochem. Biophys. Res. Commun. **189**: 794–800.
29. MULLBERG, J., E. DITTRICH, L. GRAEVE, C. GERHARTZ, K. YASUKAWA, T. TAGA, T. KISHIMOTO, P. C. HEINRICH & S. ROSE-JOHN. 1993. FEBS Lett **332**: 174–178.
30. MACKIEWICZ, A., H. SCHOOLTINK, P. C. HEINRICH & S. ROSE-JOHN. 1992. J. Immunol. **149**: 2021–2027.
31. YASUKAWA, K., T. SAITO, T. FUKUNAGA, Y. SEKIMORI, Y. KOISHIHARA, H. FUKUI, T. MATSUDA, H. YAWATA, T. HIRANO, T. TAGA & T. KISHIMOTO. 1990. J. Biochem. **108**: 673–676.
32. SAITO, T., K. YASUKAWA, H. SUZUKI, K. FATATSUGI, T. FUKUNAGA, C. YOKOMIZO, Y. KOISHIHARA, H. FUKUI, Y. OHSUGI, H. YAWATA, I. KOBAYASHI, T. HIRANO, T. TAGA & T. KISHIMOTO. 1991. J. Immunol. **147**: 168–173.
33. TATAMURA, T., N. UDAGAWA, C. TAKAHASHI, C. MIYAURA, S. TANAKA, Y. YAMADA, Y. KOISHIHARA, Y. OHSUGI, K. KUMAKI, T. TAGA, T. KISHIMOTO & T. SUDA. 1993. Proc. Natl. Acad. Sci. USA **90**: 11924–11928.
34. NOVICK, D., L. M. SHULMAN, L. CHEN & M. REVEL. 1992. Cytokine **4**: 6–11.
35. HONDA, M., Y. YAMAMOTO, M. CHENG, K. YASUKAWA, H. SUZUKI, T. SAITO, Y. OSUGI, T. TOKUNAGA & T. KISHIMOTO. 1992. J. Immunol. **148**: 2175–2180.
36. MAY, L. T., H. VIGUET, J. S. KENNEY, N. IDA, A. C. ALLISON & P. B. SEHGAL. 1992. J. Biol. Chem. **267**: 19698–19704.
37. MAY, L. T., K. PATEL, D. GARCIA, M. I. NDUBUISI, S. FERRONE, A. MITTELMAN, A. MACKIEWICZ & P. B. SEHGAL. 1994. Blood **84**: 887–895.
38. DE BENEDETTI, F., M. MASSA, P. PIGNATTI, S. ALBANI, D. NOVICK & A. MARTINI. 1994. J. Clin. Invest. **93**: 2114–2119.
39. KISHIMOTO, T., T. TAGA & S. AKIRA. 1992. Science. **258**: 593–597.
40. KISHIMOTO, T., T. TAGA & S. AKIRA. 1994. Cell **76**: 253–262.
41. PATTERSON, P. H. 1992. Curr. Opinion. Neurobiol. **2**: 94.
42. LAYTON, M. J., B. A. CROSS, D. METCALF, L. D. WARD, R. J. SIMPSON & N. A. NICOLA. Proc. Natl. Acad. Sci. USA **89**: 8616–8620.
43. GRAF, L. H., JR., P. L. KAPLAN & S. SILAGI. 1984. Somatic Cell. Mol. Genet. **10**: 139–146.
44. GEARING, D. P., C. J. THUT, T. VANDENBOS, S. S. GIMPEL, P. B. DELANEY, J. KING, V. PRICE, D. COSMAN & M. P. BECKMAN. 1991. EMBO J. **10**: 2839–2848.
45. ROSE-JOHN, S., E. HIPP, D. LENZ, L. LEGRES, H. KORR, T. HIRANO, T. KISHIMOTO & P. C. HEINRICH. 1991. J. Biol. Chem. **266**: 3841–3846.
46. ROSE-JOHN, S., G. RINCKE & F. MARKS. 1988. Gene **74**: 465–471.
47. HIRANO, T., K. YASUKAWA, H. HARADA, T. TAGA, Y. WATANABE, T. MATSUDA, S. KASHIWAMURA, K. NAKAJIMA, K. KOYOMA, A. IWAMATU, S. TSUNASAWA, F. SAKIYAMA, H. MATSUI, Y. TAKAHARA, T. TANIGUCHI & T. KISHIMOTO. 1986. Nature **324**: 73–76.
48. GEARING, D. P., N. M. GOUGH, J. A. KING, D. J. HILTON, N. A. NICOLA, R. J. SIMPSON, E. C. NICE, K. KELSO & D. METCALF. 1987. EMBO J. **6**: 3995–4002.
49. FIORILLO, M. T., C. TONIATTI, J. VAN SNICK & G. CILIBERTO. 1992. Eur. J. Immunol. **22**: 799–804.
50. SAITO, M. K., K. YOSHIDA, M. HIBI, T. TAGA & T. KISHIMOTO. 1992. J. Immunol. **148**: 4066–4071.

51. FEINBERG, A. P. & B. VOGELSTEIN. 1983. Anal. Biochem. **132:** 6–13.
52. AARDEN, L., E. R. DE GROOT, O. L. SCHAAP & P. M. LANSDORP. 1987. Eur. J. Immunol. **17:** 1411–1416.
53. KOJ, A., J. GAULDIE, G. D. SWEENEY, E. REGOECZI & D. N. SAUDER. 1985. J. Immunol. Meth. **76:** 317–327.
54. VAN DAM, M., J. MULLBERG, H. SCHOOLTINK, T. STOYAN, J. P. J. BRAKENHOFF, L. GRAEVE, P. C. HEINRICH & S. ROSE-JOHN. 1993. J. Biol. Chem. **268:** 15285.
55. INGOLD, A. L., C. LANDDEL, C. KNALL, G. A. EVANS & T. A. POTTER. 1991. Nature **352:** 721–723.
56. ZIJSTRA, M., M. BIX, N. E. SIMISTER, J. M. LORING, D. H. RAULET & R. JAENISCH. 1990. Nature **344:** 742–746.
57. PAWLOWSKI, T., J. D. ELLIOTT, D. Y. LOH & U. D. STAERZ. 1993. Nature **364:** 642–645.
58. HENDRICKSON, E. A. 1993. Am. J. Pathol. **143:** 1511–1522.
59. UTSUMI, K., Y. TAKAI, T. TADA, S. OHZEKI, H. FUJIWARA, T. HAMAOKA. 1990. J. Immunol. **145:** 397–403.
60. DE GIOVANNI, C., G. PALMIERI, G. NICOLETTI, L. LANDUZZI, K. SCOTLANDI, A. BONTANDINI, P. L. TAZZARI, M. SENSI, A. SANTONI, P. NANNI & P. L. LOLLINI. 1991. Int. J. Cancer **48:** 270–276.
61. LUGER, T. A., T. SCHWARZ, J. KRUTMANN, R. KIRNBAUER, P. NEUNER, A. KOCK, A. URBANSKI, W. BORTH & E. SCHAUER. 1989. Ann. N. Y. Acad. Sci. **557:** 405–414.
62. HOLSTI, M. A., J. MCARTHUR, J. P. ALLISON & D. H. RAULET. 1994. J. Immunol. **152:** 1618–1628.

DISCUSSION OF THE PAPER

J. S. WEBER (*University of California, Irvine, Clinical Cancer Center, Orange, CA*): You mentioned that fresh tumors make tons of IL-6. What exactly do you mean, and how do you know that it is coming from the tumor cells as opposed to any other tumor-infiltrating T cells or other accessory cells? And if it is coming from the non-tumor cells how do you know that it would be of any use to immunize the patients after some plasmid transfection?

A. MACKIEWICZ: I should make it clearer that after the surgery we isolate the cells and then culture them *in vitro* for a period of time when the cell number is adequate to transduce them.

J. A. ELIAS (*Yale University School of Medicine, New Haven, CT*): Do you have any knowledge from animals that develop metastases and those that do not as to what is actually going on? Is it a matter of implantation of the tumor? Do you see circulating IL-6 or sIL-6R in the animals in one group or in the other group? Do you have any idea why you are getting the results you are getting?

MACKIEWICZ: General administration of cytokines, including IL-6, to humans has no or very limited anti-tumor effect. The concept of cellular tumor vaccines is to deliver the co-stimulatory signal to T-cells locally rather than systemically. It was published last March in the *Journal of Immunology* that in the context of tumor cells IL-6 may provide such co-stimulation by directly activating CD28 molecules on T-cells omitting B-7 molecules. That eventually supports the local co-stimulation pathway concept rather than the systemic. However, Drs. Pravin Sehgal and Lester May are going to analyze IL-6, sIL6-R, and IL-6/sIL-6R complexes in sera of our mice. So far we have measured acute phase proteins levels in these animals and only those which were injected with tumor cells transfected with LIF developed acute phase response. Those injected with IL-6, sIL-6R or IL-6 + sIL-6R had no increased acute phase proteins levels, suggesting that these factors might be consumed locally.

REVEL: Have you done experiments in mice in which you used these cells to vaccinate the animals and then challenge them?

MACKIEWICZ: Yes, such experiments were done. Animals acquired specific immunity against wild type tumor cells. In another series of experiments, animals were simultaneously injected intravenously with wild type cells and subcutaneously with transfected cells. Such a procedure inhibited the formation of metastases in lungs.

REVEL: Because, as you know, in some of these cytokine-transfected cells we can start very late after the primary tumor is established and still cure the animal or prevent metastasis in the type of system I was describing. This is really the question which should be achieved by a combination of IL-6 and sIL-6R.

MACKIEWICZ: Yes, this experiment is in progress.

P. WALLACE (*Fred Hutchinson Cancer Research Center, Seattle, WA*): Those cell lines which were MHC I negative after you introduced the IL-6 gene, would they still be MHC I negative? Have you checked for that?

MACKIEWICZ: Yes, my brother-in-law (Dr. T. Pawlowski) has done it.

WEBER: Did I see correctly that you actually induced memory in SCID mice?

MACKIEWICZ: No, there was no memory in SCID mice, but in $\beta 2$-microglobulin knockouts.

Roundtable Discussion

PARTICIPANTS: Ayad Abdul-Ahad, Heinz Baumann (Moderator, Part I), Jack A. Elias, Georg Fey, Michael S. Gordon, Peter C. Heinrich, Friedemann Horn, Aleksander Koj, Manfred Kopf, Valeria Poli, Michel Revel (Moderator, Part II), Pravin Sehgal, Philip M. Wallace, and Jeffrey S. Weber

Heinz Baumann: This roundtable discussion (although we sit here at a square table) is intended to address thoroughly two issues that came up during the lecture presentations but could not be satisfactorily solved because of time constraints. The unresolved issues fall into the category of two highly qualified investigators reporting different findings for a seemingly identical experimental system. The first issue arose from the presentations from Valeria Poli and Manfred Kopf and involves the physiologic response in the IL-6 knockout mouse, in particular, the interpretation of the data showing the effect of ovariectomy on bone loss. I was also surprised to learn that the $\alpha 2$-macroglobulin gene is IL-6 responsive in the mouse, although that regulation has been considered to be rat specific. The second issue concerns the DNA-binding protein interacting with the IL-6 responsive element of the rat $\alpha 2$-macroglobulin gene. Here the question is whether the binding complex described by Friedemann Horn is identical to the one analyzed by Georg Fey. The underlying theme of the discussion is when two or more experimenters are studying the same scientific question by using the same experimental system, be it tissue culture cells or animals, and applying equivalent (if not identical) procedures and resources would one not expect similar results? If not, does the difference one observes tell us more about the studied model and something about the importance of minor deviations in the system or procedure which we tend to overlook? It seems that finding out why the results differed is worthwhile. To start the discussion, we turn to the topic of osteoclast activity in IL-6-deficient mice and the interpretation of the data. Valeria, would you like to restate your interpretation of the data first, and Manfred will follow.

Valeria Poli: First of all, I think that one thing that has to be pointed out is that the genetic background is not identical because the ES cells were in both cases from 129SV background, but then Manfred's mice were, I believe, generated through a cross with C57/Bl6 and always crossed one to the other. So they have, let us say, 50% Bl6, more or less. However, my mice went instead through a cross with MF1 mice, which is an outbred background and then they were crossed once more with 129 so they were about 75% 129 and 25% MF. We have done subsequent experiments on mice which were 75–80% Bl6 because we were backcrossing on the Bl6 background having more or less the same results. I think what surprises me more about Manfred's data is that he showed that trabecular bone in the mutant mice is very much reduced as compared to wild-type mice, while we are pretty confident that it is slightly reduced in our mice. Maybe I can show a few slides that I did not show yesterday. These are the calculations of the trabecular bone volume or cancellous bone volume and cortical bone volume in the mutant and wild-type mice before and after ovariectomy. As you can see, at the basal level before ovariectomy the mutant mice have slightly less trabecular bone, but it is not significantly different from wild-type before ovariectomy. The bone volume of mutant mice both before and after ovariectomy was statistically higher than that of wild-type mice after ovariectomy. This particular experiment was done on 7 mice in each group; however, we looked at the basal content of trabecular bone in about 40 mutant mice and basically we do not find a significant difference. We do find significant differences in the amount of cortical bone, which is not affected by ovariectomy (at least at the length of the treatment we have used), but it is significantly lower before and after ovariectomy in the mutant mouse than in the wild-type mice. So, our conclusions would be that trabecular bone formation is not compromised, at least on the level of bone volume, but the formation of cortical bone might be somehow changed in mutant mice. Strain differences might be important, and the number of mice analyzed might be important because, at least I am told by the people who did these experiments, there is a high variability and one should analyze many mice. The other experiments which Manfred showed about osteoclastic activity were not done by us, so it might be difficult to reconcile the data. In fact, what we have done is to measure several parameters of bone formation and bone resorption. We measured osteoid surface - which is the amount of new bone formed in recent days and not yet mineralized - and the amount of new bone formed per day using fluorochromes, which we inserted into the bone. We then calculated the number of osteoblasts and the number of osteoclasts in the bone, and what we found is that sometimes these parameters such as osteoid surface and bone formation rate are higher in the mutant mice than in the wild-type mice, which would be in the same direction as Manfred's findings. However, they never change after ovariectomy and they never reach the levels reached in wild-type mice after ovariectomy. We did not do the same experiments, so they cannot be directly compared. We also looked for colony-forming units in the tibia of our mice - in female mice of about 10 weeks of age. What we found is that GM-CFU, considered as osteoclasts progenitors, are again at a higher level as Manfred showed. Several things must be considered, such as the age and sex of the mice.

BAUMANN: Manfred, would you like to respond to the points raised?

MANFRED KOPF: Bone development in our IL-6-deficient mice has been analyzed in the lab of Clemens Lowik in the Netherlands, who is an expert in this field. Of a series of experiments, there is one result which seems to be in conflict with the data of Valeria Poli and co-workers. A group of four IL-6-deficient mice had on average a 50% reduction of trabecular bone volume compared to controls, which is statistically significant. Obviously, this result is preliminary and needs to be confirmed. As I have shown, IL-6-deficient mice do have a reduction in numbers of uncommitted progenitor CFUs and of committed progenitor GM-CFUs in the bone marrow. A defective osteoclastogenesis in IL-6-deficient mice may be the result of a defect in myeloid development, since osteoclasts are derived from myeloid progenitors. [**Note added in proof:** The reduction of trabecular bone volume in IL-6–deficient mice has meanwhile been confirmed in independent experiments (Most, C. *et al.*, submitted.)]

BAUMANN: Can you address the difference in strain or the genetic background? Do you assume that that would make any contribution to the results?

KOPF: The phenotype of IL-2-deficient mice is much more severe on a Balb/c as compared to a F2 (129 × C57Bl/6) background (Horak, personal communication). I would not be surprised to find that IL-6 deficiency on different genetic backgrounds results in slightly different phenotypes. In future, the comparison of knockouts of different backgrounds will help to understand the contribution of the genetic environment to the function of a gene.

BAUMANN: So in essence, we have solved this issue.

MICHEL REVEL: Can you say which of the different parameters you have measured and shown us would be the most relevant for the clinical situation in humans?

POLI: It is hard to say; they can all be considered important parameters for different things. The number of osteoblasts and the osteoblast functionality can, of course, be very important because it might mean the possibility of making new bone once you have lost it. One should rather think what could be measured in humans in a non-invasive way. The precursors in osteoclastogenesis, although osteoclastogenesis *in vitro* of bone marrow of humans does not work as well as it does for mice. I guess these parameters would probably be the best.

MICHAEL S. GORDON: This is an important issue because it becomes the focal point in clinical medicine with osteoporosis becoming a major problem in women; in fact, there is unpublished or recently published data with IL-6 and a primate model demonstrating that IL-6 increases osteoclast activation, and there are biochemical markers in bone resorption that one can measure, and we are actually duplicating that in the clinical trial where we are using IL-6 in women with breast cancer to evaluate that. But I think that it is an important issue, and clearly the data first published in *Science* last year showed IL-6 contributing to osteoporosis development in women as they get older. So I think it is clinically important. But the model that would support it would be Valeria's in terms of what we have seen in humans thus far, and what one of the problems that you would anticipate from knocking out IL-6 if you look at how IL-6 impacts at least the development of osteoporosis.

KOPF: Taken together, our data obtained from IL-6 deficient mice suggest that blocking of IL-6 activity interferes with early hematopoiesis, acute phase responses, and oral and systemic immunity. It is noteworthy that the absence of IL-6 does not affect LPS-induced toxic shock I doubt that long-term inhibition of IL-6 activity in post-menopausal women suffering from osteoporosis would be an adequate treatment, given the negative effects on many other body systems.

BAUMANN: There is one thing which we have not addressed yet. When Manfred injected his animals with turpentine, they survived. Valeria presented data when she injected turpentine showing that the animals became so cachectic that she had to kill them. Apparently again the same treatment produced a different outcome. Can we comment on this one?

POLI: One possible difference might be the dose which was given because I do not think that it is really known what the LD50 of turpentine is. We gave 2×75 µl. So this might be one difference. And I must say that just two of the mice died, so it is not really statistically significant.

KOPF: Obviously, the question is : what is the physiological role of the acute phase proteins? IL-6-deficient mice showed dramatically reduced acute phase protein responses after injection with *Listeria monocytogenes* and after tissue damage induced by injection of 50 µl of turpentine. The defective acute phase response in IL-6 deficient mice did not cause lethality in our experiments. However, IL-6-deficient mice had problems defending against *L. monocytogenes*. Whether in this case the defects in the immune response can be linked to the defects in the acute phase response is an interesting question, which we are currently assessing. Furthermore, studies of wound healing after a sterile abcess in IL-6-deficient mice will clarify whether acute phase proteins facilitate this process.

BAUMANN: To add to the issue of turpentine: I used turpentine as an acute-phase inducing agent for many years. We do not inject more that 25 µl into each flank of a mouse because, if given higher doses, the mouse may die from the entry of turpentine into the circulation. It might be that Valeria has overdosed the animals and they turned cachetic.

PETER C. HEINRICH: We really use turpentine very rarely, but if you ask chemists they tell you that it is a terrible mixture. So there may be an Italian turpentine and a German turpentine. You buy this in a drug store.

BAUMANN: Turpentine, at least as it is available in the USA, is indeed a powerful irritant and causes an exceedingly strong acute phase response. The acute phase response has a characteristic time course of progression in the rat. Georg Fey did not use turpentine, but Freund's adjuvant to activate acute phase in the rat. He got a time course of IL-6 RE -binding protein that appeared to be the same as the transcriptional activation of acute phase plasma protein genes. In contrast, we learned from the papers by Friedemann Horn and Peter Heinrich that the activation of the IL-6 RE-binding protein, termed APRF, is a much more rapid and transient process. The most drastic difference seems to be after 24 hours of treatment when Georg observes a maximum of IL-6 REBP whereas Friedemann noted a return of APRF to the basal level. Here again, two investigators have studied the same gene and the same induction process and have used the same regulatory element as probe, but have different results. What could be the explanation? We will start the discussion with Friedemann Horn.

FRIEDEMANN HORN: I was not really surprised to see the different kinetics shown yesterday. When we look at hepatoma cells we actually end up with the same time course. We also published that last year. It is a biphasic response: very strong in the first hour, then decreasing, as Georg also told us yesterday, and then coming up again after 4 hours. So that is identical. In the rat system we have used completely different stimuli. LPS should really be the compound which is much more directly realizing cytokines in the rat, while adjuvants need more time to really build up an inflammation. So, this may also explain why the activation Georg sees is much more long lasting than ours. So this is one point. The other thing is that we do not have really clear data on whether the two proteins we observe are the same or different. This is a rather academic discussion. We should really have data on cross-reactivity with anti-APRF antibodies or anti-Stat91 antibodies; as soon as these data are available we can answer the question, of course. The peptide sequence data may be misleading; we do not know.

BAUMANN: Can you say something about the probe? Is it truly identical to the one used by Georg, or is there a difference, let's say by one nucleotide?

HORN: In the gel shift we use exactly the same probe for looking at the time course of the activation of the protein. During purification from rat liver we used a slightly different probe for good reason. We thought that we should use the perfect palindromic one to have higher affinity so we can get higher yields in affinity chromatography. However, we also used the core probe for α_2-macroglobulin promoter to purify APRF from HepG2 cells and we ended up with exactly the same protein as we were looking at in crude extract. I do not think that there is a basic difference. But let me just very briefly comment on the situation more generally. I think at the beginning when this Jak-Stat pathway came up it was very useful to really emphasize how similar and how common features are really present in all these different proteins. How the binding characteristics are really overlapping between Stat91 and APRF. Since this definitely draws attention to the point of how general the importance of this pathway is among different cytokines. But actually I think that it is a matter of common sense that this could not be the whole truth. Where would specificity be? Let me give you just one example. We published in March in *MCB* the observation that the ARF-1 element binds both Stat91 and APRF, and we even chose the provocative title "The convergence of signaling pathways to common elements between IFN-γ and IL-6." This is something which can explain some overlapping effects of different cytokines, but it cannot be a truth in general. So now, as more data are collected (such as the excellent data of Dr. Revel), today the situation is shown to be much more complex and complicated, of course. The same element that we showed that APRF and Stat91 can bind to now shows up to bind additional complexes, which are much more complicated, and may even bind more proteins. And if you look from that point of view, the same may occur with α_2-M promoter; I would not be surprised to have additional family members, additional proteins binding to this element. So from that point of view, I would not be surprised to have a protein other than APRF purified by Georg Fey.

BAUMANN: So, your point is that the application of techniques, as well as interpretation of the data presented in gel shift analysis need more refinement?

HORN: We still have to wait for hard facts. We do not know yet whether it is different or not . Maybe one comment is that, for example, the antibodies used are something of a pitfall which we have struggled with. We also got anti-Stat antibodies to the C-terminus of p-91 but did not know that those antibodies would not react with the rat protein. If you now show that these antibodies are not reacting with purified protein from rat liver, it tells you nothing. They are just not cross-reacting against the human protein.

BAUMANN: Georg, how do you explain the differences?

GEORG FEY: There are two points. What we purified was purified by DNA-affinity chromatography, and I showed a silver-stained gel with three resolved bands. We do not know how many species are under each band. It is still possible that under the 91kD band you have two different proteins. I presented peptide sequence data saying that one of the 91kD proteins gave rise to two peptides that are not p91 and not APRF from all that is known from the available published sequences. The other species that we have was APRF. That means that what we purified using such an affinity reagent were three or maybe four proteins, and a similar result was obtained by Dr. Kishimoto's group. They used an Aachen-type probe and purified proteins from mouse liver and cut some from the gel and did obtain peptide sequences. They obtained seven peptides. Two of them were AFRF/Stat3 and the rest are so-far unidentified. They did not know what they are. What you get by purifying proteins are all the proteins which are capable of binding at the site. It does not mean that the protein we have purified is physically present in the gel shift complex. You still have to make the correlation between the complex and the purified molecular species. The first question was: how do you explain the different kinetics? Dr. Horn provided a reasonable answer. We see exactly the same picture when we use HepG2 human hepatoma cells. This is displayed in the poster outside in the hall. He explained that they have used LPS but did not say whether they used it intraperitoneally or subcutaneously.

HORN: We injected intraperitoneally.

FEY: We had to try several reagents in the past to get an optimal response. We would have loved to work with turpentine, but these studies were initiated in San Diego at the Scripps Institute, and in the USA you need to have your protocol approved by the Institutional Animal Reserch Committee if you want to do animal research. Our committee requested that we should check all possible reagents to find one that caused minimal stress to the animal, and that was complete Freund's adjuvant. We would have loved to work with other more aggressive ways of producing an acute phase response, but we were not allowed to do that. Once we had started the experiments in the USA we continued over in Germany the same way.

BAUMANN: Before I close this discussion, I would like to ask Alex Koj to tell the audience about his experience regarding regulation of α_2-macroglobulin in mouse hepatocytes. I think that he is the one who knows the most about that protein.

ALEKSANDER KOJ: Just one more comment about the turpentine and mouse and rat response. Turpentine is very well tolerated by rats, but you can kill mice with a proportional dose of turpentine. So if you combine differing sensitivities with different types of turpentine oils which can be used I am not surprised that you get different results. Turpentine is such an unidentified mixture of compounds. The message, which was probably not emphasized enough here, is that in knockout mice the response to LPS is preserved but differs from the response to turpentine. There is actually very good agreement between these two groups, and I am really pleased at that outcome as starting years ago turpentine was the first reagent used to induce the acute phase response. We are now moving to knockout mice and still using turpentine as an inducer. What is also important is that the other acute phase reactants, not only α_2-M, they react similarly in both cases. What is not clear is how α_2-M can be induced in mice because the general knowledge based on Japanese studies is that mice have two macroglobulins similar to those of the rat, but that neither of them responds to inflammatory stimuli. One of them, named murino-globulin, is even slightly decreased after the challenge. So this is something not so clear with this response.

POLI: These studies with α2-M in mice, were they done on the protein level or also on the mRNA level? Because this might be one difference.

KOJ: This is a very good point. This was only studied on the protein level. I presume that you have used rat α2-M probe for mice mRNA.

POLI: Yes.

KOJ: We are quite satisfied with using cross-reactivity of rat antibodies for mouse proteins. I do not know about cDNA probes. How about using complement C3, which is responding very strongly in rat and mice to acute phase challenge?

POLI: We did not use C3, but I am quite sure that the probe we used was the rat α2-M cDNA which we received from Peter Heinrich's group. Maybe he sent us something else, but I must say that the size on the Northern blot corresponded to that one.

KOJ: Just to conclude, I would say that the problem needs reinvestigation on the mRNA and the transcription level.

FEY: It is very unlikely that the rat α2-M probe will react with something else of the same size in the mouse. If you did it the other way around, if you took the mouse probe, then you would see in the rat α2-M and the α1-inhibitor III. You would not expect the rat probe to react with mouse C3. We have done these experiments with sufficient stringency of hybridization. And Dr. Poli's blots looked very stringent.

KOJ: OK, unless you mix the probes in the refrigerator.

BAUMANN: On that note we stop here. I would like to thank all participants for their contributions and hand over the "square-table" discussion to Professor Revel.

****

REVEL: I believe that a performance as great as Dr. Baumann's is difficult to match. On the question of therapeutic uses of IL-6 and IL-6-type cytokines, everybody who knows something about clinical applications is kindly requested to participate. Pravin Sehgal will lead off the discussion with a presentation on some of the uses of IL-6 in diagnostics. I hope that diagnostic use is not the only application of IL-6 we will see in the future.

PRAVIN SEHGAL: I would like to take 7 to 10 minutes to review one clinical situation where over the last 5 years we have conducted about 3 studies and are now launching ourselves into a fourth investigation, which will be time prospective. That is, focused on the use of IL-6 measurements in diagnostics. The first comment here is that you can make use of cytokine levels either as diagnostic or prognostic tests or use cytokines as therapeutic agents, and I leave therapeutic agents to my panel colleagues around the table. I want to focus on a specific situation in clinical medicine. In collaboration with Roberto Romero, an obstetrician, then at Yale, we did a pilot study in which we discovered that IL-6 levels in the amniotic fluid of a specific class of women in preterm labor were highly elevated; these were women who delivered prematurely and had a culture-positive amniotic fluid. This was simply a pilot study where we knew in advance what the different groups were. These IL-6 differences were so huge and dramatic that we decided that this may be a circumstance where more rigorous evaluation will be worthwhile. The objective of a second study was to determine whether the amniotic fluid IL-6 determination had a role in diagnosing microbial invasion of the amniotic cavity and whether it provided any information in terms of outcome of the preterm labor. To put things in perspective, at a referral hospital like ours we see a hundred or more women with preterm labor every year who have been referred to the New York Medical College, Westchester County Medical Center. So for us this is a great problem that we need to deal with. The key question is: Is there diagnostic information or are we fooling ourselves by watching IL-6 levels going up and down? The rigorous questions are along the following lines: Is the specific test the best source of information needed, and can the cost of the test be justified? What is the information needed? The information that is needed is along the following lines: A woman in labor is brought into the Obstetrics Department; the obstetrician needs to know whether the preterm labor was triggered because of intercurrent infection, which is a common cause of preterm labor. The other information the obstetrician needs to know very rapidly is whether there is any hope of salvaging the pregnancy. Is there any hope in putting this patient on relatively toxic β-adrenergic therapy and trying to carry the pregnancy to term? If there is a test which tells the obstetrician that there is an infection and tells this information in an accurate fashion, the obstetrician can go and enhance labor and get the fetus out as rapidly as possible. Alternatively, an obstretrician can go into very conservative therapy and try to carry the pregnancy to term. The problem is that some of the β-adrenergic agents have maternal toxicity and morbidity problems and you do not want to make these decisions without a solid base. Thus far, the typical thing has been to do a Gram stain, which is a rapid test. The alternative has been to do the amniotic fluid culture, but you do not get the result until the next day. And the issue is time sensitive and information sensitive. What we did in our second study was to look at amniotic fluid of all patients admitted to the Yale New Haven Hospital in preterm labor so as to collect about 200 patients over a 2-year period. Of these 200, 146 were evaluable in the sense that every workup had been done and the results were present in the charts. And we found the usual frequency of 10-15% for positive amniotic fluid culture. And then we went on to ask what the amniotic fluid IL-6 levels were like and whether we could relate these levels to outcome. This is one of the classic problems of a Gram-stain. A Gram-stain will miss positive cultures, and this is what reduces the reliability of a Gram stain. Although if you get positive results on Gram-stain the sensitivity is 100%. Once you see the bacteria you know they are there, but if you do not see the bacteria you do not know that they are not there. The distribution of IL-6 levels was along these lines. We have a bunch of high IL-6 levels. These have been broken down to culture-positive and culture-negative. All of the culture-positives are higher than an arbitrary cut-off of 11ng/ml except this one. Now we know that this was an early infection. Here is a key problem. These amniotic fluids are culture negative but have high IL-6 levels. To make a very long story short, it turns out that all of those who had high IL-6 levels but were culture-negative delivered preterm. There was no way to salvage these pregnancies. Out of the 146 we had 136 where we knew the outcome. These were grouped into two boxes: above 6.7 ng/ml and below 6.7 ng/ml. One can arbitrarily set the cut-off points at 6.7, 11.3, and so on. The key point is: The culture-positives went into preterm delivery; the high IL-6 all went to preterm delivery; the one patient who was culture-positive but had low IL-6 also went on to preterm delivery. But out of the 115 who were culture-negative and had low IL-6 levels the salvage rate was 85%. What that says very simply is that if you have amniotic fluid IL-6 levels above 6.7 ng/ml it is almost certain that there is going to be a preterm labor no matter what you do. Whereas when the concentration is low there is an 85% chance that the pregnancy can be salvaged to term. The next question really was comparisons of sensitivity and specificity of the IL-6 measurement versus the Gram stain. The specificity of a Gram stain is 100% but the sensitivity is lower because you will miss some that are culture-positive; but this is only with respect to the culture.

But with IL-6 the sensitivity and specificity are about 90%. Our current approach is to use Gram stain and IL-6. Now, how should we deal with a formal description of outcome? This is the receiver-operator curve in which IL-6 is tested as a predictor of tocolytic failure. This is where the information becomes interesting. And it says never mind the culture, never mind the Gram stain, just based on IL-6 measurement you can predict failure to carry pregnancy to term in a very reliable fashion. This is the way it looks such that in this group of patients once IL-6 is above 11.3 ng/ml the outcome curve crashes very rapidly with delivery within 24 to 48 hours. Amniotic fluid IL-6 and Gram stain basically gives you a sensitivity of 100%. In the third study we went to an independent data set, 150-200 patients at the Hutzel Hospital in Detroit, and checked all of these parameters again. And the bottom line here was that the combination of amniotic fluid IL-6 and Gram stain had 100% sensitivity as a predictor of a positive amniotic fluid culture. For us, one of the interesting outcomes was along these lines: neonatal morbidity. Of all the indices used - IL-6, amniotic fluid white cells, glucose, Gram stain, culture - IL-6 was the best. And that starts to tell us something very interesting: some neonatal morbidity events, for example periventricular leucomalacia, are actually triggered by prior obstetric events, and it is these obstetric events that may be flagged by an IL-6 amniotic fluid IL-6 measurement. In fact, the fourth study about to be launched is a prospective real-time study of about 400 patients which will focus on monitoring neonatal morbidity using IL-6 in amniotic fluid as a marker of neonatal morbidity. From my point of view this is one situation where if you have a very rapid IL-6 assay, like a 15-minute dipstick, it can move into obstetric practice very rapidly.

GORDON: Pravin, how do they obtain amniotic fluid? Is it all in women with ruptured membranes? Or are they having amniocentesis in the emergency room?

SEHGAL: In a Tertiary Referral Center, the standard obstetric practice in the fetal-maternal department for patients in preterm is amniocentesis. All of the data I have shown you were from women with intact membranes. We have a parallel cohort of data from women with ruptured membranes. In both our hospital and in Roberto Romero's the standard protocol is that if a woman is brought in in preterm labor they have an amnio right away. Some of the fluid is Gram-stained, some of the fluid is used for culture, and the rest of the fluid is banked. This is primarily because there are other protocols going on at the same time, such as trying to test whether antibiotic treatment helps the woman. We are piggy-backing on other research protocols that are already in existence, and that sets up an amniotic fluid bank in which you can now go in and check all the samples for IL-6.

REVEL: Does anyone have any other IL-6 diagnostic applications which they want to discuss?

JEFFREY S. WEBER: How do you get amniotic fluid from someone who has already ruptured the membranes?

SEHGAL: You can collect it *per vaginam*. The route of collection is an important aspect of the story.

REVEL: An obvious question is why in this particular type of infection IL-6 could be such a good diagnostic means while in other types of infections it does not seem to be. Do you have any explanation?

JACK A. ELIAS: This is a special circumstance in which you are not asking what the person is infected with. If someone comes in with pneumonia, knowing whether they are infected is one thing, but knowing what they are infected with is as crucial a question as knowing if they are infected. You are dealing with a space that ought to be sterile. So it is a sort of special scenario different from pneumonia, cellulitis or some other infection where IL-6 would be elevated in a rather nonspecific fashion. The evidence pointed out is that the data with CSF IL-6 levels that initially were said to be specific for meningitis and then turned out to be positive in all inflammatory processes involving the meninges. This, I agree, is a special circumstance where it does not matter what the underlying reason for infection is. Whether it is viral, syphilitic or HIV does not matter. The important thing is simply to know that there is something wrong, so you do not subject the patient to the morbidity of a β-adrenergic protocol. In essence, it may be the sedimentation rate of amniotic fluid - the clinical equivalent thereof.

SEHGAL: Yes. We have gone through and have had the opportunity to compare IL-6 data with every other criterion, including cervical dilatation, age of gestation, and so on. In this situation amniotic fluid IL-6 holds up.

FEY: You said this test could rapidly become a part of clinical routine. I have a problem with understanding how in a routine clinical setting you would get amniotic fluid. Is not the procedure for removing amniotic fluid dangerous in itself?

SEHGAL: Some of us work in Tertiary Referral Centers, where there is a clinical routine of amniocentesis in preterm labor.

WEBER: How often do these women have amniocentesis anyway? Forget about the IL-6 protocol.

SEHGAL: All the women admitted in preterm labor get an amnio for other reasons. Thus far, the IL-6 measurements are simply piggy-backing on established protocols. And even in our study number 4, the IL-6 measurements will simply piggy-back on established protocols. But for the moment, none of these women are undergoing amniocentesis for the purpose of measuring IL-6. Not yet.

WEBER: I guess that Georg's point is well taken if the spontaneous abortion rate is 2% or the death rate is 2% from doing the amnio in patients who otherwise would not have had it.

SEHGAL: I am not a fetal-maternal specialist. I do not know what the morbidity rate from an amniocentesis is at the Westchester County Medical Center. All I can simply tell you is that both at Yale and at WCMC an amnio is a first routine step in the management of preterm labor.

WEBER: And the other issue is that right now you have an ELISA to determine IL-6 level, is that correct?

SEHGAL: We have ELISAs to determine IL-6 levels, but we want to make it faster.

WEBER: That is not a routine standard thing to do.

SEHGAL: We actually have an OBG fellow trained to do it in 60 minutes flat.

FEY: But there are faster IL-6 assays which do not rely on ELISAs. Functional assays for transcription induction can work in 4 hours.

SEHGAL: We really need a 15-minute assay.

REVEL: Any other idea how to use IL-6 in diagnostics that someone wants to talk about? If not, let's move to the clinical use of IL-6, IL-11, and others. I do not know how many of us also have the feeling that we are still at the beginning of a very long way with IL-6 and the other cytokine IL-11. We did not hear about the other IL-6-type cytokines in the clinic, but I still believe that it is a good time to have the experts try to assess the future.

MICHAEL S. GORDON: I will be glad to give an assessment of where things stand right now. Among the other IL-6-type cytokines I do not think that there is going to be a place for them as hematopoietic agents in the future. Those which are not yet in clinical trials will be shut out. Among the IL-6-type agents, the E. *coli*-derived product is the furthest advanced for IL-6, and IL-11 is headed toward pivotal trials. IL-11 is currently in phase II, and I would suspect that IL-6 is also. They are going to need to be significantly speeded up. The reason I pose this is because of the newest developments presented in last week's *Nature* on the true thrombopoietin. They will literally be going to rush this into clinical trials. And since there are four companies that currently have this, I suspect that anyone with a thrombopoietic agent of the IL-6 type who does not get it to market in the next year and a half will find the door shut.

REVEL: What is known about the differences and similarities of action of these thrombopoietins and the IL-6-type cytokines?

GORDON: According to the *Nature* papers it actually acts more as an immediate platelet release factor, even in non-myelosuppressed individuals, as opposed to the delayed effect that we have seen. This delay of 7 days is due to the fact that the IL-6-type-cytokines have to have this prolonged maturational effect. You cannot speed it up regardless of what you do outside of increasing the dose. The hope among the people who are studying thrombopoietin is that it is going to be the G-CSF of platelet production. The platelet response would be immediate.

REVEL: Is that what animal experiments are already showing?

GORDON: Correct.

***QUESTION: Did you ever reach MTD with your IL-11 material?

GORDON: We essentially reached MTD. We did not think to push it to 100 μg/kg. I suspect that if we had, we would only need one more grade 3 or greater toxicity to establish an MTD.

REVEL: Can you compare specific activity of IL-6 and IL-11 in an *in vitro* system? How many units do you have for μg/protein in each?

GORDON: Not being in the laboratory I cannot answer your question.

REVEL: The reason I am asking is since the 10 mg dose seems to be low it may be that you have fewer units per μg of protein in IL-11.

GORDON: Well, you may, but it would be hard if you would say that there was a 10-fold difference and 10, 25, and 50 μg was equivalent to 1, 2.5, and 5 of IL-6. I think that clearly we are seeing similar thrombopoietic effects at these doses.

ELIAS: I am intrigued by the findings of nasal congestion. Rhinoviruses are a major stimulator of IL-11 production. Did these people have symptomatology that you would call common cold in another setting?

GORDON: What we ended up with was a lot of complaints of sinus congestion and rhinorrhea in patients who were put on Sudafed™ or Actifed™ for complaints of nasal congestion. It was very reminiscent of those people who were involved in IL-4-type sinus congestion complaints.

ELIAS: Did you get any respiratory symtomatology?

GORDON: No.

QUESTION: I am interested in whether IL-11 can also increase acute phase proteins. Do you have any ideas on why it does not cause a fever like IL-6 does?

GORDON: My view on differences between the IL-6-type cytokines is that probably the cytokines themselves are very similar; as they all send a signal through gp130 they have the same post-receptor signaling and in some ways it is probably an issue of location of receptors and the binding of the ligand in different areas. IL-6 binds to the hypothalamus and causes fever while IL-11 does not cause fever. This would be my best guess in terms of why.

BAUMANN: Just to follow up on this particular question. When the data from IL-6 and IL-11 experiments are compared we predict from, let's say, tissue culture analysis that IL-11 may not be as active on liver cells as IL-6 and that is probably due to the relative amount of the receptors for the two. Is it already possible to make a judgment whether the *in vitro* data are similar to the *in vivo* data?

*** The material between the asterisks is taken from the discussion following Dr. Gordon's presentation.

GORDON: I think that it is clear when you look at the trials with IL-6 presented earlier by Dr. Weber. When you look at the degree of elevation of C-reactive protein and the acute phase proteins in IL-6 trials direct comparisons are hard to do because the patient population is somewhat different in the IL-11 trial. I think that IL-6 tends to be a more potent stimulator of the acute phase reaction and that may go along with causing fever and so on. And so, perhaps the number of receptors on liver cell is related to that.

BAUMANN: The questions arise only because we would have made the prediction that for a prominent stimulation of C-reactive protein you would probably require IL-1 + IL-6 whereas one for haptoglobin or fibrinogen IL-6-type cytokines alone would be sufficient. So one should actually be able to compare your *in vivo* analysis with *in vitro* data to see if it is truly possible to use clinical trial data to differentiate between effects caused directly by the cytokines and ones caused by systemic processes.

GORDON: One of the issues is clearly that most of the patients in cycle zero are feeling well and doing well, so any change in their acute phase proteins is generally related to the therapy itself.

BAUMANN: My last question is: Do you have normal volunteers who will actually go through the treatment?

GORDON: For IL-6 there would not be, I believe, because of the fever and the degree of toxicity. But for IL-11 I believe that there are normal volunteer studies that had been planned; I am not involved in that, however, and I cannot be sure about that.

BAUMANN: My prediction would be that it is a more gentle treatment than endotoxin for volunteers.

ELIAS: You eliminated people with cardiac disease?

GORDON: Primarily because of doxorubicin; we did not want anybody who had pre-existing cardiac dysfunction.***

REVEL: Dr. Abdul-Ahad, do you want to say anything about the CHO-cell-derived IL-6?

AYAD ABDUL-AHAD: I agree with Dr. Gordon. We are waiting to see what the true thrombopoietin turns out to be - what side effects it has and what other effects it has. I think between Sandoz and Serono we are trying to find a place for IL-6. I personally believe that the use of IL-6 is not justified unless it is used to prevent platelet transfusion. I do not know of other uses.

REVEL: There is a possibility that some combined effect of IL-6-type cytokines in addition to thrombopoietic effect might give it an advantage over thrombopoietin. We know that it is a pleiotropic cytokine and it can have effects on white blood cells that could make a difference in some conditions.

WEBER: I have a kind of mixed opinion. My feeling is that from the available data we know now that IL-6 is probably a more toxic agent though equally as effective as IL-11, and that gives IL-11 an advantage. If it turns out that you can administer IL-6 long term and get equal effects at low doses it will be a much more marketable cytokine and it will be much more useful clinically. But I would not count out IL-6 for a couple of reasons: one is that no one has completed a trial on IL-3 + IL-6, which at least in the preclinical models were synergistic. Tolerable lower doses of IL-6 can be added to the lower doses of IL-3, which are also tolerable, and you may even see a more dramatic platelet effect. In addition, if there is an early so-called true megakaryocyte colony stimulator factor that is also an early acting factor, you may also see an impressive synergy if you add that to a late-acting factor like IL-6. Lastly, with respect to IL-6 as an anti-cancer agent that is a dead issue. As a thrombopoietin it is in a little bit of danger. The kind of studies that Andrzej Mackiewicz is doing are very interesting because in every screen of transduced cytokine cells used in the mouse system as a vaccine in the immunization challenge situation, IL-6 has activity. So it may have a future not as a reagent, but as a gene that by transduction can be put into tumor cells for use as vaccines.

REVEL: I would like to take you up on whether IL-6 is a dead issue for cancer. It would be really premature to rule out the use of IL-6 on the basis of phase I studies where you did not see responses. IL-6, at least on the basis of what we know from the experience I got with M. Feldmann—and we looked at many cytokines—, has a stronger effect on metastases than other cytokines, such as IL-2 and IL-4. And, therefore, before we test in a metastatic protocol I think that it may be premature to say that it is a dead issue. I agree with you that I would like to hear if there is any simple protocol which allows you to evaluate an anti-metastatic agent. But I still would like to give as an example the IFN story. Once it was up, then it was down, and now up again. In the last few months we have heard, and hopefully it is the truth, that IFN-β, when given together with irradiation, can significantly increase the survival rate of patients with non-small cell lung carcinoma after 5 years. Now this is a situation which nobody could predict 15 years ago. And therefore one should not ignore a cytokine like IL-6 which shows, as you demonstrated yourself, a very high efficacy in animal studies.

PHILIP WALLACE: I would like to make just one comment related to what I said earlier. It is not correct that it takes a long time to make megakaryocytes. If you take primates you can do the studies where you treat them for 7 or 10 days. If you treat them for 3 days and stop, which is not something that people do normally, 5 days later they have lots of megakaryocytes. It may be a different situation in serious thrombocytopenia when you do not have any of these cells.

ELIAS: We are talking about these agents strictly as therapeutic proteins. We can shift the topic of the conversation a little bit toward the antagonists of these proteins in disease states. We have focused a lot on myeloma, but there are clearly others where IL-6 and IL-11 may be involved in pathogenesis of disease where blocking the effects would be therapeutically useful.

REVEL: Does anyone want to talk about his experience or his impression of the use of anti-IL-6 in multiple myeloma and its prospects? The pros and the cons?

SEHGAL: I think that given the very strong chaperoning effect of anti-IL-6 antibodies I simply cannot see how you can take a human being and inject anti-IL-6 antibodies. I just do not see it. I know that it has been done, but it is not flying chemically.

WEBER: I guess that my particular bias would be that what you have is a cytostatic effect, and in the cancer business a cytostatic effect is not generally sufficient to induce a clinical effect.

REVEL: What we have learned from the IL-6 knockout mice may be used in the clinic. If I understand correctly, one of the major effects is the decrease of cytotoxic lymphocyte activity and fewer T cells in animals lacking IL-6. Is it possible for there to be a good effect not as a cytostatic but as an immunostimulator? There could be applications in human cancer.

WEBER: We did see these to a small degree in some patients who were receiving IL-6 in the highest dose they could tolerate s.c. They had their tumors resected on day 7 of IL-6 therapy. And we tried to grow tumor-infiltrating lymphocytes. In one case we admittedly failed; in two cases there was no evidence of tumor specificity. So, using the crude techniques that we have of trying to reproduce in humans what we can easily do in mice, it did not work. Again, I am a little skeptical that, using it exactly as we did in the mouse, IL-6 would be utilized to grow specific CTL.

ELIAS: I have a question for Pravin. I can understand the chaperone effect if you want to give the antagonist i.v. Do you know that similar activity goes on if you apply things topically to nasal membranes? Might not it be useful to use IL-6-type cytokine antagonists topically?

SEHGAL: The most impressive chaperoning effect we have seen is using preformed complexes of IL-6 with its antibody injected i.p. It is unusual, but in the presence of antibody IL-6 appears in the circulation a lot faster than if you just inject IL-6 i.p. So our working hypothesis is that the Fc part of the Ig molecule is actually serving as some sort of delivery or entry mechanism into the peripheral circulation.

ELIAS: There are going to be other molecules that are going to be antagonists that are not necessarily going to be antibodies.

WALLACE: In the field of antibody targeting it is routinely done to accelerate the clearance by, in principle, glycosylating or biotinylating a variety of structures to allow removal of molecules. You can actually pull it out with either phoresis or some other strategies, so I do not think that that should be a concern if you really believe that getting rid of IL-6 is really sufficient.

BAUMANN: The issue has been brought up that IL-6 production by cancer is responsible for cancer cachexia. Once we know more about what IL-6 is doing and how, we may have the opportunity to control IL-6 action, not by eliminating the IL-6, but by intervening specifically with effects downstream of this cytokine. It may be desirable to remove the harmful effects but preserve the beneficial effects of IL-6.

KOJ: When listening to this discussion and the presentations today my feeling is that the problem of IL-6-type cytokines, which up to now has been studied in the laboratory has reached a new phase, and the title of the conference—**IL-6-Type Cytokines**—is fully justified, not only from the laboratory point of view, but also from that of the clinicians. When you look at the effect of IL-6 and IL-11 and compare them it is fully justified, and I would agree fully that there is no reason to stop doing clinical trials also in combination with different cytokines, with different growth factors, and with other medical procedures including chemotherapy. I think that this symposium has just raised the problem of how to use IL-6-type cytokines.

REVEL: I think that we could not find better words to close this conference. I would like to thank all the chairpersons for their efforts.

Increase of High Molecular Weight Fibrinogen after Surgery for Renal Cancer[a]

G. ADLER, W. EICHMAN, I. TARGONSKA, AND
M. SZCZEPANSKI

Department of Biochemistry
Medical Center of Postgraduate Education
Marymoncka 99
01-813 Warszawa, Poland

The fibrinogen circulating in plasma consists of three different fractions: high molecular weight fibrinogen (HMW Fb, MW 340 kD) and two low molecular weight fibrinogen fractions (LMW Fb, MW 305 kD and LMW' Fb, MW 270 kD).[1] The postoperative increase of total fibrinogen concentration is a known phenomenon and our investigations were aimed at the assessment of its fractions response to the surgery.

MATERIAL AND METHODS

Plasma samples were taken from 15 patients before and on days 1, 3, and 7 after surgery for renal cancer. The fibrinogen concentration was measured spectrophotometrically at 280 and 315 nm ($E_{1\,cm}^{0.1\%}$ 1.58).[2] As a reference the standard of plasma fibrinogen from National Institute for Biological Standards and Controls (89/644) (Hertfordshire, UK) was used. Fibrin fractions were separated by SDS electrophoresis on 5% acrylamide gel and scanned in a Pharmacia densitometer.[3]

RESULTS AND DISCUSSION

The preoperative fibrinogen fractions in our patients, expressed as a percentage of total fibrinogen concentration, were as follows: 72 ± 3% for HMW Fb, 25 ± 2% for LMW Fb and 3 ± 1% for LMW' Fb. These proportions did not differ from ones found in healthy controls. All patients were divided into two groups: 9 patients with the values of baseline fibrinogen concentration within normal range (240 ± 34 mg%) and 6 patients with elevated values (531 ± 119 mg%). In both groups the content of HMW Fb increased after surgery and reached the highest level on the 3rd day, whereas both LMW Fb's decreased and were lowest on the same day. The percentages of all fractions returned almost to the initial values on the 7th day after surgery (FIG. 1). The rise of HMW Fb was different in each of two groups. The patients with normal preoperative fibrinogen concentrations revealed an increase of 142%, whereas this increase was only 38% in patients with high preoperative fibrinogen levels. In

---

[a] Supported by Grant W-PB-4/94 from the Medical Center of Postgraduate Education, Warszawa.

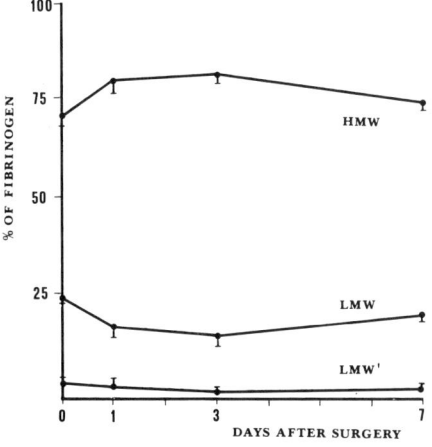

FIGURE 1. Postoperative changes of HMW Fb, LMW Fb and LMW' Fb fractions expressed, as a percentage of total fibrinogen concentration in 15 patients with renal cancer (mean values ± SD).

all patients the concentration of LMW fractions declined immediately after surgery but their later course was different in each of groups. The level of LMW Fb rose above the starting value on the 3rd postoperative day in patients with normal baseline fibrinogen, whereas in patients with high preoperative fibrinogen concentrations LMW Fb fraction reached the initial value not earlier than on the 7th day. The levels of LMW' Fb fraction were below the baseline values until the end of determinations in both groups (FIG. 2).

According to our results as well as those of others,[3,4] the higher concentration of fibrinogen in plasma after surgery is the result of the rise of the concentration of the HMW Fb. In 40% of patients with renal cancer an elevated fibrinogen level was found

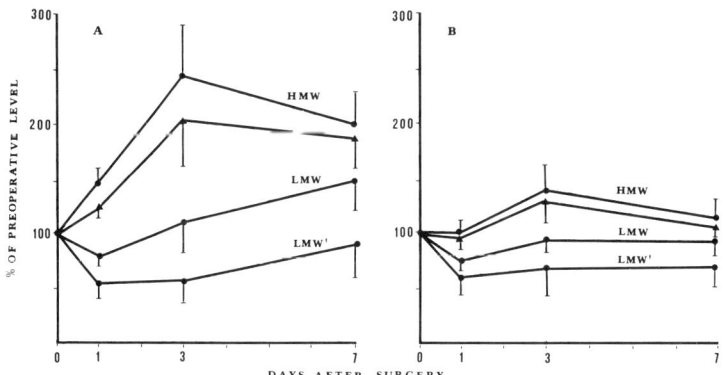

FIGURE 2. Postoperative changes in concentration of total fibrinogen *(triangles)* and its HMW, LMW and LMW' fractions *(circles)* Data of 9 patients with preoperative fibrinogen within normal range (A) and of 6 patients with elevated preoperative fibrinogen level (B). Results are presented as a percentage of a preoperative concentration of fibrinogen or of its respective fraction (mean values ± SD).

before surgery with the usual distribution of fractions. Since fibrinogen molecules are synthesized in hepatocytes, our results may suggest that these cells were already activated by the presence of cancer in some patients and that the rise of fibrinogen synthesis after surgery is smaller in preactivated hepatocytes.

REFERENCES

1. HOLM, B., D. W. T. NILSEN, P. KIERULF & H. C. GODAL. 1985. Thrombosis Res. **37:** 165–176.
2. GAFFNEY, P. & M. Y. WONG. 1992. Thromb. Hameostas. **68:** 428–432.
3. LIPINSKA, I., B. LIPINSKI, V. GUREWICH & K. HOFFMAN. 1976. Am. J. Clin. Pathol. **66:** 958–966.
4. HOLM, B. & H. C. GODAL. 1984. Thrombosis Res. **35:** 279–290.

Interleukin-6 Production in Children with Acute Lymphoblastic Leukemia[a]

A. CHYBICKA,[b] J. BOGUSLAWSKA-JAWORSKA,[b] AND
W. JAWORSKI [c]

[b]Department of Pediatric Hematology and Oncology
Faculty of Medicine
[c]Department of Pediatric Surgery
Medical Academy, Wroclaw
ul.Bujwida 44
50-345 Wroclaw, Poland

INTRODUCTION

Interleukin-6 (IL-6) is a multifunctional glycoprotein molecule that appears to be part of the cytokine network.[1] IL-6 plays a major role in host defense and hematopoiesis. In addition to its physiological properties, IL-6 is included in the pathophysiology of various neoplasias such as multiple myeloma, non-Hodgkin's lymphoma and Kaposi's sarcoma.[2] A systematic analysis of IL-6 production in children with ALL has not yet been carried out.

We have previously reported apparent deficiency of lymphocyte subsets, deficient IL-1 production, and impaired activity of natural killer cells during the whole period of cytostatic therapy in children with acute lymphoblastic leukemia.[3,4]

AIM OF STUDY

The purpose of the study was to investigate an influence of chemo- and radiotherapy on IL-6 production in children with acute lymphoblastic leukemia (ALL).

MATERIAL AND METHODS

In years 1988–1993 69 children with ALL (47 boys and 22 girls), aged from 5 to 15 years (median 9y) were treated according to the German BFM ALL 86 and 90 protocols, which consisted of aggressive chemotherapy associated with radiotherapy. All children were observed in Department of Children Hematology and Oncology, Faculty of Medicine University in Wroclaw. Twenty-five healthy children of the same age served as controls. The initial characteristics of the children are presented in the TABLE 1.

Heparinized vein blood samples were drawn from children at different stages of their disease: at the time of diagnosis, during intensive therapy (induction, consolidation), during maintenance therapy and after completion of the treatment.

Mononuclear cells were isolated on Lymphoprep (Nesco) gradient. Mononuclears were counted, resuspended in Eagle's medium containing 10% FCS and placed in an

---

[a] This work was supported by Grant 40961 91 01.

TABLE 1. Clinical Characteristics of Children with ALL

	n = 69	%
Sex		
boys	47	68
girls	22	32
Age		
<2 years	2	2.8
2–10 years	57	82.7
>10 years	10	14.5
Clinical classification		
LRG	20	29
MRG	41	59
HRG	8	12
FAB classification		
L1	57	82.6
L2	12	17.4
L3	0	
Immunological classification		
pre-B	50/58	86.2
B	—	
T	—	
non-T non-B	8/58	13.8

incubator at the concentration 2×10^6 cells/ml for 24 hours. After 24 hours of incubation the supernatants were removed. For IL-6 specific measurement commercially available antibody "sandwich" ELISA assay was used (Predicta TM Interleukin-6 Genzyme Elisa kit).

RESULTS

The results of our studies on IL-6 production are shown in FIGURE 1. At the time of diagnosis before any treatment was started and during induction therapy, we found median values of IL-6 lower when compared with the values in the control group of healthy children (450 pg/ml v 200 pg/ml v 1870 pg/ml).

IL-6 production increased after complete remission was achieved and remained high during the whole period of maintenance treatment ($p = 0.005$). After cessation of the therapy IL-6 values remained on the same level and were within normal limits or even above.

DISCUSSION

In the present study we investigated IL-6 in children with ALL before, during, and after cessation of chemotherapy. Our results revealed IL-6 production before therapy and during induction therapy lower than in control group. A number of reports have shown similar results of IL-6 studies in patients with malignancies.[7–9] The reason of decreased IL-6 production in untreated ALL patients is still not completely elucidated, though there are many data suggesting the role of suppressor cells, prostaglandins, suppressor cytokines (TGF-β, IL-10), etc.[10] Our studies revealed that IL-

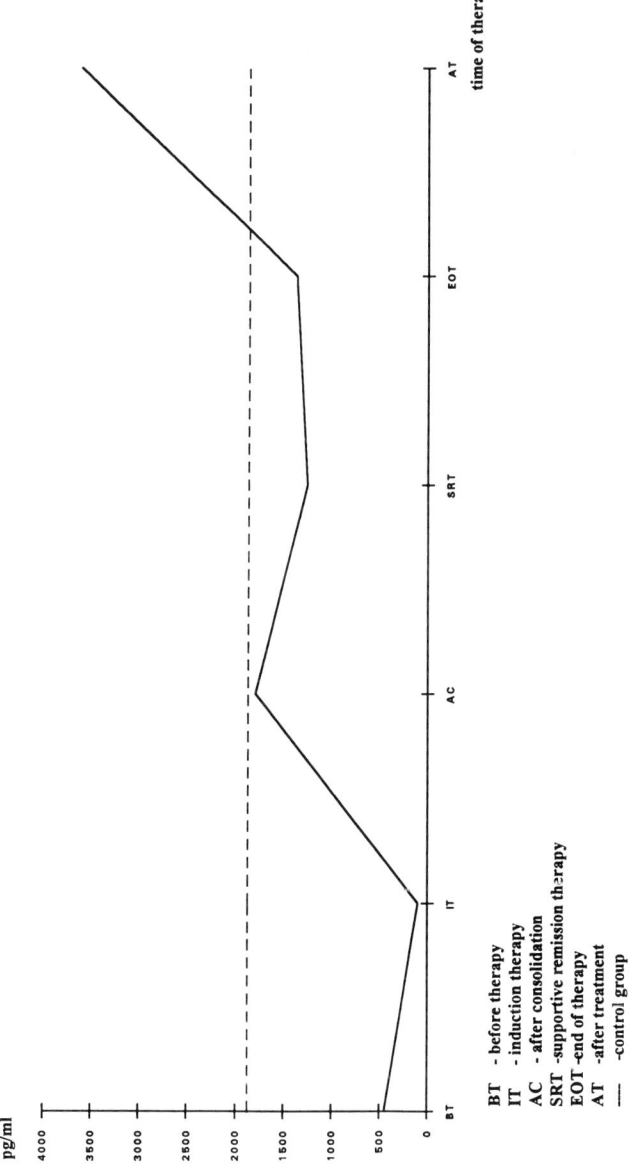

FIGURE 1. Results of IL-6 production in children with ALL (median values).

6 production during the whole period of therapy, except remission induction, was within normal limits. It should be noticed, however, that after cessation of chemotherapy the level of IL-6 production was found to be highly elevated. It has been demonstrated in other reports[11] that after completion of chemotherapy IL-6 production was rather comparable to the control values. In our studies it seems that high IL-6 activity could be explained by concomitant infection with hepatitis B and C viruses recorded in 80% of the children. However, the role of IL-6 production level after successful chemotherapy needs further studies and observation.

REFERENCES

1. WONG, G. C. & S. C. CLARK. 1988. Immunology Today **9**(5):.
2. AKIRA, S., T. KISHMOTO. 1992. Immunol. Rev. **127**: 25–50.
3. AKIRA, S. & T. KISHMOTO. 1992. Semin. Cancer Biol. **3**: 17–26.
4. FOSS, H. D., H. HERBST, E. OELMANN, et al. 1993. Br. J. Hematol. **84**: 627–635.
5. CHYBICKA, A., J. BOGUSLAWSKA-JAWORSKA. 1990. Acute Leukemia II. T. Buchner, G. Schellong, W. Hiddemann & J. Ritter. Hematol. Blood Transf. **133**: 72–75.
6. CHYBICKA, A., J. BOGUSLAWSKA-JAWORSKA, W. BUDZYNSKI, CZ. RADZIKOWSKI, W. JAWORSKI. 1992. In Acute Leukemias. Kusche and W. Hiddemann, Eds. Hematol. Blood Transf. **34**: 152–156.
7. AGUILAR-SANTELISES, M., R. MAGNUSSON, S. B. SVENSON, et al. 1991. Clin. Exp. Immunol. **84**: 422–428.
8. BAUER, J., F. HERRMAN. 1991. Interleukin-6 in Clinical Medicine. Ann. Hematol. **62**: 203–210.
9. BOER, E. C., H. W. JONG, P. A. STEERENBERG, L. A. AARDEN, et al. 1992. Cancer Immunol. Immunother. **34**: 306–312.
10. SCHINDLER, R., J. MANCILLA, S. ENDRES, R. GHORBANI & S. C. CLARK. 1990. Blood **75**(1):40–47.
11. HIRANO, T., S. AKIRA, T. TAGA & T. HISHIMOTO. 1990. Immunology Today **11**(12): 443–449.

Selectin-P (PADGEM, GMP-140)-mediated Adhesion of Human Platelets to Neutrophils *in Vitro* and Immune Complex-induced Peritonitis in Rats Is Influenced by Interleukin-8

A. DEMBIŃSKA-KIEĆ,[a] M. BURCHERT,[b] J. DULAK,[a] M. POLUS,[a]
M. PAWELEC,[a] A. SIEDLECKI,[a] AND B. A. PESKAR[c]

[a]*Department of Clinical Biochemistry*
[b]*Department of Pathomorphology*
Collegium Medicum, Jagiellonian University
31-120 Krakow, Poland

[c]*Department of Pharmacology and Toxicology,*
Ruhr University
Bochum, Germany

INTRODUCTION

Recruitment of neutrophils to the sites of inflammation occurs in several steps. Adhesion and rolling of leukocytes is suggested to be mediated by the selectin-L expressed on neutrophils, and selectin-E with selectin-P expressed on endothelium.[1]

Selectin-P is expressed on the cell membrane after stimulation with low concentrations of several agonists, such as thrombin, 5-HT, free radicals, ADP and/or PAF.[2] This selectin promotes the adhesion of activated platelets to PMNs (formation of "rosettes") as well as PMNs to endothelium.[2]

The expression of β_2-integrins on neutrophils is mediated with the endothelial cytokine: interleukin-8 (IL-8), which is released by the mitogen-stimulated T lymphocytes, cytokine-activated monocytes, and endothelial cells. IL-8 was suggested to be a promoter of inflammation by selective activation of PMNs degranulation, oxygen burst, and chemotaxis.[3]

We decided to investigate the influence of IL-8 on the selectin-P–mediated adhesion of platelets to PMNs *in vitro*, and on immune complex-induced peritonitis in rats, as a model of PMNs chemotaxis *in vivo*.

METHODS

The rosette formation assay was performed using gel-filtrated human platelets (4×10^8/ml) and human PMNs (2×10^6/ml) incubated in Ca^{++}-free Tyrode solution.[2] The number of rosettes was examined under water immersion in Zeiss Photomicroscope.

The activity of NO-synthase (NOS) in PMNs homogenates was assayed by monitoring the conversion of L-arginine-[2,3-^{3}H] to L-citrulline[2,3-^{3}H].[4] Rat peritonitis

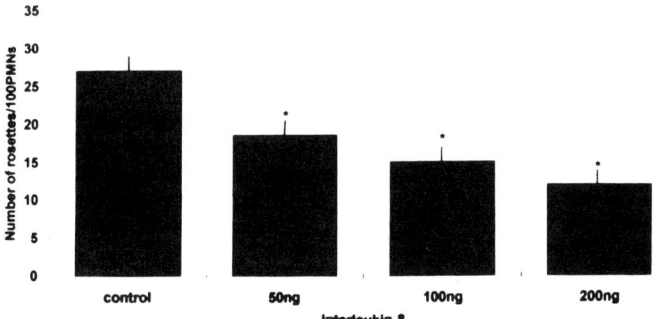

FIGURE 1. Decrease of adhesion of gel filtrated human platelets to homologous PMNs by IL-8 (50–200 ng/ml) in the presence of 30 mU thrombin (mean + SD, n = 5–11; significance $*p < 0.05$).

was induced by i.p. injection of Ova-antiOva-complexes. 1-4 hours later the abdominal PMNs were harvested for NOS activity. Occasionally IL-8 (1 µg/300 g) was given 3 min before the induction of peritonitis.

RESULTS

Co-incubation of platelets and PMNs in the presence of thrombin resulted in the increase of rosette number from 6–15 up to 30–60 rosettes/100 PMNs. The addition of anti-selectin-P Moab (kindly supplied by Prof. J. Sixma, University of Utrecht) completely prevented formation of the thrombin-stimulated rosettes and decreased the basal number of rosettes in the unstimulated cell suspension.

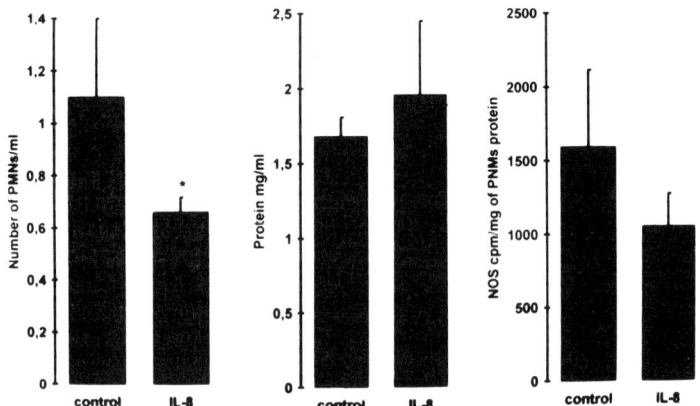

FIGURE 2. The influence of IL-8 (1 µg/300 g) given i.v. on the Ova-antiOva–induced peritonitis in rats (mean + SD; n = 3–5; significance $*p < 0.05$).

IL-8 concentration dependently decreased the number of rosettes in incubation mixtures (FIG. 1). Neither cyclooxygenase inhibitor ASA nor the NOS inhibitor L-NO$_2$-Arg influenced the inhibitory activity of IL-8 on the platelet/PMNs adhesion.

The activity of NOS of PMNs elicited from the peritoneal cavity after the immune complexes injection was relatively low (FIG. 2). IL-8 did not change the number of residual cells in the peritoneal cavity. Pretreatment of rats with IL-8 before Ova-antiOva injection resulted in a significant reduction of the number of migrating cells, and a tendency to decreased NOS activity without any influence on the protein content in exudate (FIG. 2).

CONCLUSIONS

The major finding of this study is that IL-8 inhibits the adhesion of platelets to PMNs *in vitro*, and inhibits the Ova-antiOva complex-elicited chemotaxis of PMNs, with a tendency to decrease their NOS activity.

Both the platelet adhesion to PMNs (our experimental model) and the initiation of PMNs adhesion and chemotaxis to endothelium are mediated by selectin-P. The inhibitory effect of IL-8 was related neither to the cyclooxygenase product of arachidonic acid nor to the NO, since the COX as well as NOS-inhibitors were not able to modify the inhibitory effect of IL-8.

Thus, the inhibitory effect of IL-8 on selectin-P–mediated PMNs/platelets adhesion seems to be related to the down-regulation of the selectin-L expression on PMNs membrane, as reported recently by Rot[1] and Hebert *et al.*[3]

The decrease of NO generation by PMNs after chemotaxis in rats pretreated with IL-8 was observed *in vivo*.[5] Thus, the anti-inflammatory properties of IL-8 may be related to the decrease of platelet/PMNs adhesion, the inhibition of PMNs/endothelium adhesion and chemotaxis, and to the decreased production of cytotoxic amounts of NO by PMNs.

REFERENCES

1. ROT, A. 1992. Endothelial cell binding of NAP-1/IL-8: Role in neutrophil emigration. Immunol. Today **13:** 291–294.
2. JUNGI, T. W., M. O. SPYCHER, U. E. NYDEGGER & S. BARANDUS. 1990. Platelet-leucocyte interaction. Selective binding of thrombin-stimulated platelets to human monocytes, polymorphonuclear leucocytes, and related cell lines. Blood **75:** 629.
3. HEBERT, C. A., F. W. LUSCINSKAS, J. M. KIELY, E. A. LUIS, W. C. DARBONNE, G. L. BENNETT, C. C. LIU, M. S. OBIN & J. B. BAKER. 1992. Endothelial and leucocyte forms of IL-8. Conversions by thrombin and the interactions with neutrophils. J. Immunol. **145:** 3033–3040.
4. BREDT, D. S. & S. H. SNYDER. 1990. Isolation of nitric oxide synthetase, a calmodulin-requiring enzyme. Proc. Natl. Acad. Sci. USA **87:** 682–685.
5. MCCALL, T. B., R. M. PALMER & S. MONCADA. 1989. IL-8 inhibits the formation of nitric oxide synthase in rat peritoneal neutrophils. Biochem. Biophys. Res. Commun. **186:** 680–685.

Blood Serum Concentration of C-Reactive Protein and Interleukin-6 in Diagnosis of Neonatal Infections

K. DREWS, J. SZCZAPA, J. ŻAK, R. ANDRZEJEWSKA, L. ŻAK, AND A. MACKIEWICZ

Institute of Gynecology and Obstetrics
University School of Medical Sciences
Polna 33
Poznań, Poland

Infection within the first 48 h of life is a serious condition which also occurs frequently in preterm neonates. Any delay in treatment is associated with high morbidity and mortality, but such infections are normally difficult to diagnose because the presenting features are often subtle and nonspecific. The decision to start antimicrobial therapy is therefore frequently based on clinical grounds alone. Availability of a sensitive, objective test, capable of giving results more rapidly than microbiological culture would be of considerable value in the management of this challenging clinical problem.

Among the non-specific indices of infection there has lately been a resurgence of interest in the clinical measurement of circulating acute phase proteins, especially C-reactive protein (CRP). The particular clinical value of CRP measurements results from the very low normal serum level of this protein, its extended dynamic range and the speed with which its concentration changes in response to changes in disease extent and activity. The system's reaction to infection develops into the inflammatory response leading to an enhanced vascular permeability. It finally results in the extravascular protein leakage infiltrations with leukocytes, macrophases, lymphocytes. This whole process is controlled by several humoral factors, among them cytokins. Interleukin-6 (IL-6) is the main cytokine stimulating the acute phase proteins response (CRP).

There has been considerable interest in whether this response in newborn infants can be used as an early predictor of infection.

The aim of this study was the estimation of CRP and IL-6 serum levels for diagnosis of neonatal infection. The material were blood samples from neonates treated in the Department of Neonatology, the gestational age ranged from 26 to 41 weeks, and body weight from 1120 g to 4040 g. We assigned 62 newborns in whom intrauterine (primary) or secondary (acquired during hospitalization) infection was diagnosed into separate groups. The serum CRP levels were measured by rocket immunoelectrophoresis and Il-6 concentration by enzyme immunoassay (Predicta of Genzyma Diagnostics). The 10 mg/l CRP level was accepted as normal. The first CRP and IL-6 determination was performed between the 4th and 10th days of life. Respiratory treatment time of neonates varied from 2 to 25 days.

The results of CRP determination in the infected infants has shown positive correlation between infection and high concentration of this protein. TABLE 1 gives the number of true-positive and false-negative results. Estimation of IL-6 levels in the serum of newborn infants can be useful in distinguishing intrauterine and secondary infection and can be used as a sensitive test of infection. FIGURE 1 show concentrations of IL-6 in blood serum of infected neonates (both infants infected *in utero* and those with secondary infections).

TABLE 1. Results of CRP Determination in Infected Infants

CRP	Diagnosis	Number of Neonates	Results
<10mg/l	Intrauterine infection	2	False-negative
		11	True-negative
>10mg/l	Intrauterine infection	9	True-positive
		8	False-positive
<10mg/l	Secondary infection	3	False-negative
		5	True-negative
>10mg/l	Secondary infection	7	True-positive
		2	False-positive

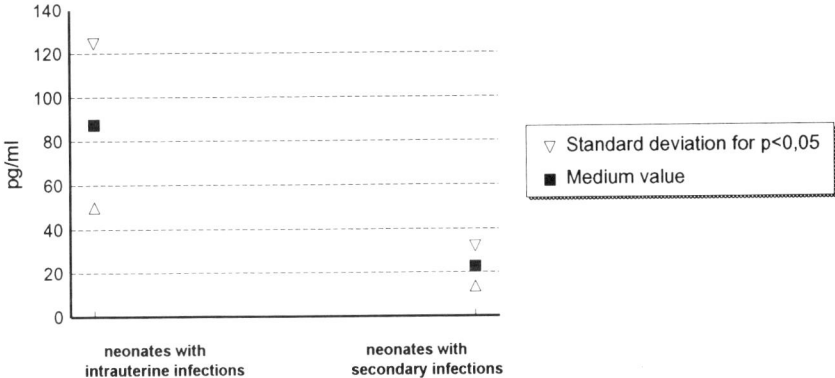

FIGURE 1. Results of IL-6 determination in primary and secondary infections.

We have found that single CRP determination is not fully reliable, as it arises from the normal range of concentration. A series of successive CRP determinations seems to be much more useful in the early detection of infection, and a single estimation of IL-6 concentration precisely indicates primary infection (confirmed by microbiological cultures).

The essential problem in neonatal pathology clinics is still early diagnosis of infection (intrauterine and or during intensive treatment), and an early administration of antibiotics for the treatment of infections. We have drawn the conclusion that CRP and IL-6 determination in neonatal blood serum is a very helpful examination in the diagnosis of infection. Il-6 determination is more sensitive and has higher value in examination of intrauterine infection and can be performed like a single estimation.

REFERENCES

1. NETTEKE, Y. N., M. D. SCHOUTEN-VAN MEETEREN & M. D. ARIENE RIETVELD. 1992. J. Pediatr. **120**: 621.
2. SHORTLAND, D., U. MACFADYEN & A. ELSTON. 1990. J. Perinat. Med. **18**: 157.
3. SOBEL, K. G. & CH. WADSWORTH. 1989. Acta Pediatr. Scand. **68**: 825.
4. VALLANCE, H. & C. LOCKITCH. 1991. Clin. Chem. **37**(No 11): 1981.
5. WASUNND, A. & A. WHITELAW. 1990. Eur. J. Pediatr. **149**: 424.

Residues 77–95 of the Human Interleuken-6 Protein are Responsible for Receptor Binding and Residues 41–56 for Signal Transduction

MARC EHLERS,[a] JOACHIM GRÖTZINGER,[a] FLORIS D.
DE HON,[b] JÜRGEN MÜLLBERG,[a] JUST P. J. BRAKENHOFF,[b]
AXEL WOLLMER,[a] AND STEFAN ROSE-JOHN[a]

[a]*Department of Biochemistry*
Rheinisch-Westfälische Technische Hochschule Aachen
Pauwelsstrasse 30
D-52057 Aachen, Germany

[b]*Department of Autoimmune Diseases*
Central Laboratory of the
Netherlands Red Cross Blood Transfusion Service
Amsterdam 1066 CX, The Netherlands

The pleiotropic cytokine Interleukin-6 (IL-6) consists of 184 amino acids and has been predicted to be a protein with four anti-parallel α-helices. The IL-6 receptor

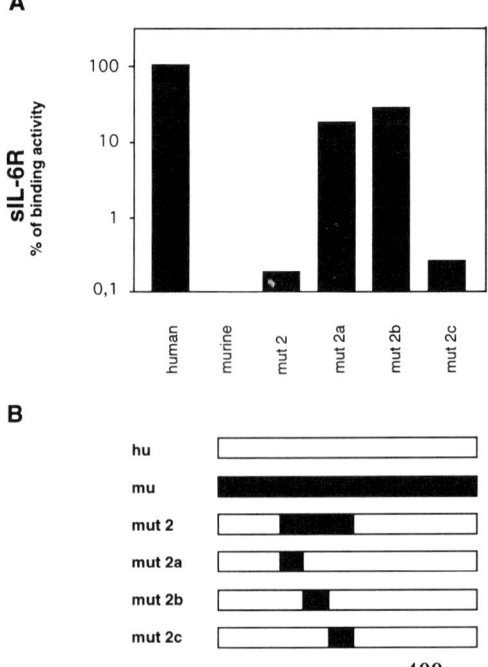

FIGURE 1. Binding of the IL-6 variants to the soluble human IL-6R. **(A)** Recombinant human soluble IL-6R (gp80) was incubated with human ^{125}I-IL-6. Binding was competed with increasing amounts of human, murine or chimeric IL-6 proteins. The soluble IL-6R/IL-6 complexes were immunoprecipitated with a sIL-6R specific antiserum and protein A Sepharose. Radioactivity was determined by γ-counting. The human IL-6 concentration which led to half-maximal competition of human ^{125}I-IL-6 was set 100%. **(B)** Schematic representation of human, murine and chimeric IL-6 proteins. Human sequences are shown as open, murine sequences as filled bars.

complex on target cells consists of two different subunits, an 80 kD ligand binding subunit (IL-6R) and a 130 kD signal-transducing protein (gp130). After the binding of IL-6 to the IL-6R protein this binary complex becomes associated with a dimer of gp130. Human IL-6 acts on human and murine cells whereas murine IL-6 is only active on murine cells. The construction of a set of chimeric human/murine IL-6 proteins has recently allowed us to define a new region (residues Lys41-Glu95: region 2) within the IL-6 molecule as important for receptor binding and biological activity.[7] We analyzed this region which mainly corresponds to the loop between the first and second α-helix of IL-6 with respect to its role in the interaction with the IL-6R and with the IL-6 signal-transducing protein gp130. By construction and analysis of human/murine chimeric IL-6 molecules with only a few amino acid residues different from human IL-6 we show that one part of this region (residues 77–95: region 2c) is responsible for receptor binding (FIG. 1) and another (residues 41–56: region 2a) for signal transduction (FIG. 2).[2] Earlier structure function analysis of IL-6 using neutralizing monoclonal antibodies had already identified two distinct sites (sites I and II) of IL-6 necessary for receptor binding or biological activity.[3,4] Site I had been shown to be the C-terminus of IL-6 and site II was mapped around residue 157. On the basis of the recently published structure of granulocyte colony-stimulating factor (G-CSF) we generated a three-dimensional model for the tertiary structure of IL-6 (see Rose-John et al., this volume). With this model we can show that site I and region 2c are in close proximity and also site II and region 2a. The separation of

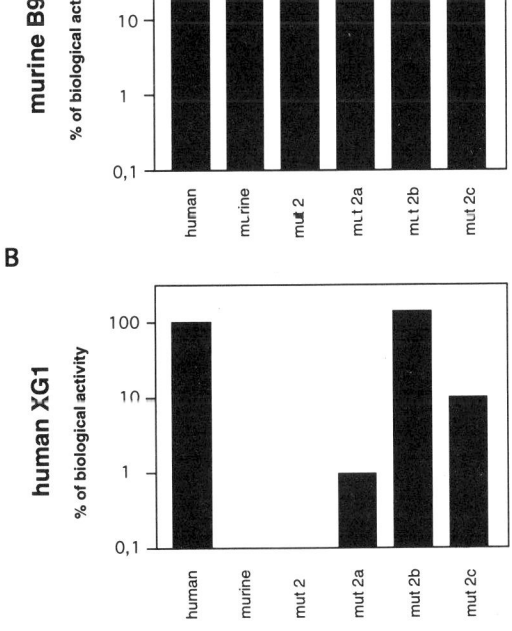

FIGURE 2. Proliferation of human and murine cells in response to IL-6 variants. Dose dependence of proliferation of murine B9 (A) or human XG-1 cells (B) in response to human, murine or chimeric IL-6 proteins. Cells were grown in the presence of increasing amounts of IL-6 variants and proliferation was measured using a colorimetric assay. The human IL-6 concentration which lead to half-maximal proliferation was set 100%.

regions within the IL-6 protein which are responsible for receptor binding and signal transduction will allow the rational design of human IL-6 receptor antagonists.

[**Note added in proof:** Recently the combination of mutations in site II and region 2a resulted in potent human IL-6 receptor antagonists on the high sensitive human myeloma cell line XG-1 (de Hon *et al.* (1994) J. Exp. Med. **180:**2395–2400; Ehlers *et al.* (1995) J. Biol. Chem. **270:**8158–8163).]

REFERENCES

1. VAN DAM, M., J. MÜLLBERG, H. SCHOOLTINK, T. STOYAN, J. P. J. BRAKENHOFF, L. GRAEVE, P. C. HEINRICH & S. ROSE-JOHN. 1993. Structure-function analysis of interleukin-6 utilizing human/murine chimeric molecules. J. Biol. Chem. **268:** 15285–15290.
2. EHLERS, M., J. GRÖTZINGER, F. D. DEHON, J. MÜLLBERG, J. P. J. BRAKENHOFF, J. LIU, A. WOLLMER & S. ROSE-JOHN. 1994. Identification of two novel regions of human interleukin-6 responsible for receptor binding and signal transduction. J. Immunol. **153:** 1744–1753.
3. BRAKENHOFF, J. P. J., M. HART, E. R. DE GROOT, F. DI PADOVA & L. A. AARDEN. 1990. Structure-function of human IL-6. Epitope mapping of neutralizing monoclonal antibodies with amino- and carboxyl-terminal deletion mutants. J. Immunol. **145:** 561–568.
4. BRAKENHOFF, J. P. J., F. D. DEHON, V. FONTAINE, E. TENBOEKEL, H. SCHOOLTINK, S. ROSE-JOHN, P. C. HEINRICH, J. CONTENT & L. A. AARDEN. 1994. Development of a human interleukin-6 receptor-antagonist. J. Biol. Chem. **269:** 86–93.

Interleukin-6 and Interleukin-6 Receptor mRNA Expression in Rat Central Nervous System[a]

R. A. GADIENT AND U. OTTEN

Department of Physiology
University of Basel
Vesalianum, Vesalgasse 1
4051 Basel, Switzerland

The multifunctional cytokine interleukin-6 (IL-6), which is a key modulator of immune and inflammatory responses, has recently been shown to exert specific functions in the central nervous system (CNS). IL-6 promotes survival of mesencephalic catecholaminergic and septal cholinergic neurons isolated from the rat postnatal brain.[1] It induces neuronal differentiation of the rat pheochromocytoma cell line PC12,[2] and significantly ameliorates the neurotoxic effects of the excitotoxic substance N-methyl-D-aspartate (NMDA) on rat striatal cholinergic neurons.[3] The physiological role of IL-6 in the CNS is still unclear. To investigate IL-6 and IL-6 receptor (IL-6R) mRNA expression in normal rat brain we used the sensitive technique of reverse transcription followed by the polymerase chain reaction (RT-PCR).[4] Our results indicate that both mRNAs are expressed in normal rat brain in a region-specific manner and are developmentally regulated (FIG. 1).[5] Most pronounced expression of both genes was observed in the adult hippocampus. Lower levels were seen in the hypothalamus and the striatum. During postnatal development a positive correlation between IL-6 and IL-6R mRNA levels was observed in the hippocampus and the striatum, whereas the hypothalamus the opposite was found. The greatest changes in both transcripts occurred in the striatum between postnatal day 2 and day 20. To investigate the cellular localization of the IL-6 mRNA a sensitive non-radioactive *in situ* hybridization technique was established.[6] As shown in FIGURE 2a, a strong IL-6 mRNA signal is visible in the hippocampus, whereas the sense control (FIG. 2b) shows no staining, indicating the specificity of the IL-6 mRNA signal. Pronounced IL-6 mRNA expression is seen in the hypothalamus (FIG. 2c) and in the striatum (FIG. 2d). In normal rat brain IL-6 mRNA seems to be predominantly expressed by neuronal cells, including the pyramidal and granular cells of the hippocampus. However, the possibility that glial cells also express IL-6 mRNA under physiological conditions cannot be excluded. To clarify this, we are currently combining *in situ* hybridization with immunohistochemistry.

In conclusion, we found that IL-6 and IL-6R mRNAs are expressed in normal rat brain in a region-specific manner and are developmentally controlled. *In situ* hybridization studies reveal that IL-6 mRNA is predominantly located in neurons, indicating that IL-6 may have a specific role in neuronal functions such as differentiation or survival.

---

[a] This study was supported by the Swiss National Foundation for Scientific Research (Grant 31-39121.93) and by grants of the Roche Research Foundation and Stiftung E. Guggenheim-Schnurr, Basel.

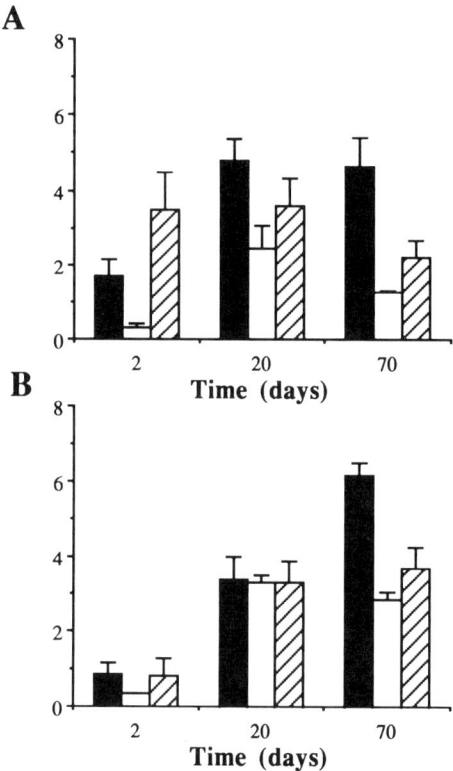

FIGURE 1. Developmental expression of IL-6 and IL-6R mRNAs in different rat brain regions. Densitometric quantification of IL-6 **(A)** and IL-6R mRNA **(B)** signals in the hippocampus *(full bars)*, in the striatum *(open bars)* and in the hypothalamus *(striped bars)*. Data are corrected for the ribosomal S12 mRNA signal and are expressed in arbitrary units. Each time point has been measured at least in triplicate; error bars represent standard error of the mean (SEM).

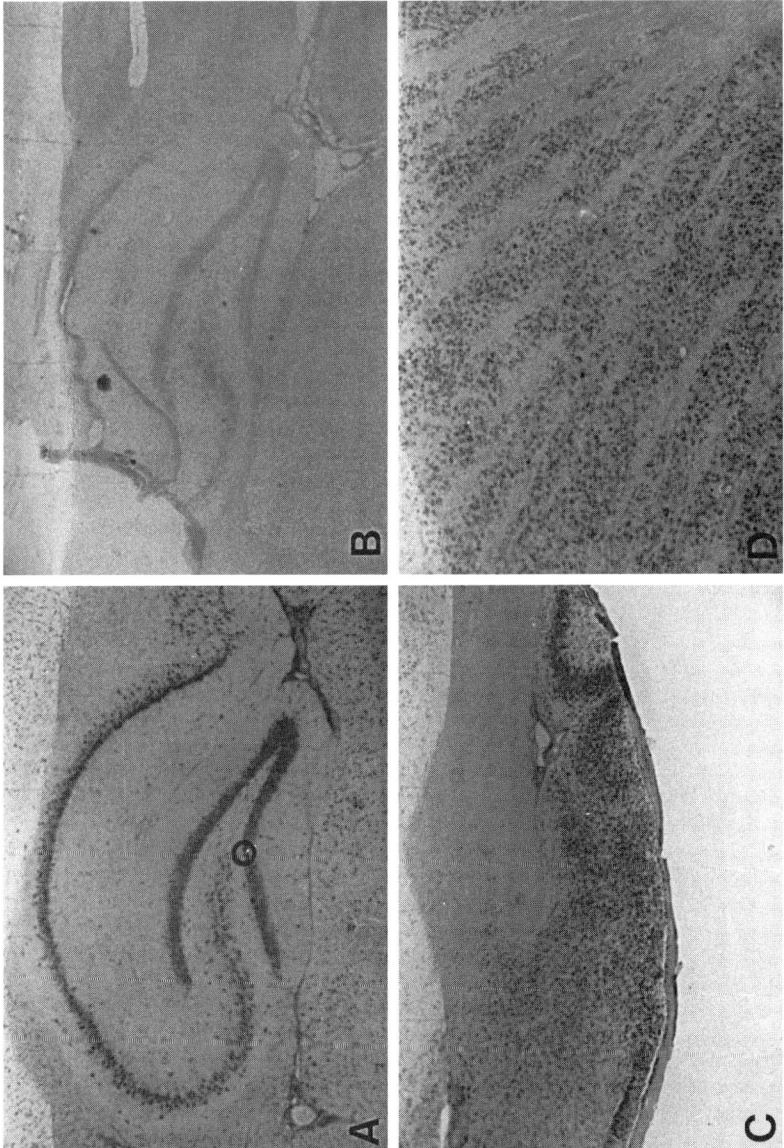

FIGURE 2. Localization of IL-6 mRNA in different regions of the adult rat brain. IL-6 mRNA was detected by hybridization with a IL-6-specific digoxigenin-labeled cRNA probe. (A, C and D) were hybridized to the antisense probe and (B) to the sense probe. Regions shown: hippocampus (A and B), hypothalamus (C) and striatum (D).

REFERENCES

1. HAMA, T., Y. KUSHIMA, M. MIYAMOTO, M. KUBOTA, N. TAKEI & H. HATANAKA. 1991. Interleukin-6 improves the survival of mesencephalic catecholaminergic and septal cholinergic neurons from postnatal two-week-old rats in cultures. Neuroscience **40:** 445–452.
2. SATOH, T., S. NAKAMURA, T. TAGA, T. MATSUDA, T. HIRANO, T. KISHIMOTO & Y. KAZIRO. 1988. Induction of neuronal differentiation in PC12 cells by B-cell stimulatory factor 2/interleukin-6. Mol. Cell. Biol. **8:** 3546–3549.
3. TOULMOND, S., X. VIGE, D. FAGE & J. BENAVIDES. 1992. Local infusion of interleukin-6 attenuates the neurotoxic effects of NMDA on rat striatal cholinergic neurons. Neurosci. Lett. **144:** 49–52.
4. GADIENT, R. A. & U. OTTEN. 1993. Differential expression of interleukin-6 (IL-6) and interleukin-6 receptor (IL-6R) mRNAs in rat hypothalamus. Neurosci. Lett. **153:** 13–16.
5. GADIENT, R. A. & U. OTTEN. 1994. Expression of interleukin-6 (IL-6) and interleukin-6 receptor (IL-6R) in rat brain during postnatal development. Brain Res. **637:** 10–14.
6. GADIENT, R. A. & U. OTTEN. 1994. Identification of interleukin-6 (IL-6)-expressing neurons in the cerebellum and hippocampus of normal adult rats. Neurosci. Lett. **182:** 243–246.

ELISA Detection of Circulating Levels of LIF, OSM, and CNTF in Septic Shock

CATHERINE GUILLET, MARYVONNE FOURCIN,
SYLVIE CHEVALIER, ANNICK POUPLARD,
AND HUGUES GASCAN

INSERM U298, CHRU Angers
Angers 49033, Cedex, France

INTRODUCTION

Il-6, Il-11, OSM, CNTF and LIF belong to the same family of cytokines using gp130/Il-6 protein transducer as a part of their receptors.[1] Circulating Il-6 in inflammatory and neoplastic pathologies has been well documented. We have recently developed sensitive ELISAs allowing the detection of Il-11, OSM, CNTF, and LIF in biological fluids and analyzed the circulating levels of these cytokines.

MATERIALS AND METHODS

Anti-Il-11 monoclonal antibodies were a kind gift of K. Turner (Genetics Institute), Il-6 ELISA and B-R3 anti-gp130 antibody were courtesy of J. Wijdenes (Innotherapie), and CNTF was kindly given by G. D. Yancopoulos (Regeneron). Polyclonal antibodies against CNTF and LIF were generated in rabbit by intra-lymphnode immunization. Anti-OSM antibodies were purchased from R&D System. Antibodies were coated at a concentration of 10 μg/ml, and after an overnight incubation of the samples, the biotinylated detector, polyclonal or monoclonal, antibody was added at 1 μg/ml for 4 hours, followed by an avidin peroxydase step and visualization with ABTS. The TF1 proliferation assay was carried out by incubating the cells in the presence of serial dilutions of serum samples and the appropriate blocking antibodies. After 60 hours, the cells were pulsed with ^{3}H-thymidine and the incorporated radioactivity determined.

RESULTS AND DISCUSSION

We have developed specific and sensitive ELISAs allowing the respective detection of 1 pg/ml of LIF, and 10 pg/ml of OSM, CNTF or IL-11. These tools were used

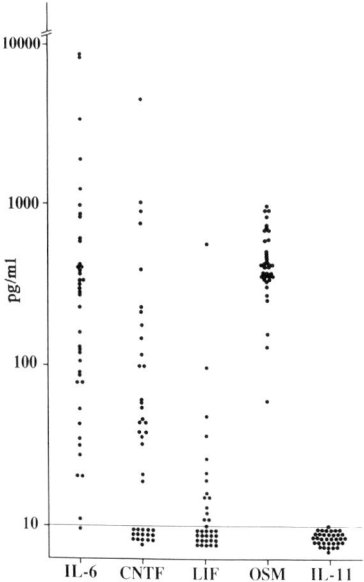

FIGURE 1. Peripheral blood concentrations of Il-6, CNTF, LIF, OSM and Il-11 determined by ELISA in patients suffering from septic shock.

to look for the presence of this cytokine family in the sera of patients suffering from septic shock. In addition to Il-6, circulating levels of LIF, OSM and CNTF were observed (FIG. 1). CNTF and LIF were found in 60% and 40% of the cases (n = 40), respectively, with concentrations ranging from 10 to 1000 pg/ml. No circulating levels were detected in normal individuals, with the exception of marginal concentrations of OSM (mean value = 30 pg/ml). In all the patients, OSM levels were increased to reach an average value of 360 pg/ml (n = 40). The sera were then tested in the TF1 cell line proliferation assay. FIGURE 2 shows that the proliferative response of the TF1 line to a serum displaying high concentrations of OSM, LIF and CNTF, but no Il-6, was entirely due to gp130 ligands, since a blocking antibody directed against this component completely abrogated the signal. Similarly, addition of the appropriate blocking antibody, to sera mainly containing only one of the studied cytokines, led to a specific decrease of the TF1 response. Since very high concentrations of CNTF were required to trigger the TF1 proliferation (>10 ng/ml),[3] only marginal responses to CNTF were observed. These results demonstrated the functional relevance of the cytokines detected by ELISA in septic shock. No correlation between Il-6, OSM, CNTF, or LIF levels could be established. We also failed to detect circulating Il-11, but we cannot rule out the possibility that Il-11 is masked by some circulating components interfering with the ELISA. Interestingly, despite the lack of signal peptide in CNTF and a neural localization of its production, septic shock represents a unique situation where we could detect this cytokine in a circulating form. This could reflect nerve injuries. Collectively these results indicate that, along with Il-6, LIF, CNTF and OSM can be detected in a pathological situation, and might participate to the evolution of the disease.

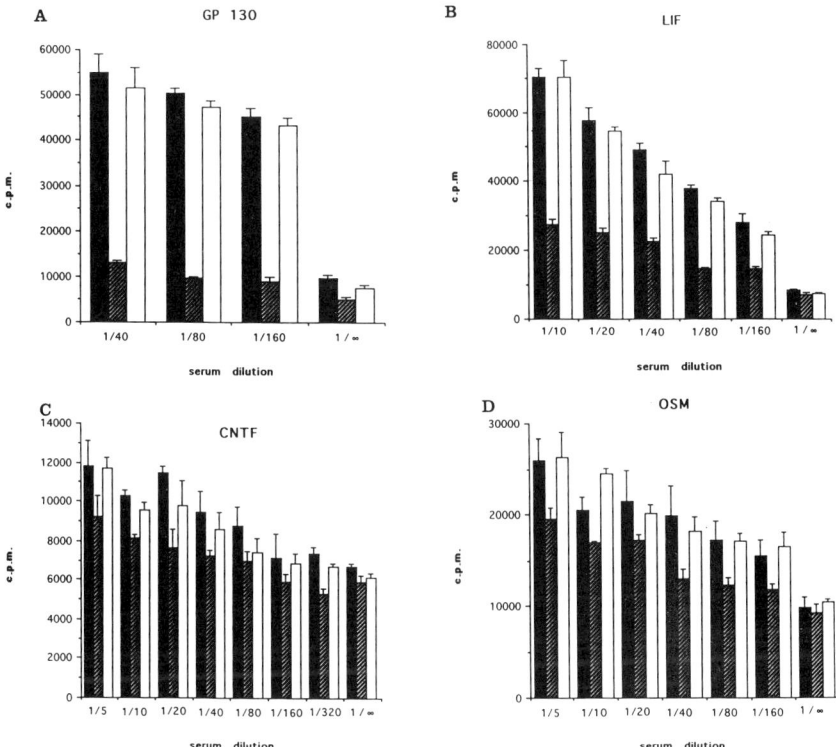

FIGURE 2. Proliferative response of the TF1 cell line to sera from patients suffering from septic shock. 2×10^4 cells were incubated for 60 h in triplicate in the presence of serial dilutions of serum alone *(black bars)*, by adding a blocking antibody (10 μg/ml) *(hatched bars)*, or a control antibody (10 μg/ml) *(open bars)*. Incorporated radioactivity was measured after a 4 h pulse with ^{3}H thymidine. **A:** Abrogation of the proliferative response to a non-Il-6 containing serum by the B-R3 anti gp130 blocking antibody. **B:** TF1 cell line response to a LIF-containing serum. **C:** TF1 cell line response to a CNTF containing serum. **D:** TF1 cell line response to an OSM-containing serum.

REFERENCES

1. GEARING, D. P., S. F. ZIEGLER, M. R. COMEAU, *et al.* 1994. Proc. Natl. Acad. Sci. USA **91:** 1119.
2. KISHIMOTO, T., S. AKIRA & T. TAGA. 1992. Science **258:** 593.
3. DAVIS, S., T. H. ALDRICH, N. Y. IP, M. STAHL, S. SCHERER, T FARRUGGELLA, P. S. DISTEFANO, R. CURTIS, N. PANAYOTATOS, H. GASCAN, S. CHEVALIER & G. D. YANCOPOULOS. 1993. Science **259:** 1665.

A Region within the Cytoplasmic Domain of the Interleukin-6 Signal Transducer gp130 Important for Ligand-induced Endocytosis of the IL-6 Receptor

ELKE DITTRICH, CLAUDIA GERHARTZ, STEFAN ROSE-JOHN,
JÜRGEN MÜLLBERG, TANJA STOYAN, PETER C. HEINRICH,
AND LUTZ GRAEVE[a]

Institut für Biochemie
Rheinisch-Westfälische Technische Hochschule Aachen
Pauwelsstrasse 30
D-52057 Aachen, Germany

Interleukin-6 (IL-6) acts via a cell surface receptor complex that is composed of two subunits: an 80 kD IL-6 binding protein (IL-6 receptor) and a 130 kD signal-transducing protein, gp130. After binding to its receptor, IL-6 is rapidly internalized and degraded by rat hepatocytes and human hepatoma cells HepG2.[1,2] In HepG2 cells this internalization leads to a loss of IL-6 binding sites at the cell surface. This finding indicates that the IL-6 receptor is down-regulated by its ligand. A ligand-induced down-regulation has been described for a number of other receptors, *i.e.* the insulin receptor, the platelet-derived growth factor receptor and the epidermal growth factor receptor. This process might play an important role as a protection against overstimulation. The mechanism leading to surface receptor down-regulation is still under investigation. One likely mechanism is that after binding of the ligand the rate of endocytosis of the receptor is increased resulting in a net loss of binding sites at the surface.

For a number of receptor transmembrane proteins, *e.g.* transferrin, the low density lipoprotein, and the asialoglycoprotein receptor, it has been shown that specific sequences within the cytoplasmic domain that contain a tyrosine are important for efficient internalization. The substitution of single amino acids within such sequence motifs and structural predictions implied that an important characteristic of such motifs is the formation of a "tight β-turn." This structure is probably recognized by adaptor proteins which mediate the accumulation of these receptors in clathrin-coated pits.[3] A different class of sequence motifs important for internalization and lysosomal targeting were found in the intracellular domains of the γ- and δ-chain of the T-cell receptor complex, the cation-dependent mannose-6-phosphate receptor, the cation-independent mannose-6-phosphate/IGF II receptor, and the interferon γ-receptor. These motifs are characterized by a leucine-leucine or a leucine-isoleucine sequence (di-leucine-motif).[3]

---

[a] Author to whom correspondence should be addressed: Institut für Biochemie, Rheinisch-Westfälische Technische Hochschule Aachen, Pauwelsstrasse 30, D-52057 Aachen, Germany. Tel: 0241-8088837; Fax: 0241-8888428.

In order to elucidate the molecular mechanism of ligand-induced internalization and down-regulation of the IL-6 receptor, we asked whether there are internalization sequences in the cytoplasmic domains of the IL-6 receptor and/or the signal transducer gp130.

In order to answer this question we transfected cDNAs coding for wild-type and mutant forms of the IL-6 receptor and gp130 together into COS-7 cells and studied the internalization of IL-6 and the down-regulation of the IL-6 receptor using ^{125}I-IL-6 (FIG. 1). When both wild-type proteins were expressed an efficient internalization of IL-6 was observed (42% of initially bound IL-6 was internalized within the first 30 min). This endocytosis was accompanied by a receptor down-regulation of about 50%. When the IL-6 receptor was expressed alone the rate of internalization was low (9% as compared to 42%) and no down-regulation was observed. This clearly indicates that expression of gp130 is crucial for the efficient endocytosis of IL-6.

We next analyzed if the cytoplasmic domains of either the IL-6 receptor or gp130 are important for this process. The results clearly show that the cytoplasmic tail of the IL-6 receptor is not important (FIG. 1). In contrast, a mutant of gp130 lacking the 136 carboxy-terminal amino acids was not able to direct efficient internalization (FIG. 1). Since a mutant lacking only 126 amino acids behaved like wild-type gp130 we conclude that the ten amino acid sequence TQPLLDSEER contains a putative internalization motif.[4] Since this sequence contains a di-leucine motif it is very likely that this motif directs the efficient internalization (and probably also the targeting to the lysosomes) of the IL-6 receptor complex. Recent experiments in which this motif has been deleted and mutated supported this notion.

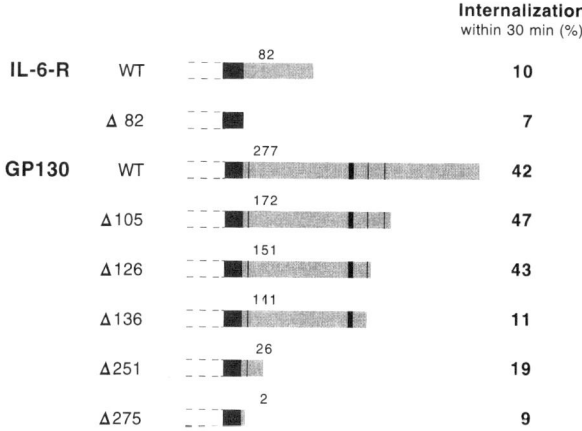

FIGURE 1. Internalization of IL-6 receptor complexes consisting of wild-type IL-6-R and gp130 or different deletion mutants. The extracellular domain is indicated by dotted lines. The black box represents the transmembrane domain. The cytoplasmic domain is shown as a grey box. Numbering of the cytoplasmic amino acids started after the transmembrane domain. The thick and thin bars within the cytoplasmic tail are locations of putative internalization sequences. *Thick, black bar:* tyrosine containing motif; *thin, black bars:* di-leucine motifs. Internalization was measured by binding 1 nM ^{125}I-IL-6 to cells at 4°C for 2h and shifting to 37°C for 30 min. Internalized IL-6 was measured after stripping surface bound IL-6 with a high salt/low pH wash. Internalized IL-6 is indicated as percentage of initially bound IL-6. The values are the mean from two to four independent experiments.

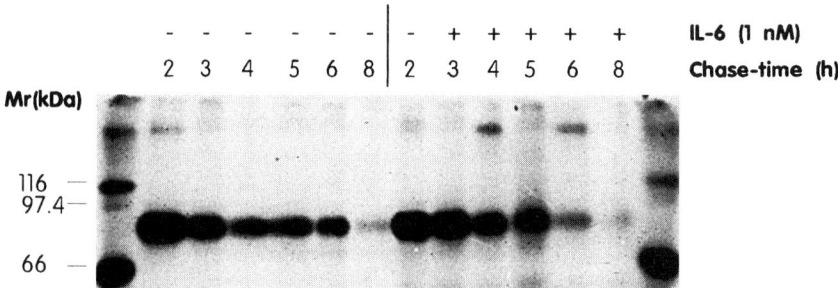

FIGURE 2. The half-life of the IL-6 receptor in MDCK-gp80 cells. Subconfluent MDCK-gp80 cells were metabolically labeled for 2 h and chased for the times indicated with or without 1 nM IL-6. The cells were lysed, the IL-6R was immunoprecipitated and analyzed by 10% SDS-PAGE and fluorography.

In many cases the ligand-induced down-regulation is accompanied by an increased rate of degradation of the respective receptor. Surprisingly, when we analyzed by pulse-chase experiments the half-lifes of gp80 in stably transfected Madin-Darby canine kidney cells (which contain endogenous gp130) and of gp130 in HepG2 cells we could not detect an increased rate of degradation of either in the presence of IL-6 (FIG. 2).[5] This indicates that the transport to and the degradation within the lysosomes is slow compared to the increased rate of endocytosis.

REFERENCES

1. NESBITT, J. E. & G. M. FULLER. 1992. Dynamics of interleukin-6 internalization and degradation in rat hepatocytes. J. Biol. Chem. **267:** 5739–5742.
2. ZOHLNHOEFER, D., L. GRAEVE, S. ROSE-JOHN, H. SCHOOLTINK, E. DITTRICH & P. C. HEINRICH. 1992. The hepatic interleukin-6 receptor. Down-regulation of the interleukin-6 binding subunit (gp80) by its ligand. FEBS Lett. **306:** 219–222.
3. TROWBRIDGE, I. S., J. F. COLLAWN & C. R. HOPKINS. 1993. Signal-dependent membrane protein trafficking in the endocytotic pathway. Annu. Rev. Cell Biol. **9:** 129–161.
4. DITTRICH, E., S. ROSE-JOHN, C. GERHARTZ, J. MÜLLBERG, T. STOYAN, K. YASUKAWA, P. C. HEINRICH & L. GRAEVE. 1994. Identification of a region within the cytoplasmic domain of the interleukin-6 signal transducer gp130 important for ligand-induced endocytosis of the IL-6 receptor. J. Biol. Chem. **269:** 19014–19020.
5. GERHARTZ, C., E. DITTRICH, T. STOYAN, S. ROSE-JOHN, K. YASUKAWA, P. C. HEINRICH & L. GRAEVE. 1994. Biosynthesis and half-life of the interleukin-6 receptor and its signal transducer gp130. Eur. J. Biochem. **223:** 265–274.

Interleukin-6-Type Cytokines Affect Glycosylation of Acute Phase Proteins *in Vitro*[a]

KATARZYNA GRYSKA,[b] ARTUR SLUPIANEK,[b] MARIA LACIAK,[b]
HEINZ BAUMANN,[c] AND ANDRZEJ MACKIEWICZ[b]

[b]*Department of Cancer Immunology, Chair of Oncology*
Academy of Medicine
Garbary 15
Poznań, Poland 61866

[c]*Department of Molecular and Cellular Biology*
Roswell Park Cancer Institute
Buffalo, New York 14263-0001

Changes in pattern of glycosylation of acute phase proteins (APP) belong to the events occurring during acute phase response. Two types of glycosylation alterations in patient sera are observed. Type I, seen in acute inflammatory processes, is characterized by relative decrease of branching of complex type N-glycans linked to APP and type II is observed in a number of chronic inflammatory states characterized by relative increase of branching of N-glycans of APP.[1] Glycosylation changes of APP in serum result from alterations occurring within hepatocytes on the biosynthetic pathway and are regulated by cytokines independently from mechanisms governing gene expression of these proteins.[2] A number of cytokines including IL-6, LIF, IFN-γ or TGFβ were reported to be involved in these processes. Moreover, other factors such as glucocorticoids or soluble IL-6 receptor are directly or indirectly controlling glycosylation of APP.[3] Here we report that other cytokines which belong to the group of IL-6-type cytokines, namely IL-11, oncostatin M (OSM) and ciliary neurotrophic factor (CNTF) also affect glycosylation of APP *in vitro*.

Human (Hep G2) and rat (H-35) hepatoma cell lines were used in these studies. Cells were cultured in the presence of cytokines and/or dexamethasone (dex) for 48 h with change of medium every 24 h. Media collected at final 24 h were analyzed. Since base line production of α_1-acid glycoprotein (AGP) in H-35 cells is very low and IL-6-type cytokines when used alone are not able to evoke significant induction of its synthesis cells were always maintained in the presence of IL-1 and dex. Glycosylation changes of α_1-protease inhibitor (PI) secreted by Hep G2 cells and AGP secreted by H-35 cells were studied by means of crossed affinity immunoelectrophoresis (CAIE) with a lectin Concanavalin A (Con A) as a ligand. In CIAE glycoproteins interact with Con A and depending on the number of biantennary N-glycans on the molecule are separated into glycoforms. CIAE revealed 3 glycoforms of human PI: 0–non-reactive with Con A (containing only triantennary structures); 1–weakly reactive (containing one biantennary structure); and 2–reactive with Con A (with 2 biantennary glycans) and 5 glycoforms of rat AGP where forms 0–2 corresponded to those of PI and forms 3 and 4 containing relatively more biantennary glycans. In

---

[a] Supported in part by M. Skłodowska-Curie II Fund (MZ/HHS-92-104) and Academy of Medicine, Poznań (grant No. 501-1-007).

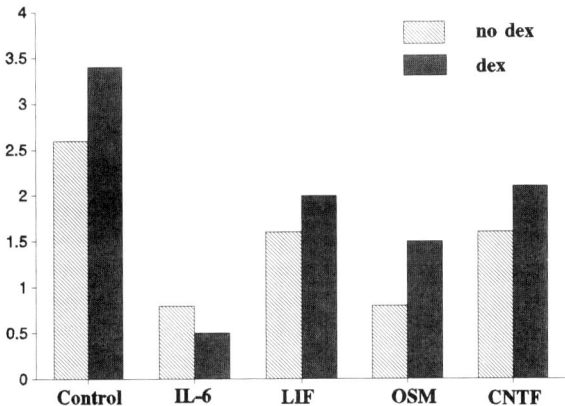

FIGURE 1. Glycosylation pattern of α_1-proteinase inhibitor secreted by Hep G2 cells stimulated with cytokines in presence and absence of dexamethasone. Results expressed as reactivity coefficients.

order to express PI and AGP glycosylation profile in numbers, reactivity coefficient (RC) was calculated according to the formula (sum of Con A reactive glycoforms)/non-reactive. In Hep G2 cells OSM and CNTF similarly as IL-6 and LIF caused relative increase of Con A non-reactive forms of PI. Effectiveness of OSM was comparable to IL-6 while CNTF had an effect similar to LIF. Moreover, dex added to the culture influenced the effect of OSM or CNTF on PI glycosylation similarly as it did for LIF; however, the effect was the opposite of that for IL-6 (FIG. 1). In H-35 cells IL-11 caused relative increase of rat AGP-Con A reactive forms as do IL-6 and LIF. The extent of change was comparable to that evoked by LIF (FIG. 2). In conclusion,

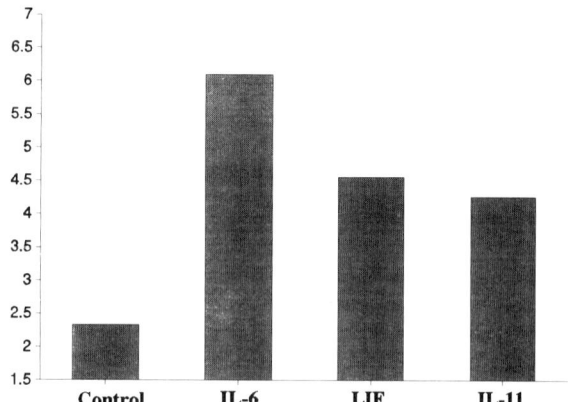

FIGURE 2. Glycosylation pattern of α_1-acid glycoprotein secreted by H-35 cells incubated with cytokines. IL-1 and dexamethasone was always present in the culture medium. Results expressed as reactivity coefficients.

all so-far recognized members of the family of IL-6-type cytokines are able to affect the profile of glycosylation of APP *in vitro*.

REFERENCES

1. MACKIEWICZ, A. & I. KUSHNER. 1989. Affinity electrophoresis for studies of mechanisms regulating glycosylation of plasma proteins. Electrophoresis **10**: 830–835.
2. MACKIEWICZ, A., M. K. GANAPATHI, D. SCHULTZ & I. KUSHNER. 1987. Monokines regulate glycosylation of acute-phase proteins. J. Exp. Med. **166**: 253–258.
3. VAN DIJK, W. & A. MACKIEWICZ. 1993. Control of glycosylation alterations of acute phase glycoproteins. *In* Acute Phase Proteins: Molecular Biology, Biochemistry and Clinical Applications. A. Mackiewicz, I. Kushner & H. Baumann, Eds. Boca Raton, FL: CRC Press.

Cytokines and the Activity of Tyrosine Aminotransferase and Superoxide Dismutase in Rat Hepatoma Cells in Culture[a]

AMALIA GUZDEK, KRYSTYNA STALIŃSKA,
AND JOANNA BERETA

Institute of Molecular Biology
Jagiellonian University
31-120 Kraków, Poland

INTRODUCTION

The regulation of acute phase protein synthesis by cytokines in hepatic cells in culture is very well documented,[1,2] but less is known about the influence of cytokines on liver cell metabolism. In our experiments the influence of TNF, IL-1β, IL-6 and hepatocyte growth factor (HGF) on the activity of tyrosine aminotransferase (TAT EC 2.6.1.5) and superoxide dismutase (SOD EC 1.15.1.1) in rat hepatoma FAO cells in culture were analyzed. Tyrosine aminotransferase is a liver-specific enzyme and its gene is regulated by endocrine hormones like insulin and glucocorticoids. The involvement of superoxide dismutase in inflammatory processes was demonstrated earlier.[3]

METHODS

Rat hepatoma FAO cells were cultured in DMEM supplemented with 5% FCS. After they reached the stage of subconfluent monolayer, they were rinsed with serum-free DMEM and cultured for additional 16 h in this medium.

For estimation of TAT activity, each well received 1 ml of serum-free medium with insulin (INS), dexamethasone (DX), HGF, TNF, or IL-6. The cells were cultured for 6, 12, 24, and 48 h and then scraped and TAT activity was evaluated according to the method of Granner and Tomkins.[4]

SOD activity was estimated in FAO cells cultured for 24 h in the presence of HGF, TNF, IL-1 and IL-6 (FIG. 1). The cells were scraped in Tris-HCl buffer, and after four cycles of freezing and thawing dialyzed overnight. For activity measurements the method described by Paoletti and Mocali[5] was chosen. To distinguish between

---

[a] This work was supported by Grant 2238/4/91 from the State Committee for Scientific Research (KBN, Warsaw, Poland).

Cu/ZnSOD and MnSOD, activity of the enzyme in cytosol and mitochondrial fractions was also evaluated.

RESULTS AND DISCUSSION

Similar to results of others[6] it was found (FIG. 2, a and b), that insulin and dexamethasone enhanced TAT activity in FAO cell. Moreover all cytokines tested decreased activity of this enzyme at least during first 12 h after cytokine supplementation (FIG. 1, c and d). On the contrary, cytokines TNF, IL-1, IL-6 and HGF slightly increased the SOD activity and especially the activity of the enzyme present in the mitochondrial fraction (MnSOD). It seems that cytokines could influence liver cell metabolism by changing activity of some liver enzymes.

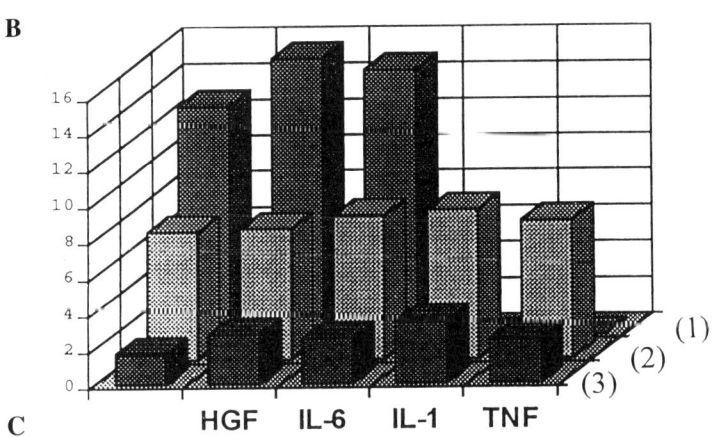

A		C	IL-1	IL-6	HGF	TNF	IL-1 +IL-6
	[U/mg protein]	25,1+2,6	39,9+5,8	38,2+7,1	33,8+6,4	33,1+4,3	41,2+9,9
	% of control	100	159	152	135	133	164

FIGURE 1. The activity (U/mg protein) of superoxide dismutase in FAO cells cultured for 24 h with IL-1 (100 units/ml), IL-6 (10 ng/ml), TNF (10 ng/ml) and HGF (20 ng/ml) (A) and (B) the SOD activity (Units in whole fraction) in the cell homogenate (1), cytosolic (2) and mitochondrial (3) fractions.

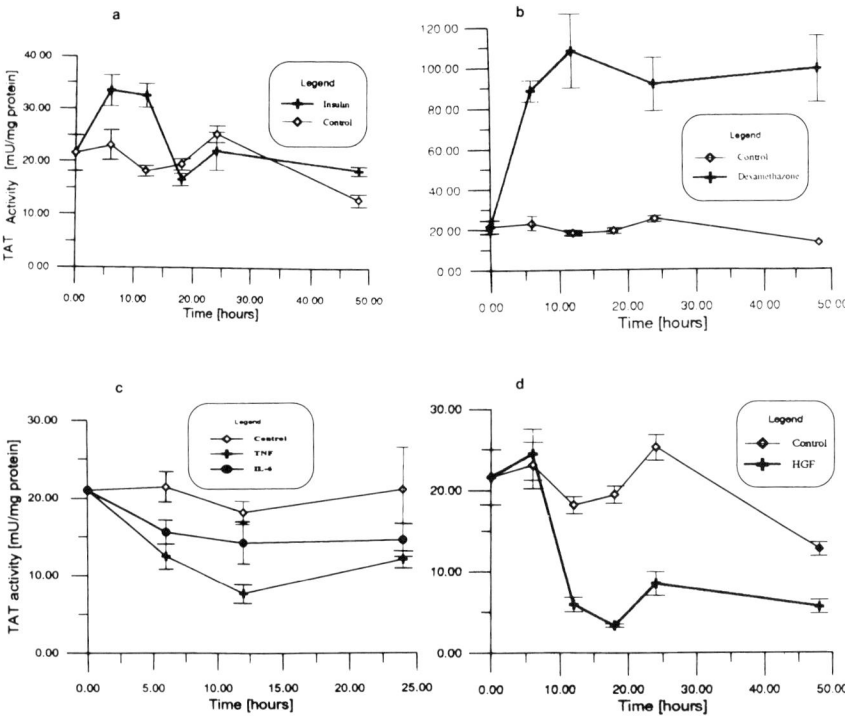

FIGURE 2. The influence of insulin (100 μM) **(a)**, dexamethasone (1μM) **(b)**, TNF (10 ng/ml), IL-6 (10 ng/ml) **(c)**, and HGF (20 ng/ml) **(d)** on the activity of tyrosine aminotransferase in FAO cells cultured for 6, 12, 24 and 48 h with tested factors.

ACKNOWLEDGMENT

The authors are grateful to Dr. T. Nakamura for providing HGF.

REFERENCES

1. BAUMANN, H., K. K. MORELLA & G. H. W. WONG. 1993. J. Immunol. **151:** 4248–4257.
2. KOJ, A., J. GAULDIE & H. BAUMANN. 1993. *In* Acute Phase Proteins, Molecular Biology, Biochemistry and Clinical Applications. A. Mackiewicz, I. Kushner, and H. Baumann. Eds: 275–287. Boca Raton, FL: CRC Press.
3. ONO, M., H. KOHDA, T. KAWAGUCHI, M. OHIRA, C. SEKIYA, M. NAMIKI, A. TAKEYASU & N. TONIGUCHI. 1992. Biochim. Biophys. Res. Commun. **182:** 1100–1107.
4. GRANNER, D. K. & G. M. TOMKINS. 1970. Meth. Enzymol. **17A:** 633–677.
5. PAOLETTI, F. & A. MOCALI. 1991. Meth. Enzymol. **186:** 209–220.
6. CRETTAZ, M., D. MULLER-WIELAND & C. R. KAHN. 1988. Biochemistry **27:** 495–500.

Effects of HGF and RA on the Class 1 and Class 2 Rat Acute Phase Proteins[a]

AMALIA GUZDEK AND ALEKSANDER KOJ

Institute of Molecular Biology
Jagiellonian University
31-120 Kraków, Poland

INTRODUCTION

The regulation of liver acute phase response is a complex process in which several cytokines, hormones and growth factors are involved.[1,2] Previously it was found that hepatocyte growth factor (HGF) and retinoic acid (RA) modulate cytokine-induced synthesis of some proteinase inhibitors in human hepatoma HepG2 cells.[3] Here, the modulatory effects of HGF and RA on the action of IL-6 and IL-1 or both cytokines, in rat hepatoma cells H-35 were analyzed.

METHODS

Rat hepatoma H-35 cells were cultured in the presence of IL-1, IL-6, HGF, RA, and combinations of these factors for 24 or 48 hours. Six serum proteins in the resulting supernatants were assessed by rocket immunoelectrophoresis.[4] Moreover, fibrinogen (FBG), α_2 macroglobulin (A2M) and C3 component of the complement (CC3) mRNA levels were evaluated by Northern analysis.[5,6]

RESULTS AND DISCUSSION

The synthesis of class 1 rat acute phase proteins CC3 and α_1-acid glycoprotein (AGP) was induced by IL-1 and IL-6 and the mixture of these two cytokines, whereas synthesis of class 2 rat acute phase proteins A2M, FBG, thiostatin (TST) and α_1-proteinase inhibitor (API) was enhanced by IL-6 only, and simultaneous addition of IL-1 suppressed IL-6 action. In the presence of IL-6 HGF increased and RA decreased A2M synthesis. Both factors exerted opposite effects on CC3 synthesis. Class 1 APP responded to the analyzed factors similarly. Class 2 APP response was more variable: HGF enhanced FBG and A2M response to the mixture of IL-1 and IL-6 but decreased that of API and TST (FIG. 1). The tested factors influenced mRNA amount of analyzed proteins in the H-35 cells. HGF, in the presence of IL-6 enhanced and RA diminished A2M mRNA. Also, the enhancement of IL-6–induced synthesis of CC3 by RA observed at the protein level was in agreement with the contents of mRNA (FIG. 2). It seems that HGF and RA affect the expression of APP genes in H-35 cells mainly at the transcriptional level, but modulation of translation should be also taken into account, because some discrepancies between the amount of mRNA and protein

---

[a] This work was supported by Grant 2238/4/91 to A. K. from the State Committee for Scientific Research (KBN, Warsaw, Poland).

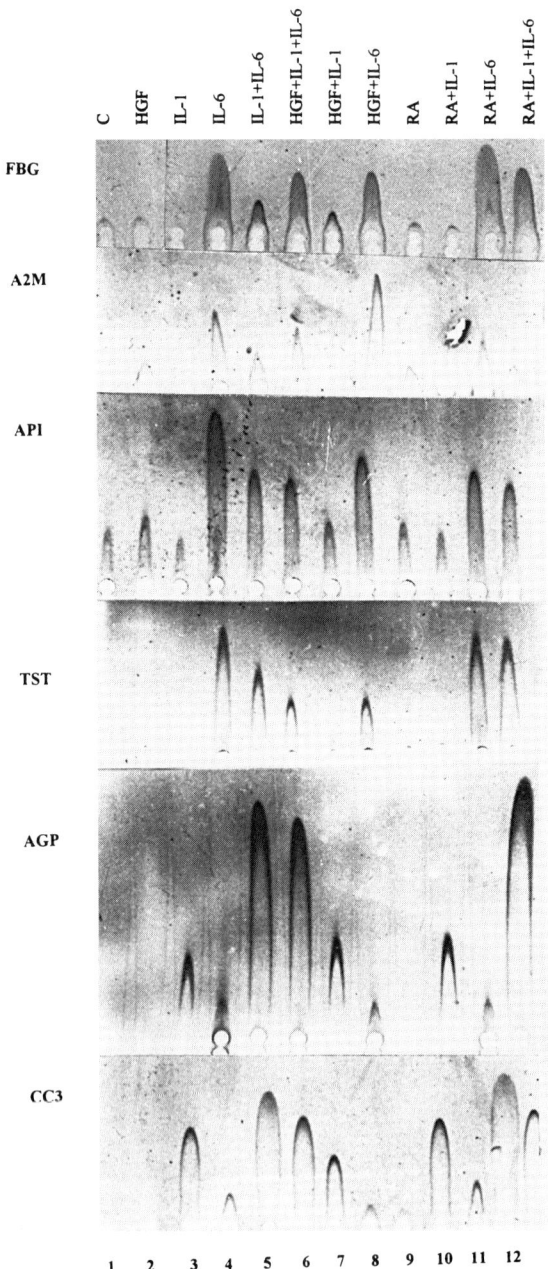

FIGURE 1. Effects of hepatocyte growth factor, retinoic acid and two cytokines on the synthesis of fibrinogen (FBG), α_2-macroglobulin (A2M), α_1-proteinase inhibitor (API), thiostatin (TST), α_1-acid glycoprotein (AGP) and C3 component of the complement (CC3) by H-35 cells. The proteins were determined in the media by electroimmunoassay after 2 days of culture of subconfluent monolayer with the following factors. HGF (20 ng/ml), IL-1β (100 units/ml), IL-6 (10 ng/ml) and retinoic acid (300 ng/ml).

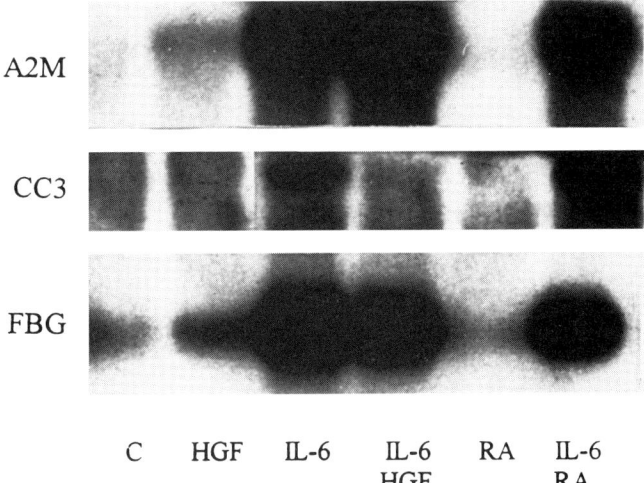

FIGURE 2. Abundance of mRNA in H-35 cells culture for 24 h with IL-6 (10 ng/ml), HGF (20 ng/ml), RA (300 ng/ml) and the mixture of IL-6 and tested factors. C, control culture. Total cellular RNA was isolated and 5 μg used for Northern blot analysis with appropriate cDNA probes.

secretion exist. For example, the content of fibrinogen mRNA was enhanced by HGF but in the presence of IL-6 both HGF and RA showed a slight inhibitory effect.

It seems, that HGF and RA may exert their modulatory effects either directly on the appropriate genes of class 1 and class 2 acute phase proteins, or indirectly by influencing transcriptional machinery and the efficiency of expression of these genes stimulated by cytokines.

ACKNOWLEDGMENTS

The authors are grateful to Dr. H. Baumann for providing H-35 cells and α-fibrinogen chain cDNA probe, to Dr. G. Fey for cDNA probes for α_2-macroglobulin and C3 complement, and to Dr. T. Nakamura for HGF.

REFERENCES

1. BAUMANN, H. & J. GAULDIE. 1990. Mol. Biol. Med. **7:** 147–159.
2. CAMPOS, S. P., Y. WONG, A. KOJ & H. BAUMANN. 1993. J. Immunol. **151:** 7128–7137.
3. KOJ, A., E. KORZUS, H. BAUMANN, T. NAKAMURA & J. TRAVIS. 1993. Biol. Chem. Hoppe-Seyler **374:** 193–201.
4. KOJ, A., J. GAULDIE, G. D. SWEENEY, E. REGOECZI & D. N. SAUDER. 1984. Biochem. J. **224:** 505–514.
5. ROSE-JOHN, S., A. DIETRICH & F. MARKS. 1988. Gene **74:** 465–471.
6. FEINBERG, A. P. & B. VOGELSTEIN. 1983. Analyt. Biochem. **132:** 6–13.

Structural and Biological Characterization of Murine-Human Interleukin-6 Chimeras

A. HAMMACHER,[a] L. D. WARD,[a,c] J. WEINSTOCK,[b] AND R. J. SIMPSON[a]

[a]*Joint Protein Structure Laboratory, Ludwig Institute for Cancer Research Walter and Eliza Hall Institute of Medical Research*
[b]*Ludwig Institute for Cancer Research Parkville, Victoria, Australia 3050*

Interleukin-6 (IL-6) is a polyfunctional cytokine that plays an important role in the immune response, acute-phase reaction and hematopoiesis (reviewed in ref. 1). IL-6 initiates its effects on target cells by binding to a specific ligand-binding subunit, the IL-6 receptor (IL-6R). The IL-6/IL-6R complex associates with gp130, resulting in high affinity binding and signal transduction across the cell membrane. We have shown that the stoichiometry of the high affinity complex is 2:2:2 with respect to IL-6, the IL-6R and gp130.[2]

We showed previously that the five C-terminal residues of mIL-6 are critical for bioactivity and conformational stability, as measured by far ultraviolet circular dichroism (far UV CD). Truncation of these residues resulted in drastically decreased mitogenicity on murine 7TD1 cells and stability to urea unfolding.[3] Using NMR spectroscopy, we found that the truncation influenced residues surrounding Tyr 22, suggesting that residues at the N- and C-terminii of mIL-6 are in close proximity.[3] Interestingly, substitution of the five C-terminal residues of mIL-6 for the corresponding amino acids of hIL-6 yielded similar bioactivity, but significantly increased conformational stability, compared to mIL-6.[3]

In this study, to elucidate the structure-function relationships of IL-6, we have generated murine/human IL-6 chimeras with the aim of probing the C-terminal region of hIL-6 for involvement in binding to the hIL-6R. The primary sequence homology between human and murine IL-6 is 42%. Whereas hIL-6 binds both the murine and the human IL-6R, mIL-6 only binds the mIL-6R. The rationale for the design of the chimeras was based on the four α-helical bundle structure of IL-6, as predicted by Bazan[4] (FIG. 1). The chimeras were generated by introducing restriction endonuclease sites at corresponding locations in the cDNA:s of m- and h-IL-6 followed by "domain swapping."[5] Recombinant hIL-6 and the chimeras were purified to >95% homogeneity from bacterial inclusion bodies as β-galactosidase fusion proteins.[5] Our data showed that 1) all chimeras were active on murine 7TD1 cells, 2) chimeras containing the seven C-terminal residues of hIL-6 (residues 178-184) displayed binding to the hIL-6R and 3) a chimera containing residues 63-113 of hIL-6 displayed significant hIL-6R-binding and activity on human HepG2 cells (TABLE 1). The results also suggested that the N-terminal region of mIL-6 can interact with the substituted

---

[c] *Current address:* AMRAD Laboratories, Hawthorn, Australia 3122.

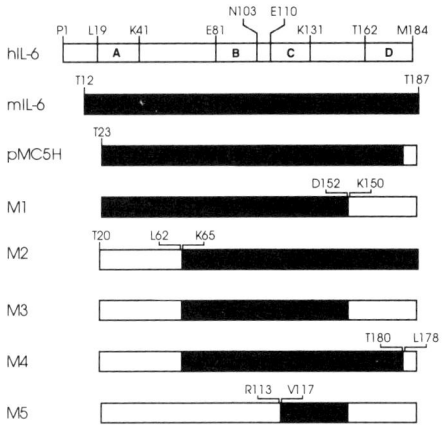

FIGURE 1. Schematic of IL-6 and murine-human IL-6 chimeras. The N- and C-terminal residues (single letter code) of each protein or section are given only when differing from previous proteins. The chimeras contain no internal deletions or additions, but are truncated at their N-terminii. The human and murine regions of the IL-6 chimeras are depicted in white and black, respectively. Superimposed on hIL-6 (boxes A-D) is a linear representation of predicted α-helices in hIL-6.[4]

TABLE 1. Summary of Receptor Binding and Bioassay Data

Sample	Mitogenic Activity on Murine 7TD1 Cells EC_{50} (pg/ml)	Competition with ^{125}I-hIL-6 for Binding to:		Fibrinogen Induction from Human HepG2 Cells EC_{50} (ng/ml)
		Human U266 cells IC_{50} (ng/ml)	shIL-6R IC_{50} (ng/ml)	
hIL-6	60	17	20	1.5
mIL-6	2	ND[a]	ND	ND
pMC5H	2	>50,000	5,000	780
M1	7	30,000	16,000	3,000
M2	400	ND	ND	ND
M3	13	6,000	2,200	>50,000
M4	18	10,000	5,000	>50,000
M5	1000	150	200	150

[a] ND = not demonstrable at 50 µg/ml.

C-terminal region of hIL-6 (cf. M1 and pMC5H), but that the converse interaction does not apply (cf. M2) (FIG. 1). The inactivity of chimera M2 in bioassays and receptor-binding could, in part, be explained by its significant loss of α-helical content (decrease in ellipticity at 220 nm relative to hIL-6), as measured by far UV CD.

We conclude that at least two regions of hIL-6, residues 178-184 and 63-113, are critical for efficient binding to the hIL-6R. Moreover, that interactions between amino acids in the N- and C-terminal regions of hIL-6 are important for the conformational stability and, therefore, biological activity of hIL-6. Our studies suggest that the interhelical interactions in hIL-6 differ from those in mIL-6, and that this should be taken into account when interpretating the results from chimeric analysis.

REFERENCES

1. AKIRA, S., et al. 1993. Adv. Immunol. **54:** 1–78.
2. WARD, L.D., et al. 1994. J. Biol. Chem. **269:** 23286–23289.
3. WARD, L.D., et al. 1993. Protein Sci. **2:** 1472–1481.
4. BAZAN, J. F. 1991. Neuron. **7:** 197–208.
5. HAMMACHER, A., et al. 1994. Protein Sci. **3:** 2280–2293.

Renal Mesangial Cells Have the Capacity to Synthesize and React to Leukemia Inhibitory Factor

A. HARTNER,[a,c] M. GOPPELT-STRÜBE,[a] G. M. HOCKE,[b]
G. H. FEY,[b] AND R. B. STERZEL[a]

[a]*Medizinische Klinik IV*
[b]*Department of Genetics*
University of Erlangen-Nürnberg
D-91058 Erlangen, Germany

So far little is known about the role of interleukin-6 (IL-6)-like cytokines in the kidney and especially in renal diseases, though IL-6 has been discussed as a mitogen for mesangial cells and a potential promoter of mesangioproliferative glomerulonephritis.

We examined the presence of leukemia inhibitory factor (LIF) and its potential involvement in the regulation of renal mesangial cell (MC) behavior by studying the expression of LIF mRNA and protein in early primary cultures of rat and human MCs and in freshly isolated glomeruli after stimulation with LPS,[1] as well as the response of MCs to exogenous LIF. Growing or growth arrested MCs and freshly isolated glomeruli constitutively expressed very low levels of LIF mRNA. Strong induction of LIF mRNA expression was caused by IL-1β (10 ng/ml), FCS (10%) and LPS (200 ng/ml), as determined by Northern blot analysis for rat MCs (FIG. 1) and glomeruli, and RT-PCR for human MCs. The induction was transient with a peak at 3–5 hours. LIF mRNA is not very stable. In response to the addition of actinomycin D (10 μg/ml) to cells stimulated with LPS for 4 hours, the LIF mRNA level was reduced to background after 45 minutes. LIF itself or IL-6 had no effect on LIF mRNA expression (FIG. 1). A similar induction pattern was observed for the expression of IL-6 mRNA. LIF protein was detected by specific ELISA in the supernates of human MCs stimulated with LPS or IL-1β. Evidence for the rat LIF receptor on MCs was obtained by detection of its mRNA in RT-PCR. The expression of LIF receptor mRNA was not changed by a stimulation of LIF or LPS for 3–5 hours. In addition, the existence of the binding protein for the IL-6/LIF responsive element[2] could be shown in a gel shift assay. Upon induction with LIF or IL-6 for 4 hours the binding of the protein in the gel shift could be augmented. Recombinant LIF effectively induced transient expression of the immediate early genes, c-fos, jun-B and egr-1 in rat MCs, with a maximum at 30–60 minutes. Also, LIF (500 U/ml) and IL-6 (200 U/ml) induced an increase in monocyte chemotactic protein-1 (MCP-1) mRNA, with a maximum at 1–3 hours, while resting and growing MCs showed only weak expression of MCP-1 (FIG. 2). Costimulation with LIF and IL-6 led to an additive MCP-1 signal. In contrast, no induction or inhibition of the expression of RANTES mRNA could be detected after LIF and IL-6 stimulation for a time period of 30 minutes up to 30 hours. (RANTES is another chemokine activating eosinophils, basophils and monocytes). While LIF by itself was not mitogenic for MCs, it slightly augmented the ³H-thymidine uptake at 24 hours induced by 25 ng/ml PDGF (1.32

---

[c] Author to whom correspondence should be addressed.

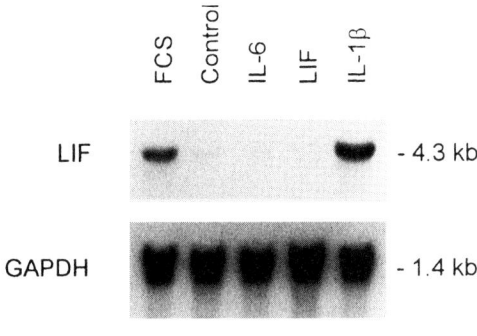

FIGURE 1. Induction of LIF mRNA in rat mesangial cells. Growth-arrested mesangial cells were incubated with IL-1β (10 ng/ml), IL-6 (200 U/ml), LIF (500 U/ml) and FCS (10%) for 3 hours; *control lane:* cells incubated with PBS/0.1% BSA. Northern blot analysis was performed with cDNA probes for LIF and GAPDH with GAPDH confirming equal loading of the gel.

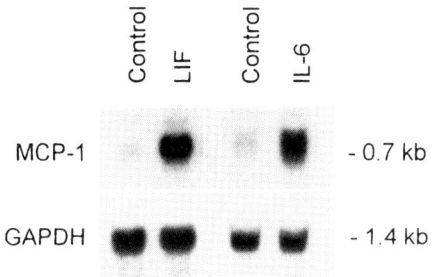

FIGURE 2. LIF and IL-6 induced expression of MCP-1 mRNA in mesangial cells. Resting mesangial cells were incubated with LIF (500 U/ml) or IL-6 (200 U/ml) for 2 hours. Northern blots were probed with MCP-1 cDNA.

± 0.06-fold, n = 5, $p < 0.001$) and 10^{-7} M serotonin (1.19 ± 0.13-fold, n = 5, $p < 0.05$). LIF had no significant effect on total protein synthesis of rat MCs as determined by leucine incorporation. Our findings indicate that glomerular mesangial cells produce and react to LIF. As a cytokine with autocrine/paracrine potential, LIF may play a role in the regulation of the glomerular inflammatory response, for example by promoting the local production of chemokines, such as MCP-1.

REFERENCES

1. HARTNER, A., R. B. STERZEL, N. REINDL, G. M. HOCKE, G. H. FEY & M. GOPPELT-STRUEBE. 1994. Cytokine-induced expression of leukemia inhibitory factor in renal mesangial cells. Kidney International **45:** 1555–1561.
2. HOCKE, G. M., M. Z. CUI, J. A. RIPPBERGER & G. H. FEY. 1993. Regulation of the rat α_2-macroglobulin gene by interleukin-6 and leukemia inhibitory factor. *In* Acute Phase Proteins: Molecular Biology, Biochemistry, Clinical Applications. A. Mackiewicz, I. Kushner, and H. Baumann. Eds.:467–494. Boca Raton, FL: CRC Press.

The LIF-Response Element Confers LIF-induced Transcriptional Control in P19 Embryonal Carcinoma Cells[a]

GERTRUD M. HOCKE

Department of Genetics
University of Erlangen-Nürnberg
D-91058 Erlangen, Germany

Leukemia inhibitory factor (LIF) is a cytokine with pluripotent functions.[1] It either acts as a growth- or differentiation-promoting agent for a variety of cell types. On cultured embryonal stem cells (ES cells) LIF has a differentiation-inhibiting activity (DIA) and is an essential growth factor. It was shown that the typeII interleukin-6 (IL-6)-response element (IL-6-RE) of the rat α_2 macroglobulin (α_2-M) gene, which mediates IL-6- and LIF-responses in hepatic cells,[2] also functioned as a LIF-response element (LIF-RE) in ES1 embryonal stem cells.[3] A characteristic DNA binding activity (complex II) interacting with the LIF-RE was induced by treatment of these cells with LIF. It had electrophoretic mobility, sequence-specificity and kinetics of induction similar to the corresponding LIF-response factor (LIF-RF) from hepatic cells.[3] Several embryonal carcinoma cells differ from embryonal stem cells, because they do not require LIF as an essential growth factor. Three different murine embryonal carcinoma (EC) cell lines, known not to depend on LIF to proliferate, were treated with LIF. We wanted to determine whether these LIF-independent cell lines still are able to activate the LIF-signal cascade after exposure to LIF.

The cells were treated with LIF, nuclear extracts were prepared and analyzed by gel mobility shift assays with the TB2 probe representing two copies of the LIF-RE (FIG. 1). In the P19 and the PC13.2 cell lines the ability to form complex II was indeed induced by LIF (FIG. 1, tracks 1,2). The PMSB[5,6] cell line showed no response to LIF. With extracts from PMSB cells complex II was formed both before and after LIF treatment. (FIG. 1, tracks 3,4). Thus, in the P19 cell line the specific DNA binding ability of the LIF-RF was induced by LIF.

Transfection studies were performed to investigate, whether the LIF-RE from the rat α_2-M gene was also able to mediate induction of transcription by LIF in embryonal cells. P19 cells were transiently transfected with luciferase reporter constructs containing copies of the LIF-RE directing various promoters.[4] Luciferase activity of P19 cells transfected with these constructs increased severalfold after a 4-hour incubation with LIF (FIG. 2). Only a marginal increase in reporter activity due to LIF treatment occurred in cells transfected with the positive control pSV2A.LUC or with the plasmid m205TK.LUC, containing a mutated LIF-RE. Thus, the LIF-RE of the α_2-M gene

---

[a] This work was supported by a grant from the DFG (Deutsche Forschungsgemeinschaft) to G. H. (Hi 291/5-4 TP6).

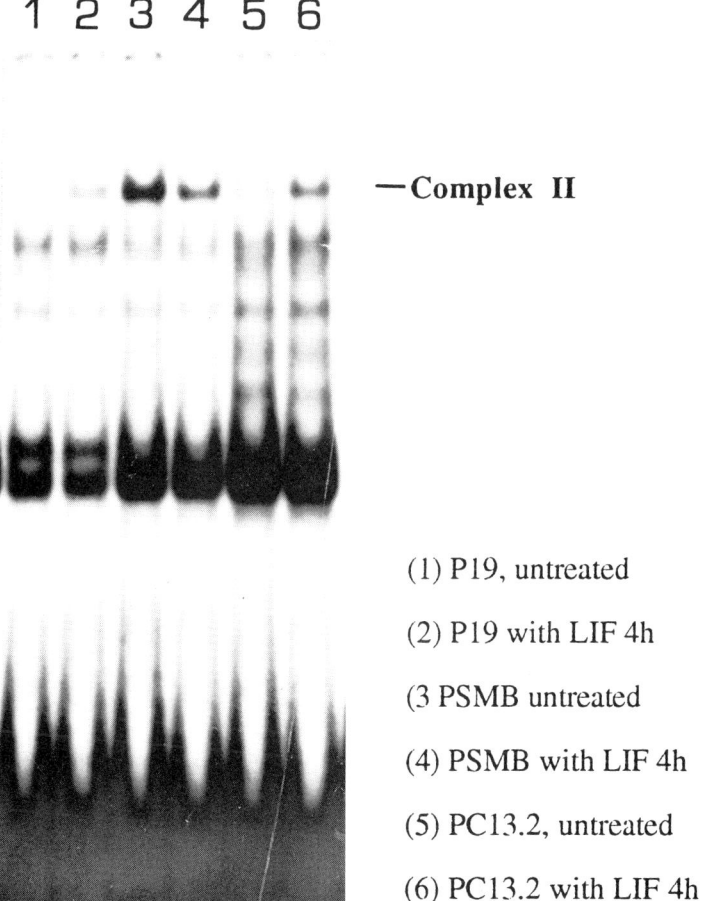

FIGURE 1. Nuclear extracts from LIF-treated P19 embryonal carcinoma cells form complex II. Gel mobility shift experiments were performed with nuclear protein extracts from P19, PSMB, and PC13.2 embryonal carcinoma cells with and without LIF treatment. The radiolabeled probe TB2, carried two tandem copies of the LIF-RE.

indeed mediated transcriptional induction by LIF in P19 embryonal carcinoma cells. Therefore, a functional LIF signal cascade ending in the activation of the LIF-RF must have been operative in P19 embryonal carcinoma cells.

This report demonstrates, that the typeII IL-6-response element of the rat α_2-macroglobulin gene, which mediates IL-6- and LIF-responses in hepatic cells, also functioned as a LIF-RE in P19 embryonal carcinoma cells. Although these cells do not depend on LIF treatment to proliferate, a functional LIF cascade is inducible in these cells.

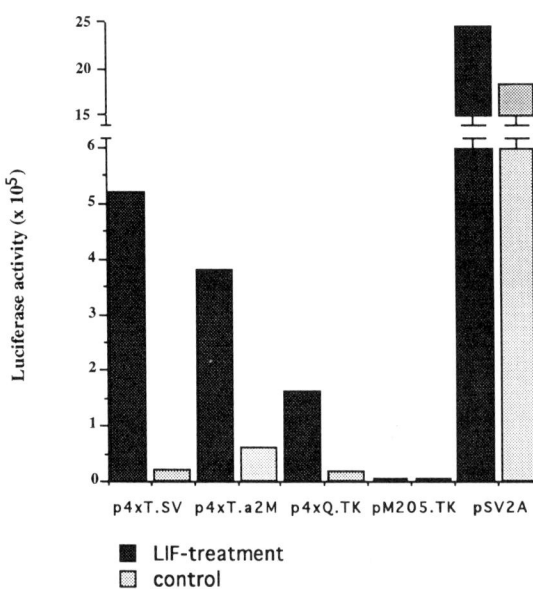

FIGURE 2. The LIF-RE confers LIF-responsiveness in P19 embryonal carcinoma cells. P19 cells were transfected with various reporter constructs, containing 4 copies of the LIF-RE of the rat α_2-M gene. In these constructs the LIF-RE directed either the enhancerless minimal promoter from the herpes simplex virus thymidine kinase (TK) gene, from the simian virus (SV40) or from the α_2-macroglobulin (α_2-M) gene, which in turn controlled the transcription of a cDNA coding for the firefly luciferase reporter gene.[4] As a negative control the construct pm205TK.LUC containing a functionally inactive LIF-RE core site (m205) was transfected. The plasmid pSV2A.LUC containing a cytokine-independent enhancer and promoter was used as a positive control. Luciferase activity was measured after a 4-hour incubation with LIF. Experiments were performed at least in duplicate with essentially reproducible results. Data are from one representative experiment.

REFERENCES

1. HILTON, J. D. 1992. LIF: Lots of interesting functions. TIBS **17:** 72–76.
2. HOCKE, G. M., M. Z. CUI, J. A. RIPPERGER & G. H. FEY. 1993. Regulation of the rat α_2 macroglobulin gene by interleukin 6 and leukemia inhibitory factor. *In* Acute Phase Proteins: Molecular Biology, Biochemistry, Clinical Applications. A. Mackiewicz, I. Kushner, and H. Baumann, Eds.: 467–494. Boca Raton, FL: CRC Press.
3. HOCKE, G. M., M.-Z. CUI & G. H. FEY. 1995. The LIF-Response Element of the α_2 macroglobulin gene confers LIF-induced transcriptional activation in embryonal stem cells. Cytokine. In press.
4. HOCKE, G. M., D. BARRY & G. H. FEY. 1992. Synergistic action of Interleukin-6 and glucocorticoids is mediated by the interleukin-6 response element of the rat alpha-2 macroglobulin gene. Mol. Cell. Biol. **12:** 2282–2294.

Pituitary Glycoprotein Hormones and Interleukins Secretion

In Vitro and *in Vivo* Human Study

J. KOMOROWSKI, M. PAWLIKOWSKI, AND H. STĘPIEŃ

Institute of Endocrinology
University School of Medicine
Dr. Sterling Str. 3
Łódź, Poland 91-425

Immune system function is under the influence of various neuromodulators and endocrine peptides. The pituitary gland, being the source of trophic hormones, plays an important role in the physiological integration of the neuro-immuno-endocrine axis. This *in vitro* study[1] describes the stimulatory effects of thyroliberin (TRH) on thyrotropin (TSH) secretion (FIG. 1) from human peripheral blood monocytes (PBM) and of pituitary glycoprotein hormones (TSH, LH, FSH) on interleukin-2 (IL-2) release from cultured human peripheral blood lymphocytes (PBL). LH and FSH increased also the secretion of IL-1β and IL-6 from PBM (FIGS. 1 and 2). *In vivo*, the increased mobilization of IL-2 during the standard TRH test in case of normal volunteers, as well as, the high IL-2 plasma levels in primary hypothyroid patients with increased TSH serum concentrations have been revealed (FIG. 1). IL-1β, IL-2, IL-6 concentrations were measured in supernatants from cell cultures and blood plasma by RIA [Amersham (England) kits], TSH by MEIA [Abbott (Germany)].

During the administration of TRH (pGlu-His-Pro-NH_2) or physiologic surges of TRH from hypothalamus, prolactin (PRL) and TSH are released immediately from lactotrophs and thyrotrophs as a result of binding of above neuropeptide to the pituitary TRH receptors. Both pituitary hormones enhance the immune system activation. TSH augments splenic B cell proliferation and antibody production as well as T-lymphocyte–dependent and –independent antibody responses. Results of our study have clearly shown that TSH stimulates IL-2 secretion from PBL in a dose dependent manner. The results presented above indicate that the patients with primary hypothyroidism and high TSH serum levels have had increased blood plasma IL-2 concentrations. Also PRL enhances the immune system activation; however, pronounced but short-term (2 h) increments of serum prolactin mobilization during oral MCP test in normal human subjects did not exert any detectable effect on IL-2 blood concentrations similar to the one observed during TRH test.[2] Although the immunostimulatory effect of TRH *in vivo* could be mediated by TSH or prolactin or both, it seems that TSH mediation is rather more probable. Also, the production of IL-2 by human pituitary cells itself has been demonstrated and we cannot entirely exclude the direct central stimulation of IL-2 release from pituitary by thyroliberin. Moreover, results obtained by us revealed the pronounced role of TRH and T_3 in the local regulation of TSH release from activated monocytes. This mechanism looks analogical to the one observed in hypothalamic-pituitary-thyroid axis. Also, gonadotrophins (LH and FSH) activated human monocytes to direct IL-1β and IL-6 release and lymphocytes to direct IL-2 secretion, as observed by us. This observation suggests the close relationship between the immune system and hypothalamo-pituitary-gonadal axis. Others have reported that human thymocytes store and secrete LH-like peptide, which acts as an autocrine/paracrine growth factor modulating T-cell proliferation. LH seems to exert the modulatory effect on cytokines and gamma-globulin secretion also in mice by binding to the specific receptors localized on macrophage and T-cells. In turn, IL-1 and IL-2 themselves are able to affect gonadotrophin regulation by the direct action on Gn-RH neurons in hypothalamus, and exhibit either stimulatory or inhibitory effect on gonadal steroids production. Both mentioned interleukins may potentiate IL-6 production. Castration or menopause is accompanied by increased levels of gonadotrophins, leading to significant rise in IL-1 and IL-6 release from monocytes, the rise being reversed in women treated with estrogen/medroxyprogesterone acetate. Although PBM contain estrogen receptors and estradiol can by itself modulate IL-1 and IL-6 production in human monocytes, macrophages and osteoclasts, we believe that also both gonadotrophins themselves may augment the secretion of both interleukins from monocytes. The abnormal IL-6 production by immune cells can play a critical role in a number of diseases and aging processes (arteriosclerosis, osteoporosis, increased hepatic lipogenesis). Normal aging has been recently shown to be accompanied by increased IL-6 levels in most serum samples obtained from "normal" elderly humans. The proinflammatory cytokines (IL-1, IL-6) may stimulate *in vitro* bone resorption and inhibit bone formation, as observed in osteoporosis. The above described situation *in vivo* is present at post-menopausal or ovariectomized women with

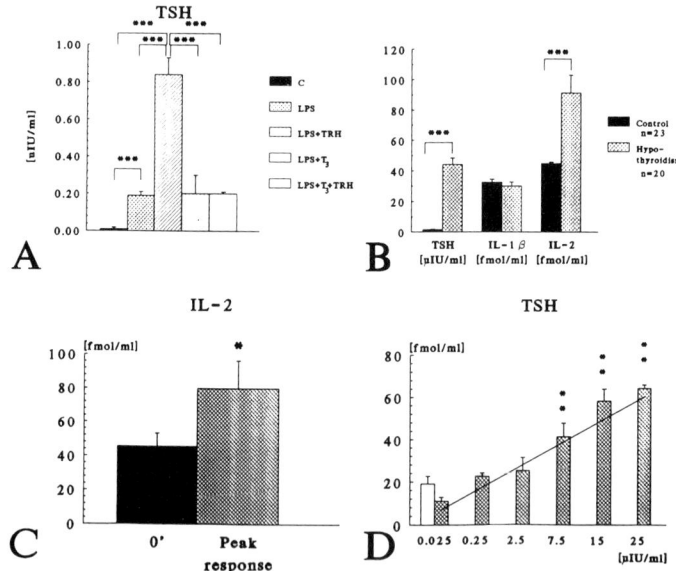

FIGURE 1. A: Effects of TRH (10^{-8}), T_3 (2×10^{-8}) and T_3 + TRH on LPS activated TSH secretion from human peripheral blood monocytes (PBM) cultured *in vitro*. **B:** *In vivo*, increased IL-2 blood plasma levels of patients with primary hypothyroidism. **C:** Results of IL-2 blood mobilization during standard TRH intravenous test (peak response) in 8 healthy subjects. **D:** Stimulatory effect of TSH on PHA activated IL-2 release into supernatants from human peripheral blood lymphocytes (PBL) cultured *in vitro* (*open bar*–PHA activation only; *hatched bars*–PHA + TSH stimulation). Mean ± SEM; *$p < 0.05$; **$p < 0.01$; ***$p < 0.001$.

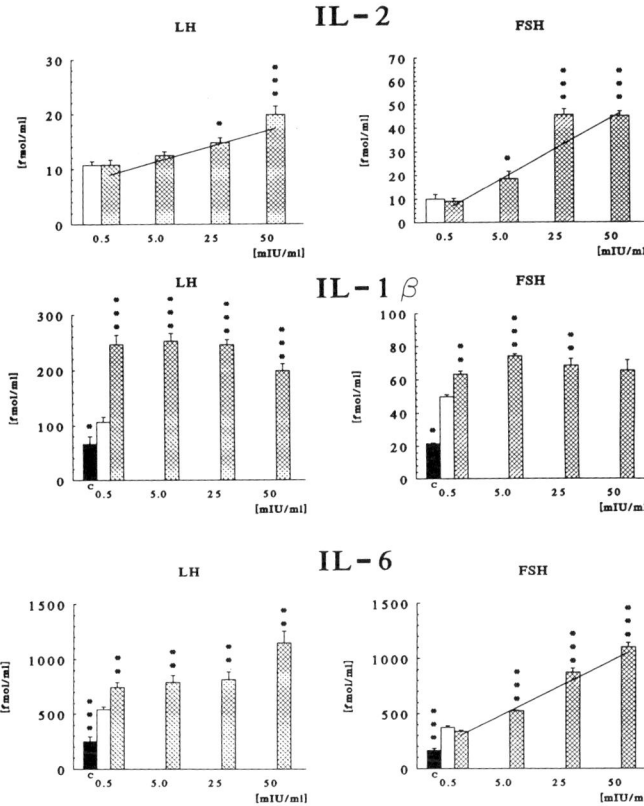

FIGURE 2. Effects of gonadotrophins (LH, FSH) on PHA activated IL-2 release from human peripheral blood lymphocytes (PBL) into supernatants and effects of LH and FSH on LPS activated IL-1β or IL-6 secretion from human peripheral blood monocytes (PBM) cultured *in vitro* (*black bars*–unstimulated monocytes (c); *open bars*–PHA or LPS stimulation; hatched bars–PHA or LPS + LH or FSH stimulation. Mean ± SEM; $*p < 0.05$; $**p < 0.01$; $***p < 0.001$.

advanced osteoporosis, therefore the high levels of gonadotrophins in blood circulation may also be the cause of aging and osteoporosis in humans.

In conclusion, the all presented data suggests that the pituitary glycoprotein hormones (TSH, LH, FSH) and TRH exert a stimulatory effect on the human immune system.

REFERENCES

1. BOYUM, A. 1969. Isolation of mononuclear cells and granulocytes from human blood. J. Clin. Lab. Invest. **21** (Suppl. 97): 77–89.
2. KOMOROWSKI, J., H. STĘPIEŃ & M. PAWLIKOWSKI. 1994. Increased interleukin-2 levels during standard TRH test in man. Neuropeptides **27**: 151–156.

Serum Levels of IL-6 in Mycosis Fungoides, Psoriasis, and Lichen Planus

B. TORUNIOWA,[a] D. KRASOWSKA,[a,c] M. KOZIOŁ,[b]
A. KSIĄŻEK,[b] AND A. PIETRZAK[a]

[a]*Department of Dermatology*
[b]*Department of Nephrology*
Medical Academy in Lublin
Radziwiłłowska 13
20-080 Lublin, Poland

IL-6 is a multifunctional cytokine that participates in the inflammatory and immune response with a number of biological activities. It is produced by activated monocytes, macrophages, endothelial cells, a variety of tumor cells, fibroblasts, keratinocytes, activated T and B cells in response to induction by a variety of stimuli which include other cytokines. A role for IL-6 in cutaneous disease is prominent. Elevated levels have been detected in lesional skin from patients with psoriasis, Kaposi sarcoma, chronic urticaria, scleroderma, mycosis fungoides, and atopic dermatitis.[1,2] IL-6 and IL-1 are chemotactic for T-cells *in vitro*, thus they can provide the directed migrational stimulus to attract T-cells to the epidermis.[3]

The aim of the study was to investigate serum concentration of IL-6 in patients with mycosis fungoides, psoriasis, and lichen planus. The proliferation of keratinocytes and/or migration of T-cells into skin are characteristic findings in these diseases.

The serum concentrations of IL-6 in 4 patients with mycosis fungoides, 20 with acute psoriasis, 36 with lichen planus, and 14 in the control group were determined. From all the patients blood samples were taken during the active phase of the disease.

The serum concentrations of IL-6 were determined using kits for ELISA assay (Genzyme Corporation, USA).

All the examined groups displayed mean values significantly higher than the controls, and the values in mycosis fungoides were also much higher compared to the ones in other diseases (TABLE 1; FIG. 1). It was only in cases of limited lichen planus that higher serum concentration of IL-6 were not displayed.

The higher concentrations of IL-6 have been found both in skin lesions and serum from active phase of psoriatic patients.[4] Ohta *et al.*[5] emphasized that IL-6 and IL-6R expression correlate well with the lesion-forming process in psoriasis. External stimuli applied to the skin can stimulate IL-6 production, and IL-6R receives IL-6 to initiate psoriatic epidermal proliferation. Mycosis fungoides (MF) is a T-cell lymphoma in which the abnormal T cells are localized in the early stages in the skin. In fully developed lesions, histology shows a dense lymphocytic infiltration in the papillary dermis that extends inside the epidermis. Lawlor's group described significantly elevated biologically active IL-6 in lesional samples of mycosis fungoides. Both Lawlor's and our results showing increased serum concentration of IL-6 should suggest that this cytokine may be involved in the pathogenesis of MF.[6] The lower serum

---

[c] Author to whom correspondence should be addressed.

TABLE 1. The Mean Serum Concentration of IL-6 in Investigated Diseases and Controls

Group	n	M	SD	SE	V%	Differences With Controls p	Differences Between Groups	p
M	4	77.40 d	8.40	4.20	10.9	<0.001	M-P	<0.03
P	20	60.76 c	12.81	2.86	21.1	<0.001	M-LPg	<0.01
LPg	20	52.17 bc	14.79	3.31	28.4	<0.002	M-LPl	<0.01
LPl	21	47.76 ab	17.28	3.77	36.2	>0.10	P-LPg	≈0.06
C	14	41.07 a	9.60	2.55	23.4	—	P-LPl	<0.01
							LPg-LPl	>0.30

M—mycosis fungoides; P—psoriasis; LPg—lichen planus generalized; LPl—lichen planus limited; C—controls; n—number of patients; M—average; SD—standard deviation; SE—mean error of the average; V%—individual variability.

concentration of IL-6 has been reported in oral lichen planus (LP).[7] Our results point to the higher serum concentration of IL-6 in generalized LP with no changes in limited LP. It seems that IL-6 is produced in local skin lesions in great amounts and then can be readily found in the peripheral circulation.[8]

In conclusion the results of our investigation indicate to the important role of IL-6 in the pathogenesis of mycosis fungoides, psoriasis, and lichen planus. Significantly higher serum concentrations of IL-6 in lichen planus generalizatus ($p < 0.02$) with no changes in limited lichen planus ($p > 0.10$) means that the extensiveness of the disease may influence IL-6 serum levels.

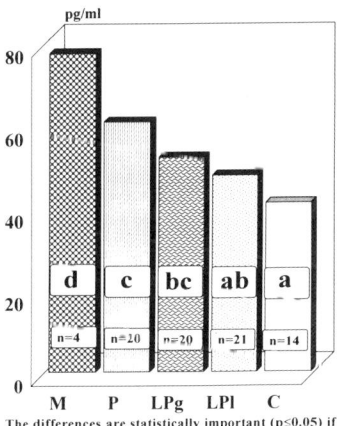

FIGURE 1. The mean serum concentrations of IL-6 in investigated diseases and controls.

REFERENCES

1. SEHGAL, P. B. 1991. Interleukin-6-acute phase response. Interferons Cytokines **19**: 29–32.
2. FLEMING, T. E., W. S. MIRANDO, L. F. SOOHOO, B. W. COOPER, M. T. ZAIM, H. M. LAZARUS & C. A. ELMETS. 1994. An inflammatory eruption associated with recombinant human IL-6. Br. J. Dermatol. **130**: 534–536.
3. BARKER, J. N. W. N. & D. M. MACDONALD. 1991. Cutaneous lymphocyte trafficking in the inflammatory dermatoses. Br. J. Dermatol. **126**: 211–215.
4. CASTELLS-RODELLAS, A., J. V. CASTELL, A. RAMIREZ-BOSCA, J. F. NICOLAS, F. VALCUENDE-CVAVERO & J. THIVOLET. 1992. Interleukin-6 in normal skin and psoriasis. Acta. Derm. Venereol (Stockh) **72**: 165–168.
5. OHTA, Y., I. KATAYAMA, T. FUNATO, H. YOKOZEKI, S. NISHIYAMA, T. HIRANO, T. KISHIMOTO & K. NISHIOKA. 1991. In situ expression of messenger RNA of interleukin-1 and interleukin-6 in psoriasis: Interleukin-6 involved in formation of psoriatic lesions. Arch. Dermatol. Res. **283**: 351–356.
6. LAWLOR, F., N. P. SMITH, R. D. R. CAMP, K. B. BACON, A. K. BLACK, M. W. GREAVES & A. J. H. GEARING. 1990. Skin exudate levels of interleukin 6, interleukin 1 and other cytokines in mycosis fungoides. Br. J. Dermatol. **123**: 297–304.
7. YAMAMOTO, T., K. YONEDA, E. UETA, J. HIROTA & T. OSAKI. 1991. Serum cytokine levels in patients with oral mucous membrane disorders. J. Oral. Pathol. Med. **20**: 275–279.
8. SEHGAL, P. B. 1990. Interleukin-6: Molecular pathophysiology. J. Invest. Dermatol. **94**: 2s–6s.

Interleukin-6– and Interleukin-4–related Proteins (C-reactive Protein and IgE) Are Prognostic Factors of Asbestos-related Cancer[a]

A. LANGE, L. KARABON, AND J. TOMECZKO

Institute of Immunology and Experimental Therapy
K. Długski Hospital
Czerska 12
53-114 Wrocław, Poland

INTRODUCTION

Lung cancer and mesothelioma are the most important asbestos-related causes of death among exposed individuals. However, cancers at other sites have also been shown to be associated with asbestos exposure. Therefore, it seems that not only the direct effect of asbestos fibers upon the target organ plays a role in carcinogenesis, but there is also some general effect on the organism's integrity making exposed individuals more prone to cancer. Known data about the relationship between asbestos exposure, humoral hyperreactivity, and anergy appear to support the hypothesis that these abnormalities contribute to the failure of the immune surveillance of neoplasms in asbestos-exposed individuals. However, our earlier studies show that humoral hyperreactivity and anergy are associated rather with a fibrotic process in the lung than with cancer.[1] The present study was undertaken to investigate this topic further.

SUBJECTS AND METHODS

Between 1981–1987 all workers employed in an asbestos-textile factory were invited for a routine medical check-up which included immunological blood work. All collected sera were frozen. Two hundred and one workers responded to the invitation; 111 of them were followed from 4 to 10 years after this primary examination. In 11 cases asbestos-related cancers became clinically apparent between 0.25–7 years after this examination. Twenty-five workers showed lung X-rays consistent with asbestosis. Therefore, all cases were described at the beginning of the follow-up with some immunological parameters and the presence or absence of asbestosis; none of them had clinically apparent cancer. In 1991 all frozen sera, collected at the primary observation, were tested for the level of IgE and CRP. ELISA for serum IgE: Nunc MaxiSorp plates were coated with monoclonal anti-human IgE Dε2 epitope antibody (Dianova, FRG), 1:10 diluted serum samples and serial dilutions of standard human IgE (gift from Dr. Haas, Borstel, FRG) were then added. Immobilized IgE was detected with the use of a sandwich technique which involved: biotin-labeled anti-human IgE anti-

---

[a] This work was supported by a grant from the Research Council (Polish, KBN)

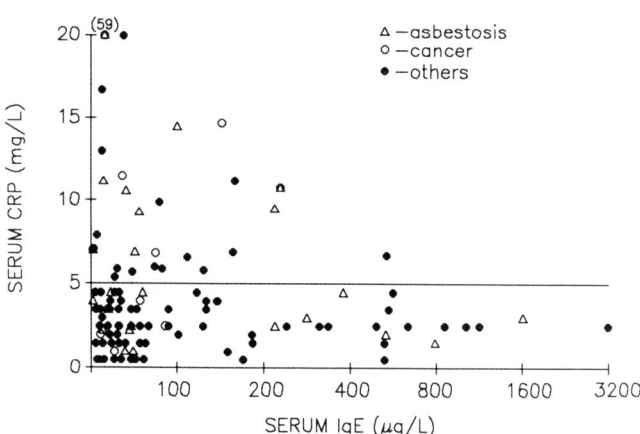

FIGURE 1. CRP and IgE levels in sera of asbestos workers. (△) workers with asbestosis at the time of CRP and IgE measurements; (○) workers without cancer at the time of these measurements who, however, developed cancer during a follow-up; (●) workers with no clinically apparent cancer either at the time of these measurements or during a follow-up.

body (Tago, USA), streptavidin-alkaline-phosphatase (SAVAP, Dianova, USA) and finally alkaline phosphatase substrate (Behring, FRG).

C-reactive protein (CRP) serum levels were determined with the use of the nephelometric NA Latex CRP assay kit (Behring, Marburg, FRG). The limit of normalcy was considered to be 5 mg/L of serum CRP.

RESULTS AND DISCUSSION

In 22 out of 111 asbestos workers IgE level exceeded 200 μg/L, being in 14 cases highly elevated (>400 μg/L) (FIG. 1). Asbestotic cases more frequently had serum IgE level above 200 μg/L as compared to workers without asbestosis (0.32 vs 0.16), but this difference was not statistically significant. Sex distribution, age and time of exposure were also not correlated with IgE elevation. The only significant association was that between serum IgE levels and the appearance of cancer during a following observation. In 11 cases cancer became clinically apparent from 0.25 and 7 years after collection of sera for IgE level measurements. Only one out of these 11 cases had IgE level higher than 200 μg/L at the time of serum IgE measurements, i.e., before cancer became clinically apparent. In contrast, elevation of serum CRP was significantly more frequent in asbestos workers who developed cancer during a following observation (FIG. 2). CRP serum level is largely governed by IL-6 production. IL-6 is produced by several cells including monocyte/macrophages and fibroblasts. These cells are triggered in asbestos-exposed people; alveolar macrophages are loaded with fibers and fibroblasts are involved in fibrotic process. IL-6 is a growth factor for some cancers.[2] Therefore, the association between CRP elevation prior to the cancer's becoming clinically apparent suggests that IL-6 plays a role promoting carcinogenesis in asbestos-exposed people. Notably, we found that the elevation of CRP and IgE (read-out proteins for IL-6 and IL-4, respectively) is mutually exclusive in the studied

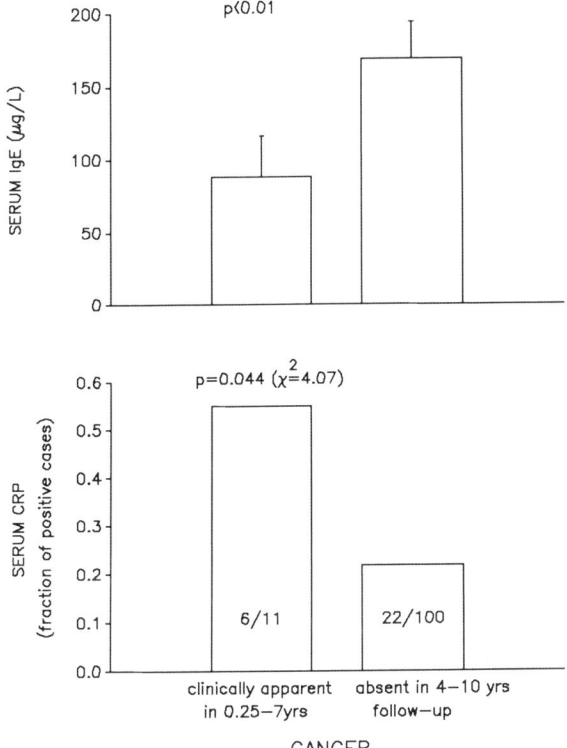

FIGURE 2. Serum IgE (mean ± SEM) and fraction of CRP positive (serum level > 5 mg/L) cases in asbestos workers groups consisting of workers who developed cancer in 0.25 to 7 years, and those not developing cancer during a 4- to 10-year follow-up after IgE and CRP measurements.

population (FIG. 1). Therefore, it appears that asbestos workers with CRP elevation are more and those with IgE elevation less susceptible to asbestos-related cancer. This is a novel observation which illustrates the possible role of cytokines as positive and negative regulators of tumor promotion and progression.[3] The associations found between a risk of cancer and levels of CRP and IgE is rather a direct association but not merely due to the correlation of these two proteins with an asbestotic process itself which is correlated in turn with cancer. Both studied proteins (CRP and IgE) are similarly frequently elevated in asbestotic cases and as it is in the whole population their levels are negatively correlated.

REFERENCES

1. LANGE, A., C. ŁABA, D. GARNCAREK-LANGE, J. TOMECZKO, H. MATEJ & B. NOWAKOWSKA. 1989. Risk factors of asbestos-related cancers. *In* Effects of Mineral Dusts on Cells. B.

T. Mossman & R. O. Begin, Eds. NATO ASI Series Vol. **H30:** 445–454. Berlin-Heidelberg: Springer-Verlag.
2. BLAY, J. Y., S. NEGRIER, V. COMBARET, S. ATTALI, E. GOILLOT, *et al.* 1992. Serum level of interleukin 6 as a prognosis factor in metastatic renal cell carcinoma. Cancer-Res. **52(12):** 3317–22.
3. MICHIEL D. F. & J. J. OPPENHEIM. 1992. Cytokines as positive and negative regulators of tumor promotion and progression. Semin. Cancer Biol. **3(1):** 3–15.

IL-6 Is Present in Sera of Bone Marrow–transplanted Patients in Aplastic Period and High Levels of IL-6 during Acute Graft-versus-Host Disease Are Associated with Severe Gut Symptoms[a]

L. KARABON, A. MONIEWSKA, A. LABA, C. SWIDER, AND
A. LANGE

Bone Marrow Transplantation Unit
K. Dłuski Hospital
Institute of Immunology & Experimental Therapy
Grabiszyńska 105
53-439 Wrocław, Poland

INTRODUCTION

Interleukin-6 (IL-6) participates in the regulation of non-adaptive and adaptive immunity and hematopoiesis and exerts an effect upon the neural system. This cytokine appears in serum when the integration of the human homeostasis is altered.[1] The survival of bone marrow transplantation (BMT) patients largely depends on the non-adaptive immune system at the time of aplasia, rapid hematological reconstitution, and a well-balanced reconstitution of the immune system. In all these areas IL-6 plays a key role. In the present study we are focusing on the relationship between serum levels of IL-6 and the location and severity of acute graft versus host disease (aGvHD).

PATIENTS AND METHODS

Twenty-three patients were allografted between 1992 and 1993; 18 patients developed aGvHD and 13 of them with hematological malignancies were studied. They belonged to two groups. Group 1 consisted of 7 patients (4 females and 3 males aged 23–41 yrs) with the skin as a main target organ for aGvHD. All of them responded well to steroids and there was no aGvHD life-threatening complications. Group 2 consisted of 6 patients (3 females and 3 males aged from 15–43 yrs) with severe gut aGvHD (5 patients—grade 4 and 1 patient—grade 3). None of them responded to high dose prednisone therapy or anti-thymocyte serum. Characteristics of Group 1 and [Group 2]: early/more advanced stage of disease: 4/3 [1/5], Cyclophosphamide (Cyc), Busulfan (Bu)/Cyc Bu Vepesid (VP-16): 3/4 [2/4], Cyclosporin A (CsA)/CsA with Methotrexate 1/6 [2/4].

---

[a] This work was supported by a grant from the Research Council (Polish, KBN).

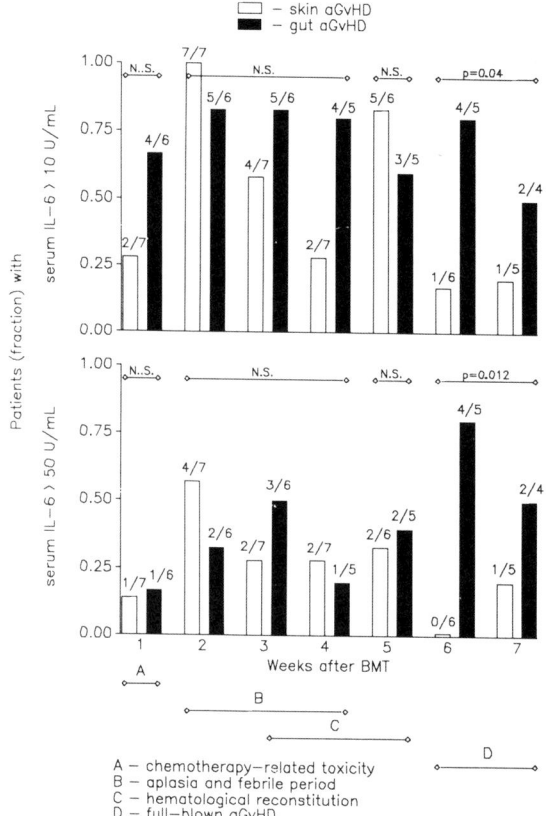

FIGURE 1. Fractions of allogeneic BMT patients with serum IL-6 level above 10 U/mL (*upper panel*) and above 50 U/mL (*lower panel*) at different intervals after BMT ((□) skin; and (■) gut aGvHD).

Serum samples for IL-6 and C-reactive protein (CRP) measurements were collected twice weekly beginning the first week after transplantation (as long as patients were hospitalized). In the present work data collected during the first 7 weeks is presented. CRP serum levels were determined with the use of the nephelometric NA Latex CRP assay kit (Behring, Marburg, Germany). Normal values < 5 mg/L. IL-6 bioassay: proliferative assay based on the mouse hybridoma IL-6 dependent cell line 7TD1. Serial dilutions of sera (started from 1:10) and standard (LPS-stimulated P388 cell culture supernatant containing a known amount of IL-6) were applied to flat-bottom culture plate wells containing 2500 7TD1 cells/well. After 4 days culture (37°C, 5% CO_2) the cells were incubated with MTT. The absorbance of lyzed material was read at 540 nm.

RESULTS AND DISCUSSION

During the first week after chemotherapy only 2 patients had relatively high levels of serum IL-6. One patient with an outstandingly high level (430 U/mL) showed

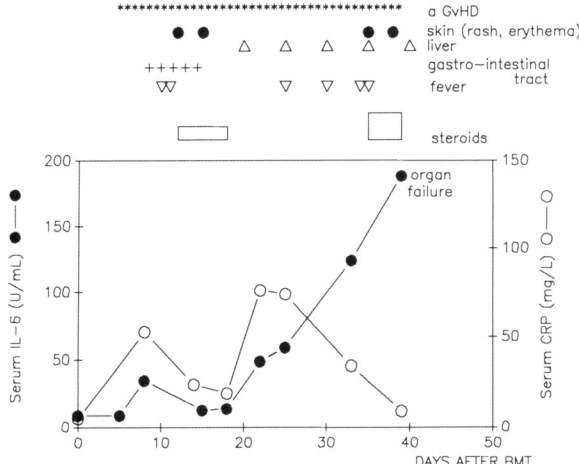

FIGURE 2. Profile of serum IL-6 and CRP levels after BMT (UPN 47) in relation to clinical symptoms.

symptoms of CNS toxicity (UPN 38). The proportion of patients with IL-6 detectable in their blood increased during the aplastic period, and at the beginning of hematological recovery. All patients had in one or more determinations IL-6 above 10 U/mL (FIG. 1). Higher values were less frequent, and the fractions of positive cases were similar in both groups, irrespective of whether the patients developed severe or mild aGvHD during the following days. Also, at the time when the first symptoms of aGvHD appeared, there was no significant difference in proportions of cases having either moderate or high level of serum IL-6 between Group 1 (skin aGvHD, symptoms started from 11 to 34 days after BMT) and Group 2 (severe gut aGvHD, symptoms started from 10 day to 30 days after BMT). The situation changed dramatically at the time interval 6 to 7 weeks after BMT. At this time aGvHD abated in the skin aGvHD Group (Group 1) but was full-blown in cases which failed to respond to the therapy (Group 2). The latter patients had severe gut GvHD and ultimately 5 out of 6 these patients died due to aGvHD-related complications (liver-kidney failure in all cases with VOD (FIG. 2) or CMV pneumonitis in two cases). These patients showed significantly higher levels of serum IL-6 (FIG. 1) with the highest values one or two weeks before death (FIG. 2). This is in line with previous reports on the association between high levels of serum IL-6 and hepato-renal complications[2] and a rapidly fatal outcome.[3] The present study demonstrates that IL-6 is present in sera of allogeneic BMT patients prior to engraftment, and the level of IL-6 had no prognostic power with respect to the severity of aGvHD. However, it is clear from our study that the level of IL-6 tends to increase when aGvHD is not controlled by therapy, and constitutes a risk factor for a fatal outcome.

REFERENCES

1. KISHIMOTO, T. 1989. The biology of interleukin-6. Blood **74:** 1–10.
2. SYMINGTON, F. W., B. E. SYMINGTON, P. Y. LIU, H. VIGUET, U. SANTHANAM & P. B. SEHGAL. 1992. The relationship of serum IL-6 levels to acute graft-versus-host disease

and hepatorenal disease after human bone marrow transplantation. Transplantation **54:** 457–462.
3. CHASTY, R. C., W. R. LAMB, H. GALLAT, T. E. ROBERTS, P. E. C. BRENCHLEY & J. A. LIU YIN. 1993. Serum cytokine levels in patients undergoing bone marrow transplantation. Bone Marrow Transplantation **12:** 331–336.

Plasma Acute Phase Proteins and Metalloproteins in Children with Neuroblastoma at Diagnosis

L. LIPIŃSKA,[a,c] T. IZBICKI,[b] T. LASKOWSKA-KLITA,[a] AND D. PEREK[b]

[a] *Department of Biochemistry*
[b] *Clinical Oncology*
National Research Institute of Mother and Child
l. Kaspzaka 17A
Warsaw, Poland 01211

INTRODUCTION

The acute-phase proteins alter their blood concentration in response to stimuli induced by many forms of tissue injury. Gerson et al.[1] reported that the serum levels of haptoglobin (Hp) and α_1 protein inhibitor (α_1PI) accurately reflected the clinical status of neuroblastoma (NBL) patients. The same was observed in the case of serum ferritin (Ft).[2] Our preliminary studies also showed that in neuroblastoma the serum acute phase proteins (App)[3] and metalloproteins (Mp)[4] are altered. The present report confirms our earlier findings in a larger population of patients. The methods used in presented paper were the same as previously described.[3,4]

RESULTS AND DISCUSSION

Previously we found that the level of serum Hp, α_1PI, ceruloplasmin oxidase activity (Cp-Ac), ceruloplasmin (Cp) and Ft increased, whereas transferrin (Tf) decreased in infants in comparison with older NBL patients. The same was recorded for patients with stage II and IV S versus patients with stage III and IV. It is commonly known that metabolism of serum proteins is age-dependent, especially in small infants.[5,6] The differences in serum proteins of patients divided into age-groups are shown in TABLE 1. Mean and median levels of serum Hp, α_1PI, Cp-Ac, Cp and Ft were lower and Tf was higher in patients younger than 1 year in comparison with older, even when data of children with physiologically expected changes in serum proteins were excluded (TABLE 1). Relation between stage of disease and the levels of measured serum proteins are shown in TABLE 2. Children under one year of age were excluded. Numerous studies showed that neuroblastoma cells contain, synthesize, and secrete ferritin and it is believed that extra Ft in sera of NBL patients is of tumor origin.[7–9] As it can be seen in TABLE 2, Ft levels were about 20 times higher in sera of patients with advanced stages (III and IV) of disease as compared to those with localized disease (II). The serum levels of other proteins also changed in response to severity of disease. These changes were not however as pronounced as in the case of ferritin. Hp, α_1-PI and

---

[c] Author to whom correspondence should be addressed.

TABLE 1. Age-dependent Levels of Serum Proteins in Neuroblastoma Patients before Treatment

	Age of Patients at Diagnosis									Kruskal-Wallis Analysis of Variance
	1–3 Months			4–12 Months			Over 12 Months			
	Mean	Median n = 5	SD	Mean	Median n = 6	SD	Mean	Median n = 33	SD	
Haptoglobin (mg/dl)	52	48	41	82	82	47	206	188	143	$p = 0.0046$
α_1-Proteinase inhibitor (mg/dl)	170	165[a]	38	188	178[b]	27	283	252	102	$p = 0.0075$
Ceruloplasmin oxidase activity (U/l)	89	80	30	189	182	35	235	238	60	$p = 0.0004$
		n = 5			n = 8			n = 41		
Ceruloplasmin (mg/dl)	25	22	7	44	44	7	55	55	14	$p = 0.0002$
Transferrin (mg/dl)	210	202	44	348	294	109	255	240	79	$p = 0.0063$
Ferritin (ng/ml)	126	138	56	35	21	28	249	90	487	$p > 0.05$

[a] Patients aged 3–6 months.
[b] Patients aged 1–3 months.

TABLE 2. Stage-dependent Levels of Serum Proteins in Neuroblastoma Patients before Treatment

	Stage of Disease									Kruskal-Wallis Analysis of Variance
	II			III			IV			
	Mean	Median n = 3	SD	Mean	Median n = 8	SD	Mean	Median n = 19	SD	
Haptoglobin (mg/dl)	91	80	26	156	153	91	256	268	162	$p = 0.0178$
α_1-Proteinase inhibitor (mg/dl)	170	199	59	245	232	74	323	342	106	$p = 0.0413$
Ceruloplasmin oxidase activity (U/l)	151	156	52	233	235	48	245	239	59	$p = 0.03$
		n = 4			n = 9			n = 25		
Ceruloplasmin (mg/dl)	42	44	12	52	54	8	60	60	15	$p = 0.0234$
Transferrin (mg/dl)	344	348	59	212	214	77	246	222	69	$p = 0.0211$
Ferritin (ng/ml)	16	15	14	433	108	743	248	105	427	$p = 0.0493$

Cp increased with stage of disease. Cp-Ac was lower and Tf was higher in sera of patients with stage II in comparison with stage III or IV patients (TABLE 2).

In conclusion, we may confirm our earlier suggestions that serum App and Mp measurements before treatment are valuable clinically in patients with neuroblastoma.

REFERENCES

1. GERSON, J., et al. 1977. Cancer **40**: 1655–1658.
2. HANN, H. L., et al. 1980. Cancer Res. 40: 1411–1413.

3. LIPIŃSKA, L., et al. 1992. Folia Histochem. Cytobiol. **30(4)**: 205–206.
4. LIPIŃSKA, L., et al. 1993. In Biologie Prospective: Comptes Rendus du 8E Colloque de Pont-A-Mousson, pp. 335–338. London-Paris: John Libbey.
5. FINCH, A., et al. 1986. West. J. Med. **145**: 657–663.
6. HITZIG, W. H. & P. W. JOLLER. 1983. In Proteins in Body Fluids, Amino Acids, and Tumor Markers, pp. 1–52. New York: Alan R. Liss, Inc.
7. BLATT, J., et al. 1990. Cancer Biochem. Biophys. **11**: 169–176.
8. IANCU, T. C. 1989. Ultrastructural Pathology **13**: 573–584.
9. HANN, H. W., et al. 1986. JNCI **76(6)**: 1031–1033.

The Value of Determining the Interleukin-6 Levels in Epithelial Ovarian Cancer

J. MARKOWSKA, K. WIKTOROWICZ, Z. SZEWIERSKI, AND R. MĄDRY

Department of Oncology
School of Medicine
Łąkowa 1/2
61-878 Poznań, Poland

Studies by Watson et al.[1] and those of Kutteh and Kutteh[2] have shown that ovarian cancer cells are capable by themselves of producing and releasing interleukin-6 (IL-6) both in cultures and *in vivo*. Berek et al.[3] have detected a correlation between IL-6 level in 36 patients with ovarian cancer on one hand and clinical status of the patients or their survival time on the other.

AIMS

The study aimed at determining IL-6 levels in serum, ascitic fluid, and in the material obtained upon surgery from neoplastic cysts.

MATERIAL AND METHODS

Patients

The analysis included patients admitted to the department for treatment after diagnosis elsewhere and patients in whom the tumor was diagnosed and resected in the department. In each patient, blood was sampled before surgery and before chemotherapy. Ascitic fluid was sampled during its evacuation. The fluid from neoplastic cysts was obtained during surgery.

Material

The obtained material was left until clotted and, then, centrifuged for 5 min at 3000 rpm. The serum or other fluids were frozen until assayed using standard ELISA-PREDICTA tests (Genzyme Diagnostics).

RESULTS

IL-6 was estimated in 16 patients with malignant tumors of the ovary. Serum IL-6 was estimated in 15 patients (one sample was accidentally destroyed during assay

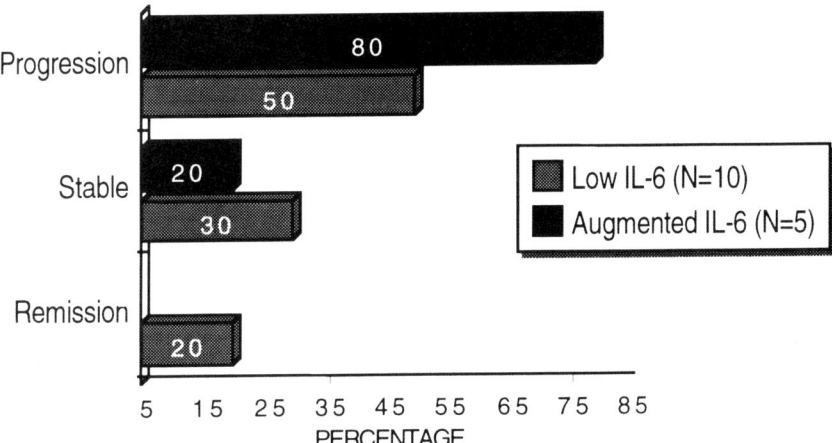

FIGURE 1. Correlation between serum IL-6 level and clinical status. Out of 10 patients with normal serum IL-6 levels 2 patients remained in remission (20%), 3 patients (30%) remained stable, and 5 patients (50%) were at the stage of progression. In 5 patients with augmented IL-6 levels in the serum, one case (20%) was stable and in the remaining 4 cases (80%) progression was established.

preparations). In 10 patients (66%) IL-6 level was below 30 pg/ml (range: 0 to 30 pg/ml), averaging 15 pg/ml. In 5 patients (33%) the IL-6 level was raised with a mean level of 600 pg/ml (range: 300 to 1000 pg/ml). In the ascitic fluid, IL-6 was estimated in 11 patients. In 5 patients (45%) the level did not exceed 30 pg/ml averaging 24 pg/ml (range: 20 to 30 pg/ml) while in 6 patients (54%) the level was augmented to a mean of 660 pg/ml (range: 150 to 1000 pg/ml). In the fluid of neoplastic cysts IL-6 was estimated in 4 patients. In three patients the level did not exceed 25 pg/ml with a mean of 15 pg/ml (range: 0 to 25 pg/ml). In one patient the level of IL-6 in the tumor cyst fluid was 750 pg/ml.

The analysis included clinical status of the patients and selected laboratory results (blood platelets, serum protein level) in two group of patients: those with low IL-6 levels and those exhibiting enhanced IL-6 levels in serum or ascitic fluid. Correlation between serum IL-6 level and clinical status is shown in FIGURE 1. FIGURE 2 shows correlation between ascitic fluid IL-6 level and clinical status. Among 3 patients with normal IL-6 level in the fluid of neoplastic cysts, 2 patients were in remission and one showed a stable process. The patient with augmented IL-6 levels in the fluid showed stable process.

Patients with low as compared to those with high levels of IL-6 did not differ in total serum protein level (mean of 7.75 g/dl, range: 5.58–9.2 g/dl) or in blood platelet level (272.1 G/l vs 271.2 G/l). No correlation was observed between IL-6 level and histological pattern of the tumor or stage of clinical advancement.

Out of 8 patients with augmented IL-6 levels both in the serum and in ascitic fluid, two (25%) were stable while 6 (75%) showed progression of the neoplastic disease. In the course of observation 4 patients died, all exhibiting progression of the disease. In all of the patients IL-6 level was augmented, in three of them both in serum and in ascitic fluid, in one in ascitic fluid.

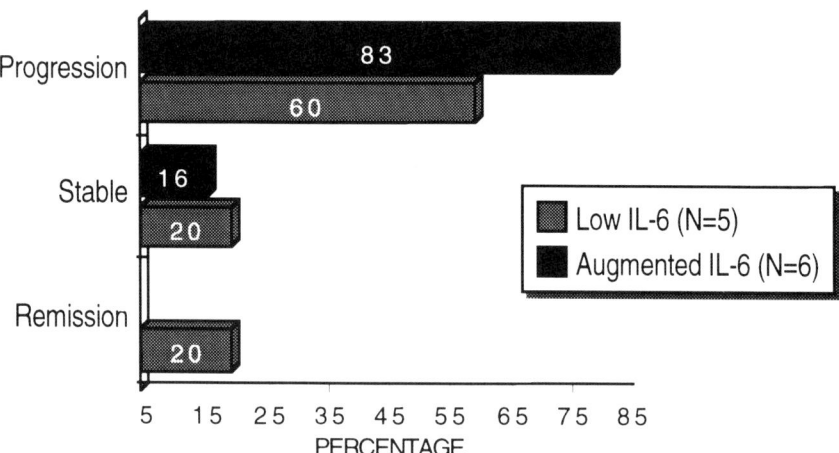

FIGURE 2. Correlation between ascitic fluid IL-6 level and clinical status. Out of 5 patients with normal IL-6 level one (20%) showed remission, one (20%) was stable, and three patients (60%) showed progression. In 6 patients with augmented IL-6 levels in the fluid one (16.6%) was stable while 5 (83%) exhibited progression.

DISCUSSION

In our studies we have demonstrated elevated IL-6 levels in the serum of 33% of patients and in ascitic fluid in 54% patients with ovarian cancer, in accordance with results of other authors.[1,3,4] IL-6 level has seemed to correlate with clinical condition of the patients which in our group has been most evident in the ascites group (83% patients with elevated IL-6 level manifested progression of the neoplastic process as compared to 60% patients with low IL-6 levels). The duration of our observation has been too short to analyze survival times, as conducted by Berek[3] but all of our patients who died in the course of the study have shown elevated IL-6 levels (in three cases both in the serum and in the ascitic fluid, in one case in ascitic fluid). In contrast to Gastl,[5] in our studies we have noted no relationship between IL-6 levels and the blood platelet levels. The role of IL-6 in ovarian cancer awaits clarification. IL-6 can stimulate proliferation of ovarian tumor cells[6] and may act as an autocrine growth factor for ovarian cancer cells.[7] Inhibition of IL-6 gene expression by exposure to IL-6 antisense oligonucleotides resulted in greatly decreased cellular proliferation. The addition of exogenous IL-6 failed to restore the proliferation of the antisense-treated cells. These results suggest that IL-6 does not directly induce the proliferation of ovarian cancer cells although endogenous IL-6 production is needed for optimal cell growth.

REFERENCES

1. WATSON, J. M., J. L. SENSINTAFFAE, J. S. BEREK & O. MARTINEZ-MAZA. 1990. Cancer Res. **50:** 6959–6965.
2. KUTTEH, W. H. & C. C. KUTTEH. 1992. Am. J. Obstet. Gynecol. **167:** 1864–1869.

3. BEREK, J. S., C. CHUNG, K. KALDI, J. M. WATSON, R. M. KNOX & O. MARTINEZ-MAZA. 1991. Am. J. Obstet. Gynecol. **164:** 1038–1043.
4. MORADI, M. M., L. F. CARSON, J. B. WEINBERG, A. F. HANEY, L. B. TWIGGS & S. RAMAKRISHNAN. 1993. Cancer **72:** 2433–2440.
5. GASTL, G., M. PLANTE, C. L. FINSTAD, G. Y. WONG, M. G. FEDRICI, N. H. BANDER & S. C. RUBIN. 1993. Br. J. Haematol. **83:** 433–441.
6. WU, S., K. RODABAUGH, O. MARTINEZ-MAZA, J. M. WATSON, D. S. SILBERSTEIN, C. M. BOYER, W. P. PETERS, J. B. WEINBERG, J. S. BEREK & R. C. BAST. 1992. Am J. Obstet. Gynecol. **166:** 997–1007.
7. WATSON, J. M., J. S. BEREK & O. MARTINEZ-MAZA. 1993. Gynecol-Oncol. **49:** 8–15.

Immunohistochemical Localization of Interleukin-6–like Immunoreactivity to Peripheral Nerve-like Structures in Normal and Inflamed Human Skin

K. NORDLIND,[a] C. LIBING,[b] A. A. AHMED,[b] A. LJUNGBERG,[b] AND S. LIDÉN[b]

[a]*Department of Dermatology*
Academic Hospital
Uppsala, S-751 85, Sweden

[b]*Department of Dermatology*
Karolinska Hospital
Stockholm, Sweden

IL (interleukin)-6 is a multifunctional cytokine, which may play a regulatory role in host defense mechanisms through immune and nervous systems. It is secreted by a wide range of cells including microglia and astrocytes.[1] IL-6 has also been detected in the cerebrospinal fluid in diseases with inflammation.[2,3]

Biopsy specimens were taken from positive epicutaneous patch-test reactions to metal salts as well as from lesional and control skin in patients with atopic eczema, neurodermatitis, prurigo nodularis, lupus erythematodes discoides and psoriasis; they were then fixed in phosphate buffered, 10% formaldehyde with 0.2% picric acid, rinsed in 0.1 M Sörensen's buffer containing 5% sucrose, and sectioned on a cryostat. The sections were incubated overnight at +4°C with a primary monoclonal antibody against IL-6 and then with a secondary rhodamine-conjugated antibody for 30 min at 37°C.

The inflamed and control skin showed IL-6–like immunoreactivity distributed to nerve-like structures in the arrector pili muscles, in vessel walls, and in the other parts of the dermis (FIG. 1). A few slender fibers were seen running to the outer part of the epidermis. The nonlesional skin in the different diseases also contained a few epidermal fibers. In lesional skin of prurigo nodularis there were clusters of fibers in the dermis, attaching the epidermis. After adsorption of the monoclonal antibody with denaturated antigen the immunoreactivity was lost.

The findings with IL-6 positive nerve-like structures in the vessel walls and in the arrector pili muscles, indicate the presence of IL-6 in autonomic as well as in sensory nerves. The clusters of IL-6–positive fibers in prurigo nodularis lesions might support a trophic effect for IL-6 on nerves. A rat pheochromocytoma cell line, PC12, was earlier reported to be differentiated into neuronal cells by human IL-6.[4]

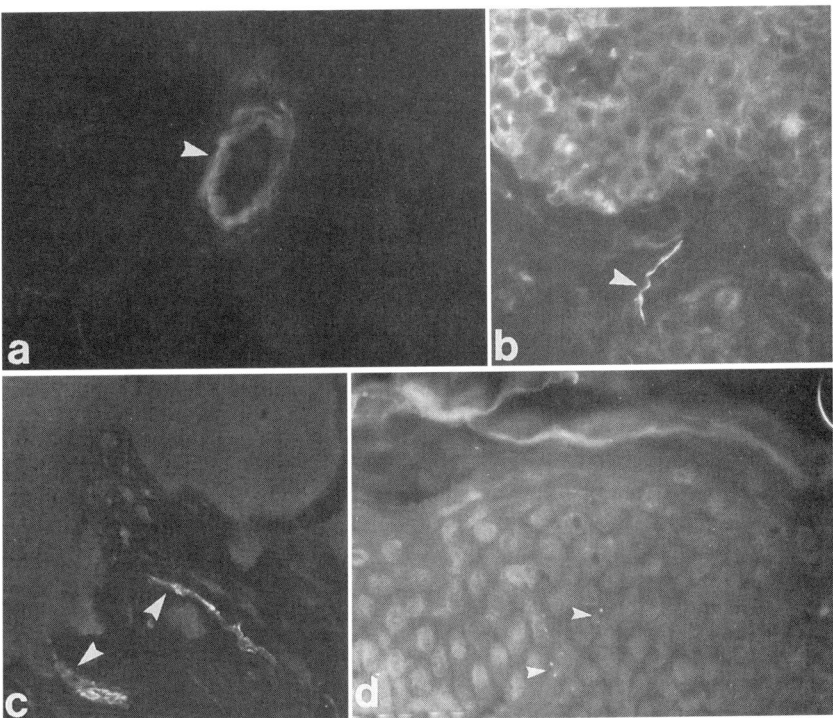

FIGURE 1. Immunoreactivity to IL-6 in nerve-like structures in a vessel wall (**a**) and other part of the dermis (**b**) in normal skin, in the dermis in lesional skin of prurigo nodularis (**c**) and in the epidermis of contact eczematous skin (**d**). Arrowheads point at nerve-like structures. (a, c ×200; b, d ×400)

REFERENCES

1. RIGHI, M., L. MORI, G. DE LIBERO, M. SIRONI, A. BIONDI, A. MANTOVANI, S. D. DONINI & P. RICCIARDI-CASTAGNOLI. 1989. Eur. J. Immunol. **19:** 1443–1448.
2. FREI, K., T. P. LEIST, A. MEAGER, P. GALLO, D. LEPPERT, R. M. ZINKERNAGEL & A. FONTANA. 1988. J. Exp. Med. **168:** 449–453.
3. HOUSSIAU F. A., K. BUKASA, C. SINDIC, J. M. VAN DAMME & J. VAN SNICK. 1988. Clin. Exp. Immunol. **71:** 320–323.
4. SATOH, T., S. NAKAMURA, T. TAGA, T. MATSUDA, T. HIRANO, T. KISHIMOTO & Y. KAZIRO. 1988. Mol. Cell. Biol. **8:** 3546–3549.

Kinetics of the Activation of the LIF-Response Factor in M1 Myeloid Leukemic Cells[a]

R. P. PIEKORZ, R. BLÄSIUS, G. H. FEY, AND G. M. HOCKE

Department of Genetics, Institute for Microbiology, Biochemistry, and Genetics
University of Erlangen-Nürnberg
Staudtstrasse 5
D-91058 Erlangen, Germany

LIF (leukemia inhibitory factor) functions as a cytokine with diverse effects on different types of target cells. It induces differentiation of M1 murine myelomonocytic leukemia cells and thus blocks their proliferation. LIF belongs to the family of IL6-type cytokines.[1]

Several important components of the IL6- and LIF-induced intracellular signaling cascades in hepatic cells have recently been described.[1] The IL6- and LIF-response elements (REs) of the prototype class II acute phase gene, the rat α_2-macroglobulin (α_2-M) gene, have been shown to be identical. In response to IL6 and LIF, a characteristic protein-DNA complex (complex II) was assembled over the IL6/LIF-RE with nuclear extracts from hepatic cells and other cell types.[2] This complex was visualized by gel mobility shift experiments with IL6/LIF-RE probes and probably plays a key role in the cytokine induced transcriptional activation of specific target genes. One of the DNA-binding components of this complex is referred to as the LIF-response factor (LIF-RF).

Here we report on: a) the correlation between the induction of differentiation and proliferation arrest in M1 cells by various agents and the concomitant generation of complex II, and b) the kinetics of appearance of complex II after treatment of M1 cells with LIF.

Induction of differentiation was monitored by the appearance of morphological features characteristic of macrophage-like cells and the ability to phagocytose latex beads. Several reagents, including LIF, IL1α, LPS, *all*-trans retinoic acid (ATRA) and lithium chloride caused reduced proliferation of M1 cells to various extents (FIG. 1). Of all these reagents, only LIF caused differentiation as judged by these parameters and induced the appearance of complex II. Thus, the activation of the signal pathway that generates complex II is closely correlated with the ability to induce differentiation in M1 cells.

Complex II was induced rapidly after a one time addition of LIF and stayed detectable for at least 6 hours as indicated (FIG. 2). Formation of the "early" complex II (up to 1 hour) was independent of ongoing protein synthesis (resistant to cycloheximide). Appearance of the "late" complex required ongoing protein synthesis (R. Piekorz *et al.*, unpublished data).

---

[a] This work was supported by a research grant from Deutsche Forschungsgemeinschaft (DFG) awarded to G.M.H. (Hi 291/5-4 TP6).

FIGURE 1. Growth inhibitory effect of Leukemia Inhibitory Factor (LIF) and other agents on M1 myeloid leukemic cells. Recombinant human LIF was the supernatant from LIF-secreting CHO- (Chinese Hamster Ovary) cells stably transfected with a human LIF-expression cDNA construct (Genetics Institute). Concentrations used were as follows: LIF: 3 ng/ml; IL1α: 10^{-10} M; lipopolysaccharide (LPS): 100 ng/ml; *all*-trans retinoic acid (ATRA): 10^{-6} M; and lithium chloride: 10 mM. After stimulation for 90 hours numbers of viable cells were determined by trypan blue exclusion and standardized against untreated control cells. Data represent means of two independent experiments.

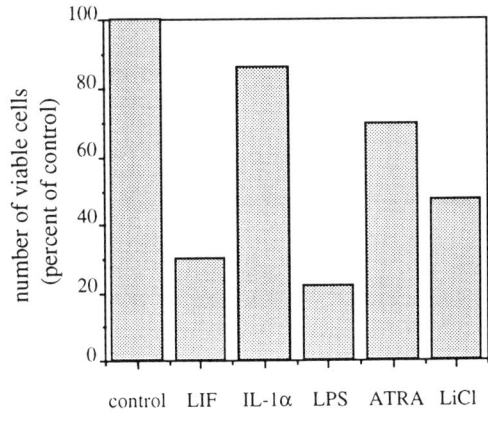

FIGURE 2. Time course of activation of the LIF-RF in LIF-treated M1 cells. M1 cells were stimulated with LIF for the indicated times; nuclear extracts were prepared and analyzed by electrophoretic mobility shift assays using an oligonucleotide with two core-elements of the LIF-RE as a probe (II: Complex II; F: free probe).

In summary, M1 cells exhibited a complex II of indistinguishable mobility after treatment with LIF of that observed in cytokine-treated hepatic cells and others. However, the characteristic property of M1 cells was that the ability to be induced to differentiate was correlated with the ability to induce this complex formation.

REFERENCES

1. KISHIMOTO, T., T. TAGA & S. AKIRA. 1994. Cytokine signal transduction. Cell **76:** 253–262.
2. HOCKE, G. M., M.-Z. CUI, J. A RIPPERGER & G. H. FEY. 1992. Regulation of the rat a_2 macroglobulin gene by interleukin 6 and leukemia inhibitory factor. *In* Acute Phase Proteins: Molecular Biology, Biochemistry, Clinical Applications. A. Mackiewicz, I. Kushner and H. Bainmann, Eds.: 467–494. Boca Raton, FL: CRC Press.

Interleukin-6 Levels in Sera and Bronchoalveolar Lavages of Patients with Selected Disorders

Z. POJDA,[a] J. STRUŻYNA,[b] M. MARUSZYŃSKI,[b] T. PŁUSA,[c] AND
A. JUNG[d]

[a]Department of Radiation Hematology WIHiE
[b]Institute of Surgery
[c]Institute of Internal Medicine
[d]Department of Pediatrics CSK WAM
ul.Kozielska 4
01-163 Warsaw, Poland

In healthy persons IL-6, according to our prior observations[1] is undetectable in serum at the level of test sensitivity. In some diseases, however, this cytokine is present in blood in relatively high concentrations.[2–4] We have examined the presence and kinetics of changes of concentrations of IL-6 in blood serum and in bronchoalveolar lavages (BAL) of patients with selected disorders. The samples of collected material were frozen at $-80°C$ until evaluation. Depending on the patient's disease and status, IL-6 level measurements were performed at 2-day intervals up to 45 days and the kinetics of IL-6 concentration changes was compared with such events as surgical trauma, fever, peripheral blood cellularity and the disease outcome. Quantitative measurements

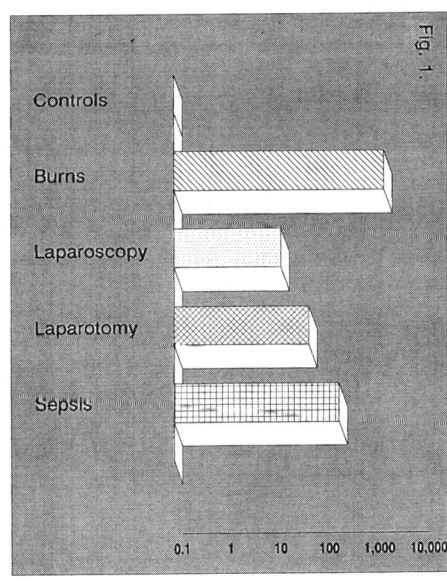

FIGURE 1. Average concentrations of IL-6 in sera of control healthy persons (30), burned patients (11), patients undergoing cholecystectomy via laparoscopy (14) or laparotomy (11) or having diagnosed sepsis episodes (15). Means of the peak values of serum IL-6 levels were calculated for each group.

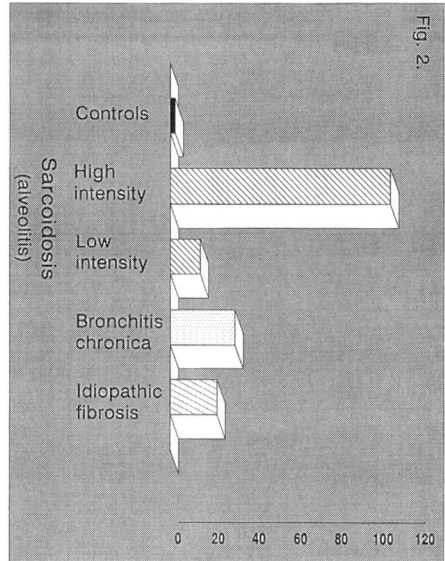

FIGURE 2. Average concentrations of IL-6 in BAL of control healthy persons (4), patients with diagnosed sarcoidosis with high (5) or low (4) intensity alveolitis, bronchitis chronica (4) or idiopathic fibrosis (2). Means of the values calculated for each group are presented.

of IL-6 concentrations were performed using commercially available ELISA kits (Amersham) and computerized reader (Hamilton). Test sensitivity was above 2 pg/ml of IL-6. We have observed elevated serum levels of IL-6 (FIG. 1) in burned patients, patients undergoing surgical operations, and at the time of massive bacterial infections. IL-6 was present in BALs (FIG. 2) of patients with pulmonary dysfunctions (sarcoidosis, bronchitis chronica, idiopathic fibrosis). In sera of the normal healthy controls IL-6 was undetectable, and in BALs in control group its concentration was very low, close to the limit of test sensitivity. We have observed positive correlation between the IL-6 concentration and the extent of surgical trauma. In septic patients the increase of IL-6 serum concentration peaked 12–24 h after manifestation of the other symptoms (fever). It may be concluded, that the examination of IL-6 concentrations in the body fluids may be the useful diagnostic and prognostic factor in selected disorders.

REFERENCES

1. STRUŻYNA, J., Z. POJDA, et al. Prognostic significance of the serum cytokine levels in burned patients. Burns. In press.
2. LAHAT, N., A. Y. ZLOTNICK, et al. 1992. Serum levels of IL-1, IL-6, and tumor necrosis factor in patients undergoing coronary artery bypass grafts or cholecystectomy. Clin Exp. Immunol. **89:** 255–260.
3. UEYAMA, M., I. MARUYAMA, et al. 1992. Marked increase in plasma interleukin-6 in burn patients. J. Lab. Clin. Med. **120:** 693–698.
4. TILG, H., J. NORDBERG, et al. 1992. Circulating serum levels of interleukin-6 and C-reactive protein after liver transplantation. Transplantation **54:** 142–146.

IL-6-Receptor–mediated Growth Inhibition by *All*-trans Retinoic Acid but Not by Interferon-α in Human Myeloma Cells

KARI PULKKI,[a,c] MARKO NEVA,[a,c] KARI KOSKELA,[b,c] HANNA OLLIKAINEN,[a,c] KARI REMES,[b] AND TARJA-TERTTU PELLINIEMI [a]

[a]*Central Laboratory*
[b]*Department of Medicine*
Turku University Central Hospital
Kiinamyllynkatu 4-8
FIN-20520 Turku, Finland

[c]*Medicity Research Laboratory*
University of Turku
Turku, Finland

INTRODUCTION

Multiple myeloma is a malignant disease of plasma cells. The biological characteristics of myeloma cells include high bcl-2 expression, high incidence of p53 mutations, secretion of interleukin-6 (IL-6) and expression of IL-6 receptors.[1] These characteristics may contribute to the low proliferative activity of the malignant cell. Also the treatment with cytotoxic drugs does not lead to a complete remission. IL-6 is suggested to function either as an autocrine or paracrine growth factor for myeloma cells *in vitro*.[2,3] The pretreatment serum IL-6 concentration is a prognostic factor for myeloma patients.[4] Therefore, we aim to study the association of IL-6 receptor expression and the therapeutic response. *All*-trans retinoic acid (ATRA) is a vitamin A derivative with growth inhibitory activities. As ATRA has been shown to inhibit IL-6 receptor expression,[5] we wanted to study the effects of ATRA and interferon-α (IFN) on human myeloma cell growth, IL-6 and soluble IL-6 receptor secretion.

RESULTS AND DISCUSSION

As experimental models for multiple myeloma, four human myeloma cell lines and one cell line started from a myeloma patient were studied. Two of the cell lines (U-266 and RPMI 8226) and the patient cells secreted soluble IL-6 receptors. Two cell lines (HS-Sultan and MC/CAR) did not secrete IL-6 nor express IL-6 receptors. The effects of ATRA, IFN, and dexamethasone (DEX) on the proliferative activity of the

TABLE 1. Growth, IL-6 and IL-6 Receptor Secretion of Human Myeloma Cells by Various Treatments[a]

	3H-Thymidine Incorp (%)[b]			IL-6 ng/l[c]			IL-6 Receptor (μg/l)[c]		
	ATRA[d]	IFN[e]	Dexa[f]	C	ATRA[d]	IFN[e]	C	ATRA[d]	IFN[e]
U-266	58	58	59	10.1	5.0	17.1	9.7	7.4	10.3
RPMI	26	59	30	4.9	2.4	3.5	1.5	0.8	1.8
HS-Sult	98	100	26	ND	ND	ND	ND	ND	ND
MC/CAR	103	96	70	ND	ND	ND	ND	ND	ND
Patient	57	70	—	—	—	—	5.0	3.0	4.0

[a] Myeloma cell culture after 48 h at 4×10^4 cells/well, means of triplicate measurements are shown.
[b] Six hour labeling after 48 h, 1 uCi/well, percentage of the control.
[c] Protein concentration in the culture medium as measured with sandwich-type ELISAs.
[d] 10^{-5} M all-trans retinoic acid.
[e] 50 U/ml interferon α.
[f] 10^{-5} M dexamethasone.
ND = not detected.

four myeloma cell lines and patient cells are shown in TABLE 1. The results indicate that ATRA treatment inhibits the secretion of soluble IL-6 receptors. The addition of exogenous IL-6 abolished part of the inhibitory effect of ATRA on the proliferation of RPMI 8226 and U-266 cell lines. Interferon-α inhibited the growth of the same cell lines as IFN, but did not show any inhibitory effect, but rather a stimulatory effect on soluble IL-6 receptor and IL-6 secretion. The effects of combined treatment with ATRA and DEX on the growth inhibition of most cell lines were additional, also at suboptimal doses. ATRA or DEX did not induce any detectable increase in the percentage of apoptotic cells as measured with flow cytometry of propidium iodide-stained cells.

As ATRA inhibits the growth and IL-6 receptor expression of human myeloma cells *in vitro*, we conclude that ATRA is a potential candidate for the therapy of myeloma patients.

REFERENCES

1. NIESVIZKY, R., D. SIEGEL & J. MICHAELI. 1993. Biology and treatment of multiple myeloma. Blood Reviews 7: 24–33.
2. BARUT, B. A., L. ZON, M. C. COCHRAN & S. R. PAUL. 1992. Role of interleukin 6 in the growth of myeloma cells-derived cell lines. Leuk. Res. 16: 951–959.
3. KLEIN, B., X-G. ZANG, M. JOURDAN, J. CONTENT, F. HOUSSIAU, L. AARDEN, M. PIECHARCZYK & R. BATAILLE. 1989. Paracrine rather than autocrine regulation oF myeloma-cell growth and differentiation by interleukin-6. Blood 73: 517–526.
4. TIENHAARA, A., K. PULKKI, K. MATTILA, K. IRJALA & T.-T. PELLINIEMI. 1994. Serum immunoreactive interleukin-6 and C-reactive protein levels in patients with multiple myeloma at diagnosis. Br. J. Haematol. 86: 391–393.
5. SIDELL, N., T. TAGA, T. HIRANO, T. KISHIMOTO & A. SAXON. 1991. Retinoic acid-induced growth inhibition of a human myeloma cell line via down-regulation of IL-6 receptors. J. Immunol. 146: 3809–3814.

Purification of the Interleukin-6–inducible Complex II Reveals Two Proteins Capable of Binding to the IL-6–Response Element[a]

J. A. RIPPERGER, S. FRITZ, G. M. HOCKE, AND G. H. FEY

Department of Genetics
University of Erlangen-Nürnberg
Staudtstrasse 5
D-91058 Erlangen, Germany

During an inflammatory process a cocktail of specific cytokines is secreted by macrophages and fibroblasts into the bloodstream. In response to this signal the liver produces a set of acute phase plasma proteins. The class 2 acute phase genes are regulated mainly by interleukin-6 (IL-6) or combinations of IL-6 + glucocorticoids, and other members of the IL-6–type family, *e.g.* leukemia inhibitory factor.[1] An IL-6-response element (IL-6RE) has been mapped in the promoter region of the α_2-macroglobulin gene, a prototype rat class 2 acute phase gene. Gel-shift experiments with this element yielded a typical complex II, which was shown to be sequence-specific and inducible by IL-6 in different systems.

To define the protein(s) binding to the IL-6RE two different approaches were taken. An initial characterization was performed by UV-crosslinking experiments (FIG. 1). The protein/DNA complex formed with one core site of the IL-6RE was covalently linked by irradiation with UV-light and then separated on a denaturing SDS polyacrylamide gel. Two major species of crosslinked DNA/protein complexes with apparent molecular weights of 70 and 80 kD and a minor species of 190 kD were observed. The intensity of the 190 kD species was greatly enhanced when higher doses of UV-light were used, indicating progressive crosslinking of two proteins as a dimer (data not shown). Thus at least two proteins capable of binding to the IL-6RE were detected.

As a second approach complex II was purified from acute phase rat livers. An acute phase response was induced by intraperitoneal injection of complete Freund's adjuvant (0.4 ml/100 g body weight). Twelve hours later livers were excised and nuclear extracts prepared. Using standard chromatographic procedures and DNA-affinity chromatography a more than 6000-fold purification was achieved.[2] Three proteins were identified in the final complex II containing fractions: A 86 kD protein and a pair with approximately 91 and 92 kD (FIG. 2). Sequencing of all three polypeptides is in progress to determine their identity and their relationship with other known IL6-response factors.

Two IL-6–inducible transcription factors capable of specific binding at type II IL-6-response elements have so far been reported: Stat1/p91Stat[3] and Stat3/APRF.[4] Recent observations suggest, that these factors dimerize upon induction and also form heterodimers.[3] The reported molecular weights of these proteins are very similar to

---

[a] This work was supported by a research grant from Deutsche Forschungsgemeinschaft (DFG) awarded to G. H. Fey (Grant # Hi 291/5-4 TP2).

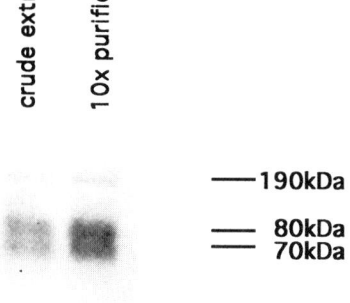

FIGURE 1. The complex built over one ^{32}P-labeled core site of the IL-6RE was irradiated with UV-light (254 nm) and the band was excised. The DNA/protein complexes were then separated on a 9% denaturing SDS polyacrylamide gel and autoradiographed. The molecular weights of three obtained complexes are indicated on the right. These numbers are not corrected for the contribution of the DNA to the mobility of the crosslinked complexes.

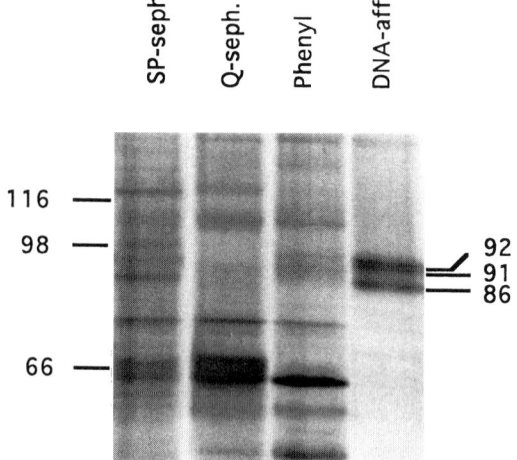

FIGURE 2. 7.5% denaturing SDS polyacrylamide gel monitoring progressive stages of purification of the IL-6RE binding proteins (silver stained). SP-seph., Q-seph., Phenyl: Protein fractions binding to the IL-6RE eluted from SP-sepharose, Q-sepharose and Phenyl-sepharose. DNA-aff.: Eluate from specific DNA chromatography showing three purified proteins of 86, 91 and 92 kD.

those obtained in our purification. The precise degree of their relatedness is under current investigation.

REFERENCES

1. HOCKE, G. M., M.-Z. CUI, J. A. RIPPERGER & G. H. FEY. 1992. Regulation of the α_2 macroglobulin gene by interleukin 6 and leukemia inhibitory factor. *In* Acute Phase Proteins: Molecular Biology, Biochemistry, and Clinical Applications. A. Mackiewicz, I. Kushner, and H. Baumann, Eds.: 467–494. Boca Raton, FL: CRC Press.
2. RIPPERGER, J. A., S. FRITZ, F. LOTTSPEICH, G. M. HOCKE & G. H. FEY. In preparation.
3. DARNELL, J. E. JR., I. M. KERR & G. R. STARK. 1994. Jak-STAT pathways and transcriptional activation in response to IFNs and other extracellular signaling proteins. Science **264:** 1415–1421.
4. AKIRA, S., Y. NISHIO, M. INOUE, X.-J. WANG, S. WEI, T. MATSUSAKA, K. YOSHIDA, T. SUDO, M. NARUTO & T. KISHIMOTO. 1994. Molecular cloning of APRF, a novel IFN-stimulated gene factor 3 p91-related transcription factor involved in the gp130-mediated signaling pathway. Cell **77:** 63–71.

TIMP-1 Protein Expression Is Stimulated by IL-1β and IL-6 in Primary Rat Hepatocytes

ELKE ROEB,[a] LUTZ GRAEVE,[b] JÜRGEN MÜLLBERG,[b]
SIEGFRIED MATERN,[a] AND STEFAN ROSE-JOHN[b]

[a]*Medizinische Klinik III*
[b]*Institut für Biochemie*
RWTH Aachen
Pauwelsstrasse 30
D-52057 Aachen, Germany

Alterations in the balance between synthesis and degradation of extracellular matrix may result in tissue sclerosis and fibrosis. The interaction between metalloproteinases and their inhibitors, the tissue inhibitors of metalloproteinases (TIMP), modulates the rate of matrix degradation and accumulation in, for example, glomerulosclerosis or liver fibrosis as well as in rapid matrix destruction occurring during arthritis (for review see ref. 1). Murine TIMP-1 is a secreted glycoprotein of 184 amino acids (Mr = 28 kD) with a high sequence identity to rat and human TIMP-1. By forming a tight complex of 1:1 stoichiometry with the target matrix metalloproteinases, TIMP-1 regulates the breakdown of collagen and basement membrane components. In murine fibroblast cells the expression of TIMP-1-mRNA is induced by serum, 4β-phorbol-12-myristate-13-acetate, fibroblast growth factor, and platelet-derived growth factor. In rat hepatocytes TIMP-1-mRNA is upregulated by inflammatory cytokines, IL-6, IL-1, IL-11, and CNTF, for example.[2]

We expressed the murine TIMP-1 protein in *E. coli* and prepared a polyclonal antiserum against the recombinant protein (FIG. 1). Using this antiserum we studied the biosynthesis and glycosylation of murine TIMP-1 protein in COS-7 cells transfected with a TIMP-1 expression plasmid. Upon metabolic labeling it turned out that TIMP-1 although it contains a signal peptide is found in both, cell lysates and culture supernatants. Indirect immunofluorescence studies with the same cells revealed that cell-associated TIMP-1 protein could be detected on the surface of non-permeabilized cells. Moreover we could demonstrate that our antiserum does not cross-react with human TIMP-1 protein (data not shown).

In order to observe the regulation of TIMP-1 in a physiological system and since we already know that TIMP-1-mRNA is upregulated in liver cells under acute phase conditions[2,3] we immunoprecipitated TIMP-1 from stimulated rat hepatocytes in primary culture. Rat hepatocytes were incubated for 12 h with recombinant human IL-1β, IL-6, or conditioned medium from human monocytes stimulated with LPS as indicated in FIGURE 2. The newly synthesized and secreted proteins were analyzed by SDS-polyacrylamide gel electrophoresis after immunoprecipitation with the antiserum against murine TIMP-1. In primary rat hepatocytes we show for the first time that TIMP-1 protein expression is upregulated upon stimulation with IL-1β and IL-6. Taken together with the finding that TIMP-1 is elevated in serum of patients with chronic liver diseases[4] TIMP-1 could possibly be involved in the pathogenesis of liver fibrosis.

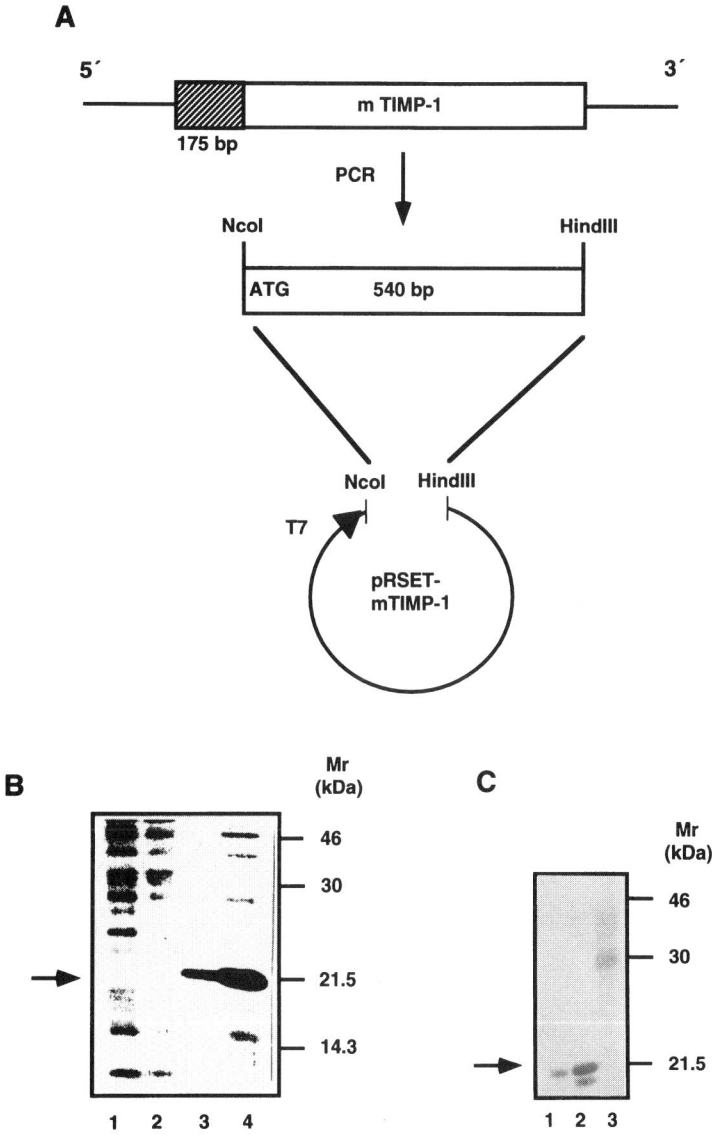

FIGURE 1. Bacterial expression of murine TIMP-1. **A:** Construction of the bacterial murine TIMP-1 expression vector: A cDNA insert coding for murine TIMP-1 without signal peptide was constructed by polymerase chain reaction and inserted into the expression vector pRSET5d. **B:** SDS-PAGE of proteins from bacteria transformed with the empty expression vector pRSET *(lane 1)*, the murine TIMP-1 vector before induction with IPTG *(lane 2)* and 1 μg *(lane 3)* and 5 μg *(lane 4)* inclusion bodies of the same cells. The arrow indicates the position of TIMP-1 expressed by transformed bacteria. **C:** Detection of murine TIMP-1 inclusion bodies by Western blotting. 1μg *(lane 1)* and 5 μg *(lane 2)* of inclusion bodies in lysis buffer were electrophoresced on a 13% SDS-polyacrylamide gel and analyzed by Western blotting using a polyclonal murine-TIMP-1-antiserum obtained as described in MATERIALS AND METHODS. The arrow indicates the position of TIMP-1 expressed by transformed bacteria.

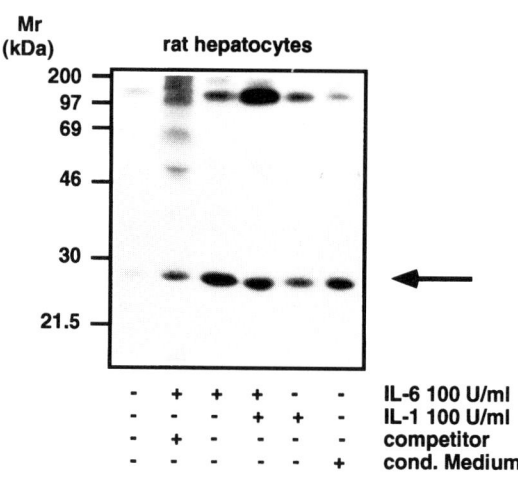

FIGURE 2. Immunoprecipitation of TIMP-1 from supernatants of rat hepatocytes in primary cultures. Rat hepatocyte primary cultures (4×10^6 cells per dish) were incubated in the presence of IL-1β, IL-6 and 1 ml of conditioned medium from LPS-stimulated human monocytes (1 μg/ml for 18 h) for 12 h before labeling with 200 μCi Tran[^{35}S]label in methionine/cysteine-free medium for 3 h. After 2 h of chasing supernatants were immunoprecipitated with murine-TIMP-1-antiserum A and analyzed by SDS-PAGE and fluorography. 100 ng of murine TIMP-1 expressed in *E. coli* was added as competitor before immunoprecipitation as indicated in the figure. The arrow indicates the position of TIMP-1.

So far, for the mouse or rat system no antisera have been described to detect the TIMP-1-protein. With the antiserum described in this study it will be possible to detect local changes in TIMP-1-protein expression in murine and rat models for tumor metastasis, fibrosis or pathological tissue breakdown like arthritis.

REFERENCES

1. DOCHERTY, A. J. P., J. O'CONNELL, T. CRABBE, S. ANGAL & G. MURPHY. 1992. Tibtech **10:** 200–207.
2. ROEB, E., L. GRAEVE, R. HOFFMANN, K. DECKER, D. R. EDWARDS & P. C. HEINRICH. 1993. Hepatology **18:** 1437–1442.
3. KORDULA, T., I. GUTGEMANN, S. ROSE-JOHN, E. ROEB, A. OSTHUES, H. TSCHESCHE, A. KOJ, P. C. HEINRICH & L. GRAEVE. 1992. FEBS Lett. **313:** 143–147.
4. MURAWAKI, Y., H. YAMAMOTO, H. KAWASAKI & H. SHIMA. 1993. Clin. Chim. Acta **218:** 47–58.

Changes in IL-6 Receptor Subunit mRNA Expression in Primary Mouse Hepatocyte Cultures and Murine and Rat Hepatoma Cell Lines

HANNA ROKITA, PIOTR PIERZCHALSKI, AND KRYSTYNA STALIŃSKA

Institute of Molecular Biology
Jagiellonian University
3, Mickiewicza Avenue
31-120 Kraków, Poland

The gp80 and gp130 encode the receptor subunits for interleukin-6 (IL-6).[1] The receptor systems for leukemia inhibitory factor (LIF), interleukin-11, oncostatin M, and ciliary neurotrophic factor employ gp130 as one of the subunits, which explains redundancy observed in the biological activities of the cytokines.[2,3] Our recent results on the mRNA expression of IL-6 receptor subunits in primary mouse hepatocyte cultures and murine and rat hepatoma cell lines are presented.

Primary cultures of mouse hepatocytes were prepared by the collagenase method from CBA mice. Murine hepatoma cell line, Hepa1b, and rat hepatoma cell line Fao, were obtained from Drs. G. Darlington and H. Baumann, respectively. Recombinant human IL-6 was the gift of Dr. P. C. Heinrich, IL-1β was provided by Dr. G. Wong through Dr. J. D. Sipe. LIF was kindly donated by Dr. H. Baumann and HGF by Dr. T. Nakamura. Total RNA was extracted from cultured cells using standard phenol-chloroform method and LiCl precipitation. Specific mRNAs were detected by hybridization at 65°C in 10% dextran sulfate, 1 M NaCl and 1% SDS, with EcoRI-BamHI fragment of the pMR301I (for murine gp80) and BamHI-BamHI fragment of the pSVLmgp130 (for murine gp130, both donated by Drs. T. Kishimoto and T. Taga) labeled with ^{32}P-dCTP by random priming. Equal loading with total RNA was verified by hybridization with human GAPDH (PstI digested pHcGAP).

In primary mouse hepatocyte cultures the amount of IL-6 binding subunit (gp80) mRNA does not change after LIF, IL-6 or IL-1 addition (FIG. 1A). Gp130 mRNA concentrations, not changed at 3 h, were upregulated by LIF and IL-1 at 24 hours. The ligand, IL-6, does not influence the mRNA of its receptor subunits. In the murine hepatoma cell line, Hepa 1b, interleukin-6 transiently, at 3 h, stimulated gp80 mRNA (FIG. 1B). Gp130 mRNA was slightly upregulated by IL-6 at 3 h and downregulated by IL-1. In the absence of dexamethasone, downregulation of gp130 mRNA is found.

In the rat hepatoma cell line, Fao, HGF in the presence of dexamethasone stimulated gp130 mRNA levels and higher molecular weight transcripts were found. HGF had no effect on gp80 mRNA (FIG. 2). IL-6 upregulated solely gp130 mRNA and in the presence of dexamethasone higher molecular weight transcripts were also found. In the other hepatoma cell line, H-35.19, no significant changes in the level of both receptor subunits mRNAs were observed (data not shown).

Thus, our results shows moderate effect of IL-6 in dexamethasone-dependent manner and are similar to findings by Schooltink in the human HepG2 cell line.[4]

A MOUSE HEPATOCYTES

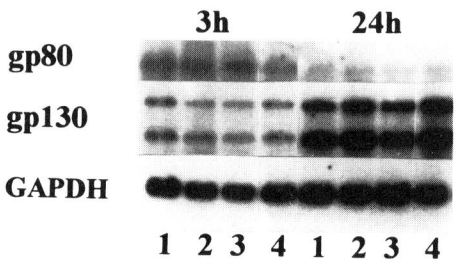

B MURINE HEPATOMA

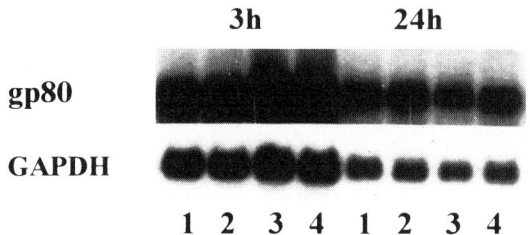

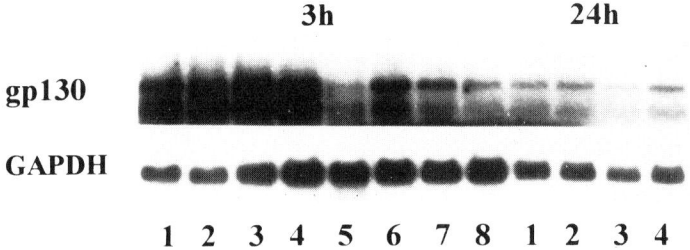

FIGURE 1. Northern blot analysis of IL-6 and LIF effects on gp80 mRNA and gp130 mRNA concentrations in CBA mice cultured hepatocytes (**A**) and the murine hepatoma cell line Hepa1b (**B**). **A:** *lane 1*—RNA from control cells; *lane 2*—LIF-treated cells; *lane 3*—IL-6-treated cells and *lane 4*—IL-1β-treated cells. **B:** *lane 1*—control cells; *lane 2*—LIF-treated; *lane 3*—IL-6-treated; *lane 4*—LIF plus IL-6-treated, 5—IL-1-treated, 6—IL-1 plus IL-6-treated, 7—IL-1 plus LIF-treated, and 8—control cells, without dexamethasone. Two species of gp130 mRNA (7 and 10 kb) are found in murine hepatocytes and the murine hepatoma cell line. Equal loading with 10 μg of RNA was verified by hybridization with GAPDH (glyceraldehyde phosphate dehydrogenase) cDNA probe.

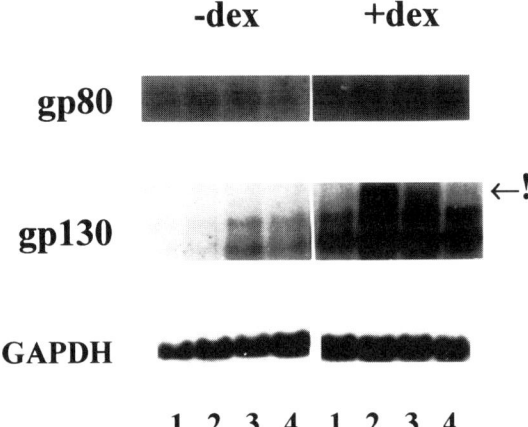

FIGURE 2. Northern blot analysis of IL-6, HGF and dexamethasone effects on interleukin-6 receptor subunits mRNA in the rat hepatoma cell line Fao. *Lane 1*—control cells; *lane 2*—HGF-treated cells (10 ng/ml); *lane 3*—IL-6-treated cells (50 ng/ml); and *lane 4*—HGF plus IL-6-treated cells. Dexamethasone concentration was 1 μM. (!)—higher molecular weight transcripts of gp130 mRNA.

REFERENCES

1. TAGA, T., M. HIBI, Y. HIRATA, K. YAMASAKI, K. YASUKAWA, T. MATSUDA & T. KISHIMOTO. 1989. Interleukin-6 triggers the association of its receptor with a possible signal transducer, gp130. Cell **58**: 573–581.
2. GEARING, D. P., M. R. COMEAU, D. J. FRIEND, S. D. GIMPEL, C. J. THUT, J. MCGOURTY, K. K. BASHER, J. A. KING, S. GILLIS, B. MOSLEY, S. F. ZIEGLER & D. COSMAN. 1992. The IL-6 signal transducer, gp130: An oncostatin M receptor and affinity converter for the LIF receptor. Science **255**: 1434–1437.
3. IP, N. Y., S. H. NYE, T. G. BOULTON, S. DAVIES, T. TAGA, Y. LI, S. J. BIRREN, K. YASUKAWA, T. KISHIMOTO, D. J. ANDERSON, N. STAHL & G. D. YANCOPOULOS. 1992. CNTF and LIF act on neuronal cells via shared signaling pathways that involve the IL-6 signal transducing receptor component gp130. Cell **69**: 1121–1132.
4. SCHOOLTINK, H., H. SCHMITZ-VAN DE LEUR, P. C. HEINRICH & S. ROSE-JOHN. 1992. Upregulation fo the interleukin-6-signal transducing protein (gp130) by interleukin-6 and dexamethasone in HepG2 cells. FEBS Lett. **297**: 263–265.

Diurnal Variations of Plasma Interleukin-6 in Man: Methodological Implications of Continuous Use of Indwelling Cannulae

WALTHER SEILER,[a] HILDEGARD MÜLLER,
AND CHRISTOPH HIEMKE

Department of Psychiatry
University of Mainz
Untere Zahlbacher Str. 8
D-55131 Mainz, Germany

Like other cytokines, interleukin-6 (IL-6) is currently attracting much attention. This and the constantly improving supply of commercially available cytokine assay kits have encouraged many nonimmunologists to work on possible links between their genuine area of research and the immune system. Following such an approach in a previous study, highly suspicious results of basal IL-6 time courses were found,[1] which prompted the present study.[2]

From six healthy volunteers (five males, one female, aged 28–45 years) blood was drawn from the antecubital vein into NH_4-heparinized monovettes. Sampling was performed at 0, 3, 6 and 9 h after cannula placement, using a static PVC-free indwelling Teflon cannula (Braun, Melsungen, Germany). At 9 h post cannula placement an additional sample was taken from the contra-lateral arm immediately after puncturing its antecubital vein. Plasma was separated (3000 × g, 15 min, 4°C) immediately and stored at −20°C until assayed. Levels of IL-6 were determined with an enzyme immunoassay (Quantikine, R&D Systems, Minneapolis, MN, USA). The manufacturer claims parallelism with the NIBSC/WHO interim standard 88/514 and that the assay is insensitive to the addition of the recombinant form of the IL-6 soluble receptor. The readings and the analyses were run on a PC-supported microtiter plate photometer (Titertek Multiskan MCC/340 MK II, Flow Lab., Meckenheim, Germany). The samples were processed in two analytical runs, with all samples of a particular subject included in the same assay. Intra- and inter-assay CVs were respectively below 5.0 and 8.0% for the concentration range used for calibration (0–100 ng/L). The detection limit was <0.4 ng/L.

Plasma IL-6 in samples withdrawn immediately after venipuncture were ≤0.5 ng/L. The subsequent time-dependent changes in plasma IL-6 after cannula placement were similar in all subjects, with a successive increase up to 2.4–15.3 ng/L after nine hours, equivalent to a 6- to 75-fold increase compared with initial values or with the detection limit, respectively. In contrast, IL-6 concentrations in plasma collected 9 h after cannula placement from the contra-lateral arm immediately after its puncturing were indistinguishable from the basal initial values (FIG. 1).

Since all blood samples of this study were processed in the same way, these results

---

[a] *Current address:* PAREXEL GmbH, Klinikum Westend, Spandauer Damm 130, D-14050 Berlin, Germany.

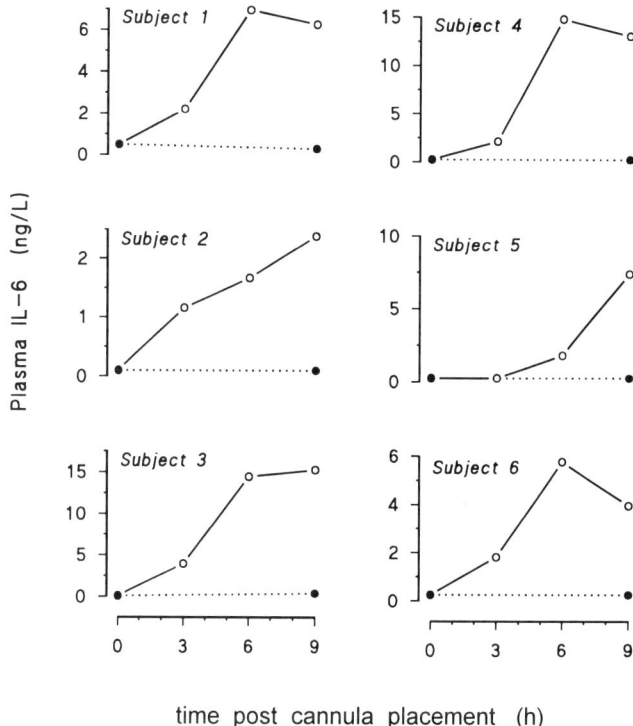

FIGURE 1. Interleukin-6 (IL-6) levels in plasma collected via two different sampling routes in six healthy volunteers: *Solid lines:* via a static indwelling cannula positioned up to 9 h before sampling; *Broken lines:* via cannula immediately after its positioning at 0 h or via newly puncturing the contra-lateral arm at 9 h. Note the different ordinate scales. Subject 5 was a woman, the others were men. (After reference 2.)

very likely reflected the *in vivo* situation rather than *ex vivo* or *in vitro* alterations post sampling (*e.g.* ref. 3). Hence, IL-6 concentrations found in plasma collected via the use of a static indwelling cannula for more than a short period reflected locally increased rather than systemically increased concentrations. The exact duration of this period, as well as the validity of the picture found in this study for other cytokines, is subject to assay sensitivities. Thus, the currently ongoing developments of ultrasensitive assays for cytokines (*e.g.* ref. 4) are likely to increase the demands imposed on data collection and interpretation in the area of immunological parameters. Reports on time courses of plasma IL-6 published so far (*e.g.* refs. 5 and 6) are likely to need re-evaluation. As long as the shortcomings of this sampling method remain unresolved, the use of static indwelling cannulae as the generally accepted method of choice to monitor time courses of blood derived parameters should be rejected for measurements of systemic profiles of IL-6 and possibly other cytokines. Repeated re-puncturing of the vein at an upstream site or of a different vessel might be a better, albeit harmful and inconvenient, way of obtaining reliable results.

Elucidation of the exact mechanism by which this increased IL-6 release was stimulated is beyond the scope of this paper. Nonetheless, the present results demonstrate that, even in the blood vessel system, drastically increased IL-6 levels can be maintained in a locally restricted area. The level of this regional focusing of protective activity undertaken by the immune system cannot be assessed on the basis of the present data.

REFERENCES

1. SEILER, W., H. MÜLLER, H. WETZEL, A. HILLERT & C. HIEMKE. 1993. Plasma levels of prolactin and interleukin-6 after acute neuroleptic doses—methodological implications of continuous use of indwelling catheter. Exp. Clin. Endocrinol. **101:** 165 (Abstract).
2. SEILER, W., H. MÜLLER & C. HIEMKE. 1994. Interleukin-6 in plasma collected with an indwelling cannula reflects local, not systemic, concentrations. Clin. Chem. **40:** 1778–1779.
3. THAVASU, P. W., S. LONGHURST, S. P. JOEL, M. L. SLEVIN & F. R. BALKWILL. 1992. Measuring cytokine levels in blood—Importance of anticoagulants, processing, and storage conditions. J. Immunol. Methods **153:** 115–124.
4. BRAILLY, H., F. A. MONTERO-JULIAN, C. E. ZUBER, S. FLAVETTA, J. GRASSI, F. HOUSSIAU & J. VAN SNICK. 1994. Total interleukin-6 in plasma measured by immunoassay. Clin. Chem. **40:** 116–123.
5. GUDEWILL, S., T. POLLMÄCHER, H. VEDDER, W. SCHREIBER, K. FASSBENDER & F. HOLSBOER. 1992. Nocturnal plasma levels of cytokines in healthy males. Eur. Arch. Psych. Clin. Neurosci. **242:** 53–56.
6. BAIGRIE, R. J., P. M. LAMONT, D. KWIATKOWSKI, M. J. DALLMAN & P. J. MORRIS. 1992. Systemic cytokine response after major surgery. Br. J. Surg. **79:** 767–780.

Stoichiometry of the Interleukin-6 High Affinity Receptor Complex

L. D. WARD,[a,c] G. J. HOWLETT,[b] A. HAMMACHER,[a] R. L. MORITZ,[b] AND R. J. SIMPSON[a]

[a]*Joint Protein Structure Laboratory*
Ludwig Institute for Cancer Research (Melbourne)
Walter and Eliza Hall Institute of Medical Research
Post Office Royal Melbourne Hospital
Parkville, Victoria 3050, Australia

[b]*The Department of Biochemistry*
The University of Melbourne
Parkville, Victoria 3052, Australia

Interleukin-6 (IL-6) is a poly functional cytokine that can have growth promoting, growth inhibiting, and differentiation effects depending on the nature of the target cell. IL-6 exerts these effects by binding to a specific cell surface receptor (IL-6R) which in turn promotes the association of the β- or signaling subunit gp-130.[1] Although IL-6 does not appear to bind to gp-130 in the absence of the IL-6R, gp-130 regulates the affinity status of the IL-6R. An extracellular or soluble form of the IL-6R (sIL-6R) when complexed with IL-6 can stimulate target cells lacking the IL-6R but expressing gp-130 suggesting that the IL-6R/IL-6 complex interacts with gp-130 through the extracellular domain.[1] Although gp-130 appears to homodimerize in the high affinity state,[2] the stoichiometry of IL-6 and the respective subunits in the complex are unknown. By purifying the soluble domains of IL-6R and gp-130 we have used a combination of size-exclusion chromatography and analytical ultra centrifugation to probe the stoichiometry of the high affinity signaling unit.[3]

Under the conditions employed IL-6, sIL-6R and sgp-130 were monomeric as judged by size-exclusion chromatography (FIG. 1) and analytical ultracentrifugation (TABLE 1). These values agree with those determined by SDS-PAGE but are higher than those calculated by amino acid composition. These data imply that the Chinese hamster ovary cell–derived proteins are glycosylated. The low affinity sIL-6R/IL-6 complex was determined by incubating the sIL-6R with molar excess of IL-6 and fractionating the complex by size-exclusion chromatography. Its molecular weight of 67,100 (TABLE 1) compares favorably with the predicted value of 71,500 if sIL-6R binds one IL-6 molecule.

Similarly, the high affinity IL-6 receptor complex was prepared by incubating sgp-130 with a molar excess of both sIL-6R and IL-6. The individual components were separated by size-exclusion chromatography. Three discrete peaks were observed (FIG. 1E), two being readily ascribed to IL-6 (14.44 min) and the IL-6·IL-6R complex (12.15 min), respectively. A higher M_r species, which corresponds to the IL-6·sIL-6R·sgp 130 complex, was also observed (elution volume, 9.16 min). When subjected to analytical ultracentrifugation (TABLE 1) this species yielded a molecular weight of 320,000.

[c] *Current Address:* AMRAD Biopharmaceutical Research Laboratory, 3 Guest Street, Hawthorn, Victoria 3122, Australia.

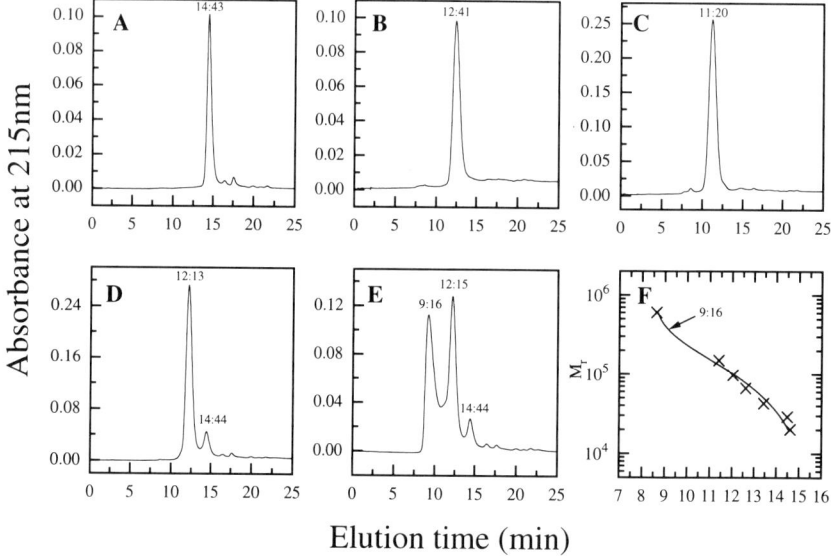

Elution time (min)

FIGURE 1. Size-exclusion chromatography of the low and high affinity IL-6 receptor complexes. Sample load, approximately 1–6 μg protein. The elution times, in minutes, are indicated for each protein peak. **A:** IL-6; **B:** sIL-6R; **C:** sgp-130; **D:** IL-6/sIL-6R complex; **E:** IL-6/sIL-6R/sgp-130 complex and **F:** Dependence of elution time upon apparent molecular weight (M_r) using standard proteins (soybean trypsin inhibitor, M_r 20,100; carbonic anhydrase, M_r 29,000; ovalbumin, M_r 42,700; bovine serum albumin, M_r 66,400; phosphorylase b, M_r 97,060; human immunoglobulin, M_r 150,000; thyroglobulin dimer, M_r 602,000). The elution position of the IL-6/sIL-6R/sgp-130 ternary complex (9:16 min) is indicated by the arrow. The theoretical relationship (indicated by solid line) was calculated assuming a linear response of M_r upon elution position.

TABLE 1. Determination of the Molecular Weights of IL-6, sIL-6R, the Low Affinity IL-6/sIL-6R Complex sgp-130 and the High Affinity IL-6/sIL-6R/sgp-130 Complex by Sedimentation Equilibrium[a]

Species	$M(1-\bar{V}\rho)$[b]	$\bar{V}$[c]	Molecular Weight[d]	Predicted Molecular Weight[e]
IL-6	5960	0.72	21,300	
sIL-6R	15500	0.69	50,200	
sIL-6R + IL-6	20220	0.70	67,400	71,500
sgp-130	23610	0.71	81,400	
sgp-130 + sIL-6R + IL-6	96070	0.70	320,000	305,800

[a] All analyses were performed in PBS buffer containing 0.02% Tween-20.
[b] Values of $M(1-\bar{V}\rho)$ were determined from sedimentation equilibrium data.
[c] The value of $\bar{V}$ for IL-6 was calculated from the amino acid composition. The values of $\bar{V}$ for sIL-6R and sgp-130 were calculated as described previously[4] using the amino acid composition, sedimentation equilibrium data and an assigned value of 0.61 ml/g for the carbohydrate component. Values of $\bar{V}$ for the complexes were calculated on the basis of zero volume change on association and assuming equimolar ratios of the components.
[d] M_W values are calculated from the measured values of $M(1-\bar{V}\rho)$ and the assigned values of $\bar{V}$.
[e] The predicted molecular weights are calculated from the molecular weights of the individual components. For the high affinity IL-6/sgp-130/sIL-6R complex a stoichiometry of 2 has been assumed for each component.

Both the sedimentation equilibrium and size-exclusion chromatographic studies support a model where the high affinity complex consists of two molecules of each sgp-130, IL-6 and sIL-6R, that is, two IL-6·IL-6R·gp-130 complexes homodimerize in the high affinity state (theoretical molecular weight, 305,800). In contrast, a model where a single IL-6·sIL-6R complex induces the homodimerization of gp-130 leads to a molecular weight of only 234,300. This is the first direct demonstration of a higher order arrangement for receptor cytokine interactions that exhibit both high and low affinity complexes.

REFERENCES

1. AKIRA, S. *et al.* 1993. Advances Immunol. **54:** 1–78.
2. MURAKAMI, M. *et al.* 1993. Science **260:** 1808–1810.
3. WARD, L. D. *et al.* 1994. J. Biol. Chem. **269:** 23286–23289.
4. WARD, L. D. *et al.* 1995. Biochemistry. **34:** 2901–2907.

Interleukin-6 Serum Levels in Depressed Patients before and after Treatment with Fluoxetine

A. SŁUŻEWSKA,[a,b,e] J. K. RYBAKOWSKI,[a] M. LACIAK,[c]
A. MACKIEWICZ,[c] M. SOBIESKA,[d] AND K. WIKTOROWICZ[d]

[a]Department of Psychiatry
Medical Academy
Bydgoszcz, Poland

[b]Department of Pharmacology
[c]Department of Cancer Immunology
[d]Department of Rheumatology and Immunology
University School of Medicine
Poznań, Poland 61-701

Major depression may be accompanied by many alterations in cell-mediated and humoral immunity. Of the various acute phase proteins (APPs) measured in depression, the most prominent changes were found in the serum levels of haptoglobin,[1] and α_1-acid glycoprotein (AGP);[2,3] and there were also alterations in AGP microheterogeneity.[3] Interleukin-6 (IL-6) is the major immune and inflammatory mediator and plays a key role in human APPs synthesis. This interleukin has been reported to be elevated in depression.[4,5]

In this study we have observed changes in serum levels of IL-6 as well as levels of C-reactive protein (CRP), AGP and its microheterogeneity (AGP-RC) in 22 inpatients from Department of Psychiatry in Bydgoszcz, before and after treatment with fluoxetine 20 mg daily (TABLE 1). The length of the study was 8 weeks. Diagnosis were assessed according to DSM-III-R criteria: MDD UP—100%. Patients who had been treated with antidepressants before hospitalization were withdrawn for all drugs for at least 7 days prior to the studies. They were medically healthy as screened by physical examination. Patients were free of chronic illnesses known to affect the immune status and of acute infections or allergic reactions for at least 2 weeks prior to the study. Blood samples and clinical status: Hamilton Depression Rating Scale (HDRS) 17 item version were performed before and after 8 weeks treatment with fluoxetine. IL-6 concentration (pg/ml) in serum was determined using enzyme-linked immunosorbent assay (ELISA), concentrations of CRP and AGP were measured by rocket immunoelectrophoresis and reactivity coefficient of its microheterogeneity—AGP-RC by crossed-affinity immunoelectrophoresis (CAIE) with free Con A as a ligand. At baseline elevated IL-6 serum levels were found in 6 out of 22 depressives. IL-6 levels did not show correlations with the severity of depression. Patients with elevated IL-6 levels compared with the remaining ones also had increased AGP serum levels (1391 ± 350 mg/l vs 1151 ± 338 mg/l), lower values of AGP-RC (1.12 ± 0.35 vs 1.34 ± 0.30) and higher CRP levels.

No correlations between the severity of depression and AGP levels was observed

---

[e] Address correspondence to Dr. Służewska at the Department of Pharmacology.

TABLE 1. Clinical and Laboratory Data of Depressed Patients with Elevated and Non-elevated IL-6 Levels and in Healthy Control Subjects

	Patients with Elevated IL-6 Levels (n = 6)	Patients with Non-elevated IL-6 Levels (n = 16)	Healthy Controls (n = 11)
Gender M/F	0/6	2/14	3/8
Age (years)	40.6 ± 2.5	42.5 ± 6.4	39.2 ± 4.2
HDRS	24.6 ± 2.8	22.7 ± 3.5	
IL-6 (pg/ml)	17.4 ± 5.5[b,d]	1.34 ± 0.3	1.26 ± 0.32
AGP (mg/l)	1391 ± 350[d]	1151 ± 338	757 ± 104
AGP-RC	1.12 ± 0.35	1.34 ± 0.3	1.35 ± 0.24
CRP (mg/l)	13.8 ± 3.6[a,b]	6.8 ± 2.1	5.0 ± 1.0
Monocytes (10^9/l)	0.42 ± 0.12[a,c]	0.26 ± 0.06	0.28 ± 0.05

All results are expressed as mean (±SD)
Difference vs patients with non-elevated IL-6 significant: [a] $p < 0.05$, [b] $p < 0.001$. (Mann Whitney test).
Difference vs healthy controls significant: [c] $p < 0.05$, [d] $p < 0.001$. (Mann Whitney test).

(TABLE 2). Eight weeks of treatment with fluoxetine resulted in decreased concentration of IL-6 and AGP. During the treatment with fluoxetine we have observed normalization of pathological glycosylation profiles to the profiles observed in the healthy controls. Whether or not IL-6 may be involved in the pathogenesis of depression remains to be elucidated.

CONCLUSIONS

The results obtained may suggest that fluoxetine treatment resulted in normalization of pathologically elevated IL-6 and AGP levels and in AGP-RC glycosylation profiles.

TABLE 2. Studied Laboratory Data in Depressed Patients Treated with Fluoxetine 20 mg Daily

	Patients with Elevated IL-6 Levels (n = 6)		Patients with Non-elevated IL-6 Levels (n = 16)	
	Before	After 8 Weeks of Treatment	Before	After 8 Weeks of Treatment
IL-6 (pg/ml)	17.4 ± 5.5	1.24 ± 0.1**	1.34 ± 0.3	1.13 ± 0.3
AGP (mg/l)	1391 ± 350	917 ± 186*	1151 ± 338	922 ± 248
AGP-RC	1.12 ± 0.35	1.24 ± 0.22	1.34 ± 0.3	1.25 ± 0.31
Monocytes (10^9/l)	0.42 ± 0.12	0.31 ± 0.14*	0.26 ± 0.06	0.25 ± 0.07

All results are expressed as mean (±SD).
Difference between before and after treatment significant: * $p < 0.05$, ** $p < 0.001$ (Wilcoxon test).

REFERENCES

1. MAES, M., J. DELANGHE, S. SCHARPE, H. Y. MELTZER, P. COSNYS, E. SUY & E. BOSMANS. 1994. Haptoglobin phenotypes and gene frequencies in unipolar depression. Am. J. Psychiatry **151**(1): 112–116.
2. NEMEROFF, CH. B., R. R. KRISHNAN, D. G. BLAZER, D. KNIGHT, D. BENJAMIN & L. R. MEZERSON. 1990. Elevated plasma concentration of alpha-1-acid glycoprotein, putatitve endogenous inhibitor of tritiated imipramine binding site in depressed patients. Arch. Gen. Psychiat. **47**: 337–340.
3. SŁUŻEWSKA, A., J. K. RYBAKOWSKI, M. SOBIESKA & K. WIKTOROWICZ. 1993. Altered microheterogeneity of alpha-1-acid glycoprotein in endogenous depression. Eur. Neuropsychopharmacol. **3**: 342–343.
4. FRONBERGER, U., P. HASELBAUER, A. FRAULIN, J. BAUER & M. BERGER. 1994. Interleukin-6 (IL-6) serum levels in depression and schizophrenie. *In* Proceedings of C.I.N.P. Workshop—Critical Issues in the Treatment of Affective Disorders. Paris 1994: 123. Basel: S. Karger A. G.
5. MAES, M., H. Y. MELTZER & E. BOSMANS. Immune alterations in major depression: Increased plasma concentrations of interleukin-6, soluble interleukin-6, soluble interleukin-2 and transferrin receptors. In press.

Possible Relationship between Interleukin-6 and Response of Immunoglobulin E to Surgical Trauma

ANDREW SZCZEKLIK,[a,c] JACEK JAWIEŃ,[a] BEDA M. STADLER,[b]
JADWIGA RADWAN,[a] WIESŁAWA PIWOWARSKA,[c] AND
ANTONI DZIATKOWIAK[d]

[a]*Department of Medicine*
[c]*Department of Coronary Disease*
[d]*Department of Cardiac Surgery*
Jagiellonian University School of Medicine
Kraków, Poland

[b]*Institute for Clinical Immunology*
Inselspital
Bern, Switzerland

We have recently observed[1] that acute myocardial infarction is associated with an immunological response characterized by a consistent pattern of change in serum IgE. We wondered whether this response is specific for myocardial infarction or whether it reflects a more generalized phenomenon, perhaps triggered by tissue injury. We, therefore, made a prospective study on patients undergoing various surgical procedures, including coronary artery bypasses.

PATIENTS

We studied 116 surgical patients (35 women, 81 men, age range 24–75 years, mean 55 years). They were divided into 3 groups:

Group A

Patients undergoing coronary artery bypass graft operations (CABG) who developed perioperative myocardial infarction (PMI)—(31 men and 8 women, average age 56 years).

Group B

Patients subjected to coronary artery bypass grafting who did not develop PMI (10 women and 32 men, mean age 58 years).

---

[c] Address correspondence to Dr. Szczeklik at the Department of Medicine, Jagiellonian University School of Medicine, Skawinska Str. 8, 31-066 Kraków, Poland; Tel: (0048 12) 56-28-40; FAX (0048 12) 56-57-86.

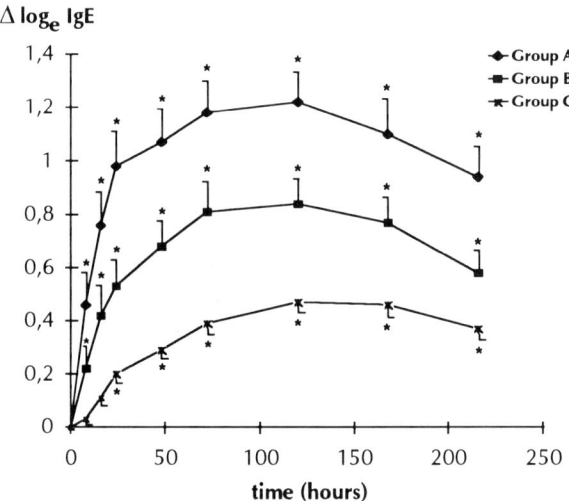

FIGURE 1. Behavior of IgE in three studied groups, expressed as the increase of the logarithmically transformed geometric means ± SEM, in relation to the initial levels. (Group A—CABG with PMI; Group B—CABG without PMI; Group C—abdominal surgery.) $*p < 0.05$, compared to the initial level; analysis by paired t-test for the logarithmically transformed values.

Group C

Patients undergoing abdominal surgery operations: cholecystectomy or repair of inguinal hernia (17 women and 18 men, mean age 53 years).

METHODS

Blood samples were drawn by venipuncture before the operation and then after the operation at the following times: 8 hours, 16 h, 24 h, 48 h, 72 h, 120 h (the fifth day), 168 h (the seventh day), and 216 h (the ninth day). In all samples concentrations of serum immunoglobulins E, G, A and M were determined using nephelometry (Behring, Germany). Serum levels of interleukins 4, 6 and interferon-γ were measured by ELISA (Genzyme Diagnostics, USA) in the same series of 9 blood samples obtained from 20 randomly selected patients subjected to coronary artery bypasses.

RESULTS

Mean serum IgE level increased gradually after the operations, becoming significantly different from pre-operative values at 8 h in groups A and B, and at 24 h in group C. It reached a peak by day 5 and then began gradually to decline. The most pronounced increase was observed in group A, followed by group B, and finally C (FIG. 1).

This behavior of IgE serum level was in striking contrast to that of the remaining

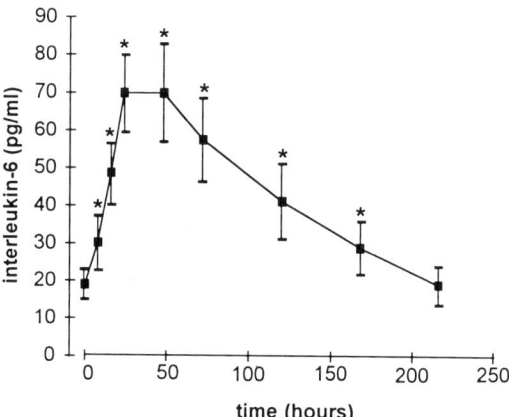

FIGURE 2. Behavior of interleukin-6 in the group of 20 patients undergoing coronary artery bypass graft, before and after operation, expressed as the arithmetic means ± SD. $*p < 0.05$, compared to the initial level; analysis by paired t-test.

serum immunoglobulins which showed a rapid fall after surgical interventions, followed by a gradual return to the initial values. Serum interleukin 6 increased early after cardiac surgery, reaching peak values 24 hours after trauma and returning to the initial level on the ninth postoperative day (FIG. 2). Serum interleukin 4 levels were undetectable in our patients, whereas serum levels of interferon-γ were very low, and did not change significantly.

DISCUSSION

We describe a general humoral immune response to tissue injury. The change in serum IgE was the hallmark of the response. Serum level of this immunoglobulin is known to be fairly constant in individual subjects. In our patients the serum level was very characteristic: it began to rise after surgical operations, continued to increase over the following days, reached a peak by the fifth day, and then gradually declined. It was, however, in contrast to other serum immunoglobulins which shortly after the operation became markedly depressed and subsequently took over a week to return to the initial values. Endogenous IL-6, the levels of which increased dramatically in our patients, is critical for induction of IgE synthesis by hydrocortisone and IL-4; *in vitro* anti-IL-6 antibody strongly inhibits IgE production by hydrocortisone and IL-4 (2). We hypothesize that the stimulation of hypothalamus—adrenal axis and/or release of glucocorticosteroids, interacting with newly synthesized interleukin-6, could explain the complex and characteristic immunological response to tissue injury.

REFERENCES

1. SZCZEKLIK, A., K. SLADEK, A. SZCZERBA & J. DROPINSKI. 1988. Serum immunoglobulin E response to myocardial infarction. Circulation 77: 1245–1249.
2. JABARA, H. H., D. J AHERN, D. VERCELLI & R. S. GEHA. 1991. Hydrocortisone and IL-4 induce IgE isotype switching in human B cells. J. Immunol. 147: 1557–1560.

Molecular Cloning and Functional Expression of Mouse cDNAs Encoding the Membrane Receptor and the Soluble Receptor for D-Factor/LIF

MIKIO TOMIDA

Saitama Cancer Center Research Institute
818 Komuro, Ina
Saitama 362, Japan

We and others have previously shown that the soluble differentiation stimulating (D)-factor/LIF (leukemia inhibitory factor) receptor is present in normal mouse serum and that it increases in the late stages of pregnancy.[1,2] In the present study, we isolated three different cDNAs for D-factor/LIF receptor from a cDNA library prepared from the liver of a pregnant mouse.[3] The mouse cDNA encoding the membrane receptor (MDR in FIG. 1) had a marked homology with its human counterpart. A second form of cDNA with a 501 bp insertion was isolated (MSDR2). The insertion introduced a stop codon (TAA) so that the mRNA encoded the soluble receptor lacking transmembrane and intracellular domains. Because the insertion contained polyadenylation signals, two different sizes of mRNA encoding the soluble receptor were produced, dependent on signal utilization. Transcripts utilizing these signals were 3 kb in size (MSDR1), and were very abundantly present in the liver, but not detectable in other tissues examined. The pregnancy-related change in the expression of the 3 kb mRNA in the liver was parallel with the change in the level of the D-factor-binding protein in the mouse serum.[4] These results suggest that the liver is the primary source of the circulating soluble receptor for D-factor/LIF.

Next, cDNAs encoding the D-factor/LIF receptor and the soluble receptor were expressed in COS-7 cells (TABLE 1). Specific binding of [^{125}I]D-factor/LIF to COS-7 cells increased 80-fold after transfection of the cDNA (MDR) into the cells. On the other hand, recombinant soluble receptors were prepared by transfection of the cDNA (MSDR1) into the cells. Conditioned medium from the transfected cells competed with the binding of human [^{125}I]D-factor/LIF to COS-7/MDR cells and mouse myeloid leukemia M1-T22 cells. Binding of the soluble receptor to human D-factor/LIF and mouse D-factor/LIF was examined by the polyethylene glycol precipitation

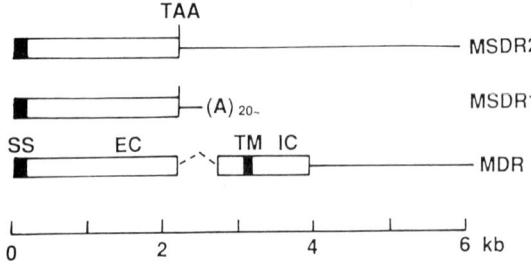

FIGURE 1. Schematic representation of three different cDNAs encoding mouse D-factor/LIF receptor. SS, signal sequence; EC, extracellular region; TM, transmembrane domain; IC, intracellular region.

TABLE 1. Expression of D-Factor/LIF Receptor cDNA and the Soluble Receptor cDNA in COS-7 Cells

Cells	Competitors	^{125}I-D-Factor–bound (cpm)
COS-7	None	4,079
COS-7	D-factor/LIF	2,078
COS-7/MDR	None	163,937
COS-7/MDR	D-factor/LIF	3,257
COS-7/MDR	Control CM (25%)	150,565
COS-7/MDR	MSDR CM (25%)	9,273
M1-T22	None	6,324
M1-T22	D-factor/LIF	371
M1-T22	MSDR CM (5%)	1,157
M1-T22	Mouse serum (0.4%)	379

COS-7 cells were transfected with a plasmid containing mouse D-factor/LIF receptor cDNA(MDR) or the soluble receptor cDNA(MSDR1). After 3 days, these COS-7 cells expressing MDR(COS-7/MDR) were incubated with human [^{125}I]D-factor/LIF in the absence or presence of competitors. The competitors were 50-fold excess of unlabeled D-factor/LIF, conditioned medium (CM) from untreated COS-7 cells and CM from the COS-7 cells transfected with MSDR1. M1-T22 cells were incubated with human [^{125}I]D-factor/LIF in the presence of serum from a pregnant mouse.

method and analyzed by the Scatchard plot. Strangely however, the affinity of mouse soluble receptor to human D-factor/LIF is 50 times higher than that to mouse D-factor/LIF. The dissociation constants of the soluble receptor for human D-factor/LIF and mouse D-factor/LIF are 267 pM and 12 nM, respectively.[5] These values are consistent with those of the D-factor-binding protein in the mouse serum.[1] The result supports that the binding protein in the serum is a soluble D-factor/LIF receptor. The mouse soluble receptors are able to compete effectively with the binding of human [^{125}I]D-factor/LIF to high-affinity cellular receptors (TABLE 1). Although the affinity of the soluble receptor to mouse D-factor/LIF is low, concentration of the soluble receptor in the mouse serum is very high (10^{13} molecules/ml). Therefore, the soluble receptor may block the systemic effect of locally produced D-factor/LIF. Alternatively, it may have a role as the carrier protein for D-factor/LIF *in vivo*.

REFERENCES

1. YAMAGUCHI-YAMAMOTO, Y., M. TOMIDA & M. HOZUMI. 1993. Pregnancy associated increase in differentiation-stimulating factor (D-factor)/leukemia inhibitory factor (LIF)-binding substance(s) in mouse serum. Leukemia Res. **17**: 515–522.
2. LAYTON, M. J., B. A. CROSS, D. METCALF, L. D. WARD, R. J. SIMPSON & N. A. NICOLA. 1992. A major binding protein for leukemia inhibitory factor in normal mouse serum: Identification as a soluble form of the cellular receptor. Proc. Natl. Acad. Sci. USA **89**: 8616–8620.
3. TOMIDA, M., Y. YAMAMOTO-YAMAGUCHI & M. HOZUMI. 1994. Three different cDNAs encoding mouse D-factor/LIF receptor. J. Biochem. **115**: 557–562.
4. TOMIDA, M., Y. YAMAMOTO-YAMAGUCHI & M. HOZUMI. 1993. Pregnancy associated increase in mRNA for soluble D-factor/LIF receptor in mouse liver. FEBS Lett. **334**: 193–197.
5. TOMIDA, M. 1995. Analysis of recombinant soluble mouse D-factor/LIF receptor. J. Biochem. **117**: 1228–1231.

Monoclonal Antibodies Define Different Functional Epitopes on gp130 Signal Transducer

SYLVIE CHEVALIER,[a] CLAUDE CLEMENT,[b]
OLIVIER ROBLEDO,[a] BERNARD KLEIN,[c] HUGUES GASCAN,[a]
AND JOHN WIJDENES[b]

[a]*INSERM U298*
CHRU Angers
49033 Angers Cedex, France

[b]*INNOTHERAPIE*
1 Bd. Fleming
25020 Besançon, France

[c]*Institut de Génetique Moléculaire*
BP 5051
34033 Montpellier, France

INTRODUCTION

Il-6, Il-11, OSM, CNTF and LIF belong to the same family of cytokines displaying some rundancies in their biological properties. This is partially explained by the common use of gp130 protein transducer as a part of their receptors.[1] In addition to gp130, LIF receptor/gp190 is also involved in the composition of the common OSM/LIF receptor and CNTF receptor.[2] In this latest case a third specific binding subunit is required to generate a high affinity CNTF receptor.[3] We have generated monoclonal antibodies directed against gp130 and analyzed their functional potentialities.

MATERIALS AND METHODS

Balb/c mice were immunized with soluble gp130 and the Baf/3 cell line stably transfected with a cDNA encoding for human gp130. Spleen cells were fused to the X63 myeloma according to the conventional protocols, and the IgG-producing clones screened for specific antibody production. For soluble gp130 ELISAs, antibodies were coated at a concentration of 10 μg/ml, and after a overnight incubation of the samples, the biotinylated detector antibody was added at 1 μg/ml for 4 h, followed by an avidin peroxydase step and visualization with ABTS. Immunofluorescence competion experiments were performed following the usual procedures and the cells analyzed on a Facscan. The TF1 and A375 proliferation assays were carried out by incubating the cells in the presence of serial dilutions of antibodies and a saturating concentration of cytokine. After 60 h, or 96 h for A375, the cells were pulsed with ^{3}H-thymidine and the incorporated radioactivity determined. Hep-G2 hepatoma cells were plated in the presence of 10^{-6}M dexamethasone, saturating concentrations of cytokines and serial dilutions of antibodies. After 24 h, the conditioned media were harvested and tested for their haptoglobin concentration by ELISA.

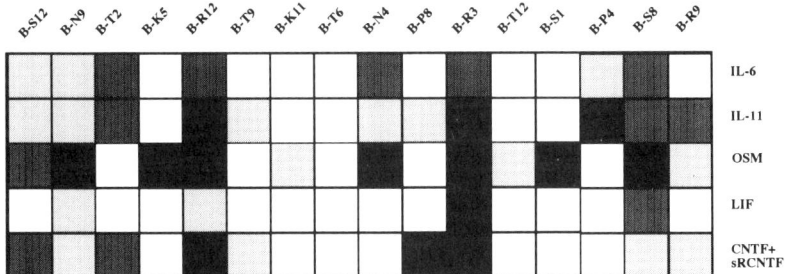

FIGURE 1. Inhibition of TF1 cell line proliferation by different anti-gp130 antibodies in response to IL-6, IL-11, OSM, LIF, and CNTF + soluble CNTF receptor. The TF1 cell line was plated at a concentration of 15×10^3 cells per well in RPMI containing 10% FCS and fixed concentration of Il-6 (20 ng/ml), Il-11 (100 ng/ml), OSM, (10 ng/ml). LIF (50 ng/ml), or CNTF (20 ng/ml) plus soluble CNTf receptor (100 ng/ml). Serial dilutions of antibodies were added in triplicate in the assay and the cells incubated for 72 h. 0.5 μCi 3HTdr were added in each well for the last 4 h of the culture and the incorporated radioactivity determined. The table summarizes the inhibition of proliferation observed for an antibody concentration of 50 μg/ml *(light grey)*, 10 μg/ml *(dark grey)*, 2 μg/ml *(black)*, or the absence of blocking effect in the presence of 50 μg/ml of antibody *(white)*.

RESULTS AND DISCUSSION

Among more than 30 generated antibodies, 16 of them were selected and analyzed by competition and blocking studies. Competition experiments analyzed by Facs defined 4 major epitopes on gp130. Two of the epitopes were consistent with the results obtained by performing bioassays on the TF1, A375 and Hep-G2 cell lines. The B-R3 type antibodies blocked all the biological responses independently of the cytokine added in the assay or the test cell lines used (FIG. 1). The B-K5 type antibodies

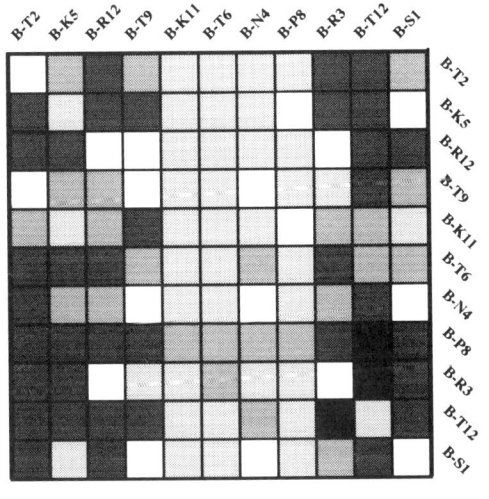

FIGURE 2. Detection of soluble gp130 by ELISA. Antibodies were coated in 100 mM carbonate buffer, pH 9.6 for 6 h at a concentration of 10 μg/ml. After saturation with 0.1 M Tris, 20% sucrose, pH 7.7, serial dilutions of a pool of human sera were incubated overnight at 4°C. After washes, the biotinylated detector antibodies were added at a concentration of 1 μg/ml for 4 h. Detection was achieved by using the avidin-peroxydase system, and ABTS as substrate. In *black:* detectable signal for 10^{-3} dilution; *dark grey:* detectable signal for 10^{-2} dilution; *light grey:* detectable signal for 10^{-1} dilution; *white:* no detectable signal.

interfered only with the OSM response of the TF1, A375 and HepG2 cell lines, but did not affect the biological properties of Il-6, Il-11, LIF or CNTF. Beside these two groups of antibodies, the biological assays defined close, but different subgroups which did not exactly fit with the competing experiment performed by Facs. The B-P8 antibody mainly affect the CNTF responses; whereas the B-P4 specifically abrogated the Il-11 driven proliferation of the TF1 line, without affecting any other response. Non-inhibiting antibodies which did not interfere with the receptor activations, such as B-T6, were also generated. We have also developed an ELISA to detect a circulating form of gp130 in human serum. A combination of the B-R3, as coating antibody and B-T12 as indicator antibody, still allowed the detection of soluble gp130 at a 1/1,000 dilution of normal human serum, with a limit of sensitivity of 20 pg/ml (FIG. 2). Interestingly, we analyzed the circulating levels of gp130 in sera of patients suffering of multiple myeloma or septic shock, where soluble Il-6 receptor levels were increased, but we failed to observe any significant variation of circulating gp130 when compared to the normal values. In summary, our results indicate that gp130/Il-6 transducer displays several functional epitopes implicated in its homodimerization or interactions with different receptor subunits and ligands.

REFERENCES

1. KISHIMOTO, T., S. AKIRA, T. TAGA. 1992. Science **258**: 593.
2. GEARING, D. P., S. F. ZIEGLER, M. R. COMEAU, et al. 1994. Proc. Natl. Acad. Sci. USA **91**: 1119.
3. DAVIS, S., T. H. ALDRICH, N. Y. IP, M. STAHL, S. SCHERER, T. FARRUGGELLA, P. S. DISTEFANO, R. CURTIS, N. PANAYOTATOS, H. GASCAN, S. CHEVALIER, G. D. YANCOPOULOS. 1993. Science **259**: 1665.

Functional Reconstitution of IL-6 Signaling in a Myeloid Leukemic Cell Line[a]

P. WULF, R. P. PIEKORZ, AND G. M. HOCKE

Department of Genetics
University of Erlangen-Nürnberg
Staudtstrasse 5
D-91058 Erlangen, Germany

Reactions controlled by cytokines of the interleukin 6 (IL-6) family play an important role in the control of hematopoesis. A key characteristic of leukemic cells is a block at an intermediate stage of differentiation in conjunction with aberrant proliferation and a loss of responsiveness to inducers of differentiation.[1] It had previously been reported, that the murine myeloid leukemic cell line M1 can be induced to differentiate in culture by treatment with IL-6–type cytokines. An important question was, whether this effect is unique for M1 cells or a general property of a majority of myeloid leukemic cells. Therefore, a significant number of independently established murine myeloid leukemic cell lines were investigated. Surprisingly, the M1 line was unique in this response (Piekorz, Hocke *et al.*, unpublished data). Consequently, we asked, whether the non-responsiveness to IL-6 of the other lines was due to a loss of the IL-6 receptor or another component of the IL-6–signal cascade. The receptor consists of two different subunits: a gp80 ligand-binding chain and a gp130 signal-transducer chain.[2]

The murine myeloblastic C cell line established by transformation with Friends Murine Leukemia Virus (F-MuLV) was provided by Dr. Brigitte Sola, Paris.[3] It had been shown, that this line did not respond to IL-6 treatment. Northern blot analysis revealed that the cells from this line contained greatly reduced levels of gp80 mRNA (Piekorz, Hocke *et al.*, unpublished data). Therefore the question was asked, whether in this line the reduced expression of gp80 mRNA was the sole cause of the observed non-responsiveness to IL-6. If so, then transfection of expression constructs for gp80 would be expected to functionally reconstitute the response to IL-6 in this cell line. Thus, IL-6–nonresponsive C-cells were co-transfected with an expression construct pcDLSRα296RIL6RC.21.ex for rat gp80[4] and the neomycin (G418) resistance plasmid pRSVneo at a ratio of 10:1. Transfection was performed by electroporation and mRNA from mass cultured stable subclones was prepared for Northern blot analysis. Subclone CSK3 of the C cell line displayed successful expression of exogenous gp80 mRNA (FIG. 1).

Consequently, CSK3 cells were tested for response to IL-6, in order to evaluate the functional reconstitution of the IL6 signal cascade. Their proliferation was blocked by addition of IL-6 (FIG. 2).

In summary, the IL-6-nonresponsive murine myeloid leukemic C cell line displayed reduced mRNA levels, which were the main cause of their observed non-responsive-

---

[a] This work was supported by a research grant from Deutsche Forschungsgemeinschaft (DFG) awarded to G. M. Hocke (Hi 291/5-4 TP6).

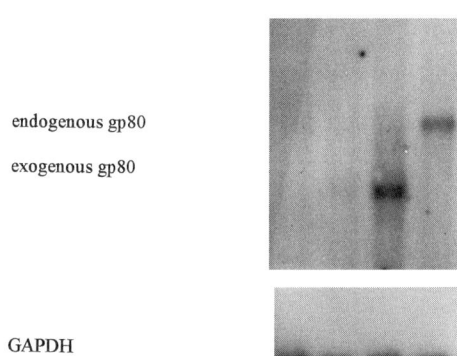

FIGURE 1. Expression of mRNA for the transfected rat IL-6 receptor ligand binding chain. Northern blot analysis with RNA from the subclone CSK3 of cell line C demonstrated successful expression of exogenous gp80 mRNA; CMK: pool of C cells transfected with gp80 cDNA after 14 days of selection in G418, prior to subcloning; C-: recipient C-cell line transfected with expression vector without insert. Hybridization Probes: *top panel:* radio-labeled cDNA for murine gp80; *bottom panel:* cDNA for rat glycerol-aldehyde-3-phosphate dehydrogenase (GAPDH) as a loading control.

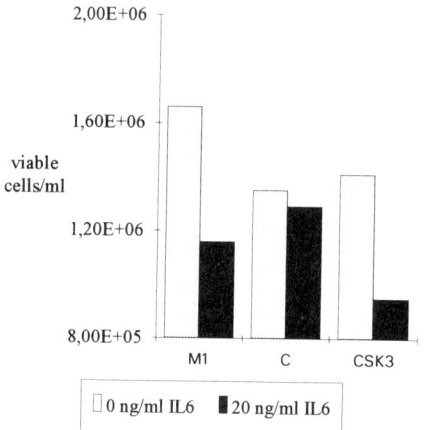

FIGURE 2. Functional reconstitution of IL6 signaling. Cells were treated with 0 or 20 ng/ml of purified recombinant murine IL-6 (Gibco). After 92 hours the number of viable cells was counted (trypan blue exclusion) in duplicate culture wells. Treatment of responsive cells led to decreased proliferation as shown for the M1 standard line *(left two bars)*. The C cell line was non-responsive to IL-6 *(middle two bars)*, whereas the reconstituted line CSK3 showed a decrease in its rate of proliferation *(right two bars)*.

ness to IL-6. Substitution of the missing gp80 mRNA by transfection, successfully reconstituted the IL-6-response in this cell line.

The successful reconstitution of the C-line opens the possibility of a broader use of differentiation induction by triggering the cascade through gp130.

REFERENCES

1. SACHS, L., 1990. The proteins that control haemopoesis and leukaemia. Ciba Foundation Symposium. **148:** 5–24.

2. KISHIMOTO, T., T. TAGA & S. AKIRA. 1994. Cytokine signal transduction. Cell **76:** 253–262.
3. SOLA, B., S. FICHELSON, D. BORDEAUX, P. TAMBOURIN & S. GISSELBRECHT. 1986. Fim1 and fim2: Two new integration regions of Friend Murine Leukemia Virus in myeloblastic leukemias. J. Virol. **60:** 718–725.
4. BAUMANN, M., H. BAUMANN & G. FEY. 1990. Molecular cloning, characterisation and functional expression of the rat liver interleukin 6 receptor. J. Biol. Chem. **256:** 19853–19862.

Lesion-induced Interleukin-6 mRNA Expression in Rat Sciatic Nerve

JIAN ZHONG AND ROLF HEUMANN

Molecular Neurobiochemistry
Ruhr University Bochum
D-44780 Bochum, Germany

INTRODUCTION

Interleukin-6 (IL-6) is an acute phase protein coordinating the immune activities of liver cells, macrophages, and lymphocytes.[1] In addition, IL-6 promotes fiber outgrowth in NGF-responsive PC12 cells[2] and shares the receptor subunit gp130 with ciliary neurotrophic factor (CNTF).[3] We are therefore investigating whether IL-6 may play a role in peripheral nerve development and regeneration. In the present study we have demonstrated IL-6 mRNA expression *in vitro* and *in vivo* in response to peripheral nerve injury.

METHODS

For the *in vitro* studies sciatic nerves from adult Wistar rats were dissected and placed in 1 ml of Eagle's basal medium without serum and incubated at 37°C in 10% CO_2. For the *in vivo* studies the rats were anesthesized and the sciatic nerve cut unilaterally with fine scissors at the sciatic notch.[4] After various time intervals the

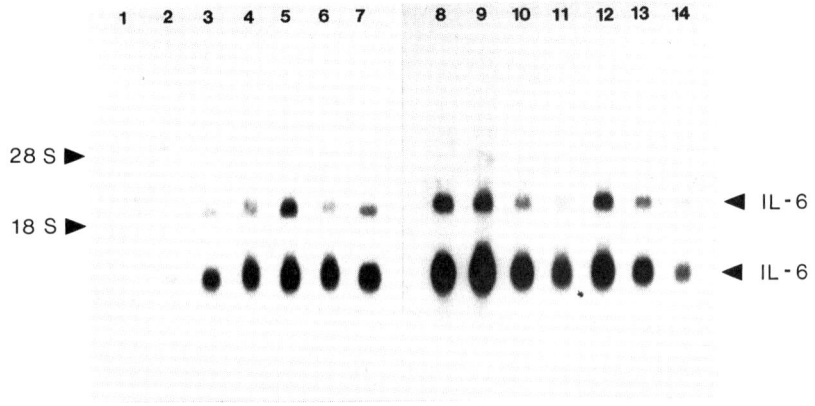

FIGURE 1. Induction of IL-6 mRNA in organ culture. Northern blot showing IL-6 mRNA at selected time points: 1) 0h, 2) 1.5 h, 3) 3 h, 4) 6 h, 5) 9 h, 6) 12 h, 7) 15 h, 8) 18 h, 9) 21 h, 10) 24 h, 11) 27 h, 12) 30 h, 13) 36 h, and 14) 48 h after dissection.

animals were killed and 10 mm segments of the nerve distal and proximal to the cut site were removed. Total RNA was isolated by the method of Chomczynski and Sacchi. Gel runs and Northern blotting onto Hybond N nylon membrane were performed as described.[5] Blots were probed with a 901 base rat IL-6 cRNA labeled with [32]P.[6]

RESULTS

No IL-6 mRNA was detected in the intact nerve (FIG. 1). A dramatic increase of IL-6 mRNA expression was observed within 3 h in organ culture, reaching maximal

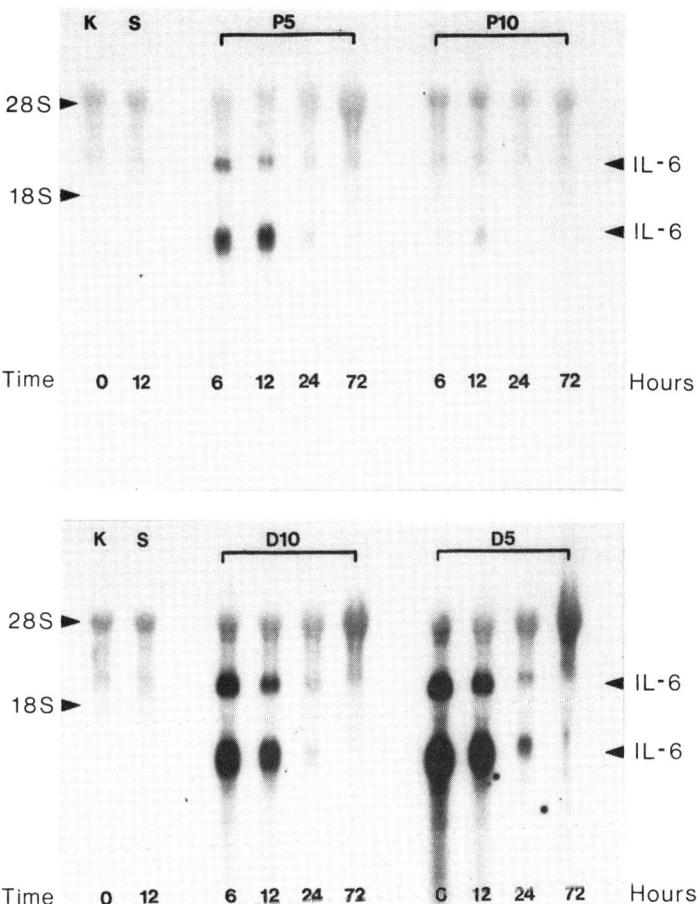

FIGURE 2. Induction of IL-6 mRNA in response to injury. Northern blot showing IL-6 mRNA at selected time points after transection. K: control, S: 12 h after sham lesion, D10: segments 5–10 mm distal to cut site, D5: segments 0–5 mm distal to cut site, P5: segments 0–5 mm proximal to cut site and P10: segments 5–10 mm proximal to cut site.

levels at about 18 h, and persisting for at least 48 h. *In vivo* a similar increase of IL-6 mRNA after transection was seen (FIG. 2). In the proximal stump, the intense IL-6 mRNA expression was confined to the region directly adjacent to the lesion site. Very slight expression was found in proximal segments further from the cut. In the distal stump the whole nerve was affected. Again the greatest increase in IL-6 mRNA was observed immediately adjacent to the transection site. Surprisingly, and quite different from the time course seen in organ culture, this high level of IL-6 mRNA declined within 24 h.

CONCLUSIONS

Thus, unlike CNTF,[7] the IL-6 mRNA level in peripheral nerve increases rapidly in response to injury. IL-6 could therefore be a "neurotrophic cytokine" involved in peripheral nerve regeneration. The difference between the *in vitro* and *in vivo* time courses indicates that unknown factors, possibly secreted by invading macrophages, must function in this down-regulation.

REFERENCES

1. KISHIMOTO, T. 1989. The biology of interleukin-6. Blood **74**: 1–10.
2. SATOH, K., *et al.* 1988. Induction of neuronal differentiation in PC12 cells by B-cell stimulatory factor 2/interleukin 6. Mol. Cell. Biol. **8**: 3546–3549.
3. IP, N. Y., *et al.* 1992. CNTF and LIF act on neuronal cells via shared signaling pathways that involve the IL-6 signal transducing receptor component gp130. Cell **69**: 1121–1132.
4. HEUMANN, R. *et al.* 1987. Changes of nerve growth factor synthesis in nonneuronal cells in response to sciatic nerve transection. J. Cell Biol. **104**: 1623–1631.
5. CHOMCZYNSKI, P. & N. SACCHI. 1987. Single-step method of RNA isolation by acid guanidinium thiocyanate-phenol-chloroform extraction. Anal. Biochem. **162**: 156–159.
6. NORTHEMANN, W. *et al.* 1989. Structure of the rat interleukin-6 gene and its regulation in macrophage-derived cells. J. Biol. Chem. **264**: 16072–16082.
7. SENDTNER, M., K. STÖCKLI & H. THOENEN. 1992. Synthesis and localization of ciliary neurotrophic factor in the sciatic nerve of the adult rat after lesion and during regeneration. J. Cell Biol. **118**: 139–148.

Effect of Interferon-α on Mitotic Index and Corticosterone Secretion in Early Stage of Adrenal Cortex Regeneration

WOJCIECH ZIELENIEWSKI

Institute of Endocrinology
Sterlinga 3
91425 Łódź, Poland

Adrenal cortex is capable to regenerate, but little is known about this process. Various mechanisms including neural pathways and humoral factors were shown to influence adrenal regeneration.[1,2] On the other hand, there is a lot of evidence that the endocrine and immune systems are closely interconnected.[3] Hence the effect of interferon-α (IFN-α) on adrenal regeneration has been investigated.

The study was performed on adult male Wistar rats subjected to adrenal enucleation combined with contralateral adrenalectomy. Half of the animals received subcutaneously human recombinant IFN-α (Roferon, Roche) 10^5 U/rat daily, and the other half served as controls. The rats were killed 4 days (highest proliferation ratio) and 8 days after operation (beginning of zonation). The adrenocortical cell growth has assessed by mitotic index and plasma corticosterone was determined radioimmunologically.

It was found that IFN-α did not alter the very early stage of adrenal regeneration. However, the mitotic activity and corticosterone output were significantly inhibited by IFN-α 8 days after operation (TABLE 1 and 2).

This study has revealed that although IFN-α is believed to stimulate adrenal ste-

TABLE 1. Mean Mitotic Index Values ± SEM

Group	Adrenal Regeneration	
	Day 4	Day 8
Interferon	10.30 ± 0.72*	3.61 ± 0.53**
Control	11.71 + 0.41	8.40 ± 0.44

* Not significant; ** $p < 0.001$ in comparison with controls.

TABLE 2. Corticosterone Plasma Concentration (ng/ml)

Group	Adrenal Regeneration	
	Day 4	Day 8
Interferon	24.87 ± 3.11*	29.71 ± 2.75**
Control	23.34 ± 1.04	72.34 ± 6.14

* Not significant; ** $p < 0.001$ in comparison with controls.

roidogenesis *in vitro*,[4] the *in vivo* effect on the hypothalamo-pituitary-adrenal axis could be different.[5]

REFERENCES

1. GRAGG, R. D. & K. F. A. SALIMAN. 1993. Life Sci. **53:** 275–282.
2. ZIELENIEWSKI, W. & J. ZIELENIEWSKI. 1993. Cytobios **74:** 163–166.
3. REICHLIN, S. 1993. New Engl. J. Med. **329:** 1246–1253.
4. GISSLINGER, H., T. SVOBODA, M. CLODI, B. GILLY, H. LUDWIG, L. HAVELEC & A. LUGER. 1993. Neuroendocrinol. **57:** 489–495.
5. SAPHIER, D., J. E. WELCH & H. E. CHULUYAN. 1993. Eur. J. Pharmacol. **236:** 183–191.

Acute Phase Proteins and Interleukin-6 Serum Levels in Patients with Chronic Arterial Occlusion

WACLAW MAJEWSKI,[a] RYSZARD STANISZEWSKI,[a]
ARTUR SLUPIANEK,[b] ALEKSANDER GORNY,[b] AND
ANDRZEJ MACKIEWICZ[b,c]

[a]*Clinic of General and Vascular Surgery*
[b]*Department of Cancer Immunology, Chair of Oncology*
Academy of Medicine
15 Garbary Street
61-866 Poznań, Poland

Recent studies have shown that serum C-reactive protein (CRP) and α_1-acid glycoprotein (AGP) levels are elevated in acute[1] and chronic[2] ischemia of lower limbs and the increase is proportional to the degree of ischemia. Moreover, these studies have demonstrated clinical usefulness of both APP in monitoring of patients undergoing surgery.[1,2] A number of studies have established the relationship between the IL-6 response and the elicitation of APP in man. The increase of IL-6 serum levels preceded or was simultaneous with the increase of serum CRP concentration.[3] Accordingly, we undertook current studies to elucidate relationship between IL-6, CRP, and AGP levels in sera of patients with chronic arterial occlusion of lower limbs and to evaluate clinical applicability of serial IL-6 measurements for monitoring of patients after surgery.

CRP and AGP levels were studied in sera of 71 patients (36–78 years of age). IL-6 was measured using ELISA (Genzyme Corp., Cambridge, MA) in sera of 12 patients. Depending on the degree of ischemia patients were divided into three groups: grade I (intermittent claudication and ankle pressure above 60 mmHg)—14 patients; II (rest pain with or without focal necrosis and ankle pressure between 40–60 mmHg)—14; III (extensive necrosis and ankle pressure below 40 mmHg—28). Reconstructive surgery was performed in 53 patients and primary major amputation in 18 cases. Blood samples were collected before surgery and serially up to 20 days following operation.

The mean concentration values of CRP and AGP in sera of patients with I, II and III grade of ischemia prior surgery were significantly different ($p < 0.001$). In most cases on days 1–3 following surgery levels of both APP increased dramatically and after 7–10 days declined. In cases in which necrosis progression after surgery was observed CRP and AGP concentrations on days 7–10 remained elevated. Surprisingly, IL-6 was detectable in sera of 4 out of 12 patients prior surgery only (FIG. 1). Following surgery in these cases IL-6 serum levels declined. In sera of remaining 8 patients in which IL-6 was not found surgery did not cause detection of the cytokine in serum.

Recently, May *et al.*[4] demonstrated that IL-6 present in circulation may be complexed with other proteins one of which is soluble IL-6 receptor (sIL-6R). Such complexed IL-6 is not always detectable by ELISA technique probably owing to the

[c] Author to whom correspondence should be addressed.

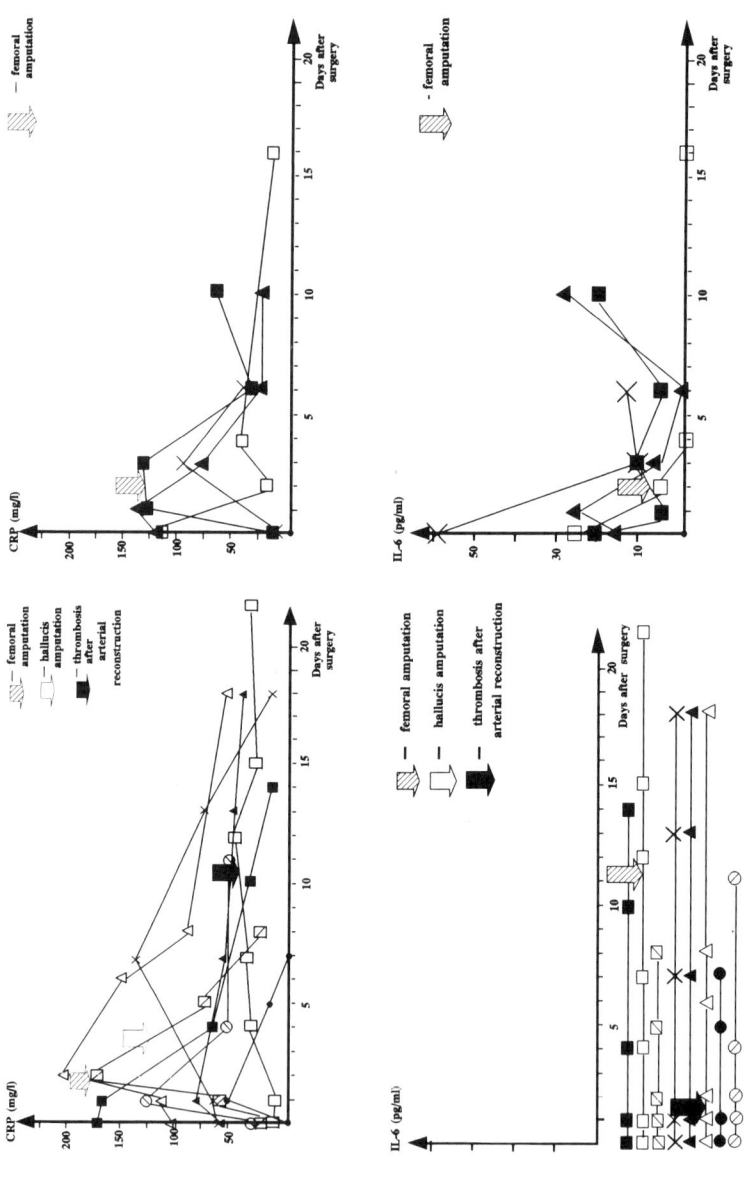

FIGURE 1. CRP and IL-6 levels in sera of patients with chronic arterial occlusion. *Left panel*: 8 patients with no detectable IL-6 in serum (1 patient with grade I of ischemia; 5 with grade II and 2 with grade III). *Right panel*: 4 patients with detectable serum IL-6. Primary surgery was performed on day 0 (1 patient with grade I of ischemia; 2 with grade II and 1 with grade III). Arrows indicate reoperations.

competition between monoclonal antibodies and sIL-6R since most of the specific antibodies are neutralizing antibodies binding to the same epitop as sIL-6R. Since, only in ⅓ of studied patients IL-6 was detected in serum such a possibility needs to be taken into consideration while evaluating obtained results. However, it is also possible but highly unlikely that in some cases of tissue necrosis IL-6 is not released into the circulation. Accordingly, in order to verify clinical usefulness of IL-6 determination in chronic arterial occlusion further studies using techniques utilizing other antibodies are necessary.

REFERENCES

1. MAJEWSKI, W., M. LACIAK, R. STANISZEWSKI, A. GORNY & A. MACKIEWICZ. 1991. Eur. J. Vasc. Surg. **5:** 641–645.
2. MAJEWSKI, W., A. ZIELINSKI, M. LACIAK, R. STANISZEWSKI, A. GORNY, S. ZAPALSKI & A. MACKIEWICZ. 1993. Eur. J. Vasc. Surg. **7:** 628–632.
3. SEHGAL, P. B. 1993. *In* Acute Phase Proteins: Molecular Biology, Biochemistry, Clinical Applications. A. Mackiewicz, I. Kushner & H. Baumann, Eds.: 621–632. Boca Raton, FL: CRC Press, Inc.
4. MAY, L. T., H. VIGUET, J. S. KENNEY, N. IDA, A. C. ALLISON & P. B. SEHGAL. 1992. J. Biol. Chem. **267:** 19698–19704.

Inflammatory Cytokines in Peritoneal Fluid of Women with Endometriosis

J. SKRZYPCZAK,[a] P. JEDRZEJCZAK,[a] M. KASPRZAK,[b] E. PUK,[a] AND M. KURPISZ[b,c]

[a]Institute of Obstetrics and Gynaecology
Academy of Medicine
Poznań, Poland

[b]Institute of Human Genetics
Polish Academy of Sciences
ul. Strzeszyńska 32
60-479 Poznań, Poland

The immunological background of endometriosis has been a puzzle for scientists. There are several isolated facts seemingly creating the hypothesis of increased numbers and activity of immunocompetent cells at the onset of the disease.[1] Furthermore, interleukin-6 (IL-6) and its elevated amounts in the first several weeks of the pathological process, as was documented in the experimental animal model,[2] can be recognized as a hallmark of the disease. These facts together, *i.e.*, increased numbers and activity of macrophages in the peritoneal fluid (PF)[3] and elevated levels of cytokines produced by mononuclear cells may indicate the particular involvement of PF monocyte/macrophages and inflammatory cytokines in the first stage of the disease. They may well be, however, non-specific factors from the immunological and/or clinical point of view. In our study therefore, we decided to identify the levels of basic inflammatory cytokines (tumor necrosis factor [TNF]-α and IL-6) in PF of women with endometriosis and to attempt to correlate its levels with number and activity of collected from the fluid monocyte/macrophages.

Peritoneal fluids were obtained from 70 women who underwent diagnostic laparoscopy to differentiate between endometriosis, infertility, and pelvic malformations. Fifty women were found to have endometriosis, which was subsequently classified into three categories according to the American Fertility Society. A control group included 20 individuals of 18–36 years of age with persistent infertility. All PF samples were evaluated for monocyte/macrophage concentration, active macrophages (PAS-staining) and IL-6 content. 25 samples with endometriosis and 12 controls were additionally screened for presence of TNFα. Cytokines were determined by using quantitative ELISA or RIA kits, respectively (IL-6, Genzyme; TNFα, Amersham Inc.).

The results are presented in TABLES 1 and 2, respectively for IL-6 and TNFα. According to the presented variations, data are not statistically significant, although the IL-6 was markedly elevated in PF's obtained from stage I and II endometriosis as compared to the control group. Monocyte/macrophage concentration was highest in the group with endometriosis classified to stage II, while macrophage activity was highest in the stage I group. In TABLE 2 where, owing to the limited numbers of analyzed samples, different stages of endometriosis were not identified, similarly we did not detect statistically significant values between control group and patients with

[c] Address correspondence to Maciej Kurpisz, M.D., Ph.D.; Fax: (4861) 233 235.

TABLE 1. IL-6 Content, Monocyte/Macrophage Number and Activity in PF from Women with Endometriosis

	Number of Individuals	IL-6 Content in pg/ml ± SD
Controls	20	49.9 ± 133.6
Endometriosis		
I stage	36	128.9 ± 284.5
II stage	10	271.6 ± 560.3
III stage	4	80.0 ± 76.2
	Number of Individuals	Monocyte/Macrophage Number in 10^5/ml ± SD
Controls	20	260.1 ± 188.3
Endometriosis		
I stage	33	294.0 ± 309.1
II stage	9	566.4 ± 674.5
III stage	4	123.1 ± 105.6
	Number of Individuals	Active Macrophages
Controls	16	10 individuals positive
Endometriosis		
I stage	29	22 individuals positive
II stage	9	6 individuals positive
III stage	4	3 individuals positive

the disorder. The TNFα levels obtained in a group with endometriosis were markedly higher than in controls; the same was true for activity of macrophages but not for their numbers. The individuals with elevated TNFα and IL-6 in PF samples were not however an overlapping population (data not shown).

On the basis of the obtained data we reached certain agreement with earlier reports that IL-6 content in PF may be rather a prognostic factor of the disease showing certain culmination in first and rather mild stage of the process.[4] This cannot be considered as the crucial factor for disease identification. IL-6 levels disappointingly did not correlate with the monocyte/macrophage content and activity (although the activity was more clearly pronounced in the milder stage of disease) as well as with TNFα presence. Both cytokines, however are known to be signals and "active partici-

TABLE 2. TNFα Content, Monocyte/Macrophage Number and Activity in PF from Women with Endometriosis

	Number of Individuals	TNFα Content in pg/ml +/− SD
Controls	12	2.1 ± 4.0
Endometriosis	25	7.0 ± 22.6
	Number of Individuals	Monocyte/Macrophage in 10^5/ml
Controls	12	210.6 ± 137.6
Endometriosis	22	260.2 ± 217.2
	Number of Individuals	Active Macrophages
Controls	11	8 individuals positive
Endometriosis	18	15 individuals positive

pants" in the inflammatory process but they may act on the different level of immune response. For example, TNFα may be more active at the enhancement of antigenic presentation; therefore, the occurrence of organ-specific or non-specific antibodies may better correspond to the elevated level of this cytokine whereas IL-6 can be enhanced in endometriosis as well as for infertile individuals.

REFERENCES

1. ROCK, J. A. & S. M. MARKHAM. 1992. Pathogenesis of endometriosis. Lancet **340:** 1264–1267.
2. LIM, Y.-T. & R. S. SCHENKEN. 1993. Interleukin-6 in the experimental endometriosis. Fertil. Steril. **59:** 912–915.
3. BRAUN, D. P., H. GEBEL, C. ROTMAN, N. RANA & W. P. DMOWSKI. 1992. The development of cytotoxicity in peritoneal macrophages from women with endometriosis. Fertil. Steril. **57:** 1203–1210.
4. RIER, S. E., A. K. PARSONS & J. L. BECKER. 1994. Altered interleukin-6 production by peritoneal leukocytes from patients with endometriosis. Fertil. Steril. **61:** 294–299.

Increased Resistance of CSF-1–deficient, Macrophage-deficient, TNFα-deficient, and IL-1α–deficient *op/op* Mice to Endotoxin[a]

MALGORZATA SZPERL,[b] AFTAB A. ANSARI,[c] ELZBIETA URBANOWSKA,[b] PRZEMYSLAW SZWECH,[b] PAWEL KALINSKI,[b] AND WIESLAW WIKTOR-JEDRZEJCZAK[b,d]

[b]Department of Immunology
Central Clinical Hospital
Military School of Medicine
ul. Szaserow 128
PL 00-909 Warsaw, Poland

[c]Department of Pathology and Laboratory Medicine
Emory University School of Medicine
Atlanta, Georgia 30322

INTRODUCTION

The release of mediators such as TNFα and IL-1α by macrophages have been implicated in the pathogenesis of postendotoxin shock and subsequent death.[1] Although this concept is supported by several lines of evidence, it has never been tested using congenitally macrophage-deficient animals, which should provide additional confirmatory evidence. The availability of *op/op* mice[2,3] provides an excellent model to test this hypothesis. These mice have a spontaneous functional knock-out of a gene for macrophage growth factor: CSF-1, which results in the total absence of this factor associated with severe deficiency of macrophages.[4,5] Therefore this mutant provides a unique opportunity to investigate the *in vivo* role of the CSF-1-dependent macrophage subpopulation in the pathogenesis of endotoxin-induced death.

MATERIALS AND METHODS

Mutant *op/op* and control mice were bred as described.[3,6] Two-month-old animals were used in the present experiments. Groups of *op/op* and control animals received i. p. injections of various doses *E. coli* LPS W 0111:B4 (Difco, Detroit, MI) dissolved in sterile saline and were observed for two weeks or until death. Separate groups of animals were used for determination of TNFα and IL-1α levels. For this experiment untreated or LPS-injected (dose of 5 μ/mouse) mice following anesthesia were bled from retroorbital plexus. LPS-injected mice were bled 30 min or 60 min after injection.

---

[a] This work was supported by grant No 413179101 from Polish Committee for Scientific Research to W. W-J.

[d] Author to whom correspondence should be addressed.

TABLE 1. Survival of Macrophage-deficient *op/op* and Control +/+ Mice Following Injection of LPS

LPS µg/g Body Weight	Number Surviving/Number Treated[a]	
	+/+	*op/op*
30	0/2	0/2
15	0/2	0/2
10	0/2	0/2
6.5	0/4	4/4
5	0/3	3/3
3.4	1/4	4/4
2.5	6/6	3/3

[a] Male mice of average weight of 20 g (4–6 months old) were used in these experiments.

The levels of TNFα and IL-1α have been determined using commercially available kits (Genzyme, Cambridge, MA).

RESULTS

As shown in TABLE 1, the *op/op* mice survived doses of LPS more than two times higher than LPS doses lethal for normal littermate mice. Death, if it occurred, was observed between 24 and 48 hours, usually during the night with *op/op* mice usually surviving a few hours longer than +/+ mice. If mice survived the first 50 hours postendotoxin injection they survived the experiment and no late deaths were observed for up to two weeks with animals behaving normally and gaining weight. In order to test whether the differences in acute phase mediators such as TNFα and IL-1α might have been responsible for this difference in LPS susceptibility, both *op/op* and littermate control mice had determined serum levels of these two mediators prior to as well as 30 or 60 min post LPS injection. As shown in TABLE 2 *op/op* mice released 4 times less TNFα and 2 times less IL-1α in response to LPS compared to control mice.

Therefore these data suggest that the reduced release of TNFα and IL-1α in response to LPS may contribute to the increased resistance of *op/op* mice to LPS. They

TABLE 2. Serum TNFα and IL-1α in Untreated and Endotoxin-injected *op/op* and Control +/+ Mice

Cytokine Tested	Time after LPS Injection	Level of Cytokine (ng/ml) Mean ± SD	
		+/+	*op/op* (N = 4)
TNFα	Untreated	0.137 ± 0.02	0.105 ± 0.02*
	30 min	0.125 ± 0.02	0.103 ± 0.03
	60 min	1.86 ± 0.45	0.46 ± 0.38**
IL-1α	Untreated	<50	<50
	30 min	193 ± 44	97 ± 37**
	60 min	472 ± 76	215 ± 62**

* Difference statistically significant at $p < 0.05$; ** difference statistically significant at $p < 0.001$.

have also provided an unquestionable evidence that the macrophages produced under the influence of CSF-1, which are by definition absent in *op/op* mice, play an important *in vivo* role in mediating lethal LPS effects. However, lethal endotoxic shock occurs in the *op/op* mice with higher LPS doses, which suggest that this role is not exclusive and other cells also contribute *in vivo* to this reaction.

REFERENCES

1. Vassali, P. 1992. Annu. Rev. Immunol. **10:** 411–452.
2. Marks, S. C., Jr. & P. W. Lane. 1976. J. Hered. **67:** 11–18.
3. Wiktor-Jedrzejczak, W., A. Ahmed, C. Szczylik & R. R. Skelly. 1982. J. Exp. Med. **156:** 1516–1527.
4. Wiktor-Jedrzejczak, W., M. Z. Ratajczak, A. Ptasznik, K. W. Sell, A. Ahmed-Ansari & W. Ostertag. 1992. Exp. Hematol. **20:** 1004–1010.
5. Naito, M., S.-I. Hayashi, H. Yoshida, S.-I. Nishikawa, L. D. Shultz & K. Takahashi. 1991. Am. J. Pathol. **139:** 657–667.
6. Wiktor-Jedrzejczak, W., A. Bartocci, A. W. Ferrante, Jr., A. Ahmed-Ansari, K. W. Sell, J. W. Pollard & E. R. Stanley. 1990. Proc. Natl. Acad. Sci. USA **87:** 4828–4832.

Characterization of the IL-6/LIF-Response Factor by Proteolytic Analysis[a]

K. SCHNEIDER, J. RIPPERGER, G. H. FEY, AND G. M. HOCKE

Department of Genetics
Institute for Microbiology, Biochemistry and Genetics
University of Erlangen-Nürnberg
Staudtstrasse 5
D-91058 Erlangen, Germany

Treatment of hepatic cells with interleukin 6 (IL-6) or leukemia inhibitory factor (LIF) causes the appearance of a cytokine-induced, sequence-specific protein-DNA complex. This complex (complex II) was visualized by gel mobility shift experiments with nuclear protein extracts and a radiolabeled double-stranded oligonucleotide probe (TB2), that contained two tandem copies of the type II IL-6/LIF-response element (IL-6RE/LIF-RE). This complex appeared with a biphasic kinetics after treatment of hepatic cells with IL-6, showing an early and a late phase. The early phase was independent of ongoing protein synthesis and not inhibited by treatment of the cells with cycloheximide.[1] The late phase required protein synthesis.[2] The current interpretation is that the early phase of the IL-6–induced complex is due to a posttranslational modification (phosphorylation) of preexisting cytoplasmic IL-6 response factor (IL-6RF).[1] Earlier studies strongly suggested that the protein component of this complex is directly involved in the IL-6–induced transcriptional activation of target genes.[2]

After 12 h of an experimental acute phase response provoked in rat livers by complete Freund's adjuvant (CFA), nuclear protein extracts were prepared. The IL-6/LIF-RF was partially purified by two consecutive steps of chromatography on different ion exchange columns (SP-Sepharose™ and Q-Sepharose™, Pharmacia). The protein was then reacted for 10 minutes with the radiolabeled TB2 oligonucleotide probe. The reactions were then incubated for 10 minutes with increasing amounts of trypsin or chymotrypsin, respectively. Reaction products were subsequently analyzed by gel mobility shift experiments.[3]

The proteolytic fragments generated with trypsin and chymotrypsin, respectively, showed interesting qualitative differences (FIGS. 1 and 2). In both cases, one major complex of faster mobility than the initial complex was generated after exhaustive proteolysis. The intermediate stages in approaching this end-point were different for both enzymes. In our interpretation this faster moving complex represents a recognizable subdomain of the IL-6/LIF-RF, that still is capable of specific DNA-binding. These minimal DNA-binding domains (MD) will facilitate the future identification of the DNA-binding domain in the primary sequence of this factor.

---

[a] This work was supported by research grants from Deutsche Forschungsgemeinschaft (DFG) Hi 291/5-4 TP2 and Hi 291/5-4 TP6.

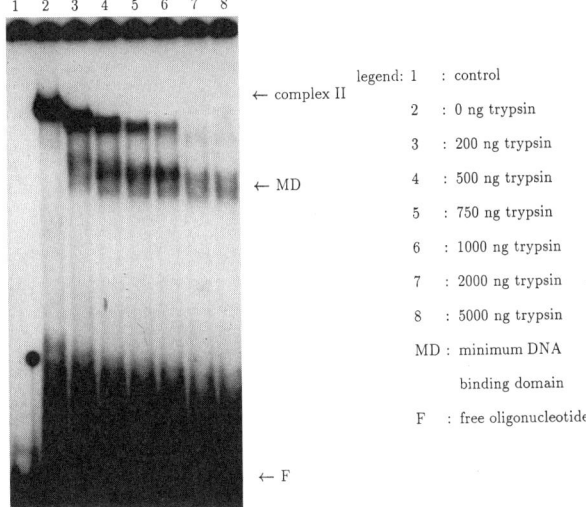

FIGURE 1. Gel mobility shift of partially purified rat acute phase protein after digestion with trypsin.

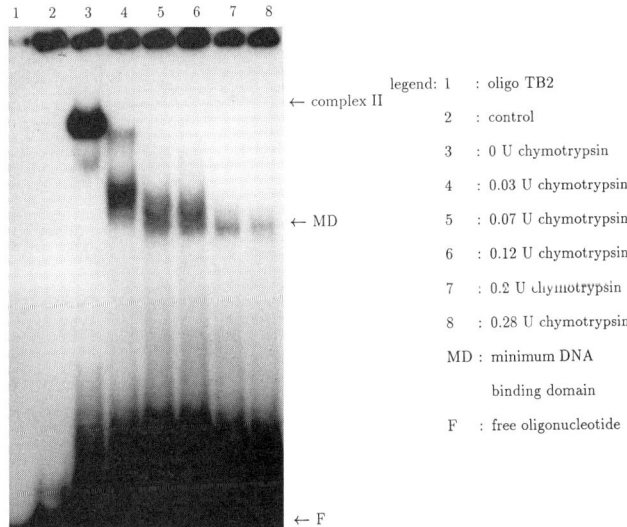

FIGURE 2. Gel mobility shift of partially purified rat acute phase protein after digestion with chymotrypsin.

REFERENCES

1. WEGENKA, U. M., C. LÜTTICKEN, J. BUSCHMANN, J. YUAN, F. LOTTSPEICH, W. MÜLLER-ESTERL, C. SCHINDLER, E. ROEB, P. C. HEINRICH & F. HORN. 1994. The interleukin-6-activated acute-phase response factor is antigenically and functionally related to members of the signal transducer and activator of transcription (STAT) family. Mol. Cell. Biol. **14:** 3186–3196.
2. HOCKE, G. M., M.-Z. CUI, J. RIPPERGER & G. H. FEY. 1993. Regulation of the rat α_2 macroglobulin gene by interleukin 6 and leukemia inhibitory factor. *In* Acute Phase Proteins: Molecular Biology, Biochemistry, Clinical Applications, A. Mackiewicz, I. Kushner & H. Baumann, Eds.: 467–494. Boca Raton, FL: CRC Press Inc.
3. SCHREIBER, E., P. MATTHIAS, M. M. MÜLLER & W. SCHAFFNER. 1988. Identification of a novel lymphoid specific octamer binding protein (OTF-2B) by proteolytic clipping bandshift assay (PCBA). EMBO **7:** 4221–4229.

Acute Phase Response and Interleukin-6 after Operative Laparoscopy and Microsurgery in Gynecology

KRZYSZTOF DREWS, KRZYSZTOF SZYMANOWSKI, JANA SKRZYPCZAK, PIOTR JĘDRZEJCZAK, AND TOMASZ ŻAK

Reproduction Clinic
Institute of Gynecology and Obstetrics
University School of Medical Sciences
ul. Polna 33
Poznań, Poland

After inflammatory stimuli and trauma the rates of hepatic synthesis of several plasma proteins, the acute phase proteins, increase dramatically while some others, most notably albumin, decrease substantially. In acute phase response the prototype of typical and most reactive protein is C-reactive protein (CRP). The stimulation process is mediated by cytokines. Interleukin 6 (IL-6) is a significant cytokine controlling the stress response induced by infection and tissue injury. Once released from the site of inflammation, it induces a wide range of systemic effects, including the hepatic acute phase response and production of CRP. The aim of our study was comparison of immunologic response to different types of gynecological operations for infertility as well as operation duration.

MATERIAL AND METHODS

Forty-four women with primary infertility, aged 24–35, underwent laparoscopy, laparoscopy with hysteroscopy, or microsurgery by laparotomy between February 1993 and May 1994. Inclusion criteria were suspicion of tubal pathology, no other causes of infertility, and former operations. Procedures were performed under general anesthesia. The blood serum samples were collected from patients at the time of anesthesia induction, and 24 and 48 h later. All the patients were given the same intravenous fluids in the perioperative period. CRP measurements were performed by rocket electrophoresis and results expressed in mg/l. IL-6 determination based on the Predicta Interleukin 6 kit of Genzyme and results expressed in pg/ml. Results were analyzed with variance analysis and Duncan's test. P-values <0.05 were considered significant.

RESULTS

Results of the CRP level estimations as well as statistical significance are shown in TABLES 1 and 2.

TABLE 1. CRP Levels (mg/l) in Blood Serum According to Length of Operation

		CRP Levels in Serum (mg/l)					
		At Anesthesia Induction (A)		After 24 h (B)		After 48 h (A)	
Number	Operation Duration (min)	Mean	±	Mean	±	Mean	±
1.	<30 n = 14	6.61 [B, C]	3.74	14.38 [A, 2, 3, 4]	8.97	14.42 [A, 2, 3, 4]	12.00
2.	31–60 n = 18	7.37	5.61	19.04 [1]	21.79	23.65 [1]	33.39
3.	61–120 n = 7	8.29	3.15	60.43 [1, 2]	57.92	50.93 [1]	52.83
4.	>121 n = 5	9.40	7.80	64.00 [1]	21.95	60.60 [1]	55.06

A, B, C, 1, 2, 3, 4 shown in brackets just below the mean value show statistical significance with the indicated ($p < 0.05$).

DISCUSSION

The most important factor influencing acute phase response is, in our study, trauma caused by laparotomy. Results vary significantly in the first and in the second postoperative day between groups, if laparotomy took place. Mean CRP value in the blood serum was after laparotomy 6- to 7-fold higher than after endoscopic operations. Operative trauma is often considered as a trigger for adhesion formation. Ryan, Grobety and Majno[15] in experimental study have shown that all the stimuli that are unavoidable during laparotomy promote adhesion formation (mechanical injury, bleeding, ischemia, introduction of foreign materials, *e.g.* talcum, bacteria). Laparoscopy minimizes all the above-listed stimuli decreasing adhesion formation as well as acute phase response. Luciano,[2] and Tavmergen, Mecke and Semm[3] have stated that adhesions after operative laparoscopy compared to laparotomy are uncommon.

CRP levels increase with the operation time also, especially in the first postoperative day and when the operation lasts over 60 minutes. We have also performed 28 estimations of IL-6 in 12 patients. Values of this cytokine ranged from 30 to 250 pg/ml.

TABLE 2. CRP Levels (mg/l) in Blood Serum According to Operation Type

		CRP Levels in Serum (mg/l)					
		At Anesthesia Induction (A)		After 24 h (B)		After 48 h (A)	
Number	Type of Operation	Mean	±	Mean	±	Mean	±
1.	Laparoscopy n = 27	6.76 [B, C]	5.15	15.25 [A, 3]	12.36	14.12 [A, 3]	10.60
2.	Laparoscopy with hysteroscopy, n = 9	6.12 [B, C]	2.74	16.78 [A, 3]	12.20	13.87 [A, 3]	5.30
3.	Laparotomy n = 10	11.20 [B, C]	6.76	75.50 [A, C, 1, 2]	42.34	88.30 [A, C, 1, 2]	59.76

A, B, C, 1, 2, 3 shown in brackets just below the mean value express statistical significance with that group ($p < 0.05$).

Concentrations of IL-6 differ dependently from the time and kind of operation, but statistical analysis was not done. We have found that CRP values had highest sensitivity for diagnosing severity of surgical trauma. Our results of IL-6 concentrations in different gynecological injury have only preliminary character and need further investigation.

CONCLUSIONS

1) Measurements of CRP levels deal with the operative trauma and may be very helpful in the clinical effect prognosis.
2) Laparoscopy compared to laparotomy cause much less immunologic response.
3) IL-6 is a good candidate for laboratory tests to explain immunological reactions caused by surgical trauma.

REFERENCES

1. Ryan, G. B., J. Grobety & G. Majno. 1971. Am. J. Pathol. **65:** 117–148.
2. Luciano, A. 1990. Treatment of Post Surgical Adhesions. New York: Wiley-Liss, Inc. pp. 35–44.
3. Tavmergen, E. N., H. Mecke & K. Semm. 1990. Zent bl. Gynäkol, **112:** 1163–1169.

Acute Phase Proteins in Endometriosis

KRZYSZTOF DREWS, JANA SKRZYPCZAK, TOMASZ ŻAK,
KRZYSZTOF SZYMANOWSKI, AND ANDRZEJ MACKIEWICZ

Institute of Gynecology and Obstetrics
University School of Medical Sciences
ul. Polna 33
Poznań, Poland

Endometriosis and other diseases of female adnexa present specific diagnostic problems and may be either symptomatic or asymptomatic. Specific diagnostic tests are not available; however, in several studies different enzymatic and immunological changes were found. In recent years we have come to appreciate that the classic powder-burn lesion, thought to be so typical of endometriosis in the past, is just one of a wide spectrum of lesions that may be visualized in the pelvis at laparoscopy. It is quite likely that, with less experienced operators performing a laparoscopy, some of less classical features of endometriosis may be missed or misinterpreted. It is established that patients with endometriosis present with a wide spectrum of symptomatology. The incidence of disease among infertile woman may be as high as 30% to 40%. Whilst it is easy to explain an association between presence of pelvic adhesions and reduced fertility potential, it is less easy to explain the association between isolated deposits of endometriosis in patients complaining of infertility but asymptomatic of the endometriotic process. The nature of relationship between endometriosis and infertility remains unresolved.

The present study was undertaken to estimate the use of determining immunoreactivity of α_1-acid glycoprotein, α_1-antitrypsin and α_1-antichymotrypsin with lectin Con A in endometriosis. All 25 observed patients were treated and diagnosed earlier (infertility). Diagnosis of endometriosis process was confirmed by histological examination (excisions of peritoneum during laparoscopy were taken). Blood serum was obtained before the operation, and peritoneal fluid was aspirated from culdesac during laparoscopy. Normal serum and peritoneal fluid samples were obtained from healthy woman. Microheterogenity of choosen acute phase proteins was determined by affinity immunoelectrophoresis with Con A as a ligand. Reactivity coefficient (Rc) was calculated. Statistical evaluation of results obtained was by Student's *t*-test.

RESULTS

Analyzing α_1-antichymotrypsin in blood serum in woman with endometriosis, we have found that Rc was significantly lower in comparison with control group (2.5 + 0.5 vs 3.1 + 1.1). In peritoneal fluid Rc was higher in endometriosis than in normal woman (3.5 + 1.2 vs 2.3 + 0.7) (FIG. 1).

α_1-Antitrypsin Rc in serum of woman with endometriosis was lower than in healthy subjects (8.6 + 2.0 vs 13.6 + 2.0) (FIG. 2). In peritoneal fluid no significant differences of Rc value were found. Reactivity coefficient calculated for α_1-acid glycoprotein in blood serum and peritoneal fluid was different in women with endometriosis and in healthy women, but without statistical significance.

Endometriosis has been known to be associated with a variety of immunological

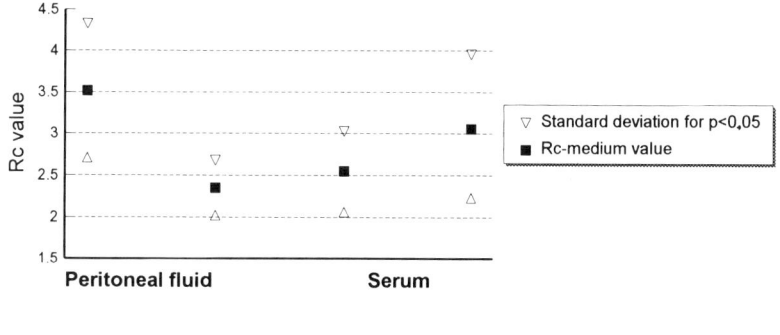

FIGURE 1. α_1-Antichymotrypsin.

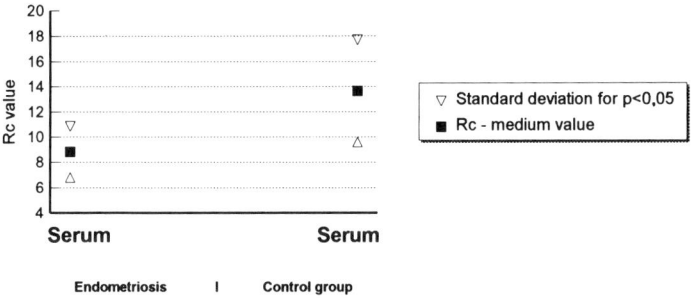

FIGURE 2. α_1-Antitrypsin.

phenomena (depressed cell-mediated immunity in peripheral blood, increased peritoneal macrophage activation). Our results may confirm the hypothesis, that endometriosis is a generalized, immunological process. We suppose, that differences found in microheterogenity of acute phase glycoproteins can be estrogen-altered. Assay of acute phase proteins in blood serum as well in peritoneal fluid need further study, and can be used as a markers of diseases and unexplained infertility.

REFERENCES

1. BROSENS, I. A. 1991. Modern Approaches to Endometriosis. London: Kluwer Academic, pp. 21–31.
2. JANSSEN. et al. 1986. J. Obstet. Gynecol. **155:** 1154–1159.
3. CORNILLIE, F. J. et al. 1990. Fertil. Steril. **53:** 989–993.
4. DMOWSKI, W. P. et al. 1981. Am. J. Obstet. Gynecol. **141:** 377–383.
5. HALME, J. et al. 1984. Am. J. Obstet. Gynecol. **148:** 85–90.
6. KENNEDY, S. H. et al. 1990. Obstet. Gynecol. **75:** 914–918.

Subject Index

Acute lymphoblastic leukemia (ALL), IL-6 production in, 391–394
Acute myelogenous leukemia (AML), 294–299
Acute phase proteins (APP). *See also* α_1 acid Glycoprotein; C-reactive protein; Serum amyloid A
 in endometriosis, 508–509
 genes of, 16
 glycosylation of
  changes in, 319–322
  cytokine regulation of, 323–325
  IL-6-type cytokines and, 413–415
  mechanism of, 325–327
  pathophysiological changes, 322–323
 induction of
  by cytokines, 15–16
  by IL-6, 313–315, 419–421
  by OSM, 47–48
  post-transcriptional mechanisms in, 102–106
 in ischemia, 493–495
 in NBL, 443–444
 synthesis of, 419–421
Acute phase response (APR)
 cytokines involved in, 2, 108–109
 hormonal modification of, 108
 in IL-6-deficient mice, 377
 LPS induction of, 108, 111–112, 114–115
 modified proteins in, 108–115
 after surgery, 505–507
 turpentine-induced, 377–379
Acute phase response elements (APREs)
 in APP genes, 16
 DNA binding factors and, 58–59
 in IL-6 signal pathway, 57
 JEBS binding of, 60–62
 NF-IL6 binding to, 17
 Stat protein recognition of, 58–59
Acute phase response factors (APRFs)
 activation of, 226–230, 377–379
 JEBS binding to, 60–62
 molecular cloning of, 20–23
 tyrosine phosphorylation of, 23–24, 229–231
Adenovirus vectors
 biological activity of, 286–290
 construction of, 284–285
 for cytokine gene expression, 282–283
Adrenocorticotrophic hormone (ACTH), IL-1/IL-6 and, 71, 79
AIDS
 anti-IL-6 therapy, 131
 IL-6 levels in, 130

ALL. *See* Acute lymphoblastic leukemia
All-trans retinoic acid (ATRA), 457–458
Alzheimer's disease, IL-6 levels in, 130
AML. *See* Acute myelogenous leukemia
Antioxidants
 and inflammatory cytokine production, 332–338
 molecular biological effects of, 336–338
Aplasia, IL-6 levels in, 439
APREs. *See* Acute phase response elements
APRFs. *See* Acute phase response factors
Asthma. *See also* Respiratory inflammation
 IL-6-type cytokines and, 89
 IL-11 in, 89–90
 respiratory viruses and, 97
ATRA. *See* *All*-trans retinoic acid

Bacterial endotoxin (LPS)
 APR induction by, 108
 IL-1/IL-6 induction by, 111–114, 222
 and inflammatory cytokine production, 332–338
 op/op mouse resistance to, 499–501
 and septic shock, 315, 336–338
BAL. *See* Bronchoalveolar lavage
BMT. *See* Bone marrow transplantation
Bone marrow transplantation (BMT), and CRP/IL-6 levels, 440–441
Bronchoalveolar lavage (BAL)
 and asthma, 89
 IL-6 levels in, 287–290, 455–456

Cachexia
 IL-6 levels in, 130–131
 OSM and, 43
Cancer. *See also specific cancers*
 asbestos-related
  CRP levels and, 435–437
  IgE levels and, 435–436
 IL-6 and, 385–387
 IL-6 serum levels in, 130, 446–448
 and post-surgical HMW Fb increase, 388–390
Cardiotrophin-1 (CT-1). *See also* IL-6-type cytokines
 and cardiac myocyte hypertrophy, 12
 and gp130, 1–2
C/EBP
 expression of, 19
 family members, 16, 19
 and IL-6 promoter induction, 2–3
 p53 and, 4–10
 tyrosine kinase activation of, 262

C/EBPβ-deficient mice
  APR in, 269–270, 377
  lymphoproliferative alterations in, 270–272
Chronic arterial occlusion. See Ischemia
Ciliary neurotrophic factor (CNTF). See also Inflammatory cytokines; Interleukin-6-type cytokines
  in APP induction, 15
  in APRF phosphorylation, 23–24
  in C/EBP family, 19
  cytokines related to, 37
  and gp130, 1–2
  in septic shock, 407–409
Ciliary neurotrophic factor (CNTF) receptor, 213–215
CNTF. See Ciliary neurotrophic factor
Corticosteroid receptors. See Glucocorticoid receptors
C-reactive protein (CRP)
  as APP, 109
  in chronic arterial occlusion, 493–495
  IL-6 induction of, 102–104, 106
  mRNA half life, 105
  in neonatal infection diagnosis, 398–399
  regulation of, 103–106
  serum levels of
    and asbestos-related cancer, 435–437
    after BMT, 440–441
    IL-6 and, 435–436
    after surgery, 505–507
CRP. See C-reactive protein
CRU. See Cytokine response unit
CSF-1. See Macrophage growth factor
CT-1. See Cardiotrophin-1
Cytokine receptors. See also Hematopoietin receptors
  SIF activation and, 196–203
Cytokine response unit (CRU)
  binding factor (YY1), 239, 241–242
    NFκB competition with, 245–249
    in SAA1-promoter repression, 242–245
  binding sites within, 239
Cytokines. See also Inflammatory cytokines; Interleukin-6-type cytokines
  and APP induction, 15–16
  and corticosteroid receptors, 71–76
  glucocorticosteroid inhibition of, 79–80
  using gp130, 1–2
  IL-6-type, 1–2
  in IL-11 regulation, 92
  induction of
    by LPS, 111–112
    by taxol, 112, 114
  in ISGF3 activation, 24–25
  and liver cell metabolism, 416–418
  in mammalian development regulation, 29
  networks of, 71, 76
    and GCSB, 73–75
    and glucocorticosteroid production, 71
    and SOD activity, 416–418
  synthesis/release of, 109, 111–115
  and TAT activity, 416–418

D

D-factor. See Differentiation stimulating D-factor
Differentiation stimulating (D)-factor/LIF receptor, 480–481
Disease, IL-6 role in, 130–131
DNA-binding factors, IL-6-induced, 58–59

E

E_2. See Estradiol
Endometriosis
  APP in, 508–509
  inflammatory cytokine levels in, 496–498
17β-Estradiol (E_2), and IL-6 gene expression, 82–84
Ets binding site (JEBS)
  APRF binding with, 60–62
  in IL-6 signal transduction, 57–58
  in JRE-IL6, 55

G

GAS. See γ-Interferon activated site
GCSB. See Glucocorticosteroid binding
Glucocorticoid receptors (GR)
  cytokine networks and, 71–76
  and gene expression, 80–81
  and NF-κB, 81, 84
  p65 and, 82
  and transcription factors, 80
  in transcription factor superfamily, 79
Glucocorticoid response elements (GRE), 80
Glucocorticoids
  and cytokine blood levels, 71
  and IL-6 gene expression, 80–81
  immune system actions of, 79–80
Glucocorticosteroid binding (GCSB)
  basal level of, 73–75
  inflammatory cytokines and, 71, 73–76
$α_1$ acid Glycoprotein (AGP)
  in chronic arterial occlusion, 493–495
  IL-6 REs and, 16
  induction of, 422
  regulation of, 252
gp80. See also Interleukin-6 receptor
  cytokine regulation of, 465–467
gp130. See also Interleukin-6 receptor; Interleukin-6-type cytokines; Soluble gp130
  cytokine regulation of, 465–467
  functional epitopes on, 482–484
  and IL-6R endocytosis, 410–412
  in IL-11 receptor, 2
  in junB activation, 56–57
  phosphorylation of, 23–24, 231–232

SUBJECT INDEX

signal transducer function of, 55
signal transduction through, 25–26
GR. *See* Glucocorticoid receptor

H

H7-sensitive kinases. *See also* Protein kinases
  in IL-11 signaling, 33, 37
H7-sensitive pathway
  in IL-6 RE activation, 62–64
  in IL-6 signal transduction pathway, 56
  in *junB* activation, 56–57
  in signal transduction, 55–57
Hematopoietin receptors. *See also* Cytokine receptors
  APP gene regulation by, 191–194
  ligands for, 166–169
  and SIF activation, 196–203
  subunits of
    functions of, 189–190
    signaling function of, 194–196
Hepatic acute phase gene classes, 252–253
Hepatocyte growth factor (HGF)
  and APP synthesis, 419–421
  and TAT/SOD activity, 416–418
hFDGI. *See* Human fibroblast-derived growth inhibitor
HGF. *See* Hepatocyte growth factor
High molecular weight fibrinogen (HMW Fb), post-operative levels of, 388–390
Histamine, 92–93, 96
HMW Fb. *See* High molecular weight fibrinogen
Human fibroblast-derived growth inhibitor (hFDGI), IL-6 identity of, 1

I

Immunoglobulin E (IgE)
  post-surgical response of, 477–479
  serum levels of
    and asbestos-related cancer, 435–437
    IL-4 and, 435–436
Inflammatory cytokines. *See also* Ciliary neurotrophic factor; Interleukins; Leukemia inhibitory factor; Oncostatin M; Tumor necrosis factor
  antioxidants and, 332–338
  in endometriosis, 496–498
  inhibition of, 331
γ-Interferon activated site (GAS). *See also* Palindromic interferon response element
  IL-6RE binding to, 58
  Stat factor binding to, 56
Interferon-α (IFN-α)
  and adrenal cortex regeneration, 491–492
  and myeloma cell growth, 457–458

Interferon-stimulated gene factor 3 (ISGF3), 16, 24–25
Interleukin-1 (IL-1)
  and ACTH levels, 71, 79
  in AGP induction, 252
  antioxidants and, 331–338
  in APP induction, 15, 102–106
  synthesis/release of, 109, 111–115
Interleukin-1β (IL-1β)
  and GCSB, 71, 73–76
  in SAA induction, 102–105
  TIMP-1 induction by, 462–464
Interleukin-6 (IL-6)
  and ACTH levels, 71, 79
  action mechanism of IL-6, 129–130
  activity of, 55
  AGP regulation by, 252
  in ALL, 391–394
  APP induction by, 15, 102–106
  and APP synthesis
    HGF and RA influence on, 419–421
    after tissue damage/infection, 313–315
  and APR, 1–2
  in APRF phosphorylation, 23–24, 229–231
  in B cell differentiation, 311–313
  biological activities of, 129
  and cancer, 385–387
  clinical applications of, 380–383
  in CNS, 403–405
  in CRP induction, 102–105, 252
  cytokines related to, 37, 213–215, 222
  and cytotoxic chemotherapy
    clinical trails with, 357
    evaluation of, 359–360
  effect on leukemic cell lines, 294–296
  functional analysis of, 262–263
    C/EBPβ-deficient mice in, 269–272
    by gene targeting, 265–272
    IL-6-deficient mice in, 265–269
  and GCSB, 71, 73–76
  hFDGI identified as, 1
  and human myeloma cells, 132
  and IgE response, 477–479
  IL-6 mutant antagonists of, 131–132
  and IL-6R, 222–223
  induction of
    by CRP, 109
    by LPS, 111, 266
    by taxol, 112, 114
  IRF-1 gene pIRE enhancer activation by, 349–352
  junB gene induction by, 56–57
  kinase activation by, 55–56. *See also* Tyrosine kinases
  and leukemic blast cell growth, 295–296
  and leukemic cell lines, 294–295
  and LPS-induced septic shock, 315

and MDS, 299–300
mechanism of action of, 129–130
mRNA expression
  in CNS, 403–405
  lesion-induced, 488–490
multiple effects of, 55
murine-human chimeras, 422–423
in myeloid leukemic cell line M1, 485–486
myeloproliferative disease models, 301–302
in neonatal infection diagnosis, 398–399
and N-*ras* genes activation, 300
OSM induction of, 48
and osteoclast activation, 377
in osteoporosis, 212, 376–377
physiologic actions of, 282
production of
  in ALL, 391–394
  antioxidants and, 332–335
  cell types involved in, 120, 308
  inhibition of, 331–332, 338
  in PTL, 10–12
receptor-binding residues of, 400–402
regulatory actions of, 55
response modulation, 4–10
role in disease, 130–131
in SAA induction, 104–105
serum levels of
  in AIDS, 130–131
  in aplasia, 439
  in BAL, 455–456
  after BMT, 440–441
  in cutaneous disease, 432–433
  diagnostic/prognostic value of, 10–12
  diurnal variations in, 468–470
  fluoxetine treatment and, 474–475
  in ischemia, 493–495
  in ovarian cancer, 446–448
  post-operative, 506–507
  in septic shock, 407–409
signal transduction residues of, 400–402
structure-function analysis of, 131
synthesis/release of, 109, 111–115
TIMP-1 induction by, 462–464
tyrosine kinase activation by, 55
Interleukin-6 (IL-6) action
  on murine tumor models
    mechanisms of, 346–352
    metastasing tumor models, 343–346
    myeloid leukemia models, 342–343
  on transcription factor regulation, 347–349
  on tumor cells
    immune system involvement in, 346–347
    IRF-1/IRF-2 and, 347–348

Interleukin-6 (IL-6) chaperones
  antibodies as, 123–125
  in blood, 120–121
  and IL-6 masking, 121–123
  and immunotherapy-induced IL-6 levels, 125–126
Interleukin-6 (IL-6)-deficient mice. *See also op/op* mice
  APP synthesis in, 313–315
  B cell differentiation in, 311–313
  bone defects in, 267–268
  CFU-s reduction in, 309–310
  embryonic development of, 309
  generation of, 265–267, 309
  inflammatory response in, 268–269
  osteoclast activity in, 375–377
  osteoporosis in, 375–377
  ovariectomy-induced bone loss in, 375–377
  pleiotropic defects in, 308–309
  septic shock protection in, 315
  T cell growth/function in, 310–311
Interleukin-6 (IL-6) gene expression
  adenovirus vectors for, 282–290
  E2 regulation of, 82–84
  glucocorticoid repression of, 80–81
  and N-*ras* gene activation, 300
  steroid regulation of, 79–80
Interleukin-6 (IL-6) promoter
  p53 and, 5–7
  transcription factors and, 2–3
Interleukin-6/LIF response factor, 502–503
Interleukin-6-like immunoreactivity, 450–451
Interleukin-6 receptor (IL-6R). *See also* Interleukin-6-type cytokine receptors; Soluble Interleukin-6 receptor
  gp80 subunit of, 55, 465–467
  gp130 subunit of, 2, 55, 465–467
  high-affinity-complex stoichiometry, 471–473
  IL-6/IL-6R internalization, 223–224
  models of interaction of, 130
  mRNA expression, in CNS, 403–405
  and myeloma cell growth, 457–458
  signal mediation by, 64–67
  signal transduction through, 55–56. *See also* IL-6 signal transduction pathway
  soluble subunits of, 64–67
Interleukin-6 receptor (IL-6R) antagonists, 129
  development/characterization of, 131
  and IL-6 activity on myeloma cells, 132–133

SUBJECT INDEX

molecular design of, 136–137, 147–149, 215–218
IL-6 mutagenesis, 139, 142–147
and IL-6Rα/gp130 interface, 144–147
molecular modeling, 138–141
superantagonist generation, 143–144
Interleukin-6 response elements (IL-6 RE)
activation of, 56, 62–64
in APP genes, 16
DNA motifs in, 55
GAS affinity for, 58
IL-6-induced DNA binding factors and, 58–59
JEBS-APRF binding, 60–62
JRE-IL6, 55
proteins binding with, 252–253, 256–258
amino acid sequence analysis of, 255–256
purification of, 253–255
Stat protein binding to, 62, 459–461
tyrosine phosphorylation and, 62
Interleukin-6 signal transduction pathway
APRE activation by, 56, 62–64
and gp130 phosphorylation, 231–233
H7-sensitive pathway in, 56, 62–64
IL-6R and, 55–56
IL-6 RE activation by, 62–64
JEBS factors mediation of, 57–58
model of, 233
protein kinases and, 55–56
Stat protein involvement in, 55–56, 58–59
Interleukin-6-type cytokine receptors. See also Hematopoietin receptors
APP gene elements regulation by, 191–194
Interleukin-6-type cytokines. See also Cardiotrophin-1; Ciliary neurotrophic factor; Interleukin-11; Leukemia inhibitory factor; Oncostatin M
and AML, 297–299
and APP glycosylation, 319–326, 413–415
clinical applications of, 383–385
and CRP levels, 435–437
in gene therapy of melanoma, 361–371
and glycosylation regulation, 323–325
and gp130, 1–2, 23–24, 42
and IgE levels, 435–437
and leukemic cell lines, 294–295
and melanoma, 369–371
and myeloproliferative disease models, 301–303
soluble receptor subunits of, 213–215
and TAT/SOD activity, 416–418

Interleukin-8 (IL-8), and selectin-P-mediated platelet adhesion, 395–397
Interleukin-11 (IL-11)
in airway fluids, 94–95
and airways hyperresponsiveness, 95–96
in APP induction, 15
in asthma, 89–90
biologically active regions of, 152–153, 160–163
clinical applications of, 384–385
cytokine regulation of, 92
cytokines related to, 37
and gp130, 1–2, 37
histamine regulation of, 92–93
infectious agent stimulation of, 93–95
kinase activation by, 31–37
and leukemic blast cell growth, 297
and leukemic cell lines, 295, 297
lung cell production of, 91–92
mutagenesis of
and biological activity, 159–163
C-terminal alanine-scan, 155–158, 161–163
N-terminal alanine-scan, 158–163
myeloproliferative disease models, 301–302
pleotropic nature of, 90
primary response gene activation by, 36–37
in pulmonary biology/homeostasis, 96–98
in respiratory inflammation, 89–90, 96–98
in septic shock, 407–409
in signal transduction, 31
H7-sensitive kinases involved in, 33
Jak family tyrosine kinases in, 32–33
MAP kinases in, 33
protein kinases involved in, 31–34
second messenger(s) involved in, 34
src-family kinases in, 33–34
transcriptional factor(s) involved in, 34–35
tyrosine kinases in, 32–34
viral stimulation of, 93–98
Interleukin-11 receptor, and gp130, 2, 16
Interleukin-12 (IL-12), 2
actions of, 274
radioprotection by, 276–278
radiosensitization by, 276–278
Interleukins. See also Inflammatory cytokines; Interleukin-6-type cytokines
pituitary hormones and, 429–431
Ischemia
APP serum levels in, 493–495
IL-6 serum levels in, 493–495
ISGF3. See Interferon-stimulated gene factor 3

JEBS. *See* Ets binding site
JRE-IL6. *See* Interleukin-6 response elements
junB gene activation
 H7-sensitive pathway in, 56–57
 by IL-6, 56

Kaposi's sarcoma cells, OSM and, 49

Leukemia inhibitory factor (LIF). *See also* Inflammatory cytokines; Interleukin-6-type cytokines
 in APP induction, 15
 in APRF phosphorylation, 23–24
 cytokines related to, 37
 and gp130, 1–2
 and leukemic blast cell growth, 296–297
 and leukemic cell lines, 295
 in mammalian development regulation, 29
 m-hLIF hybrids
  amino acid sequences of, 166–167
  binding activity of, 165–176
  specific biological activity of, 168–169
 mLIF binding activity, 168–169
 mLIF crystal structure, 179–186
 myeloproliferative disease models, 302
 renal mesangial cells and, 424–425
 in septic shock, 407–409
Leukemia inhibitory factor receptor (LIF-R). *See also* Differentiation stimulating factor/LIF receptor
 gp130 in, 55
 hLIF binding to, 165–166
 and leukemic cell lines, 295–297
 soluble subunits of, 213–215
Leukemia inhibitory factor response element (LIF-RE)
 activation of, 452–454
 in myeloid leukemic cells, 452–454
 and P19 carcinoma cell line, 426–428
Leukemic blast cell growth, IL-6-type cytokines and, 295–297
Leukemic cell lines, IL-6-type cytokines and, 294–297
Lichen planus (LP), 432–433
LIF. *See* Leukemia inhibitory factor
LPS. *See* Bacterial endotoxin

M1. *See* Myeloid leukemic cell line
α_2 Macroglobulin (α_2M)
 as hepatic acute phase gene inducer, 252
 Stat proteins and, 58–59
α_2 Macroglobulin (α_2M) gene, IL-6 RE of, 253–255
 protein binding at, 256–258
 Stat factors and, 255–256
Macrophage growth factor (CSF-1), and LPS resistance, 499–501

MAP kinases. *See* Mitogen-activated protein kinases
MDS. *See* Myelodysplastic syndromes
Melanoma
 B-78/B-78 transfected cells
  characterization of, 364–365
  tumor growth of, 365–369
 gene therapy of, 361–363
 IL-6-type cytokines and, 362, 369–371
Mitogen-activated protein kinases (MAP kinases). *See also* Protein kinases; Tyrosine kinase
 activation of, 18, 33
 IL-6 and, 18
 in IL-11 signaling, 33, 37
 in NF-IL6 phosphorylation, 18
Multiple myeloma. *See* Myeloma cell growth
Mycosis fungoides (MF), 432–433
Myelodysplastic syndromes (MDS), 294
 IL-6 involvement in, 299–300
Myeloid leukemic cell line (M1)
 LIF-RE activation in, 452–454
 reconstituted IL-6 response in, 485–486
Myeloma cell growth
 ATRA and, 457–458
 IL-6 activity and, 131–133
 inhibition of, 457–458
Myeloproliferative disease models, 294
 IL-6/IL-11 excess, 301–302
 LIF excess, 302

NBL. *See* Neuroblastoma
Neuroblastoma (NBL)
 APP levels in, 443–444
 metalloproteins, 443–444
NF-IL6
 in APP gene regulation, 16–17
 in C/EBP family, 16–17
 in gene expression, 20
 IL-6RE binding with, 17
 macrophage-specific expression of, 17–18
 NF-IL6 -/- mouse generation, 20
 phosphorylation of, 18–19
NF-κB, 3
 in gene expression, 20
 as GR target, 81
 steroid receptor antagonism with, 84
 YY1 competition with, 245–249
N-*ras* genes
 IL-6 and, 300
 in MDS, 300

Oncostatin M (OSM). *See also* Inflammatory cytokines; Interleukin-6-type cytokines
 APP induction by, 15, 47–48
 in APRF phosphorylation, 23–24
 blood clearance of, 43–45

SUBJECT INDEX

cytokines related to, 37, 42
expression in AML, 299
and gp130, 1-2, 42
IL-6 induction by, 48
and Kaposi's sarcoma cells, 49
and leukemic cell lines, 295
n vivo properties of, 42-49
properties shared with other cytokines, 49
in septic shock, 407-409
therapeutic potential of, 49
thrombocytopenia palliation by, 47
thrombopoietic activity of, 45-46
tissue distribution of, 43-45
Oncostatin M (OSM) receptor
gp130 in, 2, 55
soluble subunits of, 213-215
op/op mice, LPS resistance in, 499-501
OSM. *See* Oncostatin M
Osteoporosis
gonadotrophin levels and, 431
IL-6 and, 212, 376-377
in IL-6-deficient mice, 375-376
inflammatory cytokines and, 430
ovariectomy-induced, 375-377, 431
Ovarian cancer, IL-6 serum levels in, 446-448

P53. *See also* Transcription factors
C/EBP modulation by, 4-9
and expression vectors, 6
and hepatic IL-6 response, 4-10
and IL-6 promoter activity, 5, 7, 9
mutations in, 4-6
and protein-protein interactions, 9-10
proteins binding to, 4
and reporter construct p50-2, 5-6
as transcription regulatory factor, 4-10
Palindromic interferon response element (pIRE). *See also* γ-IFN activated sequence
IL-6 activation of, 349-352
IL-6-dependent complexes with, 350-351
sequences of, 349
pIRE. *See* Palindromic interferon response element
Pituitary hormones, and interleukin secretion, 429-431
Preterm premature labor (PTL), amniotic IL-6 levels in, 10-12
Protein kinases. *See also* H7-sensitive kinases; Mitogen-activated protein kinases; Tyrosine kinases
in IL-11 signaling, 31-34
Psoriasis, 432-433
PTL. *See* Preterm premature labor

RA. *See* Retinoic acid
ras gene, IL-6 expression and, 300

Respiratory inflammation. *See also* Asthma
IL-11 in, 89-90
Respiratory viruses
and asthma, 97
and IL-11 production, 96
Retinoic acid (RA). *See also All*-trans retinoic acid
and APP synthesis, 419-421

SAA. *See* Serum amyloid A
Septic shock
IL-6-type cytokine levels in, 336, 407-409
LPS in, 315, 336-338
Serum amyloid A (SAA)
IL-6 induction of, 102, 104-106
inflammation levels of, 238
mRNA half life, 105
SIF. *See* Stat proteins
Signal transduction. *See also* IL-6 signal transduction pathway
gp130 in, 25-26
H7-sensitive pathway in, 55-57
IL-6 receptor in, 55, 64-67
IL-11-mediated
H7-sensitive kinases in, 33
and MAP kinases activation, 33
protein kinases involved in, 31-32
JRE-IL6-mediated, 64-67
Ras-independent, 55
Stat factors in, 55
tyrosine kinases in, 32-34, 262
SOD. *See* Superoxide dismutase
Soluble gp130, 207, 211
and IL-6R-IL-6 complex, 212-213
Soluble interleukin-6 receptor (IL-6R), 207, 224-226
gp130, 211
IL-6 complex with, 211-212
IL-6R protein, 208-211
and IL-6-soluble gp130 complex, 212-213
Stat proteins
activation of, 64-66
APRE recognition by, 58-59
cloned cDNA of, 60
and cytokine receptor action, 196-203
and GAS/pIRE genes expression, 349-350
as IL-6-induced DNA binding factors, 58-59
IL-6 RE binding of, 62, 459-461
in IL-6 signal transduction, 55-56
in IL-11 signaling, 31-37
and α_2M REs, 58-59
phosphorylation of, 55-56, 62, 349-350
as transcriptional factors, 34-35

Steroid receptors. *See also* Glucocorticoid
    receptors
  and gene expression, 80, 82–84
  NF-κB antagonism with, 84
  and positive transcription factors, 80,
    84–86
  synergism/antagonism models, 84–86
  transcription factors association with, 80
Superoxide dismutase (SOD), 416–418

T AT. *See* Tyrosine aminotransferase
Taxol
  acute phase cytokines induction by, 108,
    112–114
  and endotoxin-responsive gene expression,
    114
Thrombocytopenia, OSM palliation of, 47
Thrombopoiesis, OSM activity and, 45–46
TIMP-1. *See* Tissue inhibitors of
    metalloproteinases
Tissue inhibitors of metalloproteinases
    (TIMP-1)
  inflammatory cytokine induction of, 49
  interleukin induction of, 462–464
TNF-α. *See* Tumor necrosis factor
Transcription activation/repression model,
    248
Transcription factors. *See also* Acute phase
    response factors; C/EBP; CHOP-
    10; NF-IL6; NF-κB
  CRU binding with, 241–249
  as cytokine signal targets, 238–239
  estrogens modulation of, 3
  glucocorticoid modulation of, 3
  in IL-6 induction, 3
  p53 modulation of, 4–9

and steroid receptors, 80, 84–86
superfamily of, 79
Transcription factors (IRF-1/IRF-2)
  IL-6 induction of, 349–352
  and IL-6 tumor cell effects, 347–348
Tumor necrosis factor (TNF-α)
  in APP induction, 15
  in endotoxin resistance, 499–501
  and GCSB, 71, 73–76
  inhibition of
    antioxidants and, 331–338
    clinical benefits of, 331
    compounds active in, 331–332
Tyrosine aminotransferase (TAT), 416–418
Tyrosine kinases. *See also* Protein kinases;
    Tyrosine phosphorylation
  families of, 32–34, 64–65
  gp130 activation of, 56
  in IL-6R-mediated signals, 64–67
  in IL-6 signal transduction, 55–56,
    62–63
  in IL-11 signaling, 32–34
  in JRE-IL6-Stat protein complexes, 62
  and signal transmission, 55, 64–67, 262
  in Stat protein phosphorylation, 55–56
Tyrosine phosphorylation
  of APRF, 23–24, 229–231
  differences in, 37
  of gp130, 23–24, 55, 231–233
  IL-6 induction of, 55–56, 231–233
  of IL-6 RE complexes, 62
  IL-6-type cytokines induction of, 23–24
  in IL-11 signaling, 31–37
  of Stat proteins, 55–56, 62, 349–350

Y Y1. *See under* Cytokine response unit

Index of Contributors[a]

Aarden, L.A., 129–135
Abdul-Ahad, A., 359–360, *375–387*
Adler, G., 388–389
Ahmed, A.A., 450–451
Akira, S., 15–28
Ali, N., 274–281
Allison, A.C., 331–341
Altamura, S., 136–151
Andrzejewska, R., 398–399
Ansari, A.A., 499–501

Baumann, H., 189–206, 308–318, *375–387*, 413–415
Bellavia, D., 262–273
Bennett, F., 152–164
Bereta, J., 416–418
Bing, Z., 238–251
Biró, J., 71–78
Bläsius, R., 452–454
Boguslawska-Jaworska, J., 391–394
Borden, E. C., 359–360
Braciak, T., 282–293
Brakenhoff, J.P.J., 129–135, 400–402
Breitmeyer, J.B., 359–360
Brombacher, F., 308–318
Burchert, M., 395–397
Burris, H., 359–360
Burstein, S.A., 42–54

Cabibbo, A., 136–151
Campos, S.P., 189–206
Cappelletti, M., 262–273
Chebath, J., 342–356
Chevalier, S., 407–409, 482–484
Chybicka, A., 391–394
Ciapponi, L., 136–151
Ciliberto, G., 136–151
Clark, R., 165–178
Clement, C., 482–484
Costantini, F., 262–273
Cullinan, E., 29–30
Czupryn, M., 152–164

De Hon, F.D., 129–135, 400–402
Demartis, A., 136–151
Dembińska-Kieć, A., 395–397
Dittrich, E., 222–237, 410–412
Drechsler, D., 359–360
Dreier, B., 252–261
Drews, K., 398–399, 505–507, 508–509
Dube, J., 152–164
Dulak, J., 395–397
Dziatkowiak, A., 477–479

Ehlers, M., 207–221, 400–402
Eichman, W., 388–389
Einarsson, O., 89–101
Eisenbach, L., 342–356
Elias, J.A., 89–101, *375–387*
Erren, A., 222–237
Eugui, E.M., 331–341

Falus, A., 71–78
Fattori, E., 262–273
Feldman, M., 342–356
Fey, G.H., 252–261, *375–387*, 452–454, 457–458, 502–504
Fourcin, M., 407–409
Freer, G., 308–318
Fritz, S., 252–261, 457–458
Fujitani, Y., 55–70

Gadient, R.A., 403–406
Gadzinowski, J., xv
Galanos, C., 308–318
Galazka, A., 359–360
Garcia, D., 120–128
Gascan, H., 407–409, 482–484
Gauldie, J., 282–293
Gearing, D., 189–206
Geba, G.P., 89–101
Gerhartz, C., 222–237, 410–412
Goppelt-Strübe, M., 424–425
Gordon, M.S., *375–387*
Gorny, A., 493–495
Gough, N.M., 165–178
Graeve, L., 222–237, 410–412, 462–464
Graham, F., 282–293
Grant, K., 152–164
Grey, L, M., 179–188
Grossberg, S.E., 359–360
Grötzinger, J., 207–221, 400–402
Gryska, K., 413–415
Guillet, C., 407–409
Gulino, A., 262–273
Gutierrez-Ramos, J.-C., 308–318
Guzdek, A., 108–119, 416–418, 419–421

Hammacher, A., 422–423, 471–473
Hanson, M.B., 42–54
Haran-Ghera, N., 342–356
Harroch, S., 342–356
Hartner, A., 424–425
Hawley, R.G., 294–307
Heath, J.K., 179–188
Heinrich, P.C., 222–237, 361–374, *375–387*, 410–412

---

[a] Italic numbers indicate Roundtable Discussion.

Hemmann, U., 222–237
Heumann, R., 488–490
Hiemke, C., 468–470
Hirano, T., 55–70
Hocke, G.M., 252–261, 424–425, 426–428, 452–454, 457–458, 502–504
Horn, F., 222–237, *375–387*
Howlett, G.J., 471–473
Huang, J., 238–251

Inoue, M., 15–28
Izbicki, T., 443–445

Jawień, J., 477–479
Jaworski, W., 391–394
Jedrzejczak, P., 496–498, 505–507
Jiang, S.-L., 102–107
Jones, E.Y., 179–188
Jung, A., 455–456

Kalinski, P., 499–501
Karabon, L., 435–438, 439–442
Kasprzak, M., 496–498
Katz, A., 342–356
Keever, C., 359–360
Kishimoto, T., 15–28
Klein, B., 482–484
Köhler, G., 308–318
Koj, A., xiii, 108–119, *375–387*
Kojima, H., 55–70
Komorowski, J., 429–431
Kopf, M., 308–318, *375–387*
Koskela, K., 457–458
Koziol, M., 432–434
Krasowska, D., 432–434
Ksiażek, A., 432–434
Kumaki, S., 189–206
Kurpisz, M., , 496–498
Kushner, I., 102–107

Laba, A., 439–442
Laciak, M., 413–415, 474–476
Lahm, A., 136–151
Lai, C.-F., 189–206
Landry, M.L., 89–101
Lange, A., 435–438, 439–442
Laskowska-Klita, T., 443–445
Layton, M.J., 165–178
Lazzaro, D., 262–273
Li, L., 238–251
Liao, W. S.-L., 238–251
Libing, C., 450–451
Liden, S., 450–451
Lipińska, L., 443–445
Ljungberg, A., 450–451

Löchner, K., 252–261
Lottspeich, F., 252–261
Lozanski, G., 102–107
Lu, S.-Y., 238–251
Lütticken, C., 222–237

Mackiewicz, A., xiii, 308–318, 361–374, 398–399, 413–415, 474–476, 493–495, 508–509
MacMaster, J.F., 42–54
Madry, R., 446–449
Majewski, W., 493–495
Margulies, L., 1–14
Markowska, J., 446–449
Marschalek, R., 252–261
Maruszynski, M., 455–456
Matern, S., 462–464
Matsuda, T., 55–70
Matsusaka, T., 15–28
May, L.T., 120–128
McCoy, J.M., 152–164
Metcalf, D., 165–178
Metinko, A., 89–101
Moniewska, A., 439–442
Morella, K.K., 189–206
Moritz, R.L., 471–473
Müllberg, J., 207–221, 400–402, 462–464
Müller, H., 468–470

Nakae, K., 55–70
Nakajima, K., 55–70
Ndubuisi, M.I., 120–128
Neta, R., 274–281
Neva, M., 457–458
Nicola, N.A., 165–178
Nishio, Y., 15–28
Nordlind, K., 450–451
Nowak, J., 361–374

Ollikainen, H., 457–458
Otten, U., 403–406
Owczarek, C.M., 165–178

Pan, H., 1–14
Panettieri, R.A., Jr., 89–101
Paonessa, G., 136–151
Patel, K., 120–128
Pawelec, M., 395–397
Pawlikowski, M., 429–431
Pawlowski, T., 361–374
Pellniemi, T.-T., 457–458
Perek, D., 443–445
Peskar, B.A., 395–397
Piekorz, R.P., 452–454, 485–487
Pierzchalski, P., 465–467
Pietrzak, A., 432–434

INDEX OF CONTRIBUTORS

Piwowarska, W., 477–479
Płusa, T., 455–456
Pojda, Z., 455–456
Poli, V., 262–273, *375–387*
Polus, M., 395–397
Pouplard, A., 407–409
Puk, E., , 496–498
Pulkki, K., 457–458

Radwan, J., 477–479
Rákász, É., 71–78
Ramsay, A., 308–318
Ray, A., 79–88
Ray, P., 79–88
Rayanade, R. , 1–14
Remes, K., 457–458
Revel, M., 342–356, *375–387*
Richards, C.D., 282–293
Richter, K., 252–261
Rillema, J.R., 42–54
Ripperger, J., 252–261, 457–458, 502–504
Ritch, P.S., 359–360
Rivkin, S., 359–360
Robinson, R.C., 179–188
Robledo, O., 482–484
Roeb, E., 361–374, 462–464
Rokita, H., 465–467
Rose-John, S., 207–221, 462–464
Rouleau, K.A., 42–54
Rybakowski, J.K., 474–476

Salvati, A.L., 136–151
Samols, D., 102–107
Savino, R., 136–151
Schiller, J., 359–360
Schneider, K., 252–261, 502–504
Schneider-Mergener, J., 222–237
Scoble, H., 152–164
Screpanti, I., 262–273
Sehgal, P.B., xiii, 1–14, *375–387*
Seiler, W., 468–470
Sellitto, C., 262–273
Shoyab, M., 42–54
Siedlecki, A., 395–397
Siegel, M.D., 79–88
Simpson, R.J., 422- 423, 471–473
Skrzypczak, J., 496–498, 505–507, 508–509
Slupianek, A., 413–415, 493–495
Służewska, A., 474–476
Sobieska, M., 474–476
Sookdeo, H., 152–164
Stadler, B.M., 477–479
Stalińska, K., 416–418, 465–467
Staniszewski, R., 493–495
Staunton, D., 179–188

Stępien, H., 429–431
Sterzel, R.B., 424–425
Stewart, C.L., 29–30
Stiefel, S.M., 274–281
Stoyan, T., 410–412
Strużyna, J., 455–456
Stuart, D.I., 179–188
Swider, C., 439–442
Szczapa, J., 398–399
Szczeklik, A., 477–479
Szczepanski, M., 388–389
Szewierski, Z., 446–449
Szperl, M., 499–501
Szwech, P., 499–501
Szymanowski, K., 505–507, 508–509

Takeda, T., 55–70
Tanaka, T., 15–28
Targonska, I., 388–389
Tomeczko, J., 435–438
Tomida, M., 480–481
Toniatti, C., 136–151
Toruniowa, B., 432–434
Tristram, D., 89–101
Truitt, R.L., 359–360
Tweardy, D.J., 189–206

Urbanowska, E., 499–501

Vaickus, L., 359–360
Van Dijk, W., 319–330
Von Hoff, D.D., 359–360

Wallace, P.M., 42–54, *375–387*
Wang, L., 1–14
Wang, X.-J., 15–28
Wang, Y., 189–206
Ward, L.D., 422- 423, 471–473
Weber, J.S., 357–358, *375–387*
Wegenka, U., 222–237
Wei, S., 15–28
Weiergräber, O., 222–237
Weinstock, J., 422- 423
Wellıver, R., 89–101
Wijdenes, J., 482–484
Wiktor-Jedrzejczak, W., 499–501
Wiktorowicz, K., 446–449, 474–476
Witt, P.L., 359–360
Wiznerowicz, M., 361–374
Wollmer, A., 400–402
Wulf, P., 485–487

Xing, Z., 282–293

Yamanaka, Y., 55–70
Yang, Y.-C., 31–41

Yin, T., 31–41
Yoshida, N., 15–28

Żak, J., 398–399
Żak, L., 398–399
Żak, T., 505–507, 508–509

Zhang, D., 102–107
Zhang, D.-H., 79–88
Zhong, J., 488–490
Zhou, Z., 89–101
Ziegler, S.F., 189–206
Zieleniewski, W., 491–492